HANDBOOK OF MEDICAL BIOCHEMISTRY
VOLUME 2

CLINICAL APPLICATIONS AND SYSTEMIC BIOCHEMICAL PATHWAYS

Prof. Ramesh Chandra
and Dr. Heerak Chugh

ALLIED
HEALTH
PRESS

Handbook of Medical Biochemistry Volume 2

Clinical Applications and Systemic Biochemical Pathways

Authors: **Prof. Ramesh Chandra and Dr. Heerak Chugh**

Allied Health Press
4164 Lakeshore Road
Burlington ON L7L 1A4
Canada
www.alliedhealthpress.com
Email: orders@arclereducation.com

ISBN: 978-1-77956-815-1

Allied Health Press publishes wide variety of books and eBooks. For more information about Allied Health Press and its products, visit our website at www.alliedhealthpress.com

ABOUT THE AUTHORS

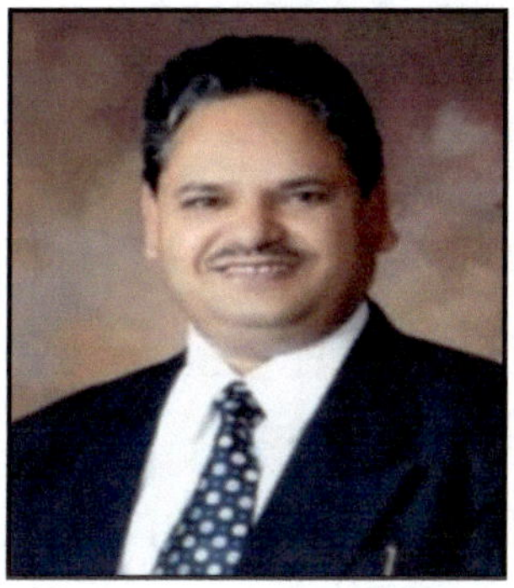

Prof. Ramesh Chandra is a distinguished scientist; Fellow of the Royal Society of Chemistry, London and an outstanding researcher in the field of Biomedical Sciences. Currently, he is the Vice-Chancellor at Maharaja Surajmal Brij University, Bharatpur, Rajasthan, and Founder Director of Dr. B. R. Ambedkar Center for Biomedical Research (ACBR), University of Delhi. He is Official resource person to the Minister and Department of Science and Technology in the kingdom of Lesotho, South Africa.

He started his research career at the University of Delhi, then at The New York Hospital-Cornell University Medical College, and The Rockefeller University, New York; State University of New York at Stonybrook, Harvard University Medical School-Massachusetts General Hospital (MGH) jointly at MIT, Cambridge, USA.

Prof. Chandra has been Vice-Chancellor, Bundelkhand University, Jhansi (1999-2005) as well as President of the Indian Chemical Society, Member, Planning Commission, Government of U.P. India; Secretary - Zaheer Science Foundation, New Delhi and Non-Official Director, Rashtriya Ispat Nigam Ltd, Government of India. He was also Head of the Department of Chemistry, University of Delhi.

He is recipient of several international recognitions: J. William Fulbright Scholarship, The Rockefeller Foundation USA-Biotechnology Career Award, Award of the Highest Honor of Soka University, Tokyo, Japan; Millennium Plaques of Honor (Life Time Achievement Award for contribution in Science & Technology) by the Indian Science Congress Association (ISCA), Lifetime Achievement Award of the Indian Chemical Society (1CS); UGC Research Scientist Award; UGC Career Award; Rajib Goyal Award for Young Scientists and others.

Prof. Chandra shows deep commitment to the cause of higher education & research and possesses in ample measure quality of dynamic leadership, vision required for building academic institutions and excelled in his academic pursuits. To illustrate, he has to his credit several international patents, 9 Books; 28 Book Chapters; and more than 400 original Scientific Research Papers in International journals of repute. He has mentored more than 100 Ph.D. students.

In recognition of his outstanding Scientific Research and Administrative Qualities, Prof Ramesh Chandra has been conferred Capital Foundation Dr A.P.J. Abdul Kalam National Award.

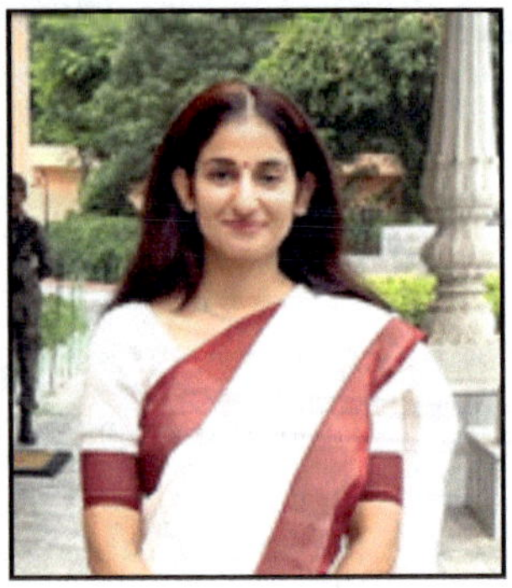

Dr Heerak Chugh is a life scientist who is currently working as a Senior Researcher funded by Indian Council of Medical Research (ICMR) at University of Delhi, Delhi. She is also teaching as an Adjunct Assistant Professor at Maharaja Surajmal Brij University, Rajasthan.

Her Research focusses on advancing our current understanding of cancer and exploring therapeutic interventions to improve treatment (patient) outcomes. She has extensive experience in Cell biology, molecular biology, biochemistry, cancer biology, chemical biology, biophysical chemistry, chemotherapeutics, drug delivery and cancer nanomedicine.

Dr Heerak Chugh completed her graduation and postgraduation in Life Science from Sri Venkateswara, University of Delhi, Delhi and Central University of Punjab, Bathinda, Punjab, respectively.

Dr Heerak Chugh developed her research interest while working as a research intern at CSIR-IGIB where she was working on synthesizing plant-based nanoparticles and cationic nanoparticles as novel anti-microbial agents. To continue her research interests, Dr Heerak Chugh joined a Ph.D. programme in University of Delhi, Drug Discovery and Development Laboratory, Department of Chemistry, University of Delhi wherein she worked on increasing the therapeutic efficacy of Noscapine, an anti-cancer agent.

Dr Chugh was awarded prestigious Prime Minister Fellowship for Doctoral Research by Science and Engineering Research Board (SERB), Government of India and Confederation of Indian Industry (CII); until now, she is the only recipient from University of Delhi. She was also awarded Junior Research Fellowship through National Eligibility Test (All India Rank 60). Further, she was also awarded Senior Research Fellowship by Indian Council of Medical Research.

During her Ph.D., she worked at Department of Biological Sciences, Purdue University, Indiana, USA as Science and Engineering Research Board, Government of India funded Overseas Doctoral Visiting Fellow where she studied HYPE protein and its role in cancer.

She was one of the subject matter experts on Voet's Biochemistry Adapted Edition 2021. She has published over a dozen research articles in various peer-reviewed International Journals, and continues to work and publish actively in the field of cancer biology and cancer therapeutics. She also serves as an invited reviewer for various international journals.

Brief Table of Contents

Getting Started with This Book

Chapter Openers

A list of Chapter Outline is presented providing a brief Introduction to what will be covered in the chapter.

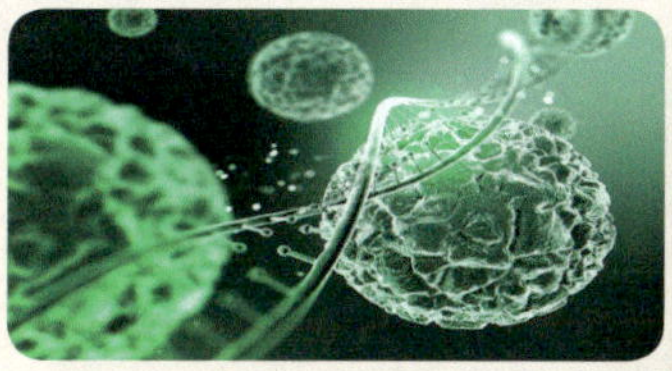

Introduction

Often referred to as the science of life, biology is a broad field of study aimed at comprehending the several kinds of life on Earth, from tiny creatures to sophisticated multicellular entities. Comprising several subfields, including molecular biology, ecology, and evolutionary biology, each of which advances our knowledge of living systems, this field clarifies the mechanisms controlling life events, including development, reproduction, and interaction with the surroundings, which is the central goal of biology. Moreover, biology fills in the void between the natural sciences and medicine by offering a necessary understanding of health, illness, and the interactions between organisms and their environments. Dealing with urgent global issues such as climate change, biodiversity loss, and new diseases depends on an awareness of these complex biological interactions, therefore highlighting the critical part biology plays in modern civilization. Fundamentally, biology explores and tests ideas about the living world using the scientific method. Through methodical observation and experimentation,

LEARNING OBJECTIVES

After studying this chapter, you will be able to:

1. Discuss the scientific method in biology;
2. Explain the cell theory;
3. Discuss the genetics and heredity;
4. Evolution and natural selection;
5. Focus on ecology and ecosystems;
6. Learn about human biology;
7. Evaluate the plant biology;
8. Explain the microbiology;
9. Focus on current trends in biology.

1.1. The Scientific Method in Biology

Learning Outcome

1. Describe the steps of the scientific method;
2. Focus on hypothesis formation;
3. Learn about experimental design.

Learning Outcomes

The beginning of each section of every chapter contains a set of Learning Outcomes that inform students of concepts they should understand. These outcomes help students understand what they should be able to do if they have mastered the material in that section.

Test Your Knowledge

Throughout each chapter, Test Your Knowledge cues you to note which topics have been covered and to self-test your understanding of the material presented.

Test Your Knowledge

1. Explain why correlation does not imply causation in scientific experiments.
2. How does the scientific method help reduce the influence of personal opinions in research?

Chapter Summary

The Summary Section appear at the end of each chapter and summarize main concepts covered throughout the chapter. These points provide key concepts in an engaging and meaningful way.

Summary

The investigation of biological principles highlights the importance of a comprehensive view of life by reflecting the intricate interactions that occur within living systems. The complexity of biology goes beyond individual species or systems, as this essay highlights; it also includes the interactions that mold ecosystems and affect biodiversity. Researchers can conduct in-depth analyses of metabolomic data using sophisticated technologies like MetaboAnalyst, which offer insights into the molecular mechanisms underlying these interactions. As demonstrated by the developments in MetaboAnalyst, for example, the integration of diverse omics data promotes a thorough understanding of metabolic pathways and helps identify important biological markers necessary for research on development and disease (Chong et al., 2018). Additionally, the phenomenon of ecological invasions is a key component of biological research and a vital field of study. The introduction of non-native species into unfamiliar habitats has significant ramifications and calls for multidisciplinary management strategies. Examining the origins and effects of these biological incursions, invasion science has become a crucial field that highlights the need to comprehend ecological dynamics and community interactions. As interest in biological invasions increases, new findings are emerging that put conventional ecological theories and practices to the test. The importance of incorporating various scientific viewpoints is shown by this developing discipline, which also highlights how invasive species shape ecosystems and advances our knowledge of ecological resilience (David et al., 2013). When taken as a whole, these discoveries from invasion science and metabolomics highlight the value of multidisciplinary biology research. Fostering cross-disciplinary collaboration and utilizing technological breakthroughs to improve our comprehension of intricate biological interactions are crucial as we look to the future of biological research. In addition to deepening our understanding of the complexities of life, this method lays the groundwork for tackling urgent environmental issues. Future studies can ensure the continued relevance of biology in a world that is constantly changing by acknowledging the interconnection of biological systems and opening the door to creative solutions that support sustainability and biodiversity conservation. We might imagine a thorough comprehension of life that serves both academia and society at large through ongoing investigation and integration of scientific knowledge.

Knowledge Assessment

The chapter includes material designed to review and reinforce each content. It includes Critical Thinking Questions to help test of your understanding of information presented in the chapter and Short answer Questions to review your understanding of the key concepts presented in the chapter.

Critical Thinking Questions

1. **Who is known as the "Father of Modern Biology"?**
   a. Aristotle
   b. Charles Darwin
   c. Gregor Mendel
   d. Louis Pasteur
2. **What is the basic unit of life?**
   a. Atom
   b. Molecule
   c. Cell
   d. Organism
3. **Which branch of biology studies the interaction of organisms with their environment?**
   a. Genetics
   b. Ecology
   c. Physiology
   d. Botany
4. **Which macromolecule is the main source of energy for living organisms?**
   a. Proteins
   b. Lipids
   c. Carbohydrates
   d. Nucleic acids
5. **DNA is primarily responsible for which function in living organisms?**
   a. Energy production
   b. Protein synthesis
   c. Storing genetic information
   d. Regulating body temperature

Short Answer Questions

1. What is biology, and why is it important to study biology?
2. What are the three main domains of life, and how are they different from one another?
3. Define homeostasis and give an example of how it works in living organisms.
4. What is the cell theory, and why is it fundamental to biology?
5. How do autotrophs and heterotrophs differ in the way they obtain energy?
6. What is the scientific method, and how is it applied in biological research?
7. Discuss how biology helps address global challenges such as climate change, disease, and food security.
8. Explain the levels of biological organization from the smallest unit to the largest. Provide examples at each level.
9. Describe the relationship between structure and function in biology, giving specific examples from cells or organs.
10. How has the discovery of genetics shaped our understanding of inheritance and variation among organisms?

Supplementary Materials

Key Terms: A list of key terms is given for quick reference

KEY TERMS FROM THIS CHAPTER

Annotation enrichment analysis	Biological structure	Cell
Cell theory	Cellular structure	Ecology
Ecosystems	Genetics	Human biology
Microbiology	Natural selection	Organism
Plant biology		

Further Resources: Recommendations for additional readings, websites, and multimedia resources.

References

1. Argelaguet, R., Velten, B., Arnol, D., Dietrich, S., Zenz, T., Marioni, J. C., Buettner, F., et al. (2018). Multi-omics factor analysis—A framework for unsupervised integration of multi-omics data sets. *Molecular Systems Biology, 14*. https://doi.org/10.15252/msb.20178124.
2. Bacher, S., Blackburn, T. M., Essl, F., & Genovesi, P. (2017). *Socio-Economic Impact Classification of Alien Taxa (SEICAT)*. https://core.ac.uk/download/286567949.pdf (accessed on 8th March 2025).
3. Barnett, R., Brace, S., Cucchi, T., & Dobney, K. (2013). *Divergent Evolutionary Processes Associated with Colonization of Offshore Islands*. https://core.ac.uk/download/20664364.pdf (accessed on 8th March 2025).

Detailed Table of Contents

CHAPTER 13

LIST OF FIGURES

PREFACE

The study of biological systems, particularly at the molecular and chemical level, continues to reveal how essential biochemical processes sustain life, regulate health, and influence disease. As our understanding advances, there is growing recognition of the significance of the effects of biochemistry on clinical outcomes, therapeutic intervention strategy, and human physiology in the fullest sense. These advances require both fundamental knowledge and current insight into topics that range across the biological and medical sciences.

Biochemistry connects the cellular and systemic levels of health so that practitioners and researchers know about physiological states in terms of chemical reactions and molecular interactions. From a knowledge of metabolic pathways to the interpretation of hormone actions and clinical biomarkers, this science supports a range of healthcare applications. Increased knowledge of these subjects not only supports research capability but also enhances diagnostic precision and treatment planning in the clinic.

This volume, *Handbook of Medical Biochemistry: Volume 2: Clinical Applications and Systemic Biochemical Pathways*, is a systematic and thorough coverage of the principal themes and developments relevant to medical biochemistry. As a sequel to the central topics covered in Volume 1, this volume presents advanced topics and system-based advances in biochemical processes. Each chapter is an equal blend of theoretical principles and practical data, enabling readers to have a better insight into the application of biochemical mechanisms in clinical and biomedical contexts. This text is intended to be a reference and an instruction guide for students, educators, clinicians, and researchers with an interest in the biochemical properties of human disease and health.

Chapter 1 presents Clinical Biochemistry and the way it is vital for disease diagnosis and surveillance. The chapter summarizes the most common biochemical markers in the clinical laboratory and explains their uses in diagnosing disorders. Glucose, lipid profiles, and enzyme activity parameters are explained in terms of their diagnostic limits, normal ranges, and clinicopathological correlations. The chapter also deals with quality control of laboratory testing and interpretation of biochemical data in patient care.

Chapter 2 addresses Liver and Kidney Function Tests and explains the role of these organs in metabolism and excretion. It explains the biochemical markers to indicate hepatic and renal function, for example, bilirubin, transaminases, urea, creatinine, and electrolyte concentrations. Pathologic changes, abnormal value interpretation, and the physiological basis for each test are detailed. The chapter emphasizes the significance of organ-specific biochemical testing in the early diagnosis and management of disease.

Chapter 3 discusses Blood Biochemistry with an emphasis on the molecular blood components and their functional implications. Hemoglobin structure and hemoglobin variants, plasma proteins, coagulation factors, and blood gas parameters are discussed, along with acid-base balance and oxygen transport discussions. Clinical abnormalities of anemia, clotting disease, and pH derangement are highlighted, as well as the importance of biochemical tests in hematology.

Chapter 4 covers Free Radicals and Antioxidants, providing an overview of oxidative stress and its role in disease. Production and elimination of reactive oxygen species (ROS) are described alongside antioxidant defense systems. The chapter discusses the role of oxidative damage in chronic diseases, including cancer, cardiovascular disease (CVD), and neurodegeneration. It also includes laboratory assays for quantifying oxidative stress and antioxidant status.

Chapter 5 treats Xenobiotics and Biotransformation, which explains how the body handles foreign chemicals like drugs, toxins, and pollutants. Biochemistry of detoxification stages, enzyme systems involved (e.g., cytochrome P450), and roles in conjugation reactions are described. Pharmacological and toxicological examples are employed to illustrate how metabolism influences drug efficacy and toxicity and offer insight into personalized medicine and risk assessment.

Chapter 6 is on Nutrition and Metabolism, in which the process of utilization and regulation of food components within the human body is explained. Macronutrient and micronutrient metabolism, energy homeostasis, and biochemical consequences of undernutrition are elaborated. Enzymatic, coenzymatic, and hormonal functions in nutrient processing and case studies of metabolic syndromes and dietary care are also explained.

Chapter 7 addresses the Metabolism of Specialized Tissues, describing the biochemical characteristics unique to organs such as the brain, muscle, adipose tissue, and skin. It describes how such tissues provide energy needs, deliver substrates, and perform specialized functions through specific metabolic adaptations. Abnormal tissue metabolism disorders are also addressed, illustrating how organ function is affected by systemic biochemistry.

Chapter 8 addresses Immunochemistry with a focus on the biochemical aspect of immunity. It addresses antigen-antibody interactions, functions of the complement system, structure of immunoglobulins, and mechanisms of signaling for immunity. Experimental techniques such as ELISA and immunoblotting are discussed further in the chapter and connected with biochemical findings and immunological and diagnostic immunopathology.

Chapter 9 discusses Endocrinology from a biochemical viewpoint, focusing on hormone secretion, transport, action, and degradation. Peptide and steroid hormones are discussed, including feedback control and receptor binding. Diabetes, thyroid disease, and adrenal imbalance are associated with their respective biochemical processes. Hormonal assays and diagnostic tests are provided to make clinical application easier.

Chapter 10 covers Techniques in Biochemistry essential for present-day laboratory research. Chapter subjects include chromatography, electrophoresis, spectrophotometry, immunoassays, and molecular techniques such as PCR and blotting approaches. Chapter 10 provides background information for the interpretation of experimental results and for understanding the technical basis of research and diagnostic protocols.

Chapter 11 covers Proteomics and Metabolomics, highlighting high-throughput analysis of proteins and metabolites in health and disease. It covers methods like mass spectrometry, 2D gel electrophoresis, and NMR spectroscopy, along with analysis software used to crack complex datasets. Disease biomarker identification, functional protein investigation, and metabolic profiling uses are also covered, reflecting the expanding contribution of bioinformatics to biochemistry.

Chapter 12 is dedicated to Epigenetics, explaining how biochemical alterations of histones and DNA influence gene expression without modifying the genetic information. It introduces methylation, acetylation, and other epigenetic changes, along with the enzymes and cofactors involved in these processes. The connection of epigenetics with diseases such as cancer, neurodegenerative diseases, and developmental disorders is explained, along with possible therapy.

Chapter 13 presents Biochemical Pharmacology, the integration of biochemical principles and pharmacological practice. It presents drug-receptor interactions, signal transduction, pharmacokinetics, and pharmacodynamics from a biochemical viewpoint. Mechanisms of drug resistance, enzyme inhibition, and targeted therapy are described in the context of their biochemical rationale. The chapter enlightens the reader on how biochemical processes regulate therapeutic action and impact drug design.

This book is planned to meet the learning and reference needs of a wide range of readers. Medical, biochemistry, and health science undergraduate students will find useful systematic explanations and clinical correlations for academic success and exam preparation. Clinicians, clinical laboratory scientists, and researchers will appreciate the detailed discussions of biochemical processes and their applications to diagnostics, therapeutics, and laboratory methods. The book is also available as a supplementary textbook in nutrition, immunology, pharmacology, and molecular biology courses, particularly in courses where more emphasis is laid on biochemical principles.

CLINICAL BIOCHEMISTRY

1

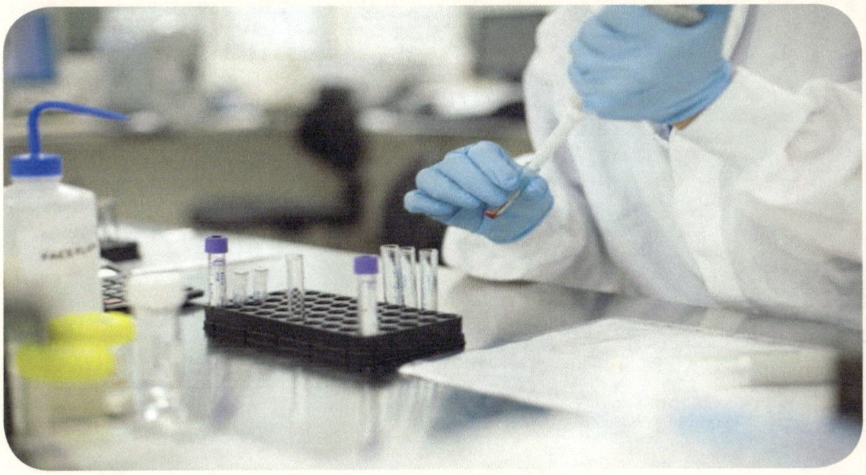

LEARNING OBJECTIVES

After studying this chapter, you will be able to:

1. Describe the laboratory techniques in clinical biochemistry;
2. Learn about clinical applications of biochemical tests;
3. Understand the biochemical markers in disease diagnosis;
4. Describe the emerging trends in clinical biochemistry.

Introduction

Clinical biochemistry appears as a required interface between the biochemistry of the body and the clinical approach of diagnosis and disease management. Clinical biochemistry involves the study of biomolecules, metabolic pathways, and how they apply to the cause and maintenance of health. Clinical biochemistry basically enlightens the functioning of the body at the molecular scale. Biochemistry of urine, blood and other body fluids can help the clinician to get valuable data about the metabolic state of the patient, hormonal state of balance and nutrition deficiency of essential nutrients. Due to these types of biochemical research, medical personnel are able to make rational decisions when managing patients, diagnosing them, and choosing the treatment option, which speaks of the role of biochemistry application in clinical practice. The best thing about clinical biochemistry is that it has an open arm policy to personalized medicine. An example of such a shift is the development of pharmacogenomics, which takes into account the contribution of genes in determining how individuals react to drugs. Physicians can provide treatment regimens tailored to each patient's genetic profile based on their understanding of genetic factors that influence drug metabolism.

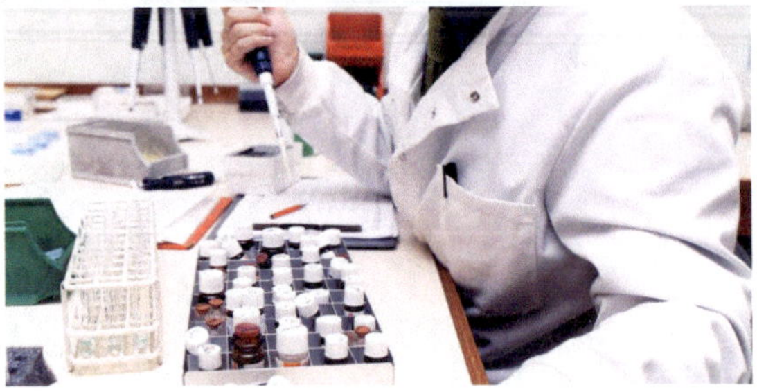

Figure 1.1. Clinical biochemistry.

Source: https://www.rcpath.org/static/e61498cd-646f-49b7-9c5bd7ac3e8917a5/standardpagepartialimagea6d87b84d50738980caee9288a67cb0a/young_man_with_trays_of_tubespipette_scans_of_a_scotts_trainees_general_lab_785x400.jpg.

As an example, the investigations of cytochrome P450 genes, which play an important role in drug metabolism, allow practitioners to determine the way a patient metabolizes drugs to enhance their effectiveness and reduce side effects. Such advancements reveal the potential of personalized medicine to achieve its highest possible patient outcome through the interactive nature of clinical biochemistry and personalized healthcare approaches (Blevins et al., 2020). Technology and big data assist the students in learning clinical biochemistry, as well, because they allow them to grasp the subjects better. The students can relate theory to practice through active learning exercises that access large databases, including those that examine the pharmacogenomics of the cytochrome P450 genes. The analysis of real data in the classroom setting, as in these cases, confirms the student's power to interpret biochemical analysis and its impact on clinical decision-making. Using case studies, including differences in responses to drugs in different patients, the faculty can underline the relevance of biochemistry to the effectiveness of treatment and the safety of patients. In addition to promoting knowledge, such an approach empowers future health care providers to prosper in an increasingly complex clinical environment (Phelps et al., 2004) (Figure 1.1).

1.1. Laboratory Techniques in Clinical Biochemistry

Learning Outcome

1. Learn about spectrophotometry and its applications;
2. Describe the chromatography methods for biomolecule separation;
3. Understand the immunoassays for disease detection.

Clinical biochemistry laboratory techniques are important in the diagnosis and monitoring of diseases. Advanced methodologies, such as enzyme-linked immunosorbent assays (ELISAs) and mass spectrometry, enable clinicians to quantify biomolecules with high sensitivity and specificity. ELISA has transformed the hormones, proteins, and antibodies detection and has given fundamental information on diseases like diabetes and autoimmune diseases. Also, mass spectrometry, the technique that accurately measures the mass-to-charge ratio of ions, is used to analyze metabolites and lipids, thus enabling the characterization of complex biological samples. This is a technological development that increases the diagnostic power of clinical biochemistry laboratories and it fills the gap between biochemical research and clinical practice. Being aware of these methods and their consequences keeps the practitioners in a position to deal with the dynamics of biochemical markers as applied in patient management. Laboratory techniques must incorporate quality control measures, which are of utmost importance in guaranteeing the reliability and validity of test results in clinical biochemistry. Regular calibration of analytical instruments and adherence to standard operating procedures (SOPs) form the foundation of consistent laboratory performance. The quality assurance procedures identify the accuracy of the test results that are essential in informing clinical decisions. In addition, inter-laboratory proficiency testing enables benchmarking and enhancement, which eventually leads to the improvement of patient safety. Laboratory personnel should understand the importance of such quality control measures and be cautious to ensure the accuracy of test results. With the growing trends in automation and digitization of laboratories, quality assurance is one of the principles that ensures the maintenance of the integrity of clinical biochemistry. New developments in laboratory methods indicate the current progress in clinical biochemistry. Innovations such as point-of-care testing (POCT) have gained traction, shifting diagnostic processes closer to the patient and expediting clinical decision-making. This move is not only associated with better patient outcomes, but it has also been seen to decrease the burden on central laboratories. Furthermore, the incorporation of next-generation sequencing (NGS) into routine diagnostics stands to revolutionize genomics and personalized medicine. NGS offers clinicians a chance to gain invaluable knowledge of hereditary diseases and response to treatment by enabling the fast and thorough analysis of genetic material. There is also an investigation of new methods in proteomics and metabolomics, which may provide new disease state and therapeutic efficacy biomarkers. As these methods are still under development, their implementation in clinical practice will further develop the sphere of clinical biochemistry, helping to treat patients more precisely and individually (Figure 1.2).

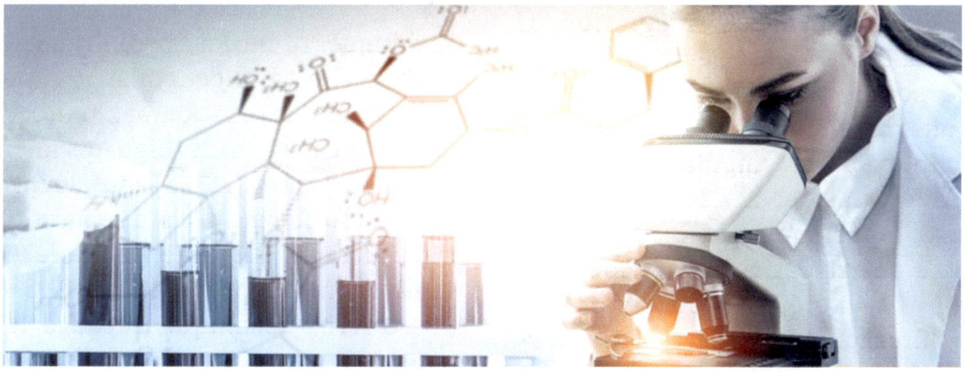

Figure 1.2. Scientist examining samples under a microscope with chemical structures and lab glassware in the background.

Source: https://www.elgalabwater.com/sites/default/files/2020-03/GettyImages-1156386832%20%282%29.jpg.

1.1.1. Spectrophotometry and Its Applications

Clinical biochemistry Spectrophotometry is a flexible analytical method that is used extensively to measure biomolecules on the basis of their light-absorbing properties. The science behind the method is based on the interaction of light and matter effect whereby the absorption spectrum of a material can be used to produce valuable data on the concentration and the molecular structure of the material. This non-destructive method is especially beneficial in clinical practice, and it is possible to quickly and reliably determine a wide range of compounds: proteins, enzymes, and metabolites. The most valuable feature of spectrophotometry is its universality in use; it is employed in the calculation of the concentrations of biomolecules that are present in complicated biological samples, which qualifies it to be more universal in both diagnostics and research fields. The development of more spectrophotometric methods also enabled the design of more advanced methodologies, such as colorimetric and chemiluminescent assays. They are based on the inherent optical properties of target analytes to enable enhanced sensitivity and specificity of clinical analysis. As an illustration, colorimetric assays usually entail the interaction of a given analyte with a chromogenic reagent to alter the absorbance characteristics of a sample so that it can be determined. These methods have enhanced the high accuracy of diagnostic devices, especially those used in point-of-care diagnostics. The integration of CMOS sensor-based technologies has further redefined the scene, providing low-cost yet high-quality alternatives to costly large-sized equipment employed for singular diagnostic techniques (Al-Rawhani et al., 2017). Besides diagnostic use, spectrophotometry is also used in routine therapeutic areas, especially in unraveling the molecular cause of the disease. The interaction of metalloinsertor-DNA experiment has provided significant data with respect to cancer treatment. For instance, certain complexes, e.g., $Rh(bpy)_2(chrysi)^{3+}$, possess selectivity for DNA damage, e.g., abasic sites and single-base bulges. Such selectivity is extremely crucial in targeted therapy designed to repair or neutralize the deleterious effects of genetic mutations (Barton et al., 2009). Spectrophotometric methods applied to the characterization of such interactions not only foster the knowledge of molecular biology but also give rise to the possibility of new diagnostic and therapeutic agents in clinical biochemistry. With further improvement that is bound to occur, one can envisage an increasingly wider sphere of applications, which will ultimately be useful to patients in the clinical environment (Figure 1.3).

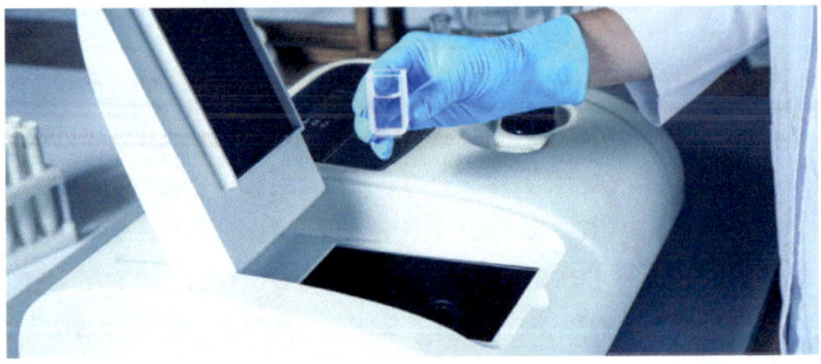

Figure 1.3. Spectrophotometers for routine to complex clinical testing.

Source: https://labdepotinc.com/media/wysiwyg/Articles/September/TLD_Blog_2024_Sept_1_Banner.jpg.

1.1.2. Chromatography Methods for Biomolecule Separation

Techniques of chromatography have now become part of clinical biochemistry, especially in the analysis and separation of biomolecules. Various techniques, such as high-performance liquid chromatography (HPLC) and gas chromatography (GC), allow for the precise separation of proteins, nucleic acids, and other biomolecules based on their chemical properties. HPLC especially, is a preferred technique because it can resolve complex mixtures within a relatively short period of time and with high resolution. Biomolecule separation can be optimized by the specificity of the stationary and mobile phases, enabling the structural, functional and interaction analysis of biomolecules. All these developments of the chromatographic methods not only help in the identification of biomarkers to diagnose diseases but also help in developing drugs and monitoring therapies, which will give a clearer picture of the clinical conditions. The hybrid hydrophobic interaction chromatography (HHIC) represents a novel evolution in biomolecular separation, particularly for therapeutic monoclonal antibodies (mAbs). The method is useful in taking advantage of the disparities in hydrophobicity between biomolecules to carry out high-resolution separations at non-denaturing conditions. By utilizing poly(alkyl aspartamide) silica columns, HHIC demonstrates the potential to improve peak capacity while minimizing the usage of organic solvents. Research outlined in relevant literature has indicated that the manipulation of mobile phase parameters, such as salt concentration and pH, greatly influences the retention and separation efficiency of mAbs and related biomolecules (Srikoti, 2020). Therefore, HHIC not only expands the chromatographic elution window but also increases the analytical usefulness of several biomolecules, thereby playing an important role in the effectiveness of the existing biochemistry applications. As well as in separation techniques, the development of virus detection by chromatographic techniques demonstrates the possibility of new methods to simplify and improve clinical biochemistry practice.

The incorporation of aqueous two-phase systems (ATPS) for virus particle purification serves as a significant development in vaccine manufacturing. By effectively partitioning viral particles away from contaminant proteins, this method can dramatically improve yield and purity without necessitating traditional chromatographic processes (Turpeinen, 2020). These separation techniques are also readily adapted in biosensing technologies , such as the application of graphene-based paper biosensors in the quick detection of viruses. These applications not only serve to illustrate the flexibility of the chromatography-related methodologies but also to highlight the importance of these methodologies in providing solutions to some of the urgent public health concerns by way of better therapeutic and diagnostic agents.

1.1.3. Immunoassays for Disease Detection

Clinical biochemistry, especially the diagnosis and treatment of most diseases, relies heavily on the use of immunoassays. Immunoassays employ the specificity of antibodies in binding to their antigens that are related to disease conditions or pathogens, and hence their usefulness as powerful tools in diagnostic and predictive practices. The scientific principle of immunoassays relies on the antigen-antibody interaction, which is quantitatively measured in different formats , such as ELISA, radioimmunoassay, and lateral flow assays. All these formats have certain sensitivity, specificity, and ease-of-use advantages and disadvantages, thereby offering a chance of a custom-made choice based on the clinical situation or analyte of interest. As the need to develop fast and precise diagnostics increases, the further development of immunoassays is bound to play a vital role in increasing our ability to diagnose disease early and achieve much better patient outcomes. Immunoassays are highly flexible and respond in a number of clinical situations and pathogens for disease detection. An example is the use of immunoassays, which have been widely used in the diagnosis of infectious diseases like HIV and hepatitis, which are utilized in screening and also for confirmation of diagnosis. Further, they have also proved useful in the quantification of chronic disease biomarkers, for instance, cardiac troponin (cTn) levels in myocardial infarction (MI). According to latest international guidelines, including the 2012 Third Universal Definition of Myocardial Infarction by the Joint ESC/ACCF/AHA/WHF Task Force, an increase in cardiac troponin (cTn) more than the 99th percentile upper reference limit (99th URL) should be considered significant, with the latter being numerically defined with an imprecision of 10% CV%. Development of reliable reference values is essential, and this underlines both the technological progress and the need for a set of strict methodological guidelines on assay usage. Although they have an enormous advantage, clinical application of immunoassays is not without its problems, especially about assay methodology and development of reference ranges. Assay performance heterogeneity is a factor of several other factors , such as demographic prevalence, physiological variability, as well as the inherent properties of the analytical procedures used. An example of such multi-factorial complexity is in attempts to find a well-defined 99th URL for cTn assays. The critical review conducted established that no common protocol is observed and regulatory agencies have not yet come up with common guidelines to aid the definition of normality in healthy groups. Such guidelines should be prepared by an expert panel comprising laboratory and clinical investigators, biomedical statisticians, and representatives of the regulatory agencies. This step would not only make immunoassays more valid but also unify their application in clinical practice, which would lead to better management of diseases and patient care (Eilerts, 2016) (Figure 1.4).

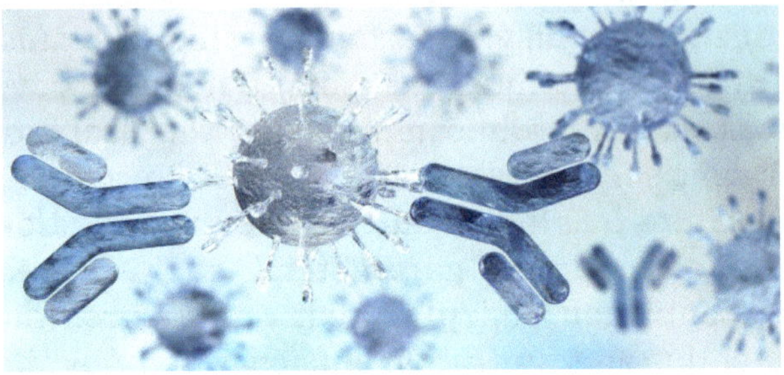

Figure 1.4. Immunoassay.

Source: https://s7g10.scene7.com/is/image/biomerieux/immunoassay%20header%203?qlt=85&wid=1600&ts=1701442243759&dpr=off.

Test Your Knowledge

1. What are the applications of spectrophotometry?
2. What are the chromatography methods for biomolecule separation?

1.2. Clinical Applications of Biochemical Tests

Learning Outcome

1. Understand the role of blood glucose monitoring in diabetes management;
2. Describe the lipid profiles in assessing cardiovascular risk;
3. Understand the liver function tests (LFTs) and their significance.

Introduction of biochemical tests in clinical practice has transformed diagnosis and treatment of different ailments. These tests promote the analysis of metabolic and physiological conditions by analyzing body fluids, mainly blood and urine. Through the measurement of the concentration of certain biomarkers, medical practitioners can detect any irregularities, which indicate the existence of either diabetes, CVDs, or liver failure. As another example, determination of the level of glucose in serum can give information about metabolic control and insulin sensitivity, which is critical in the diagnosis of diabetes mellitus. Moreover, technological developments, including high-throughput screening (HTS) and POCT, have increased the convenience and promptness of the results, enabling timely interventions, which are capable of improving patient outcomes. Biochemical tests are also considered central in the monitoring of the disease progress and the effectiveness of treatments. By routinely monitoring biomarkers, clinicians are in a position to determine how a patient responds to a particular therapy, making changes to the treatment regimens when the need arises. This is especially in the treatment of chronic illnesses, where regular checkups of enzymes and hormones can direct a shift in therapy. As an example, liver enzyme tests, including AST and ALT, present invaluable data about hepatocellular damage, which helps clinicians to make the right decisions about the intervention and lifestyle changes. Additionally, the evaluation of advanced glycation end products (AGEs) in serum serves as an important marker in conditions like insulin resistance, shedding light on metabolic health and guiding lifestyle and pharmacological interventions for improved patient management (Ekremoğlu et al., 2020).

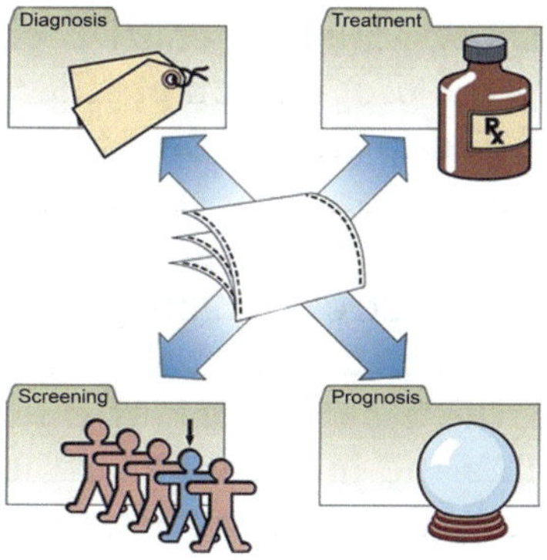

Figure 1.5. How are biochemical tests used?

Source: https://clinicalgate.com/wp-content/uploads/2015/03/B9780702051791000016_f001-002-9780702051791.jpg.

In addition, oxidative stress has led to the expansion of the clinical utility of biochemical tests because of the development of particular biomarkers of oxidative stress. Oxidative stress biomarkers give information about the redox status between ROS and antioxidants and, thereby, help to comprehend numerous pathological states. Given the potential link between oxidative stress and diseases , such as cancer, neurodegenerative disorders, and CVDs, these tests can contribute significantly to risk assessment and early diagnosis (Marrocco et al., 2017). With the field of clinical biochemistry constantly changing, the addition of these advanced tests highlights the value of a good knowledge of the underlying biochemical pathways. Such knowledge will ultimately increase the accuracy of diagnosis and lead to the era of personalized medicine, where treatments can be designed based on the individual biochemical makeup of individuals (Figure 1.5).

1.2.1. Blood Glucose Monitoring and Diabetes Management

Effective blood glucose monitoring is an important aspect of the management of diabetes, as it is one of the most important tools to measure metabolic control and avoid chronic hyperglycemia-related complications. The introduction of continuous glucose monitoring (CGM) technologies has changed patient self-management of diabetes. As opposed to the traditional methods that usually involve random blood glucose measurement, CGM devices continuously monitor blood glucose, and thus, patients can make proper food, exercise, and insulin treatment decisions. In addition to the increased patient autonomy through the feedback loop, medical staff are given useful information about a patient's trend in glycemia, ultimately resulting in more personalized therapeutic programs. By integrating these technologies into daily diabetes management, healthcare providers are able to improve treatment of the disease and restore related complications , such as CVD and neuropathy, e.g., reversing them. Glycated protein testing and, more particularly, Hemoglobin A1c (HbA1c) testing have an enormous emphasis in diabetes management. Originally used as a diagnostic test for diabetes, it is the average concentration of glucose in the blood over a period of months, which measurements of HbA1c indicate, typically two or three months. This great clinical tool has developed immense analytical improvements since its discovery in the 1970s, significantly enhancing its accuracy and dependability in monitoring the effectiveness of treatment. As the literature describes, Hemoglobin A1c testing has been taking a progressively more central role in establishing worldwide standards for blood glucose control, making it possible to treat diabetes uniformly in various clinical settings (English et al., 2014). But one must acknowledge that HbA1c may actually fail to function the same in every patient due to certain characteristics , such as variation in red blood cell (RBC) lifespan, with careful interpretation and the potential to utilize other markers , such as glycated albumin (GA) for individual patient assessment (English et al., 2014).

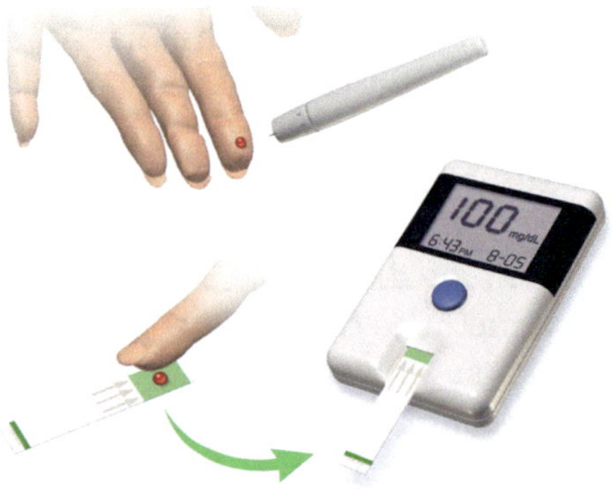

Figure 1.6. Blood glucose monitoring.

Source: https://upload.wikimedia.org/wikipedia/commons/6/62/Blausen_0301_Diabetes_GlucoseMonitoring.png.

The establishment of other markers, , such as GA, attests to the limitations of HbA1c and attests to the intricacy of the management of diabetes. GA has been touted as a satisfactory alternative for patient populations for whom HbA1c would be an unsuitable test, , such as patients with disease-modifying erythrocyte turnover or hemoglobinopathies. The strength of GA is its ability to indicate glycemic control within a limited time frame so that adjustments to therapy can be made and patient outcomes enhanced. The deliberate inclusion of both HbA1c and GA as ongoing monitoring is a tribute to the constantly developing understanding of the congenital pathophysiology of the disease. Employment of these biochemical markers gives a holistic approach towards diabetes in a way that enhances the quality of care alongside long-term health results in the patients (Abdolrahim et al., 2017) (Figure 1.6).

1.2.2. Lipid Profiles and Cardiovascular Risk Assessment

The lipid profile of individuals is a very important element of cardiovascular risk assessment, as it is closely linked with heart disease. Lipid profiles typically include measurements of total cholesterol, low-density lipoprotein (LDL), high-density lipoprotein (HDL), and triglycerides. High amounts of LDL cholesterol and triglycerides, along with low amounts of HDL cholesterol, may worsen the progression of atherosclerosis, or plaque buildup in the blood vessels. Such changes in lipid contents can cause impaired blood flow and eventually cause CVDs, including heart attacks and strokes. Lipid profiling clinical utility is established, and healthcare providers can assess the risk factors of an individual and formulate the intervention strategies that comprise lifestyle changes and pharmacotherapy to maximize heart health. Further complicating the landscape of cardiovascular risk assessment is the relationship between lipid profiles and renal health, particularly in patients with end-stage kidney disease (ESKD). It has been shown that patients who are on hemodialysis tend to have unique lipid abnormalities, with changes in cholesterol and triglyceride levels that do not always correlate with conventional cardiovascular risk factors. Polyphenol-rich intervention administration has been promising in the reduction of CVD risk factors in this population. A systematic review utilizing the Preferred Reporting Items for systematic reviews and meta-analyses (PRISMA) guidelines found that these interventions significantly improved several markers, including triglyceride levels and diastolic blood pressure, which are crucial indicators of cardiovascular health (Campbell et al., 2017). This indicates the need to have personalized medicine when it comes to the treatment because of the distinct changes in lipid profiles in patients with ESKD. Lipid profile assessment and management is an important issues in a wider personalized medicine perspective, where an individual approach to therapy is of fundamental importance. Since CVD is one of the major causes of morbidity and mortality in the world then the intricacies of lipid metabolism and what they entail are important in the prevention and treatment of the disease. Recent literature, including findings from the Journal of Lipid Research, underscores the importance of continuous research into the interactions between lipid profiles, dietary components, and lifestyle factors in cardiovascular health (Cheung et al., 2017). This involves the recognition of the effect of different interventions that can influence lipid levels and the mechanisms by which they might lower cardiovascular risk and this involves the incorporation of clinical biochemistry into a multifaceted mode of managing the patient. With the help of the lipid profile tests and their interpretation as the main priority, medical professionals will be able to develop evidence-based approaches to minimizing cardiovascular risk in a variety of populations (Figure 1.7).

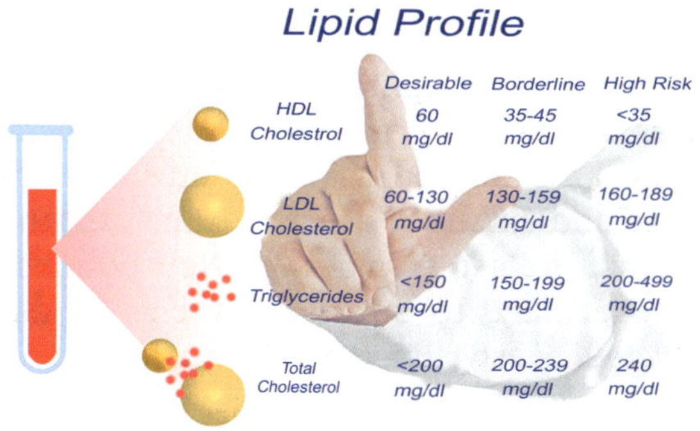

Figure 1.7. Lipid profile.

Source: https://i0.wp.com/gmdiagnosticsandpolyclinic.com/wp-content/uploads/2023/01/image.png?resize=778%2C458&ssl=1.

1.2.3. Liver Function Tests and Their Significance

Liver function tests (LFTs) are valuable clinical biochemistry investigations, which provide information regarding hepatic synthetic, metabolic, and excretory functions. Tests estimate different biochemical parameters , such as enzymes , such as alanine aminotransferase (ALT) and aspartate aminotransferase (AST), indicating hepatic cell damage, and alkaline phosphatase (ALP) and bilirubin, indicating cholestasis. Abnormal levels of such enzymes generally indicate the underlying liver disease that directs the clinicians to interventions that are indicated. Interpretation of LFT requires a profound knowledge of every marker and how it is to be interpreted in a clinical context, since an elevation or a fall in these markers may be representative of an extremely broad spectrum of conditions from acute hepatitis to chronic liver disease. LFTs are thus not only valuable in making a diagnosis but also in monitoring disease and therapeutic response, a testament to their value in patient management. Additionally, the fact that LFT levels correlate with certain liver diseases is evidence of the utility of such tests in the field. For instance, an abnormal 5′nucleotidase (5′NT) level may be indicative of bile duct obstruction or cholestasis, while elevated ALT and AST levels may indicate hepatic cell damage. In gallbladder disease, derangement in the liver function test can reflect underlying illness, as implied in studies indicating the specificity of 5′NT above ALP for cholecystitis diagnosis. Recognition of such trends and associations allows clinicians to make a proper diagnosis and treatment plan, ultimately improving patient outcomes. Finally, LFTs provide a general impression of liver function, creating a bridge between the laboratory result and clinical decision-making. In recent years, the application of LFTs to daily clinical screening has been increasingly popular, with their protective function promoted above detection of liver disease at an earlier phase.

In nonspecific abdominal complaints, extensive investigation, through the means of the assistance of LFTs, can lead to early detection of diseases , such as chronic hepatitis or even liver cirrhosis, which in some instances is associated with abnormal enzyme activity. Furthermore, continued scientific breakthrough in biochemical testing and clinical norms, e.g., those created by the European Commission, enhances the credibility of such tests in deciding the liver status. As clinical biochemistry continues to develop, there is a need for clinical professionals to keep abreast of new research and methods to be able to deliver effective and prompt patient care. The nature and degree of involvement of LFTs not only indicate their utility in the diagnosis of liver disease but also in the management and monitoring programs in clinical practice (Figure 1.8).

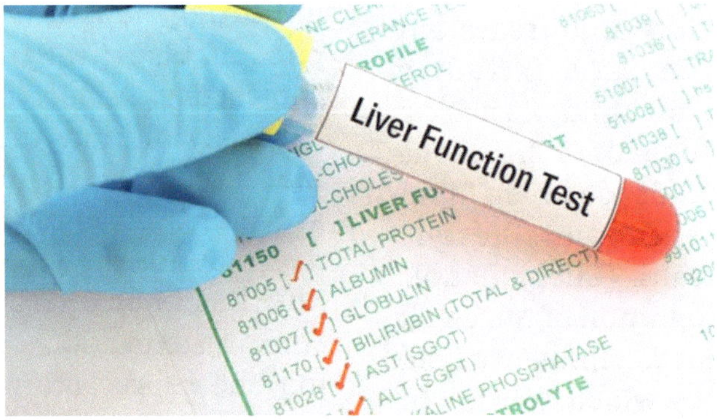

Figure 1.8. Liver tests.

Source: https://www.drpathikparikh.com/wp-content/uploads/2020/03/Liver-Test.jpg.webp.

Test Your Knowledge

1. What is the role of blood glucose monitoring in diabetes management?
2. What lipid profile is a cardiovascular risk?

1.3. Biochemical Markers in Disease Diagnosis

Learning Outcome

1. Describe the use of tumor markers;
2. Understand the role of cardiac biomarkers in diagnosing myocardial infarction;
3 Learn about hormonal assays in endocrine disorders.

Application of biochemical markers in the diagnosis of diseases is a great step in the field of clinical biochemistry, as it provides important information about the physiological and pathological conditions of a patient. These markers are normally present in blood, urine or tissue and may be used to determine the presence and extent of diseases, thus assisting in clinical decision making. Nevertheless, these tests have to be carefully chosen and interpreted. Most clinicians are guided by the idea that since a test is available, it should be used; as a result, there is a possibility of a tendency to order many tests that do not have definite diagnostic reasons. The practice has the effect of not only overwhelming clinical laboratories but also causing overdiagnosis and unnecessary treatment interventions. Therefore, it is crucial to establish a rationale based on clinical evidence and relevance to ensure that biochemical testing contributes effectively to patient outcomes (Buhagiar et al., 2005). The latest trends in the sphere of clinical biochemistry are related to the creation and approval of particular biomarkers that can increase the accuracy of diagnosis. As an example, conventional serum markers, , such as CA 15.3 and carcinoembryonic antigen (CEA), have shortcomings with regard to sensitivity and specificity in the diagnosis of early-stage diseases, including breast cancer. However, serial measurement of these markers has demonstrated potential in monitoring disease recurrence and in measuring treatment effectiveness. Conversely, the role of tissue-based markers, , such as estrogen and progesterone receptors, cannot be underestimated in terms of making a reasonable decision related to the hormone therapy of breast cancer patients. Moreover, recent advancements have introduced novel prognostic markers, , such as urokinase plasminogen activator, which can stratify node-negative breast cancer patients who may require adjuvant chemotherapy (Abraha et al., 2005). Routine clinical practice involving biochemical markers not only increases the accuracy of diagnosis but also shortens the patient management channels. With the help of evidence-based guidelines, healthcare providers may be sure that biochemical tests are ordered in a reasonable way and provide actionable information. Such rationalization of laboratory testing is necessary, particularly in an environment where healthcare resources become more and more limited by economic demands. In the long run, with the validation and uptake of new markers, the disease diagnosis paradigm will shift to allow personalized medicine where treatment modalities are selected and customized according to the biomolecular profile of individual patients. The challenge lies in balancing the need for comprehensive testing against the risks associated with unnecessary interventions, thereby optimizing patient care in the realm of clinical biochemistry (Buhagiar et al., 2005) (Figure 1.9).

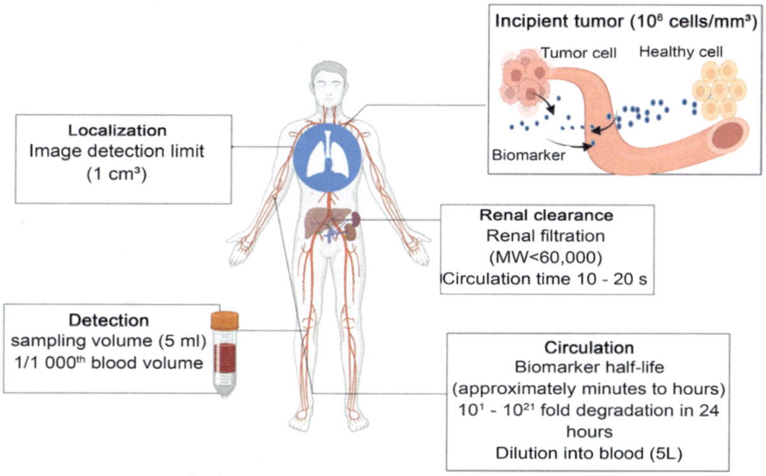

Figure 1.9. Difficulties related to the identification of tumors in their early stages.

Source: https://www.mdpi.com/sensors/sensors-24-00037/article_deploy/html/images/sensors-24-00037-g001.png.

1.3.1. Tumor Markers and Cancer Detection

The discovery and application of tumor markers are a great breakthrough in clinical biochemistry science, particularly in cancer diagnosis and management. Tumor markers are usually proteins or other substances that are released by cancer cells into the circulation or very near it, and they contain information regarding the existence and development of malignancies. Specifically, , such as CEA and CA 15-3, these clinical applications have been developed, whose sensitivity and specificity, however, can be low, precisely for the identification of early cancers. These markers, however, become significant in the assessment of the success of the therapy and recurrences, and introduce serial measurement as a method of enhancing patient outcome in cancer therapy as reasonable (Abraha et al., 2005). The therapeutic utility of tumor markers is not only their diagnostic function but also their prognostic importance for personalized therapy. Tissue-bound tumor markers have, in addition, contributed to the accuracy of cancer diagnoses and personalized treatment programs. The identification of estrogen and progesterone receptors in breast cancer patients, for example, is of particular importance in identifying appropriate candidates for hormone therapy. This personalized strategy follows the push towards precision medicine, whereby treatment protocols are formulated according to the unique composition of an individual's tumor profile. Furthermore, determination of the HER-2 protein needs to be measured in order to identify those patients who qualify for targeted therapy , such as trastuzumab. New markers like urokinase plasminogen activator have been shown to be valuable agents in the risk stratification of lymph node-negative breast cancer patients so that the clinician can recognize patients who can be spared adjuvant chemotherapy (Abraha et al., 2005). Use in everyday clinical practice attests to the increasing role of tumor markers in the optimization of cancer patient treatment. In the fluctuating setting of cancer diagnosis, microRNAs (miRNAs) are now potential tumor markers due to their stability in biological fluids and ability to reflect the molecular status of tumors. miRNAs are short, non-coding RNA molecules with regulatory functions in gene expression, with particular expression characteristics related to various types of cancers. The current research indicates the potential of miRNAs to be utilized as biomarkers for the early diagnosis of lung cancer, a condition that is usually diagnosed late due to the fact that there are no adequate screening reagents. The potential of the research on circulating miRNAs provides a less invasive procedure by which cancer diagnosis and monitoring can be done, thereby making miRNA research an economically useful tool. These new advances in miRNA biomarker identification have vast potential to revolutionize cancer treatment with treatment options earlier on, as well as with tailor-made treatment strategies that ultimately result in improved prognoses for patients (Figure 1.10).

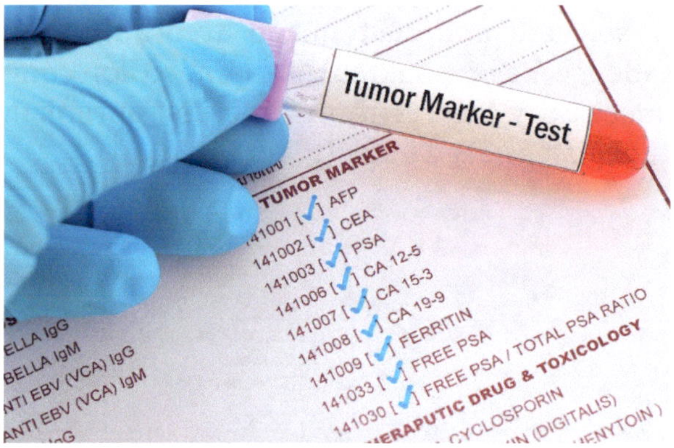

Figure 1.10. Tumor marker test.

Source: https://www.omegahospitals.com/blog/storage/2024/04/word-image-301-1.jpeg.

1.3.2. Cardiac Biomarkers in Myocardial Infarction

In the realm of clinical biochemistry, the role of cardiac biomarkers in diagnosing myocardial infarction (MI) has garnered significant attention. Cardiac troponins are among these biomarkers which have been widely acknowledged to be specific and sensitive in the detection of cardiac injury. Troponins are released into circulation when myocardial cells die (necrosis) because of lack of blood supply, thus they are a specific sign of MI. The decisive benefit of the cardiac troponin level measurement is the possibility to diagnose an acute MI within several hours and up to days after the event. This temporal feature enables the diagnosis and treatment in time, eventually enhancing the patient outcome. In light of their test accuracy, troponins have become the cornerstone of MI evaluation, often prioritized over other enzyme markers historically used in clinical practice (Abdolrahim et al., 2015). Besides, the latest developments in the methodologies, which are applied to detect troponins, have contributed to a major improvement in clinical diagnostics. Optical immunosensing technologies have undergone innovations that have offered better sensitivity and specificity that enables the quantification of cardiac troponins in the bloodstream with high accuracy. These improvements have not only sharpened the diagnostic abilities but also solved the past predicaments that were characterized by low concentration levels of troponins that required high-precision detection techniques. The availability of a large number of commercially available troponin assays has currently made it possible to better stratify patients according to the severity of myocardial damage, resulting in the targeted therapeutic approach. Furthermore, understanding the pathophysiological context surrounding elevated troponin levels is crucial, particularly when considering differential diagnoses that may yield similar biochemical profiles (Abdolrahim et al., 2015). Along with these developments, there is the need to follow the laid-down guidelines and critical levels as far as the interpretation of cardiac troponins is concerned. As emphasized in the 2012 Third Universal Definition of Myocardial Infarction, an increase in cardiac troponin levels above the 99th percentile upper reference limit (99th URL) is clinically significant. The determination of this reference limit is, however, affected by many issues, one of them being the analytical performance of the various cTn assays and the definition of a healthy reference population. The absence of standardization in the definition of these parameters creates difficulties in clinical practice in the consistent use and interpretation of cardiac biomarkers. Thus, it is crucial to develop global recommendations considering demographic factors and analysis criteria that would ensure the credible results of the diagnosis and contribute to the improved treatment of MI across populations of different patients (Figure 1.11).

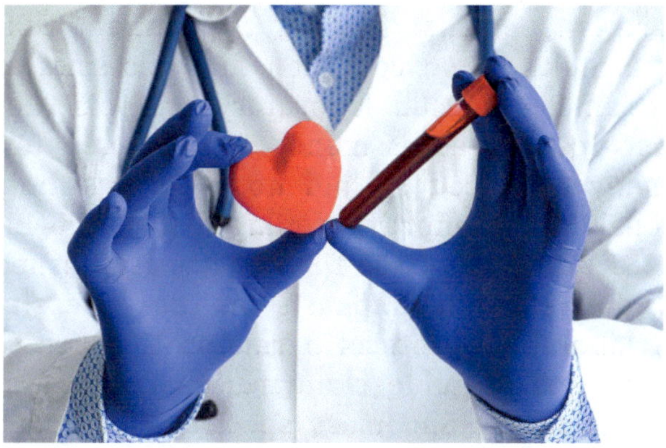

Figure 1.11. Troponins.

Source: https://www.cqssalud.com/wp-content/uploads/2022/11/Troponinas-y-otros-marcadores-cardiacos-scaled.jpg.

1.3.3. Hormonal Assays in Endocrine Disorders

Hormonal assays have become the cornerstone reagents of the diagnostic armamentarium of endocrine disease and have significantly enhanced the ability for detection and treatment of these occult diseases. Through quantitation of the level of individual hormones in biologic fluids—primarily serum, plasma, or urine—medical professionals are able to establish correlations between hormonal derangements and associated pathologies. For instance, parathyroid hormone (PTH), calcitonin, and vitamin D assays are central to the complete comprehension of calcium metabolism diseases and their implications on bone health. Novel methods that evolved in radio assay technology served to further improve the accuracy of these measures, such that more vigorous monitoring and diagnosis of disease , such as hyperparathyroidism and osteoporosis could be achieved. The integration of such hormonal screening in clinical practice allows physicians to appropriately personalize therapy to patients' needs, thereby improving patient outcomes (Potts et al.). For disease or sex development variation (DSD), tests for hormones have a further specialist field of application. DSD is a multifaceted condition that necessitates extremely focused laboratory analysis, not just routine assessment of hormones but highly advanced steroid hormone profiling. Collaborative effort, including that of the EU COST Action BM 1303 DSDnet, has established guidelines with emphasis on the necessity of laboratory protocol harmonization across Europe. The guide standardizes the use of immunoassay and mass spectrometry-based approaches in the precise diagnosis of DSD. Thus, by utilizing the guidelines, it is guaranteed that hormone testing delivers reproducible and interpretable results regardless of the laboratory performing the analysis. Lastly, all these pursuits aim to optimize patient management through the provision of continuity in diagnostic parameters and treatment regimens. The application of hormonal assays in clinical biochemistry is more than diagnostics; it is a cornerstone element in the continuous management of endocrine disease. For example, persistent monitoring of hormone levels facilitates evaluating the efficacy of treatments and the identification of potential complications arising due to diabetes or thyroid diseases. Longitudinal measurement becomes important for tailoring treatment modalities and dose adjustment of hormone replacement therapy (HRT), where optimal physiological equilibrium is obtained by the patients. With the evolving technology, innovation of point-of-care assays and non-invasive testing is the answer to expanding access to hormonal testing and enabling more advanced patient monitoring. On this premise, simulation of hormonal assays is also spearheading not only in diagnosis but in enabling proactive and personalized management of endocrine disorders (Potts et al.) (Figure 1.12).

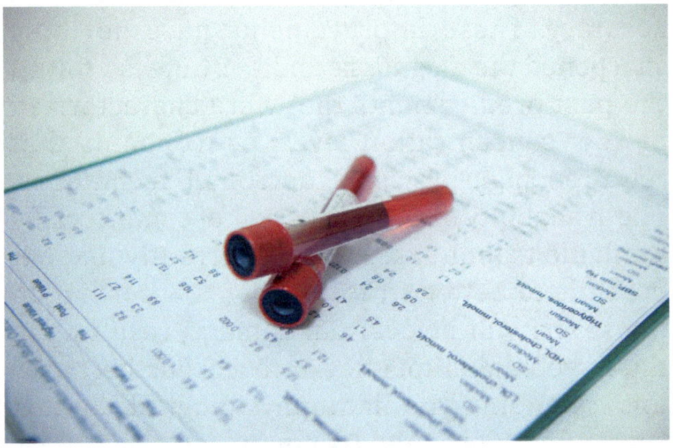

Figure 1.12. Hormonal assays test.

Source: https://healthinfo.healthengine.com.au/assets/iStock-897885224.jpg.

Test Your Knowledge

1. What are tumor markers?
2. What is the role of cardiac biomarkers in diagnosing myocardial infarction?

1.4. Emerging Trends in Clinical Biochemistry

Learning Outcome

1. Discuss advances in personalized medicine;
2. Understand the role of genomics and proteomics;
3. Integrate the artificial intelligence (AI) in diagnostics.

The face of clinical biochemistry is fast changing, and this is mainly due to the changes in technology and methods. Recently, the integration of AI and machine learning has shown promise in enhancing diagnostic accuracy and efficiency. The technologies can process large amounts of data, which a human cannot, and result in better predictive models of disease onset and progression. These innovations not only help to streamline laboratory operations but also help to personalize medicine, whereby clinicians can use these innovations to design treatments according to individual biochemical profiles. This trend underscores the need for clinical biochemists to adapt to new technologies and leverage them to advance patient care, a necessity emphasized in ongoing discourses within laboratory medicine (Fortina et al., 2015). In addition, another major trend in clinical biochemistry is the emergence of omics technologies, which include genomics, proteomics, and metabolomics. This systems approach enables the biological systems to be studied holistically at different levels and provides information that other traditional methodologies might miss. As an example, metabolomics has the potential to give a real-time snapshot of metabolic activity, which can deliver useful data on disease conditions and response to therapy. Such a multidimensional view is central to complex diseases like cancer, where dynamic interactions occur between biochemical pathways. As research continues to unfold, adapting to these omics technologies becomes essential for biochemists, aligning their practices with the increasing demand for integrative diagnostic frameworks that reflect the intricacies of patient health (Chen et al., 2011). Also of significance is the focus on social sustainability in the biotechnological innovations, especially as the health systems across the world are getting overwhelmed. The ethical connotations and social effects of the developing trends in biochemistry are important to understand in terms of building social trust and equal accessibility to the new diagnostic methods. This knowledge will guide a more concerted effort between researchers, healthcare providers, and policymakers to make sure that innovations can help different populations and do not worsen the current health disparity situation. As clinical biochemistry embraces these emerging trends, the field must navigate the delicate balance between advancing technology and maintaining human-centric values, which is vital for securing the future of laboratory medicine and its role in global health (Fortina et al., 2015) (Figure 1.13).

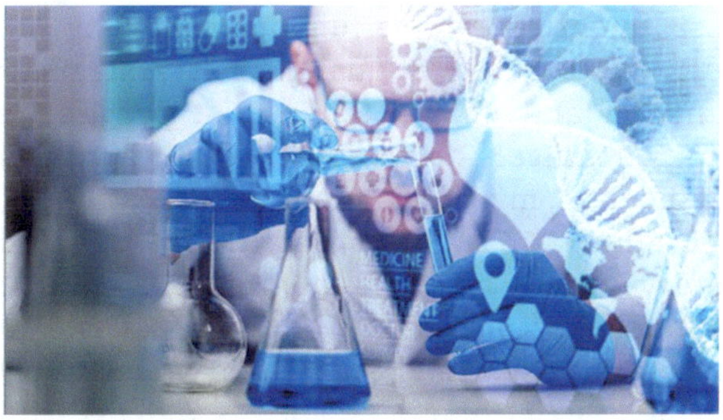

Figure 1.13. Scientist performing laboratory research with digital overlays of DNA and molecular data.

Source: https://industry.pharmafocusasia.com/articles/images/current-trends1.jpg.

1.4.1. Advances in Personalized Medicine

The evolution of personalized medicine is an epochal paradigm shift in clinical biochemistry that alters the diagnosis, treatment, and outcome strategy of clinicians. By integrating genomic, proteomic, and metabolic data, personalized medicine provides individualized therapeutic strategies that are complementary to the one-of-a-kind characteristics of every individual patient. This is brought about due to what has been attained in biochemistry and molecular biology, enabling clinicians to see with clarity the molecular cause of disease. Such specificity has been highly beneficial in oncology, where treatment is personalized according to the genetic makeup of the tumor, resulting in less toxic and more effective therapy. In addition, it can also enhance preventive interventions by assessing those at risk for diseases in biological markers, thereby leading to better long-term care outcomes and overall healthcare cost savings. Specifically, regarding CVD, MI, personalized medicine has the prime tools to perform risk stratification and individualized therapeutic regimens. Technological advancements in cardiac imaging, , such as cardiac magnetic resonance (CMR), have revolutionized the assessment of cardiac function following MI. CMR can be used to quantify left ventricular function and enable the use of prognostic biomechanical parameters. Quantification methods of myocardial contractility, stiffness, and stress are highly promising for directed intervention, which recognizes the unique response of the heart of each patient to injury. But successful integration of such new methods into clinical practice is fraught with challenges, including model validation and software-user amenability. Bridging such gaps will be through cooperative efforts by clinicians, mathematicians, and software engineers to attain improved overall patient experience and outcomes for cardiovascular wellness (Mangion et al., 2017). Moreover, the use of AI and machine learning in personalized medicine is a leapfrog advancement in clinical biochemistry. AI and machine learning can analyze large pools of data, genomic and clinical, to search for patterns and be in a position to predict the result. For instance, predictive models may improve the choice of therapeutic approaches based on patient-specific information in an attempt to achieve optimal efficacy from the treatment at the expense of minimal adverse effects. As AI continues to advance in the future, its usage in precision medicine can hopefully be able to discover novel biomarkers to extend further the horizon of precision healthcare. Besides the technological hurdle, a robust ethics development framework will be the most significant challenge that has to be bridged across data-sharing and privacy problems. With the sustained growth of personalized medicine, it can revolutionize the career of clinical biochemistry, enhance the quality of patient care, and create avenues for innovations in numerous aspects of medicine (Fortina et al., 2015) (Figure 1.14).

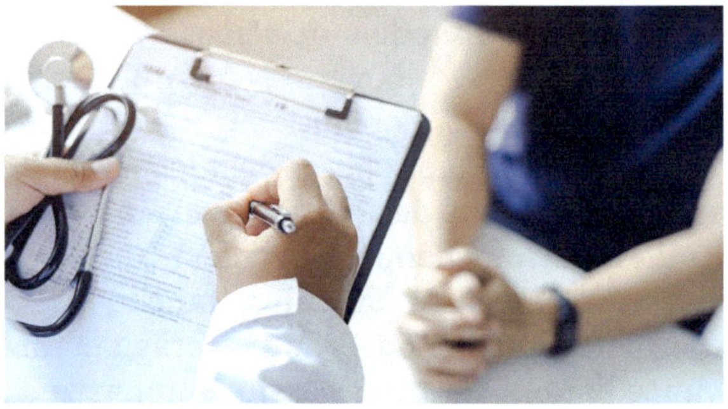

Figure 1.14. Diagnostic advances driving personalized medicine.

Source: https://assets.technologynetworks.com/production/dynamic/images/content/368595/diagnostic-advances-driving-personalized-medicine-368595-960x540.jpg?cb=12113994.

1.4.2. Role of Genomics and Proteomics

Genomics has brought sweeping changes to the discipline of clinical biochemistry, especially in the realization of the genetic basis of different diseases. Through genome mapping, scientists have discovered some vital genes that relate to pathogenicity and drug resistance. An example here is Staphylococcus aureus, an opportunistic pathogen in which genomic analysis showed clear clusters of virulent and non-virulent strains. The genomic profiling demonstrated some major differences, including allelic divergence in genes encoding established virulence factors and the existence of non-functional pseudogenes in avirulent strains. This knowledge highlights how genomic information can guide therapeutic approaches and possibly result in the emergence of personalized therapies that deal with genetic susceptibilities and microbial resistance profiles. Genomics is therefore being regarded as a tool that is almost essential in disease diagnosis and management and this is the basis of the personalized medicine projects. Proteomics, or the analysis of the complete set of proteins encoded by a genome, further supplements the genomic results and is central to clinical biochemistry. It enables the study of protein expression patterns, which might not be obvious based on the genomic data. Proteomic technologies have evolved and it is now possible to identify and quantify disease-relevant proteins in a disease pathway. As an illustration, in the case of the investigation of *S. aureus* strains, the investigators applied proteomics to clarify the variations in protein expression between virulent and non-virulent phenotypes. The results demonstrated how high expression of certain proteins, including immunoglobulin-binding protein Sbi and superoxide dismutase (SOD), might be closely connected with the pathogenicity and virulence processes. With this kind of proteomic analysis, clinicians can understand the disease process, which can help them develop new diagnostic and prognostic biomarkers. Integrating both genomic and proteomic data forms a comprehensive approach to understanding human health and disease, guiding research initiatives like the proposed human proteome project (HPP). This multidisciplinary approach provokes a discussion about the most effective approaches to proteomic investigation, where one of the debates is between a gene-based and protein-based framework. These debates are important as we aggressively attempt to explain complex biological processes at a systems level. The promised results of the large-scale proteomic efforts hold the promise of solid information about disease processes and identification of novel therapeutic targets. Genomic and proteomic technologies are converging and their combination not only increases our knowledge in the field of clinical biochemistry but also provides us with opportunities to innovate in the diagnostic and treatment approaches that represent a new paradigm in the management of health conditions (Figure 1.15).

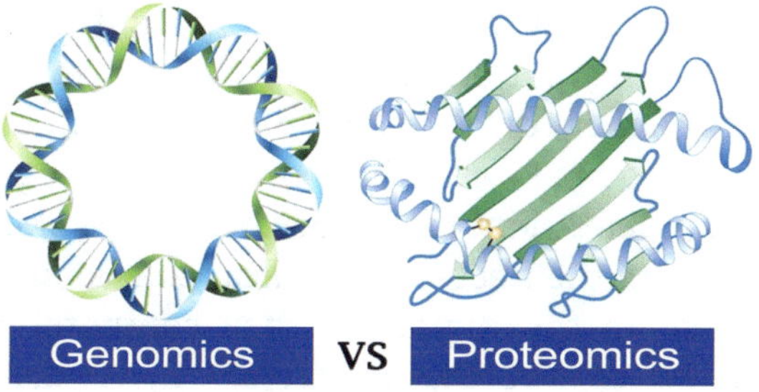

Figure 1.15. Genomics and proteomics.

Source: https://microbenotes.com/wp-content/uploads/2019/02/Difference-Between-Genomics-and-Proteomics.jpg.

1.4.3. Integration of Artificial Intelligence in Diagnostics

As clinical biochemistry continues to evolve, the position of AI in diagnosis is also becoming increasingly important. AI applications, especially founded on machine learning algorithms, can analyze vast amounts of data very quickly compared to conventional methods. This is especially useful in laboratory medicine practice, where accurate diagnosis is a matter of utmost importance. For example, AI can analyze complex biochemical pathways and laboratory results to find patterns that might otherwise go unnoticed by experienced practitioners. Such immense analytical power enables clinicians to make more informed decisions on patient care, potentially making diagnoses more precise and reducing the time it takes to arrive at a conclusion about a patient's status in the first place. Furthermore, as reasserted in the review of laboratory medicine challenges and forecasts, adopting AI may revolutionarily transform the clinical diagnostics of the future since AI provides new vistas of insight that were before partially familiar biochemical processes (Fortina et al., 2015). Notwithstanding, AI use in clinical biochemistry diagnostics comes with challenges. Ethical issues, including safeguarding data and algorithmic bias, are pre-eminent with increasing dependence on computer systems in medicine. These include navigating the thin line between using AIs potential and maintaining patient care holiness. The very practice of medical education is even needed to be brought into line with technological developments. Future doctors need to be skilled not only in the necessary clinical competencies but also in the digital literacy competencies required to operate effectively in AI-driven environments. Clinicians should critically analyze AI-generated information to preserve human clinical judgment as the key ingredient in the diagnostic process. According to recent medical literature, closing such knowledge gaps will be central to creating effective healthcare professionals who can navigate the nuances of AI in diagnostic processes (Galdames et al., 2024). In general, AI in diagnostics is a revolution in clinical biochemistry that is characterized by increased predictive power and improved patient outcomes. As AI continues to develop, its ability to read and synthesize complex biochemical data will make diagnostic procedures economical, hence saving time and resources in the clinical setting. Nevertheless, AI must go hand in hand with stringent ethics and continuous oversight in order to offset the possible risks of machine-driven decision-making. Moreover, medical school curricula must be revised in such a way that future doctors possess the ability to implement AI safely without sacrificing patient-oriented care (patient-centered care) values. AI can do wonders to transform paradigms of clinical biochemistry diagnosis, but it depends on smart use and collective efforts by healthcare providers and technology (Fortina et al., 2015; Galdames et al., 2024) (Figure 1.16).

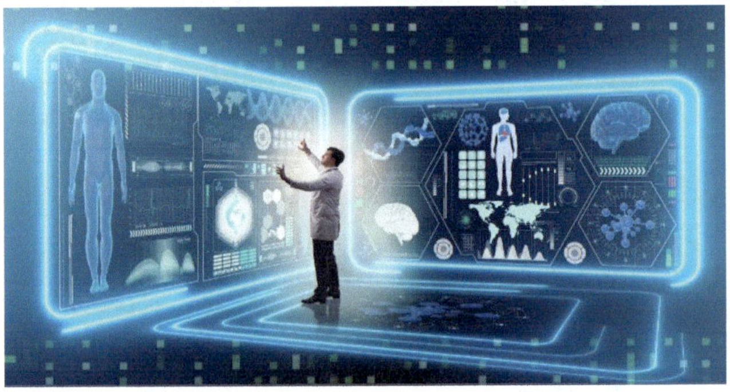

Figure 1.16. The integration of artificial intelligence in healthcare diagnostics.

Source: https://media.licdn.com/dms/image/v2/D5612AQG57Dp4DUWiTw/article-cover_image-shrink_720_1280/article-cover_image-shrink_720_1280/0/1714304280779?e=2147483647&v=beta&t=ENcL4fCENzOyvDwGS0LG2ivKpj6XrOmP-G8thxUW5os.

Test Your Knowledge

1. What are the new advances in personalized medicine?
2. What is the role of genomics?

SUMMARY

In conclusion, clinical biochemistry can be considered a pillar of human and veterinary medicine, which underlines its great diagnostic potential. Although traditionally underutilized in aquaculture, recent studies indicate the potential benefits of implementing clinical biochemistry practices within this sector, particularly for monitoring the health status of species , such as Atlantic salmon (*Salmo salar* L.). The issues that are associated with pre-analytical variables in sample collection and processing highlight the importance of the need to have standardized protocols. As we advance our understanding of biochemical analytes, the establishment of reference ranges becomes crucial, aiding veterinary practitioners and the aquaculture industry in assessing health and disease effectively (Ashby et al., 2016). Moreover, our diagnostic horizon is being transformed by the emerging technologies in clinical biochemistry, e.g., glycomics. The example of the discovery of particular glycomic patterns in liver diseases, especially in the case of patients with compensated cirrhosis, demonstrates the potential of the transformative power of biomarker development. These innovations do not only make us better in our diagnosis but also promote the aspect of early intervention, which can lead to a significant change in the outcome of patients. The integration of glycomic analysis using readily available capillary electrophoresis (CE) equipment points to a future where clinical biochemistry can offer more precise prognostic information, enhancing our understanding of disease progression (Callewaert et al., 2019). Finally, the value of clinical biochemistry is not just limited to its diagnostic usefulness; it also covers preventive health measures and therapeutic monitoring, which proves to be very crucial in both the developed and the developing markets. The mutual interaction of technology development and clinical applications has the potential of coming up with novel methodologies that transform the existing practices in the medical sector. The role of clinical biochemistry is increasingly important as the research fills the gaps and provides standardized protocols. The active attempt to combine these developments will not only help to establish healthier monitoring of aquaculture but also will add to the overall picture of clinical medicine, helping us to react to various health-related issues effectively.

The discussion of the main ideas of the field of clinical biochemistry shows the complexity of interactions between biochemical processes and clinical results. Central to this discourse is the understanding of noncoding RNAs (ncRNAs), particularly miRNAs and long noncoding RNAs (lncRNAs), which have garnered attention for their regulatory roles in vascular biology. Recent research stresses the role of ncRNAs in the pathophysiology of vascular injury, with a special focus on their role in the development of such diseases as vein graft disease and pulmonary arterial hypertension. These findings underscore the significance of ncRNAs as potential biomarkers and therapeutic targets, given their ability to mediate cell-to-cell communication and regulate cellular processes within the vascular system (Baker et al., 2016). These findings open up new avenues of novel therapeutic approaches, which may enhance patient outcomes in vascular-related pathologies. The other important issue of clinical biochemistry addressed pertains to the satisfaction of students in academic institutions, which, according to the discussion, depends on the intensity and structure of the programs, particularly those that are clinically based degrees. According to research conducted by the National Students Survey, students in clinical programs show a greater level of satisfaction, which is a result of good teaching techniques and organization of the course. This association indicates that the education standard offered in the field of clinical biochemistry is not only significant to the academic life of the students but also indicates the need to keep on improving the educational processes to make the learning experiences better. The findings demonstrate that satisfaction can be positively impacted by factors , such as institutional support and resource availability, thus shaping future educational frameworks within clinical biochemistry (Bell et al., 2018). Furthermore, the complex nature of clinical biochemistry cannot be complete without paying attention to the technological progress and the ways of using it in diagnostic and treatment approaches. Developments in molecular methods and biochemical tests are central to personalized medicine, whereby treatment can be individualized in relation to the biochemical profile of a particular person. This change in clinical biochemistry is also reflective of the wider changes in healthcare and therefore, there is a necessity to ensure that educational programs and clinical practice are constantly modified to reflect these changes. A combination of the latest research discoveries and practice-oriented methods demonstrates the active development of the sphere, contributing to a more holistic perception of the disease processes and treatment options that may substantially change the clinical course. With the help of these discussions, the topicality of clinical biochemistry is once again confirmed as one of the basic elements of contemporary healthcare practices.

KEY TERMS FROM THIS CHAPTER

Autoimmune disorders
Biomolecules
Clinical biochemistry
Diabetes
Digital technology
Drug metabolism
Gas chromatography
Hormonal balances
Immunoassays
Metabolic pathways
Next-generation sequencing
Nutrient deficiencies
Personalized medicine
Pharmacogenomics
Spectrophotometry

CRITICAL THINKING QUESTIONS

1. **Which biochemical test is used to assess kidney function?**
   a. Alanine transaminase (ALT)
   b. Blood urea nitrogen (BUN)
   c. Creatine kinase (CK)
   d. Amylase
2. **Which of the following is a diagnostic marker for liver function?**
   a. Lipase
   b. Bilirubin
   c. Creatinine
   d. Urea
3. **Which electrolyte imbalance is commonly associated with dehydration?**
   a. Hypokalemia
   b. Hyponatremia
   c. Hypermagnesemia
   d. Hypernatremia
4. **Which of the following tests is used to monitor long-term glucose control in diabetics?**
   a. Fasting blood glucose
   b. Oral glucose tolerance test (OGTT)
   c. Glycated hemoglobin (HbA1c)
   d. Random blood glucose
5. **What is HbA1c used to measure?**
   a. Short-term glucose levels
   b. Long-term glucose control over 2–3 months
   c. Insulin levels in blood
   d. Lipid profile abnormalities

Short Answer Questions

1. What is clinical biochemistry?
2. What techniques are used in the clinical biochemistry lab?
3. What are immunoassay tests used to detect?
4. What are the names of the liver function tests, with their significance?
5. What is the role of biochemical markers in disease diagnosis?

Answers to Critical Thinking Questions

1. (b); 2. (b); 3. (d); 4. (c); 5. (b)

REFERENCES

1. Abdolrahim, M., Rabiee, M., Alhosseini, S. N., Tahriri, M., Yazdanpanah, S., & Tayebi, L. (2015). Development of optical biosensor technologies for cardiac troponin recognition. *Analytical biochemistry*, *485*, 1–10. https://doi.org/10.1016/j.ab.2015.06.003(accessed on 12th June 2025).
2. Abdolrahim, M., Jazayeri, H. E., Rabiee, M., Rajab, A., et al. (2017). Evaluation of glycated albumin (GA) and GA/Hba1c ratio for diagnosis of diabetes and glycemic control: A comprehensive review. https://core.ac.uk/download/213086982.pdf (accessed on 12th June 2025).
3. Abraha, R. S., Andreasen, P. A., Arie van Dalen, ASCO Expert Panel, Barak, V., Barnes, D. M., Baselga, J., et al. (2005). Tumor markers in breast cancer–European Group on Tumor Markers recommendations. https://core.ac.uk/download/16432224.pdf (accessed on 12th June 2025).
4. Acheampong, E., Ajami, S., Aykal, M., Mattiuzzi, C., Carraro, P., Danaher, J., Lippi, G., et al. (2017). Patient and sample identification. Out of the maze? https://core.ac.uk/download/154328382.pdf (accessed on 12th June 2025).
5. Addona, T., Aicher, T., Andersen, J., Anderson, L., Anderson, N., Anderson, N., et al. (2010). Is a gene-centric human proteome project the best way for proteomics to serve biology? https://core.ac.uk/download/52693951.pdf Rabilloud, T., Hochstrasser, D., & Simpson, R. J. (2010). Is a gene-centric human proteome project the best way for proteomics to serve biology?. *Proteomics*, *10*(17), 3067–3072. https://doi.org/10.1002/pmic.201000220 (accessed on 12th June 2025).
6. Agarwal, R., Agarwal, A., Anonychuk, A., Anonychuk, D., Barlow, N., Barlow, M., Barth, J., et al. (2013). Adding value to laboratory medicine: A professional responsibility. https://core.ac.uk/download/9652177.pdf (accessed on 12th June 2025).
7. Al-Rawhani, M. A., Beeley, J., Cheah, B. C., Cumming, D., et al. (2017). Wide-range optical CMOS-based diagnostics. https://core.ac.uk/download/111557675.pdf (accessed on 12th June 2025).
8. Marrocco, I., Altieri, F., & Peluso, I. (2017). Measurement and Clinical Significance of Biomarkers of Oxidative Stress in Humans. *Oxidative medicine and cellular longevity*, *2017*, 6501046. https://doi.org/10.1155/2017/6501046 (accessed on 12th June 2025).
9. Ambrušová, K., Bartušová, M., Einspanier, R., Hanisch, C., et al. (2014). Ninety-day oral toxicity studies on two genetically modified maize MON810 varieties in Wistar Han RCC rats (EU 7th Framework Programmed project GRACE). https://core.ac.uk/download/288114335.pdf (accessed on 12th June 2025).
10. Cheung, C. M. G., Gan, A., Fan, Q., Chee, M. L., Apte, R. S., Khor, C. C., Yeo, I., Mathur, R., Cheng, C. Y., Wong, T. Y., & Tai, E. S. (2017). Plasma lipoprotein subfraction concentrations are associated with lipid metabolism and age-related macular degeneration. *Journal of lipid research*, *58*(9), 1785–1796. https://doi.org/10.1194/jlr.M073684 (accessed on 12th June 2025).
11. Ashby, A., Braceland, M., Eckersall, P. D., Haining, H., et al. (2016). Technical pre-analytical effects on the clinical biochemistry of Atlantic salmon (*Salmo salar* L.). https://core.ac.uk/download/42370197.pdf (accessed on 12th June 2025).
12. Baker, A. H., Bradshaw, A. C., & Deng, L. (2016). Role of noncoding RNA in vascular remodeling. https://core.ac.uk/download/46558277.pdf (accessed on 12th June 2025).

13. Barton, J. K., Boland, J. A., & Zeglis, B. M. (2009). Recognition of abasic sites and single base bulges in DNA by a metalloinsertor. https://core.ac.uk/download/4881218.pdf (accessed on 12th June 2025).

14. Batta, A. (2011). Cholecystitis & an enzyme study. *Int J Cur Biomed Phar Res., 1*(1), 1–5. https://core.ac.uk/download/pdf/14665.pdf (accessed on 12th June 2025).

15. Bell, A. R., & Brooks, C. (2018). What makes students satisfied? A discussion and analysis of the UK's national student survey. https://core.ac.uk/download/74206885.pdf (accessed on 12th June 2025).

16. Mangion, K., Gao, H., Husmeier, D., Luo, X., & Berry, C. (2018). Advances in computational modelling for personalised medicine after myocardial infarction. *Heart (British Cardiac Society), 104*(7), 550–557. https://doi.org/10.1136/heartjnl-2017-311449 (accessed on 12th June 2025).

17. Blevins, A. E., Foster, E. D., Harrington, M. A., Pratt, W., et al. (2020). Introducing first year medical students to personalized medicine concepts in a small group activity. https://core.ac.uk/download/322846987.pdf (accessed on 12th June 2025).

18. Buhagiar, G. (2005). Rationalization of the biochemistry laboratory: Which way forwards? https://core.ac.uk/download/46602008.pdf (accessed on 12th June 2025).

19. Callewaert, N., Geerts, A., Van Vlierberghe, H., Verhelst, X., et al. (2019). The potential of glycemic as prognostic biomarkers in liver disease and liver transplantation. https://core.ac.uk/download/287942150.pdf (accessed on 12th June 2025).

20. Campbell, K., Itsiopoulos, C., Kelly, J., Marshall, S., et al. (2017). The effect of polyphenol-rich interventions on cardiovascular risk factors in hemodialysis: A systematic review and meta-analysis. https://core.ac.uk/download/196605748.pdf (accessed on 12th June 2025).

21. Capiau, S., Stove, C., & Velghe, S. (2016). Opening the toolbox of alternative sampling strategies in clinical routine: A key-role for (LC-)MS/MS. https://core.ac.uk/download/84043363.pdf (accessed on 12th June 2025).

22. Chen, Y., & Ely, A. (2011). Health biotechnology innovation for social sustainability–A perspective from China. https://core.ac.uk/download/2731317.pdf (accessed on 12th June 2025).

23. Clerico, A., Masotti, S., Passino, C., Plebani, M., et al. (2017). The 99th percentile of reference population for cTnI and cTnT assay: Methodology, pathophysiology and clinical implications. https://core.ac.uk/download/154328384.pdf (accessed on 12th June 2025).

24. Eilerts, Diane F. (2016) "Beyond DNA: Epigenetics and Proteomics in Forensic Science," *Themis: Research Journal of Justice Studies and Forensic Science*: Vol. 4 : Iss. 1 , Article 10. DOI: https://doi.org/10.31979/THEMIS.2016.0410 https://scholarworks.sjsu.edu/themis/vol4/iss1/10(accessed on 12th June 2025).

25. Ekremoğlu, M., Pasaoğlu, H., Pasaoğlu, Ö. T., Severcan, F., et al. (2020). An investigation of acute effects at various doses of malathion on glucose homeostasis and insulin resistance in rat liver, pancreas and serum. https://core.ac.uk/download/304672915.pdf (accessed on 12th June 2025).

26. English, E., John, W. G., & Milosevich, E. T. (2014). *In vitro* determination of hemoglobin A1c for diabetes diagnosis and management: Technology update. https://core.ac.uk/download/41992337.pdf (accessed on 12th June 2025).

27. Fortina, P., Kricka, L. J., Park, J. Y., & Polsky, T. G. (2015). The future of laboratory medicine – A 2014 perspective. https://core.ac.uk/download/54509579.pdf (accessed on 12th June 2025).

28. Friedrich, A. W., Sabat, A. J., Wladyka, B., Bonar, E. A., Dubin, G., Dubin, G., Miedzobrodzki, J., et al. (2018). Joint genomic and proteomic analysis identifies meta-trait characteristics of virulent and non-virulent *Staphylococcus aureus* strains. https://core.ac.uk/download/161347738.pdf (accessed on 12th June 2025).

29. Phelps, C. L. (2004). *Advances in Teaching & Learning Day Abstracts 2005.* https://core.ac.uk/download/46714715.pdf (accessed on 12th June 2025).

30. Potts, J. T., Jr. (2025). The control of calcium metabolism by parathyroid hormone, calcitonin and vitamin D. https://core.ac.uk/download/pdf/42878870.pdf (accessed on 12th June 2025).

31. Srikoti, M. (2020). Chromatographic behavior of therapeutic monoclonal antibodies in hybrid hydrophobic interaction chromatography (HHIC). https://core.ac.uk/download/322982124.pdf (accessed on 12th June 2025).

32. Suazo Galdames, I. (2024). *De la Anatomía al Algoritmo: Alcance de las Competencias Diagnósticas Asistidas por Inteligencia Artificial en la Educación en Ciencias de la Salud.* https://core.ac.uk/download/630469681.pdf (accessed on 12th June 2025).

33. Turpeinen, D. G. (2020). Continuous viral vaccine manufacturing and viral detection strategies. https://core.ac.uk/download/346148578.pdf (accessed on 12th June 2025).

34. Xu, H., Deng, W., Deng, W., Gong, W., & Qin, X. (2014). The tumor cytosol miRNAs, fluid miRNAs, and exosome miRNAs in lung cancer. https://core.ac.uk/download/323067052.pdf (accessed on 12th June 2025).

LIVER AND KIDNEY FUNCTION TESTS

2

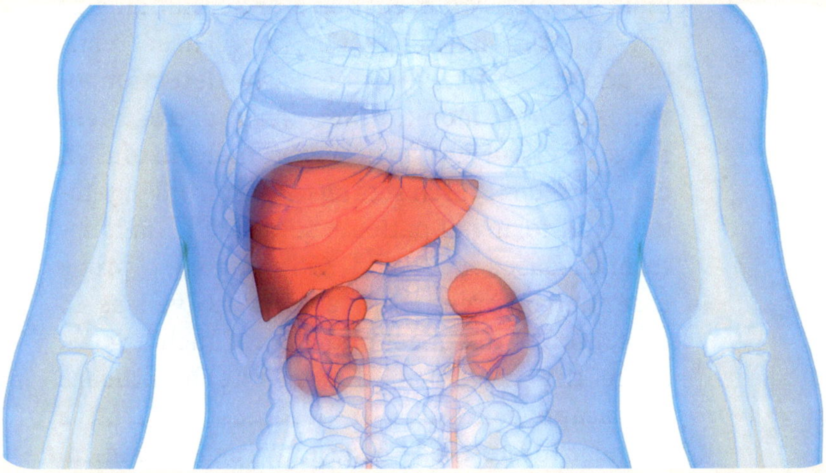

LEARNING OBJECTIVES

After studying this chapter, you will be able to:

1. Learn about the anatomy and physiology of the liver;
2. Learn about the anatomy and physiology of the kidneys;
3. Understand the common liver function tests;
4. Understand the common kidney function tests;
5. Interpret the test results for liver and kidney function;
6. Understand the clinical significance of abnormal results.

Introduction

The liver and kidney organs assume a central role in the maintenance of overall well-being by carrying out their distinct physiological roles. The liver plays the prime role of metabolizing nutrients, eliminating harmful substances from the body, and forming critical proteins like those involved in blood coagulation. The kidneys possess a specialized role of maintaining the balance of fluids in the body, electrolyte levels, and the removal of waste products via urine. It is important to understand how these organs perform their respective functions in the context of liver and kidney function tests (KFTs). These tests are crucial in describing the integrity of these organs, revealing potential dysfunction, and guiding clinical decisions in diseases , such as diabetes and chronic kidney disease (CKD), which have enormous effects on patient outcomes and quality of life (Muluye et al., 2024). The clinical significance of kidney and liver function tests (LFTs) cannot be overstated, particularly in patients at risk of metabolic disorders. For instance, derangement in liver function may result from alcoholic cirrhosis, viral hepatitis, or non-alcoholic steatohepatitis. Likewise, impaired kidney function is usually associated with hypertension and diabetes. Regular biochemical monitoring, including serum bilirubin, transaminases, and creatinine, is useful in the overall assessment of liver and renal function. Recent studies have also proven the close relationship between liver dysfunction and the risk of kidney disease, highlighting integrative approaches to patient health care (Dash et al., 2023).

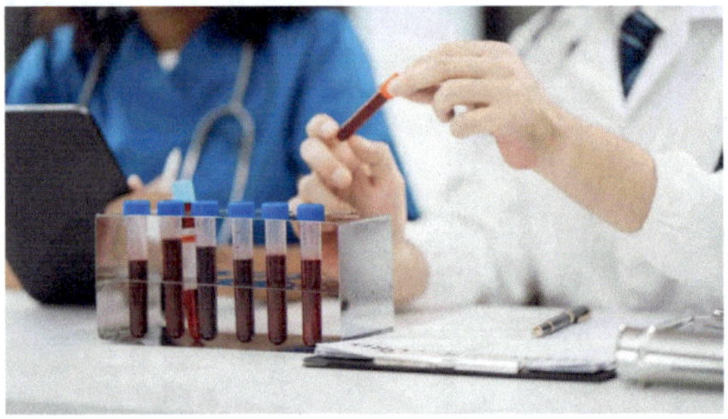

Figure 2.1. Blood test reveals information about your liver and kidney health.

Source: https://www.pasadenauc.com/wp-content/uploads/2025/02/doctor-team-analysis-the-blood-test-examination-r-2024-12-19-13-49-33-utc_11zon_11zon-1024x589.webp.

Detection of dysfunction in such organs at an early stage in the disease course allows clinicians to initiate early intervention that may stop or minimize subsequent, more severe health complications. Furthermore, technical advancements in diagnostic technology have enhanced the capability to conduct liver and KFTs with even greater accuracy and dependability. Techniques , such as serum protein electrophoresis and imaging modalities make a more comprehensive understanding of organ pathophysiology possible. These tests, in addition to facilitating early detection of abnormalities, monitor the efficacy of treatment protocols and are hence extremely useful in clinical and research settings. Apart from day-to-day monitoring of patients suffering from long-term diseases, liver and KFTs may also prove essential in pre-operative tests as well as in determining the effect of drugs on such organs. Since the transformation of the healthcare landscape continues, it becomes imperative to incorporate these tests into regular clinical practice as a priority toward better patient management and outcomes of liver and kidney health (Figure 2.1).

2.1. Anatomy and Physiology of the Liver

Learning Outcome

1. Describe the functions of the liver in metabolism;
2. Understand the role of the liver in detoxification;
3. Understand the importance of liver health in overall well-being.

The liver is a vital organ that has a complicated anatomy and physiology and is a central constituent in a number of body functions. The liver is located in the right upper quadrant of the abdomen and is subdivided into right and left lobes, which are further subdivided into smaller functional units called lobules. The lobules are made up of hepatocytes, which are the main functional cells that carry out metabolic activities like protein synthesis, storage of glucose and detoxification of toxic substances. The rich blood supply to the liver, mainly by the hepatic artery and the portal vein, enables the exchange of metabolites and waste. This dual blood supply has a special role of increasing its capacity to handle nutrients; hence the liver plays a key role in digestion and metabolism. The anatomy of the liver and the complex physiological functions it entails are important in the interpretation of LFTs, which give an insight into the wellbeing of the liver and its systemic effects. On the physiological level, the liver is part of homeostasis, which controls the biochemical balance in the body. It is important in carbohydrate metabolism, fat metabolism and protein metabolism, storing excess glucose as glycogen and releasing it as required, thereby stabilizing blood glucose levels. In addition, the liver also produces the necessary proteins, , such as albumin and clotting factors, which are important to sustain osmotic pressure and coagulation. The liver detoxification mechanisms entail biotransformation of toxins and drugs, which makes excretion possible through biliary or urinary excretion. LFTs measure various enzymes and substances in the blood, , such as bilirubin, alanine aminotransferase (ALT), and aspartate aminotransferase (AST), to assess the liver's ability to perform these critical functions. An abnormal test result may be an indication of underlying liver disease or dysfunction, which requires a closer look into the liver physiology and pathology. Liver Function and Whole-Body Health are complexly connected with each other, which is supported by interactions with other organ systems, especially the kidneys.

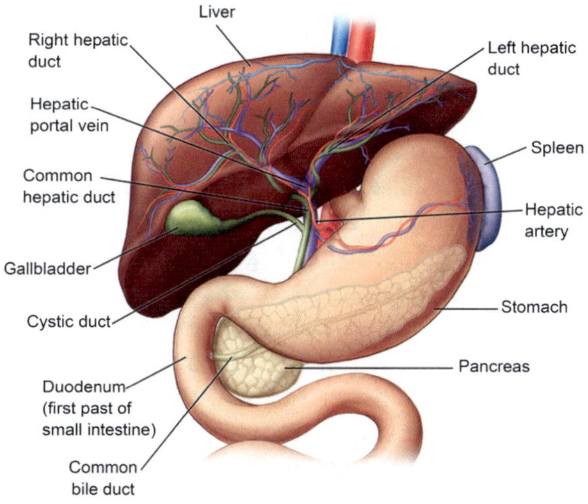

Figure 2.2. Anatomy of the liver.

Source: https://www.hopkinsmedicine.org/-/media/images/health/1_-conditions/liver-gallbladder-and-pancreas/liver-anatomy.png.

The interaction of the liver and kidneys in the physiological aspect is crucial in the body's fluid and electrolyte regulation. In the case of liver dysfunction, complications like renal impairment may arise and make the situation of assessing and treating liver disease more complicated. As an example, cirrhosis and other conditions may cause hepatorenal syndrome (HRS), in which the reduction of blood flow to the kidneys due to liver failure causes renal dysfunction. Thus, the knowledge of the anatomy and physiology of the liver is essential not only in the interpretation of LFTs but also in the prediction of the impact of liver diseases on the kidneys. Integrating knowledge of sex and gender differences in these processes is essential, as these factors influence disease progression and response to treatment, further highlighting the complexity of liver and KFTs (Mauvais et al., 2020; Hilscher et al., 2022) (Figure 2.2).

2.1.1. Functions of the Liver in Metabolism

The liver is a central organ of biochemical reactions in the body that helps in the maintenance of homeostasis. Carbohydrate metabolism is one of its major functions. Liver can also store glucose as glycogen and this process is known as glycogenesis, which can be quickly released into glucose form (glycogenolysis) when energy is required. Also, the liver is involved in gluconeogenesis, a process in which the liver converts non-carbohydrate compounds into glucose, especially in the condition of fasting or when exercising extensively. This capacity to sustain the blood sugar is very important to the overall metabolic balance. The role of the liver in carbohydrate metabolism, besides forming the basis of instantaneous energy requirements, also forms a part of long-term energy storage and retrieval, thus making the liver more significant in the maintenance of metabolic pathways that support life. Another important aspect of metabolism that is under the strong influence of the liver is lipids. Liver also produces fatty acids that are vital in many ways in the cell, like cell membrane integrity and energy metabolism. It is also involved in the catabolism of fatty acids, a process called beta-oxidation, converting lipids into forms of usable energy. Moreover, the liver is the place where lipoproteins are produced, and they play a crucial role in the distribution of lipids in the body. Abnormalities in lipid metabolism, , such as excessive lipid accumulation, can lead to conditions like non-alcoholic fatty liver disease (NAFLD), underscoring the liver's role in lipid homeostasis. Understanding the liver's function in lipid metabolism is crucial, especially when considering LFTs that may indicate metabolic dysregulation, allowing for early intervention in metabolic diseases (Singh, 2024). Liver also has a key role in protein metabolism, amino acids synthesis and degradation and control of the urea cycle.

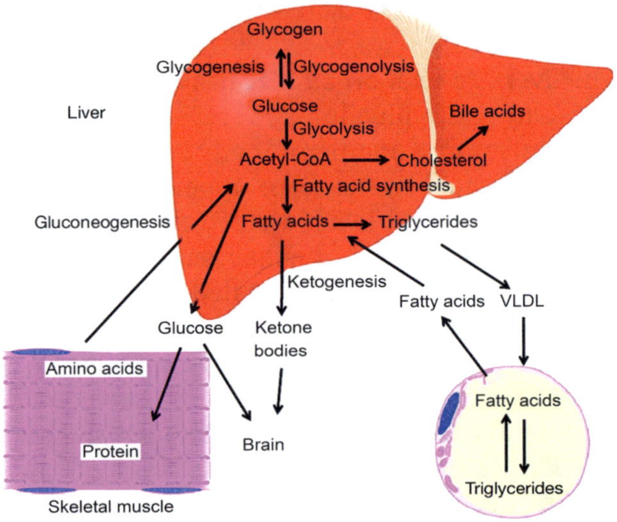

Figure 2.3. Major metabolic functions of the liver.

Source: https://www.researchgate.net/profile/John-Chiang-4/publication/271910276/figure/fig3/AS:667598400262156@1536179270549/Major-metabolic-functions-of-the-liver-During-the-fed-state-glucose-is-stored-in-the.png.

It produces vital proteins like albumin and other clotting factors that are imperative in the maintenance of osmotic equilibrium and proper hemostasis, respectively. Also, the liver can also turn the unnecessary amino acids into glucose or fatty acids, thus connecting the protein metabolism and energy production and storage. Ammonia, which is a byproduct of amino acid metabolism, is also detoxified in the liver and converted to urea to be safely excreted through the kidneys. These activities indicate the complicated interactions of the liver with various metabolic processes. As metabolic disturbances often manifest in LFTs, a deeper understanding of these processes can inform physicians about a patient's overall metabolic health (Azab, 2022) (Figure 2.3).

2.1.2. Role of the Liver in Detoxification

The liver is a detoxifying central depot that assumes the vital function of metabolizing xenobiotics and endogenous chemicals in order to counteract their potential toxicity. The organ utilizes an elaborate set of enzymatic reactions, including Phase I (oxidation, reduction, and hydrolysis) and Phase II (conjugation) reactions, to metabolize toxic substances into less toxic metabolites. Moreover, the liver secretes bile, which guarantees the discharge of such metabolites into the intestine and is responsible for detoxification. Recent studies, , such as the impact of titanium dioxide nanoparticles (TiO_2-NP) on liver physiology, demonstrate that acute exposure elevates glutathione (GSH) levels as a compensatory response to oxidative stress, while histopathological features of hepatocytes are affected. This defines the liver's vital role not just in detoxification but also in homeostasis under the influence of environmental stress (Lustosa et al., 2019). Liver enzyme systems, particularly those targeting GSTs, are vital to detoxify xenobiotics and reactive species. Enzymes facilitate the conjugation of toxic substances to make them water-soluble, so they can be eliminated. Moreover, liver metabolism for such substances as acetylcholinesterase plays a significant role in neurotransmission and can be used to illustrate how pesticide exposure impacts mechanisms of detoxification. When acetylcholinesterase activity is inhibited, , such as with certain organophosphate (OP) compounds, there is an accumulation of acetylcholine that disrupts cholinergic signal function in normal conditions. This interaction illustrates the importance of LFTs as an indicator not only of liver integrity but also of the toxicological action of numerous substances on metabolic processes, putting the liver in a central position in maintaining total well-being (Mirjana et al., 2013). Although primarily recognized for detoxification, the liver also works closely with the kidneys in the excretion of toxic metabolites. Liver injury can result in the buildup of harmful compounds that the kidneys have to metabolize, thereby adding to their workload and potentially leading to renal damage. Additionally, biochemical research on titanium dioxide in aquatic organisms has explained that both the liver and kidney are responsible for metabolizing nanoparticles, which is a demonstration of a multi-organ system strategy of detoxification. This interrelatedness places strong emphasis on detailed liver and kidney function testing as central diagnostic and monitoring tools for environmental toxin exposure. By examining the functioning of both the liver and the kidneys, medical practitioners can obtain information about the body's general ability to metabolize and excrete toxic substances, thus providing effective therapeutic interventions in patients (Lustosa et al., 2019) (Figure 2.4).

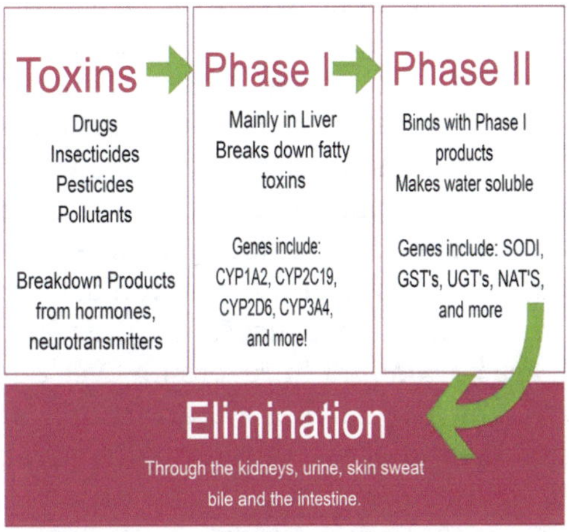

Figure 2.4. Phases of detoxification in the liver.

Source: https://vitaone.in/web/image/2127-46059a53/Detoxification-Pathways.webp?access_token=a4c32a2a-a3c1-4a12-ace8-9a5c2c805f56.

2.1.3. Importance of Liver Health in Overall Well-Being

The liver is one of the most important organs of the human body and it is instrumental in the well-being and health of the body. It also has diverse roles , such as detoxification of drugs and other harmful substances, protein synthesis, and the production of biochemicals that are required in the digestive process. Once the liver health state worsens, the outcomes may be devastating; a damaged liver may cause numerous health-related problems, including jaundice, hepatic encephalopathy, and vulnerability to developing chronic diseases. In addition, the liver plays a significant role in metabolism by controlling blood sugar levels, cholesterol, and fats and protein metabolism. Therefore, the necessity of liver health cannot be overstated; without a fully functioning liver, the body's ability to process and assimilate nutrients is significantly hindered, illustrating the direct link between liver function and overall well-being (François et al., 2019). Liver health monitoring is a part of overall wellness, not only of an individual but also of the avoidance of systemic health conditions. Liver and KFTs are important diagnostic measures, which help health care professionals to identify abnormalities in the functioning of the liver at its initial stages. The tests analyze the quantity of different enzymes, proteins, and substances contained in the blood, which gives information about the functioning of the liver and the possibility of liver disease. Early detection of liver dysfunction using these tests may result in successful interventions, which are paramount in reversing liver damage or arresting the further deterioration of the existing liver disease. Additionally, given the liver's interdependence with other organ systems, including the kidneys, the results of LFTs can inform about the broader implications on health, emphasizing the necessity of regular monitoring and proactive healthcare strategies (Levitsky, 2019). The importance of liver health cannot be underestimated further due to its immunological functions and the influence on the overall metabolic homeostasis of the body. The liver not only coordinates the activities of different biochemical pathways, but it is also a key player in immune functions and thus forms a very important part of the body's defense system. As research indicates, the liver has unique immunoregulatory properties that can mitigate the adverse effects of inflammation and infection (Levitsky, 2019). When liver functioning is poor, these protective processes may be perturbed, resulting in enhanced susceptibility to infections and chronic inflammatory diseases. This brings up a loop in which the health of the liver directly affects the immune system strength and vice versa; any damage to the liver's functioning can severely affect the wellbeing. Therefore, taking preventative care and lifestyle decisions to aid liver health is a crucial part of long-term well-being (Figure 2.5).

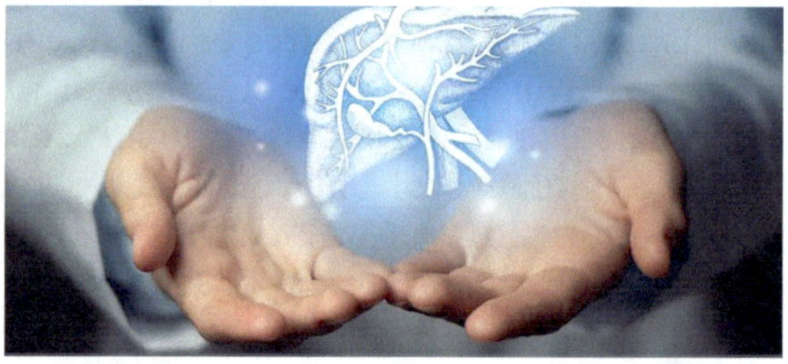

Figure 2.5. Importance of liver health in maintaining overall well-being.

Source: https://www.megawecare.com/_next/image?url=https%3A%2F%2Fcdn.megawecare.com%2FFeatured-Images%2FWcsdI8sv1jDlGq1kLbuILQMzTHCuwvTgtr30Fvrf.webp&w=1920&q=75.

Test Your Knowledge

1. What is the role of the liver in detoxification?
2. What is the importance of the liver in our body?

2.2. Anatomy and Physiology of the Kidneys

Learning Outcome

1. Know the functions of the kidneys in waste elimination;
2. Describe the role of the kidneys in fluid and electrolyte balance;
3. Understand the importance of kidney health in systemic health.

The structure of the kidneys is crucial to their physiological role because this pair of organs is largely involved in filtering waste in the blood and maintaining homeostasis since it is a vital organ. Kidneys are normally bean-shaped organs that are positioned retroperitoneally; each kidney is composed of an outer cortex and an inner medulla. Nephrons are the functional units of the kidneys, which are composed of a renal corpuscle and renal tubules. The renal corpuscle consists of the glomerulus, the place of blood filtration, and the Bowman's capsule. The renal tubule system consists of proximal convoluted tubules, loop of Henle, distal convoluted tubules and collecting ducts, which enable the reabsorption of useful nutrients and water and the secretion of waste products. The complicated structure of the kidney facilitates a very effective filtration process, which is important in the regulation of fluid and electrolyte balance in the body, which is essential to the well-being of the body in general. Physiologically, kidneys have a number of important functions that are part and parcel of homeostasis, among them being the excretion of waste, fluid homeostasis, and acid-base homeostasis. In the glomeruli, the filtration process enables the segregation of waste products, electrolytes, and water to be segregated with the bloodstream. This fluid is now called filtrate and it is converted into urine by different processes of reabsorption and secretion by the renal tubules. A very important role of the kidney functions is the maintenance of blood pressure by the renin-angiotensin-aldosterone system. Renin is an enzyme released by the juxtaglomerular cells in response to low systemic pressure, which triggers a cascade that eventually raises the systemic pressure. The kidneys also synthesize erythropoietin, which encourages the bone marrow to manufacture RBCs and therefore, is involved in oxygen transportation and metabolism in general.

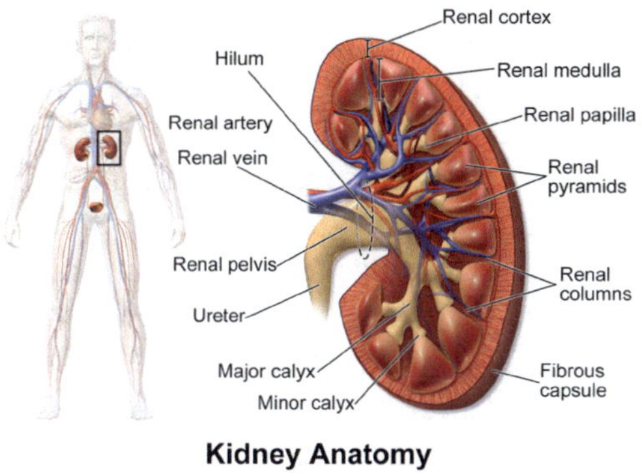

Figure 2.6. Kidney anatomy.

Source: https://upload.wikimedia.org/wikipedia/commons/d/d6/Blausen_0592_KidneyAnatomy_01.png.

The anatomy and physiology of the kidneys are very important in the interpretation of liver and KFTs because the tests help in giving information about the health and effectiveness of the organs. Blood tests commonly include the analysis of such substances as creatinine and urea nitrogen, which indicate the kidney filtration activity, and other tests determine the level of liver enzymes, providing a more comprehensive view of the hepatic and renal functionality. Furthermore, the pathophysiological alterations in the kidneys may have serious systemic consequences, such as the changes in blood constituents and pressure maintenance. As highlighted, gender and age can influence renal responses and the prevalence of kidney diseases, suggesting that both anatomical and physiological factors must be considered in clinical assessments, echoing the importance of precision medicine in healthcare (Liu et al., 2020; Mauvais et al., 2020). The combined erudition not only helps in the diagnosis but also enlightens focused therapeutic approach to kidney-related ailments (Figure 2.6).

2.2.1. Functions of the Kidneys in Waste Elimination

The kidneys are significant organs that eliminate waste, primarily through two mechanisms: filtration and secretion. Situated in the renal cortex and medulla, these organs filter blood to eliminate waste products, toxins, and excess substances, which are expelled as urine. The kidneys are supplied with blood from the renal arteries, where it is filtered within the nephron—a functional unit made up of the glomerulus and renal tubules. When blood passes through the glomerulus, water, electrolytes, and small molecules are filtered out from the blood and larger molecules , such as proteins are retained. In this way, selective filtration allows the kidneys to function in homeostasis and control fluid balance so that vital substances are reabsorbed and waste products are excreted. The efficiency of the process helps to highlight the vital role that the kidneys play in the maintenance of a stable internal environment, essential for overall health. Besides filtration, renal secretion aids in the removal of waste by actively eliminating unwanted products of metabolism from the blood into the renal tubules. Waste products of metabolism, drugs, and various ions are secreted into the tubular fluid for their removal from the body. This function allows the kidneys to regulate the blood content, clearing away substances that would accumulate to toxic levels if they were not removed. A good illustration of this is the removal of excess hydrogen ions in order to keep blood pH steady and the regulation of potassium through careful control via secretion. By effectively managing electrolyte/waste balance, the kidneys are critical to metabolic homeostasis. The reciprocal dynamic of secretion and filtration emphasizes the kidneys' intricate role in the excretion of wastes and overall bodily function, demonstrating the importance of renal status in the assessment of liver and KFTs.

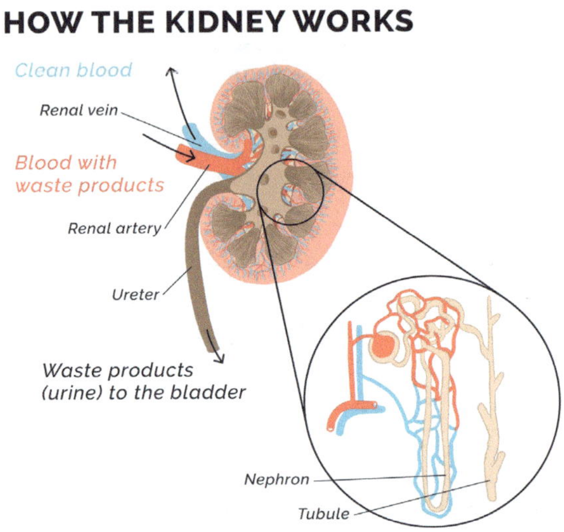

Figure 2.7. Diagram showing the role of the kidneys in waste removal.

Source: https://mosaicdx.com/wp-content/uploads/2022/09/How-The-Kidney-Works.jpg.

The implications of kidney function extend beyond waste removal; they are intimately connected with systemic health and pathologic processes. Injured renal function could lead to the buildup of toxic metabolites and metabolic waste products, and resultant conditions , such as uremia that could manifest in gastrointestinal, neurological, and cardiovascular symptoms. Besides, as observed in hemodialysis patients, the filtration capacity of the kidneys significantly influences the concentration of cardiac biomarkers , such as cTNT and NT-proBNP, which are indicators of cardiovascular function. Increased levels of these biomarkers in hemodialysis patients reflect the complex interplay between renal function and overall health outcomes, demonstrating how renal impairment can further escalate cardiovascular morbidity (Rosa et al., 2017). Therefore, regular liver and KFTs are a fundamental diagnostic tool for earlier identification and management of renal impairment, finally demonstrating the crucial role that the kidneys play in maintaining health and preventing systemic complications (Patra et al., 2018) (Figure 2.7).

2.2.2. Role of the Kidneys in Fluid and Electrolyte Balance

Kidneys are instrumental in the regulation of fluid and electrolyte balance, which is of utmost importance in homeostasis in the human body. The kidneys control the composition of blood and regulate the volume of body fluids through the processes of filtration, reabsorption, and secretion. The functional unit of the kidney is the nephron, which filters blood to create urine, which enables the elimination of unwanted water, electrolytes, and waste. It is a complex system that allows the conservation of substances, like sodium and potassium, which are needed, and the possibility of getting rid of the excess amounts. Moreover, kidneys are sensitive to many physiological stimuli, such as hormonal signals and blood pressure changes, which allow them to regulate the amount of fluid. These regulatory functions are necessary because a disruption in the kidney operation may cause a serious imbalance that threatens the general health. This is one of the most important functions of the kidneys: to be dynamic in reacting to alterations in hydration state and electrolyte requirements. As an example, during dehydration, the kidneys are able to concentrate urine, conserving water and avoiding excessive loss. On the other hand, when there is too much fluid, the kidneys are able to dilute urine in order to get rid of the excess. The kidneys also have a tight regulation of the electrolytes, especially sodium and potassium. Specific hormonal signals, such as aldosterone and antidiuretic hormone (ADH), guide the kidneys in adjusting electrolyte reabsorption or secretion based on the body's demands. This refinement is essential because an excess of sodium can cause high blood pressure, whereas a lack of potassium balance can influence heart activity, which proves the kidneys' significant importance in the balance of fluids and electrolytes in the body. Moreover, the kidneys contribute to the management of the endothelial glycocalyx layer (EGL), which plays a significant part in sustaining fluid homeostasis.

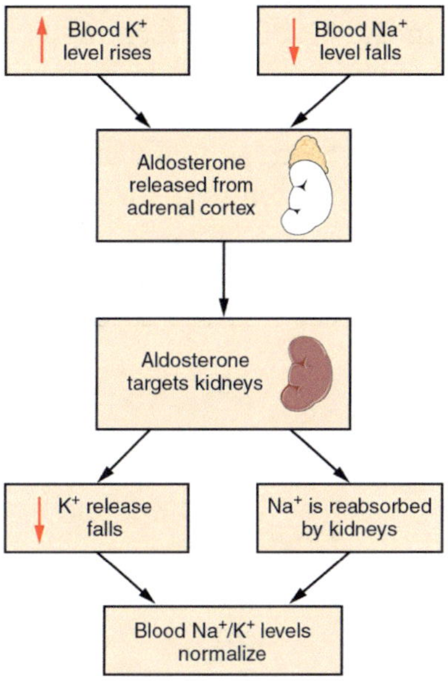

Figure 2.8. The aldosterone feedback loop: Aldosterone, which is released by the adrenal gland, facilitates the reabsorption of Na^+ and thus the reabsorption of water.

Source: https://open.oregonstate.education/app/uploads/sites/157/2021/02/2711_Aldosterone_Feedback_Loop-01-678x1024.jpg.

The vascular endothelium is covered by the EGL, which acts as a protective layer and controls fluid and solute transport. In case of impaired integrity of the EGL (which is often impaired in pathological conditions), fluid balance may be violated, and such complications as edema or cardiovascular problems may arise. Renal Function Tests are usually done not only to check the health of the kidneys but also the efficiency of the kidneys in achieving this dynamic equilibrium. This consideration becomes critical when discussing intravenous fluid management and the types of fluids administered, which should align with preserving the integrity of the EGL (Goswami et al., 2019). Conclusively, the overall role of the kidneys in fluid and electrolyte homeostasis forms a core basis in the overall assessment of health status and in the provision of medical interventions that are critical in ensuring that patients achieve the best possible outcomes (Figure 2.8).

2.2.3. Importance of Kidney Health in Systemic Health

Kidneys are very important organs, which perform a central role in ensuring the wellbeing of the system by controlling a number of body functions. In addition to their major role of filtering waste products in the blood and forming urine, kidneys also regulate fluid and electrolyte body balance, blood pressure, and produce hormones, such as erythropoietin that triggers the production of RBCs. The existence of this multidimensional interaction highlights the fact that the health of the kidneys is directly dependent on the well-being. Kidney dysfunctions are usually the reflection of more profound systemic disorders, including CVD and diabetes, which, in turn, can worsen the renal conditions. Therefore, it is imperative to take care of the kidneys not only to prevent renal disease but also to prevent the sequelae that these damages may cause in other organ systems, especially the liver and the cardiovascular system.

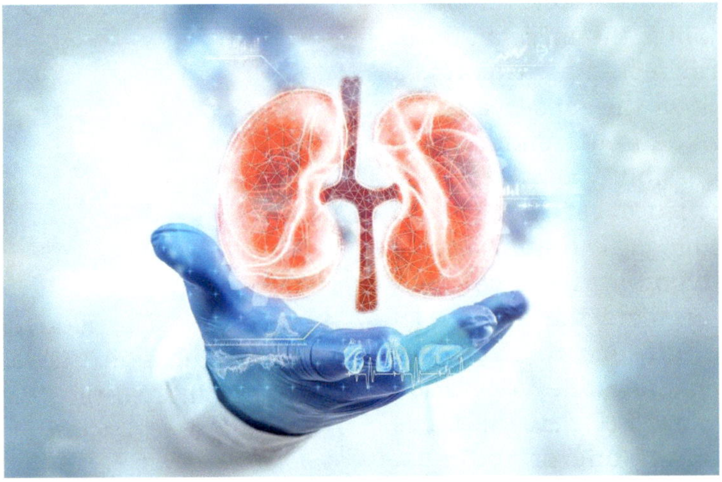

Figure 2.9. The vital role of kidney health in overall well-being.

Source: https://urocarechennai.com/wp-content/uploads/2024/03/2547597.jpg.

The mutual relationship between the kidneys and the liver is an indication of their cooperative role in the systemic health. The two organs play a role in breaking down and detoxifying substances and therefore their functioning is important in ensuring proper waste disposal in the body. Disruption in the kidney functioning may cause a build-up of toxins that may surpass the hepatic processing abilities, causing conditions , such as hepatic steatosis. As demonstrated in recent studies, conditions , such as metabolic dysfunction-associated steatotic fatty liver disease (MASLD) have emerged as significant public health concerns, significantly affecting kidney function and overall metabolic health. The health of the kidneys, therefore, must be addressed as a means of preventing or treating systemic diseases. Biomarkers , such as regular liver and kidney function tests can be used to monitor these interrelated health aspects, which helps in the early identification and intervention of any health-related problems. Moreover, the significance of kidney health can be extrapolated into the wider role of non-invasive diagnostic tools in the medical practice. There is also an emergence of literature that underlines the importance of considering kidney parameters in addition to liver tests, especially with the improvement of non-invasive methods. Amid such advancements, serology markers and imaging technologies are becoming more central to the diagnosis of kidney complications, all the time reducing the risks of invasive interventions. As an example, the definition of renal activity in the framework of MASLD can help clarify the links between liver failure and subsequent kidney distress, making it possible to perform life-saving interventions at an early stage. These methodologies are bound to change; they will demonstrate the importance of combined techniques in evaluating the health of the kidneys to promote overall systemic health, which will eventually improve patient outcomes and, at the same time, lead to a greater understanding of the interactions that occur between these critical organs (Figure 2.9).

Test Your Knowledge

1. What are the functions of the kidneys in waste elimination?
2. What is the role of the kidneys in fluid and electrolyte balance?

2.3. Common Liver Function Tests

Learning Outcome

1. Describe the alanine aminotransferase (ALT) and aspartate aminotransferase (AST);
2. Learn about alkaline phosphatase (ALP).

LFTs are critical in clinical practice, particularly in the diagnosis of hepatic diseases. LFTs under routine conditions typically include measurements of enzymes, proteins, and levels of bilirubin in blood. Certain of the significant enzymes , such as ALT and AST, are typically elevated in liver inflammation and damage. The raised ALP may indicate cholestasis, whereas gamma-glutamyl transferase (GGT) helps distinguish between bone and liver disease. The level of total bilirubin provides an idea about the capacity of the liver to conjugate and secrete waste products, and raised levels may indicate diseases , such as Gilbert's syndrome or cirrhosis of the liver. Together, these tests convey vital information regarding the pathophysiological processes within the liver, enabling clinicians to make informed decisions regarding further investigation or management. Noninvasive liver testing has, in the last decade or so, expanded the clinician's role for LFTs. These include a range of biomarkers and imaging modalities that are potentially available in addition to standard blood tests. For instance, noninvasive tests , such as fibrosis markers and elastography have come to the fore for the evaluation of conditions , such as NAFLD and its aggressive variant, NASH. The identification of these markers allows detection of liver damage at an earlier level, aiding in risk stratification for progression to advanced fibrosis or cirrhosis. This shift towards full liver assessment is in line with initiatives to maximize patient outcomes, as highlighted in organizational reports , such as those from the American Association for the Study of Liver Diseases (AASLD) on noninvasive risk assessment and management (Mary et al., 2023). Also, the integration of liver tests with kidney assessment remains important in identifying the interplay between liver and renal function. HRS is a syndrome where liver dysfunction provokes renal failure, rendering the management techniques for the concerned patients problematic. Liver enzyme and bilirubin elevation may induce renal perfusion changes, along with an impact on kidney function. Synergism among liver and kidney tests is important in practice, particularly in those with evidence of liver disease decompensation, as emphasized by current guidelines (Scott et al., 2021). Combined, this comprehensive approach enhances clinician awareness and the diagnostic model to provide patients with timely and suitable treatment of liver and kidney abnormalities (Figure 2.10).

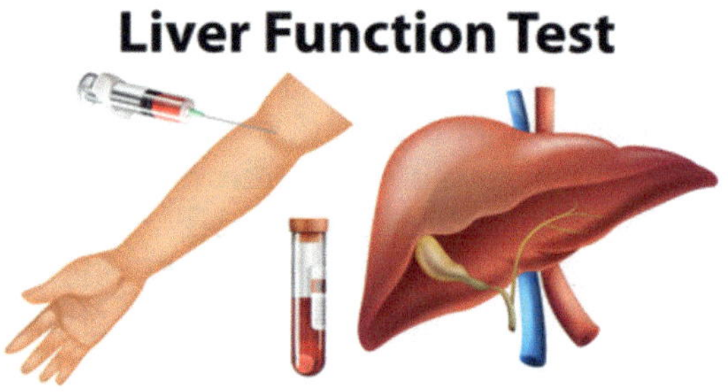

Figure 2.10. Liver function tests.

Source: https://teslascans.com/wp-content/uploads/2020/09/liver-function-test-1.jpg.

2.3.1. Alanine Aminotransferase (ALT)

In the realm of liver function assessments, ALT serves as a crucial biomarker. ALT is an enzyme that is mainly located in the liver, and its increase in serum is usually a sign of damage to liver cells. When the liver is damaged (hepatic injury), ALT is released into the blood, and as a result, the serum level of this enzyme increases and can be identified with the help of a routine laboratory test. The significance of monitoring ALT levels extends beyond simple hepatic function assessments; it is instrumental in diagnosing and managing various liver diseases, including NAFLD and hepatitis. Notably, recent studies have reported a connection between ALT levels and complications arising from chronic conditions like type 2 diabetes mellitus (T2DM), highlighting the importance of systemic evaluations of liver enzymes in clinical practice. The value of ALT in the assessment of liver functioning can also be supported by its connection with metabolic diseases. As an example, one study has shown a significant rise in the levels of ALT in patients with T2DM, indicating its association with the changed liver functioning and the possible development of NAFLD. In a study of Iraqi T2DM patients, elevated ALT levels were among multiple dysfunction markers, indicating the need for comprehensive assessments of organ function in this demographic (Matar et al., 2024). Moreover, the present study demonstrated that the deficiency of vitamin D was negatively associated with the liver functional parameters, which suggests a possible route of the regulation of liver health in diabetic individuals. These observations demand an increase in the intensity of the study of ALT as a prominent indicator since metabolic health can now be directly related to hepatic condition. Moreover, the consequences of high ALT levels enter the sphere of treatment and intervention measures. A longitudinal study exploring the effects of comprehensive care on T2DM patients demonstrated that interventions leading to weight reduction corresponded with decreased ALT levels, suggesting improved liver function (Vilar-Gomez et al., 2018). The variations of the ALT level can therefore be used as a good indicator of the success of the therapy, especially when dealing with metabolic syndromes. These results underline the necessity to include a regular monitoring of ALT as a part of the complex examination of patients with liver and kidney diseases, and, therefore, allow healthcare professionals to further customize treatment to the needs of particular patients. Finally, the overall importance of keeping the ALT levels optimal is not only associated with the health of the liver but also with the overall treatment of chronic conditions that may affect not only the liver but also kidney functions (Figure 2.11).

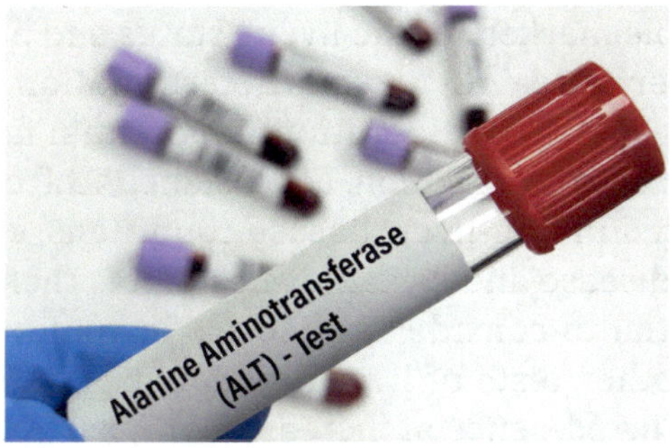

Figure 2.11. Alanine aminotransferase test.

Source: https://cdn.scope.digital/Images/Articles/alt-nedir-dusuklugu-yuksekligi-ve-tedavisi-9991676.jpg?tr=w-630,h-420.

2.3.2. Aspartate Aminotransferase (AST)

Aspartate aminotransferase (AST), also known as serum glutamic oxaloacetic transaminase (SGOT), is a crucial enzyme predominantly found in the liver, heart, and skeletal muscles. Its metabolic importance in the metabolism of amino acids, namely transaminating aspartate to yield oxaloacetate and turning α-ketoglutarate to glutamate, forms the basis of its importance in metabolic pathways. High concentration of AST in the blood is frequently an indication of damage to cells in these tissues, which is why it is a useful biomarker when assessing the health of the liver and kidneys. It is particularly relevant in the diagnosis of diseases like hepatitis, liver cirrhosis and MI since it is not only an indicator of liver damage but also an indication of the cardiac and skeletal muscle involvement due to the wide-ranging physiological significance of the enzyme. The clinical assessment of AST levels is frequently performed alongside other LFTs, such as ALT, ALP, and bilirubin. Such a multifaceted method enables medical professionals to obtain an overall picture of the functioning liver and be able to notice possible dysfunction. As an example, a considerably high level of AST, particularly in comparison with ALT, may signify alcoholic liver disease or disorders associated with muscles. On the other hand, during the interpretation of AST results, it is essential to take into account other factors like demographic and co-morbid conditions of the patient, like hypertension and diabetes, because they may affect the level of enzymes. Recent research illustrates that AST levels can be particularly revealing in the context of systemic conditions, such as COVID-19, where elevated enzyme activity has been associated with severe disease progression and liver injury in hospitalized patients (Mo et al., 2020). Besides, the applicability of AST is not limited to hepatic diseases, but it is also applicable in renal dysfunction, whereby its elevation may indicate the presence of non-hepatic factors that influence the kidney.

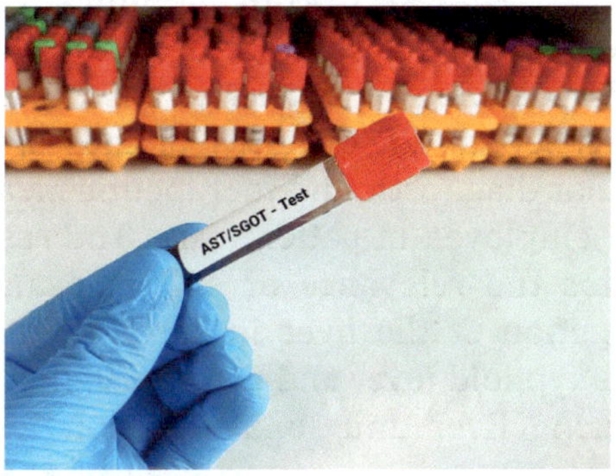

Figure 2.12. Aspartate transaminase (AST) blood test.

Source: https://www.shutterstock.com/image-photo/blood-sample-astsgot-test-liver-600nw-1839223393.jpg.

Studies have indicated that measuring AST, alongside other markers like blood urea nitrogen (BUN) and serum creatinine, provides a more comprehensive assessment of kidney health and functionality. In specific patient populations, such as trauma victims, AST levels can assist in identifying organ injuries where liver and kidney functionalities may be compromised (Kumar et al., 2012). Therefore, although AST is a major indicator of liver health, its diagnostic value in the evaluation of kidney functionality and general metabolic state highlights its versatility in medical practice (Figure 2.12).

2.3.3. Alkaline Phosphatase (ALP)

Alkaline phosphatase (ALP) is an important tissue enzyme throughout the body, including the liver, bones, kidneys, and bile ducts. Elevation of ALP typically serves as a sign of a collection of pathological conditions, primarily biliary obstruction, and liver functional disorders. Concerning LFTs, high levels of ALP by several fold can indicate cholestasis, i.e., stopped bile flow, leading to liver injury. Clinically, the measurement of ALP is important for the detection of liver disease , such as liver cirrhosis, hepatitis, and biliary tract disease. Awareness of the importance of elevated ALP is not only useful in determining hepatic pathology but also in distinguishing between hepatic and extrahepatic causes, where particular diagnostic and therapeutic measures can be employed in patient care. The research indicates the relevance of ALP in examining the function of the liver in systemic disease, such as typhoid fever and COVID-19. In a study comparing liver and renal function tests in typhoid fever patients, serum levels of ALP were significantly elevated in comparison to control groups, indicating direct influence on the liver function due to infection. This finding highlights the utility of ALP in diagnosing liver damage in infectious conditions. Similarly, research done in COVID-19 patients has also noted that high levels of ALP, as well as other liver enzymes, may signify the existence of concomitant hepatic damage based on systemic inflammation and hypoxia. All these findings strongly suggest the importance of monitoring ALP levels in patients with systemic infections since these are highly valuable markers of the liver's status and health. Furthermore, ALP levels determination calls for a general consideration of potential factors influencing its variation. For instance, ALP can be elevated in non-liver disease conditions, e.g., in bone disease and certain cancers. It is therefore essential to consider ALP levels in conjunction with other tests of liver function, e.g., ALT and AST. The presence of increased ALP, particularly in association with significant increases in ALT and AST, may suggest cholestatic liver disease. Thus, a sensitive technique of interpreting ALP results is crucial for accurate diagnosis and effective management of kidney and liver function. Continued investigation and clinical practice with the application of ALPs will enhance its utility in the interpretation of LFTs, with potential benefits for patients in a wide variety of clinical conditions (Figure 2.13).

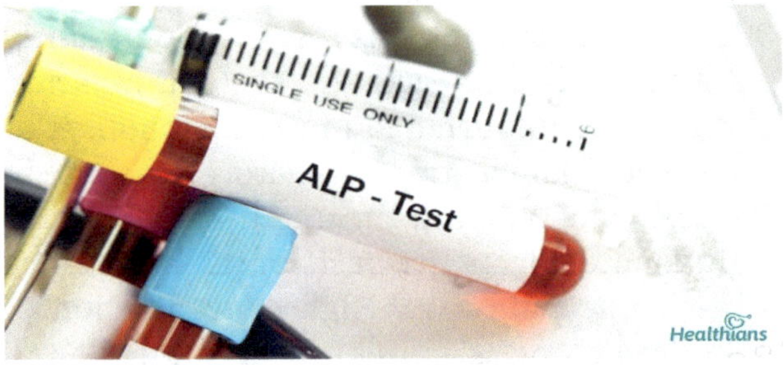

Figure 2.13. Alkaline phosphatase (ALP) test.

Source: https://cdn1.healthians.com/blog/wp-content/uploads/2020/10/1025.jpg.

Test Your Knowledge

1. What is alanine transaminase (ALT)?
2. What is aspartate transferase (AST)?

2.4. Common Kidney Function Tests

Learning Outcome

1. Describe the serum creatinine levels;
2. Learn about blood urea nitrogen (BUN);
3. Understand the glomerular filtration rate (GFR).

Renal health diagnosis and management require a thorough knowledge of the common tests of kidney functions. Key tests include serum creatinine, BUN, and the estimated glomerular filtration rate (eGFR). Serum creatinine is a by-product of muscle metabolism and when kidney function decreases, the levels of serum creatinine rise in the blood. BUN is used to quantify the nitrogen content of the blood, which is derived from urea, another product of protein metabolism. An increase in the level of BUN can be a sign of kidney malfunction or other diseases, including dehydration or excessive consumption of protein. The eGFR is a calculated value that estimates the filtering capacity of the kidneys and is critical for staging CKD and monitoring kidney function over time, thereby guiding treatment decisions. Along with the above-mentioned tests, urinalysis is also crucial in the assessment of the kidney functioning. This is a urine test to check the presence of elements like protein, sugar, and blood, which can help to understand the condition of the kidneys. An example is that the presence of protein in urine could be evidence of kidney damage or disease and glucose could be evidence of diabetes. Further, a comprehensive urinalysis will indicate an infection or other metabolic diseases. Metabolic acidosis is an important parameter to monitor in a patient with CKD or patients under dialysis. Since metabolic imbalances may lead to severe health consequences, particularly in those cases that involve hemodialysis, specific management approaches are essential. Studies have shown that addressing metabolic acidosis can lead to improved biochemical parameters and reduced hospitalization rates, demonstrating the interconnected nature of kidney function assessment and patient outcomes (Singh et al., 2024). More so, imaging tests that include ultrasound, CT scans, and MRIs are part of a comprehensive assessment of renal health. Such methodologies are frequently used to get an image of the structure of the kidneys and identify any deviations in the form of cysts, stones, or tumors. In cases of renal cell carcinoma, these diagnostic imaging techniques help inform surgical decisions and treatment plans (Ademi et al., 2024). It is important to mention that the combination of imaging studies and laboratory tests offers a solid basis for early identification and intervention of kidney diseases. By adopting a multidimensional paradigm that considers the combination of traditional KFTs with imaging techniques, healthcare professionals will have a better chance of monitoring the health of kidneys and introducing timely interventions that will prevent the further development of complications and increase the quality of life of patients (Figure 2.14).

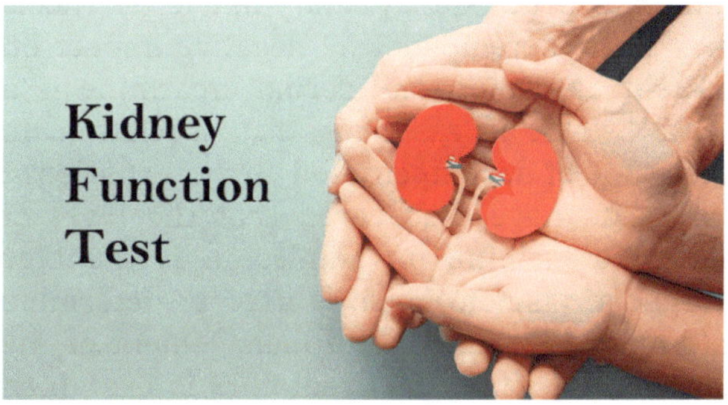

Figure 2.14. Kidney function tests.

Source: https://cdn-ildfjmj.nitrocdn.com/mwaUbGxWOcEzUDjcHGIScUjbayUTLPKI/assets/images/optimized/rev-558d84f/www.healthcareontime.com/wp-content/uploads/2025/01/kidney-function-test.png.

2.4.1. Serum Creatinine Levels

Serum creatinine concentration is an essential biomarker of renal functionality since it indicates a steady state between the generation and excretion of creatinine in the blood. Clinically, high levels of serum creatinine are usually evidence of the inability of the kidneys to perform their filtration functions, and this may occur as a result of both chronic and acute renal diseases. In particular, the determination of the level of serum creatinine will be especially important in patients with liver cirrhosis since they are highly subject to complications in the form of acute kidney injury. Studies suggest that the severity of liver disease, indicated by factors like the MELD score and child-Turcotte-Pugh (CTP) score, correlates directly with the elevation of serum creatinine levels, thus serving as a predictive marker for short-term mortality in these patients (Mukhtar et al., 2023). Therefore, the interpretation of serum creatinine level helps to give important insights into renal functioning as well as the prognosis. The relationship between liver dysfunction and increased serum creatinine levels is also explained using different clinical studies. To illustrate, acute kidney injury in liver cirrhosis may have a tremendously negative impact on patient outcomes, and serum creatinine is a critical value in assessing the association. In the study of decompensated cirrhotic patients, scientists have discovered that the level of serum creatinine on admission is a major prognostic factor, which is used to determine the line of treatment and management of the disease. When serum creatinine is examined together with other pertinent laboratory tests, e.g., prothrombin time (PT) and serum bilirubin levels, its predictive powers are increased. Indeed, these indicators collectively enhance the understanding of a patient's clinical status and help tailor appropriate interventions aimed at stabilizing renal and hepatic functions (Mukhtar et al., 2023). Additionally, the role of serum creatinine levels extends beyond traditional renal evaluation, particularly when considering its association with other systemic conditions, as seen in OP poisoning cases. In this case, serum creatinine gets checked with other lab values to decide the level of toxicity and related organ damage. Creatinine and LFTs have also been noted to be elevated in cases of moderate to severe intoxication with OP and give a thorough perspective on the status of the liver and kidneys. These observations serve to highlight the value of considering serum creatinine level as a multi-dimensional parameter to be used in diagnosis and monitoring of numerous clinical situations, emphasizing its applicability in the wider scheme of things in liver and kidney functional tests (Figure 2.15).

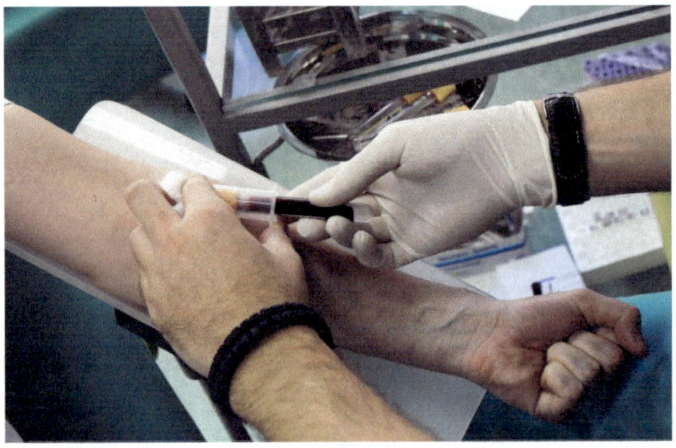

Figure 2.15. High serum creatinine levels are a potential sign of kidney disease.

Source: https://cdn-prod.medicalnewstoday.com/content/images/articles/325/325397/high-serum-creatine-levels-can-indicate-an-issue-with-the-kidneys.jpg.

2.4.2. Blood Urea Nitrogen (BUN)

Blood urea nitrogen (BUN) is a significant biomarker in assessing renal function because it quantitates the effectiveness of the kidneys in eliminating waste products from the body through the circulatory system. Measurement of BUN is included in liver and kidney function assessments, as abnormal BUN may indicate a range of medical conditions. In the clinical setting, a high BUN generally points to impaired renal function, often in the setting of acute kidney injury or CKD. Reversible increases in BUN are also observed with conditions , such as dehydration or increased catabolism of proteins without necessarily reflecting intrinsic renal illness. Therefore, once BUN is interpreted by clinicians, they must relate the result to clinical presentation and other laboratory values to reach an integrative conclusion on the renal status of the patients. Of course, BUN can also inform one about the liver function, particularly in cases of advanced liver disease. The liver plays a key role in the urea cycle process, catabolizing ammonia into urea for excretion by the kidneys. Therefore, in patients of hepatic insufficiency, i.e., cirrhosis patients, the concentration of BUN may even decrease due to the liver's reduced capacity to synthesize urea from ammonia. In a study among patients who received orthotopic liver transplantation, the co-dependence of renal and hepatic functions was emphasized; they presented with elevated levels of BUN before the transplant, representing renal stress due to compromised hepatic function. Following liver transplantation, renal function was significantly restored, highlighting the significance of BUN as a marker not only of kidney integrity but also of liver function in certain clinical conditions (Iwatsuki et al., 1973).

Besides, the correlation of BUN with inflammatory disorders highlights the biomarkers' role in disease management. Research has investigated the influence of some treatments on BUN levels in patients who have diseases like gout and arthritis, examining the impact of anti-cytokine treatment as well as conventional medication. In this context, changes in BUN levels can reflect the treatment load and success. The results indicated that while the BUN levels changed in patients under treatment, the changes were not statistically significant despite being detected. This points to the complexities of quantifying BUN levels across varied clinical settings and requires a wide-ranging approach to diagnosis and treatment, considering both liver and kidney assessment (Martini et al., 2014) (Figure 2.16).

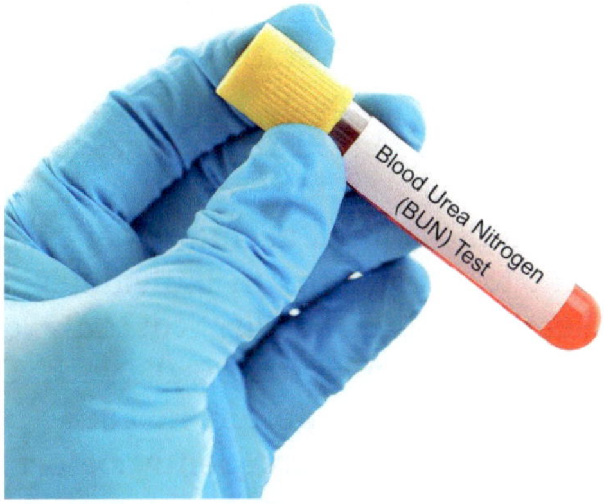

Figure 2.16. Blood urea nitrogen (BUN) test.

Source: https://labs.selfdecode.com/app/uploads/2019/10/bigstock-142429214-min.jpg.

2.4.3. Glomerular Filtration Rate (GFR)

Understanding GFR is essential in evaluating kidney function, particularly in patients with liver disease. GFR, a measure of the effectiveness of kidney filtration of blood, is a vital indication of renal health status. This value can be calculated in different ways, such as by the clearance of substances, creatinine, and cystatin C, which indicate the filtration functions of the kidneys. Creatinine levels, as commonly applied, might not necessarily reflect the true image of renal function, especially in patients with liver dysfunction. This is a critical limitation in the interpretation of liver and KFTs because varying creatinine levels may conceal an underlying GFR deterioration, which may result in erroneous diagnosis and subsequent delay in treatment. Studies have also shown that cystatin C is a better indicator of GFR, particularly in patients undergoing an orthotopic liver transplantation procedure. An example is a study that reported the correlation of serum cystatin C with GFR, as determined by iohexol plasma clearance, was much greater than that of serum creatinine. The results showcased that, in cases of moderate reductions in GFR, cystatin C levels rose sharply while creatinine levels remained in the normal range (Biancofiore et al., 2006). This difference highlights the value of cystatin Cs in identifying renal dysfunction, especially in the important first postoperative period when assessment of kidney function is vital for in-patient outcome. Additional studies on the usefulness of cystatin C point out to its benefits in individuals with liver diseases like cirrhosis. Not only does serum cystatin C correlate well with GFR, but it also performs better in identifying early renal dysfunction, frequently before the conventional markers showing problems. A study of liver transplant candidates indicated significant associations between cystatin C and calculated GFR across various estimation formulas, suggesting its superior accuracy in distinguishing mild renal dysfunction (Abo-Raia et al., 2015). Such an ability is especially relevant in the clinical environment, where timely diagnosis may enable timely interventions, thereby enhancing the management of patients and patient outcomes with regard to liver and kidney function assessment (Figure 2.17).

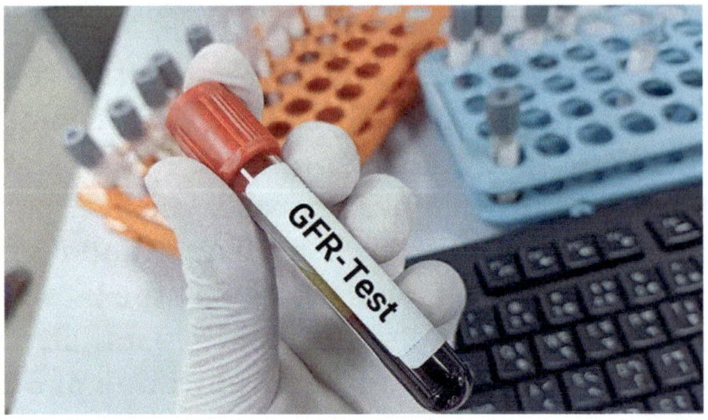

Figure 2.17. Glomerular filtration rate (GFR).

Source: https://sa1s3optim.patientpop.com/768x/filters:format(webp)/assets/production/practices/bf9c8d73f006f0bf5a5d0ab8220b944baa4725c3/images/2515012.png.

Test Your Knowledge

1. What is a blood urea nitrogen test?
2. What is the normal GFR?

2.5. Interpretation of Test Results

Learning Outcome

1. Understand the normal ranges for liver function tests;
2. Understand the normal ranges for kidney function tests;
3. Describe the factors influencing liver and kidney function test results.

Liver and kidney functional test results interpretation plays an important role in the diagnosis and treatment of numerous health disorders. Such tests involve a number of biochemical parameters that would give information about the health and functioning of the organs. For LFTs, for instance, measurements of enzymes , such as ALT and AST are essential. An increase in these enzymes may signal liver damage or inflammation. Similarly, KFTs typically involve assessing creatinine and urea levels, which reflect the kidneys' ability to filter waste products from the bloodstream. Proper interpretation of these tests not only affects clinical decision-making but also helps to determine the efficacy of the current treatments, which means that medical professionals should have a subtle understanding of these results. In addition, liver and KFTs are naturally complicated to interpret and have to take into consideration the demographics of the individual patient, including age and sex. Due to the considerable variation in laboratory values among these demographics, as noted in recent studies, the reference intervals for interpreting test results may be affected. Specifically, Jalei et al. (2024) emphasize that male participants often present higher levels of certain liver enzymes compared to females, thereby necessitating tailored reference ranges that accurately reflect these differences. These demographic factors are extremely crucial because they enable health practitioners to prevent misunderstandings that can either cause unnecessary anxiety or improper treatment of patients. Thus, medical workers should include demographic information in their analysis to give more adequate conclusions about the state of the liver and kidneys. The importance of sophisticated statistical analysis techniques and technology tools is also proving to be a major determinant in making sense of test results. The contemporary research into machine learning algorithms is becoming useful in optimizing diagnostic methods of conditions associated with liver and kidney functionality. For example, Zhang et al. (2025) discuss the application of machine learning in identifying predictive markers for attention-deficit/hyperactivity disorder (ADHD) through the analysis of blood parameters, highlighting the potential for these techniques to enhance diagnostic accuracy. With the help of modern computational power, clinicians have the opportunity to run complex data through algorithms to find subtle patterns that the human eye would not be able to recognize. Such technological incorporation is not only promoting a higher degree of accurate interpretations but is also improving the overall process of patient management and eventually giving rise to the era of better clinical outcomes and customized healthcare approach (Figure 2.18).

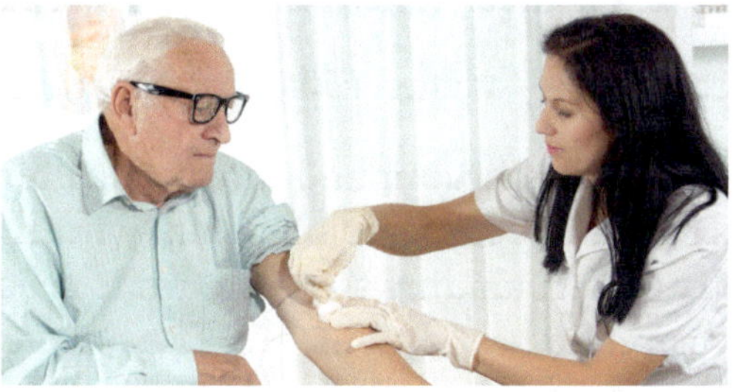

Figure 2.18. Healthcare professional performing a blood draw on an elderly patient.

Source: https://www.niddk.nih.gov/-/media/Images/Health-Information/Kidney/TW_AUG20_KidneyDisease_TwitterCard_TestingforKidneyDisease.png.

2.5.1. Normal Ranges for Liver Function Tests

Normal values for LFTs are crucial points of reference for the assessment of hepatic function and well-being. LFTs typically entail measurement of serum enzymes , such as ALT, AST, ALP, and bilirubin. Elevation of these enzymes from the normal ranges can represent hepatocellular injury, cholestasis, or bile obstruction, while decreased levels may signify dysfunction or injury to the liver. For instance, ALT reference value is typically 7 to 56 U/L, while AST reference value is typically 10 to 40 U/L.

Liver Function Test Normal Range Chart

Name: ______

Sex assigned at birth: ______ Date of test: ______

Test	Normal range	Results	Interpretation
Alanine aminotransferase (ALT)	4-36 IU/L		
Aspartate aminotransferase (AST)	5-30 IU/L		
Alkaline phosphatase (ALP)	30-120 IU/L		
Alpha-fetoprotein (AFP)	< 10 to 20 ng/mL or < 10 to 20 ng/L		
Lactate dehydrogenase (LDH)	50-150 IU/L		
Gamma-glutamyl transpeptidase (GGT)	6-50 IU/L		
Bilirubin	2-17 micromol/L		
Direct bilirubin	0-6 micromol/L		
Prothrombin time	10.9-12.5 secs		
Albumin	35-50 g/L		

Figure 2.19. Liver function test normal range chart.

Source: https://www.carepatron.com/files/liver-function-test-normal-range-chart.jpg.

The total bilirubin and direct bilirubin levels are measured to assess the capacity of the liver to excrete and conjugate bilirubin, with the normal level for total bilirubin typically less than 1.2 mg/dL. Understanding these values is crucial so that clinicians can efficiently diagnose and follow up liver-related conditions. Moreover, the clinical interpretation of these normal ranges should take into account various factors like the patient's age, sex, and ethnicity because they are known to influence enzyme levels and bilirubin content. For example, some studies identify that males have significantly higher AST and ALT levels compared to females, and this is something that clinicians should keep in mind when interpreting test results. Moreover, recent literature emphasizes the importance of the context in which the tests are taken. Presence of other diseases might complicate interpretation of LFTs; for example, elevated liver enzymes do not have to indicate hepatic impairment if the patient suffers from an acute trauma or underlying systemic condition. Such complexities call for a comprehensive approach to measurement and management so that all patient information will be utilized in making an accurate diagnosis and treatment. The correlation of LFTs with the severity of liver damage also emphasizes the importance of these markers in clinical management. Increased procollagen type III peptide levels, as documented in studies, can be correlated with liver injury severity and prognosis in patients with severe trauma, suggesting that LFTs cannot indicate the overall liver health. LFTs are made more complex by the interaction between hepatic, renal, and coagulopathy risk, as elaborated by Lockhart et al. (2003). With such intricate dynamics, a normative reference should be established not only for the diagnosis of liver diseases but also for preoperative testing and potential postoperative complications. Overall, normal values in LFTs are a foundation piece in appropriate clinical evaluation and patient care for the discipline of liver and kidney function research (Figure 2.19).

2.5.2. Normal Ranges for Kidney Function Tests

This is essential in the diagnosis and monitoring of the health of the kidneys since it gives the normal ranges of KFTs. Key indicators of kidney function include serum creatinine, BUN, and the eGFR. Serum creatinine, a byproduct of muscle metabolism, is normally in the range of 0.6 to 1.2 mg/dL in adults. An increase is often suggestive of renal impairment, but a decrease can be due to a variety of non-renal causes, including loss of muscle bulk. BUN, whose normal value is about 7 to 20 mg/dL, indicates the kidney's capacity to eliminate waste. BUN is highly variable with dehydration, intake of dietary proteins and liver functioning. Thus, clinicians use these values along with patient history and other tests to give a complete analysis of the kidney condition. The eGFR serves as a pivotal measure of kidney function, reflecting the kidneys' efficiency in filtering blood. The normal values are usually taken to be more than 90 mL/min/1.73 m 2, though this depends on age and sex. A decline in eGFR, particularly below 60 mL/min/1.73 m^2, may denote CKD, prompting further investigations into its etiology and stage. It is essential to note that the eGFR is often calculated using serum creatinine results, demographic factors, and specific formulas, such as the modification of diet in renal disease (MDRD) equation. eGFR interpretation has been found to not only assist in the diagnosis of renal dysfunction but also help to guide the clinician on the correct treatment plan, as well as help to monitor disease progression in patients, thus helping to improve management strategies. When applied to the management of kidney health, normal ranges of KFTs frequently require the incorporation of liver function testing, because the two organ systems are metabolically and pathophysiologically interrelated. As an illustration, a disease , such as diabetes and hypertension, which may influence the renal and hepatic functions, will require frequent checks of both renal and hepatic biomarkers to assess the health status holistically.

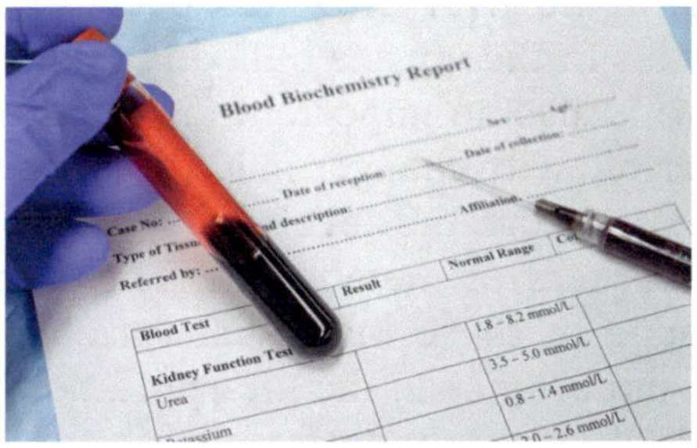

Figure 2.20. Understanding blood test results in kidney disease.

Source: https://centersurgentcare.net/wp-content/uploads/2024/11/kidney-disease-blood-test-results.png.

Successful monitoring may give an idea about the progression of conditions like diabetic nephropathy or liver complications as a result of kidney disease. Moreover, with the deterioration of renal function, the hepatic function may be impaired because of changes in drug metabolism and clearance, and this is why a holistic perspective is essential in assessing the organ functions. Understanding these interdependencies is essential for optimizing therapeutic interventions in patients with renal and hepatic concerns, as seen in studies involving metabolic regulation in conditions like type 1 diabetes, where renal function impacts treatment efficacy and safety (Tzakis et al., 1993; Bhargava et al., 2020) (Figure 2.20).

2.5.3. Factors Influencing Test Results

The accuracy of liver and KFTs is significantly influenced by biological variables, including age, gender, and body mass index (BMI). The metabolic rate and organ functionality differ in various age groups and thus may cause the test results to vary. As an example, the liver enzymes usually decrease with age, which may conceal the health problems of elderly people. Likewise, the gender difference influences the enzyme functioning; men tend to have an increased level of some liver enzymes because of the disparities in the muscle bulk and metabolism. The BMI is also an important factor, as obesity is associated with changes in kidney functioning that may distort the levels of creatinine and other markers of metabolism. Therefore, the knowledge of these biological variables is of utmost importance in the interpretation of test results and it helps in the formulation of specific diagnostic methods of liver and kidney-related diseases. In addition, extraneous factors like drugs, food and water intake play a major role in affecting the accuracy of liver and KFTs. Some medications can also raise liver enzymes, such as antibiotics and anti-inflammatories, resulting in a false interpretation of liver functioning. Eating patterns, especially a rich intake of proteins, may increase the concentration of urea and creatinine, which may indicate kidney malfunction in case of their normal functioning. Also, hydration state has a significant influence on the test outcomes; dehydration may concentrate waste products and give the impression of renal failure. Conversely, overhydration might dilute markers, masking underlying conditions. Thus, to put test results in perspective, clinicians need to examine the medication history and eating habits of a patient, as well as evaluate his or her hydration status. It is a summation of such knowledge on the external factors that can be crucial to healthcare providers in making clinical decisions regarding the wellbeing of the liver and kidneys of patients. Finally, the method of analysis and pre-analytical issues, including sample collection and storage, are important to consider when defining the validity of liver and kidney function tests. Different testing methodologies may give different results in different laboratories; thus, the need to have standardized testing methodologies to allow comparison of results. Moreover, mishandling of the samples , such as delays in sample processing or exposure to extreme temperatures, may result in degradation of some markers, giving misleading outcomes. As an example, liver enzyme levels can be artificially increased by hemolysis of samples. The appropriate method of collecting samples and maintaining high laboratory standards are the key to getting the right results in the tests. Moreover, the quality control and continuous training processes in the laboratories can lead to improved reliability of liver and kidney function tests and, consequently, to improved patient care.

Test Your Knowledge

1. What are the normal ranges for liver function tests?
2. What are the normal ranges for kidney function tests?

2.6. Clinical Significance of Abnormal Results

Learning Outcome

1. Learn about the implications of elevated liver enzymes;
2. Describe the implications of impaired kidney function;
3. Describe the potential diseases indicated by liver and kidney function test abnormalities.

Abnormal liver and kidney function test results diagnosis is crucial in in-patient health assessment and management. A raised level of liver enzymes, such as AST and ALT, can indicate liver injury or disease and requires further study and treatment. For instance, a study of typhoid fever cases revealed significantly higher LFTs when compared with healthy controls, reflecting the disease's tendency to cause hepatic dysfunction. Abnormalities are indicative of clinicians looking for etiology, assessing the severity of the condition, and taking appropriate therapeutic steps to antidote the liver damage and prevent complications arising due to deranged liver function, highlighting the clinical importance of abnormal test results (Gashaw et al., 2025). In the evaluation of kidney function, abnormal levels of creatinine are pivotal indicators of renal impairment. An increase in serum creatinine typically indicates a decrease in GFR, and investigation into the cause, such as acute kidney injury or CKD, is warranted. The findings of the research concerning the stability of kidney function in patients treated with Remimazolam mesylate confirm the importance of following renal variables during surgical procedures. The outcomes of the study's findings revealed no significant changes in renal function post-surgery, which meant that this anesthetic is safe to administer regarding renal status among the geriatric group (Zhao, 2024). Such types of findings are evidence for continued monitoring of kidney function as part of patient care, especially in susceptible populations. Aside from this, it should be remembered that abnormal findings of the kidney and LFTs do not always denote critical pathology; they can be due to transient states or drug effects. For example, fluctuation in liver enzymes following surgery can be secondary to stress and not due to chronic liver disease. An understanding of the patient's baseline state and the testing situation is necessary for proper interpretation. Clinicians will be required to integrate clinical history, risk factors, and laboratory data to make proper interpretations of test abnormalities. Therefore, a comprehensive interpretation of these findings means better patient outcomes and optimal management strategies that appropriately match individual patient requirements, thereby solidifying the role of liver and KFTs in clinical practice (Zhao, 2024) (Figure 2.21).

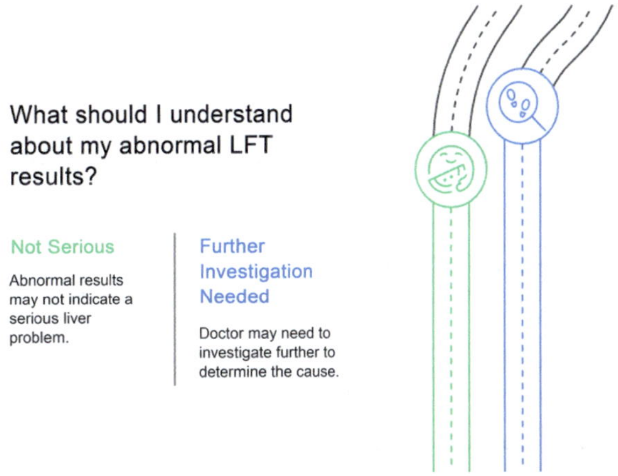

Figure 2.21. What should I understand about my abnormal LFT results?

Source: https://cdn-ildfjmj.nitrocdn.com/mwaUbGxWOcEzUDjcHGIScUjbayUTLPKI/assets/images/optimized/rev-558d84f/www.healthcareontime.com/wp-content/uploads/2025/03/What-should-I-understand-about-my-abnormal-LFT-results.png.

2.6.1. Implications of Elevated Liver Enzymes

An increase in liver enzymes is usually a sign of some form of hepatic dysfunction and as such, medical practitioners will seek to explore possible causes. Elevation of enzymes , such as ALT and AST signals hepatocellular injury, which can arise from various causes, including viral hepatitis, alcoholic liver disease, or fatty liver disease. These enzymes are used as indicators of liver inflammation and damage and thus they give important information about the health of the liver when incorporated in a panel of LFTs. Notably, the consequences cannot be reduced to the sphere of diagnosis since high liver enzymes may indicate poorer outcomes without intervention. As an example, its sustained elevation can cause chronic liver disease and, eventually, cirrhosis or liver failure in case the underlying condition is not adequately addressed, which illustrates the need to monitor its levels closely and consider therapeutic intervention in case of persistence.

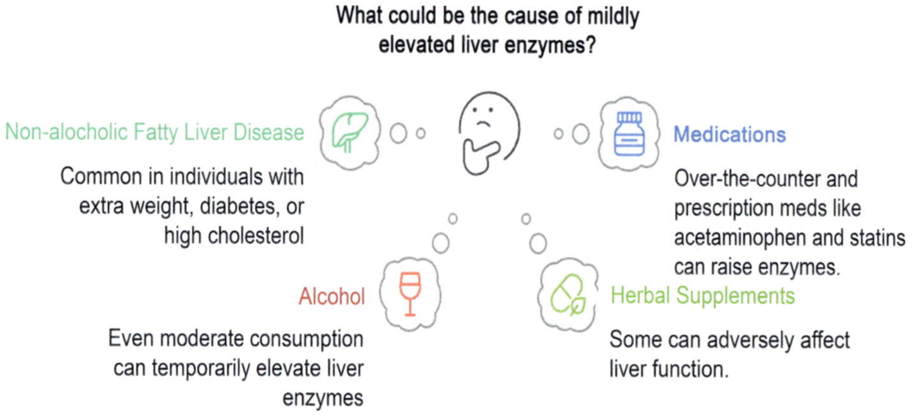

Figure 2.22. What could be the cause of mildly elevated liver enzymes?

Source: https://cdn-ildfjmj.nitrocdn.com/mwaUbGxWOcEzUDjcHGIScUjbayUTLPKI/assets/images/optimized/rev-558d84f/www.healthcareontime.com/wp-content/uploads/2025/03/What-could-be-the-cause-of-mildly-elevated-liver-enzymes.png.

The evaluation of raised liver enzymes does not only limit its investigation to the health of the liver; it can also reveal related systemic diseases. More recent research has demonstrated that raised liver enzymes in some cases may be associated with metabolic syndrome, including insulin resistance and obesity, indicating that the links between liver health and whole-body metabolism are complex. For instance, patients with conditions like hepatocyte nuclear factor 1B (HNF1B) mutations often demonstrate elevated liver enzymes alongside renal anomalies, complicating the clinical picture and requiring a more extensive evaluation of both hepatic and renal functions (Calcena et al., 2019). Besides, the presence of elevated liver enzymes can be a preemptive indication of the occurrence of disorders , such as acute hepatic porphyrias, which, when unaddressed, might lead to the development of serious acute neurological complications, making the integrated approach to the management of a patient rather important. Moreover, clinical implications of abnormal liver enzymes rise to the level of treatment patterns and patient education. Awareness of the causative mechanisms of enzyme elevation may guide personalized treatment approaches, including lifestyle changes or medical treatment to reduce liver stress. As an illustration, in NAFLD, lifestyle interventions , such as weight management and diet can be used to normalize the levels of enzymes in the body and hence prevent further damage to the liver. On the one hand, chronic diseases, like hepatitis, require frequent monitoring of complications, including the possibility of developing hepatocellular carcinoma, which creates the need to involve an interprofessional approach to patient care. Furthermore, pertinent screenings and education regarding potential triggers for exacerbating conditions, including certain medications or lifestyle choices, can empower patients to take an active role in their health management (Andant et al., 2019). It is in this complicated terrain that the interaction between raised liver enzymes and the overall health of individuals highlights the immense significance of routine checkups and a multifaceted approach to treatment (Figure 2.22).

2.6.2. Implications of Impaired Kidney Function

The consequences of compromised renal function are diverse and affect both the health outcomes of individuals and the larger health care systems. With the decrease in kidney functioning, the homeostasis and the waste products filtering capacity of the body is impaired. The dysfunction may cause a build-up of toxic substances in the blood including urea and creatinine, which are very dangerous to the overall metabolism in the body. Moreover, comorbid situations including diabetes worsen kidney damage, as manifested in the development of phenotypes, such as non-albuminuric renal impairment. As highlighted in recent research, these different pathways toward ESKD complicate management strategies, particularly in diabetic patients, where the traditional focus on albumin levels must expand to encompass deteriorating renal function independent of albuminuria (Barutta et al., 2019). Hence, diminished renal functioning needs a multifaceted mode of diagnosis and therapy that takes into consideration such intricacies. Also, the neurological consequences of poor kidney functioning cannot be underestimated. With the increase in the ammonia concentration because of the decrease in renal clearance, there is a high likelihood of developing multi-organ dysfunction. Ammonia primarily poses threats to brain function, leading to conditions like hepatic encephalopathy; however, recent findings suggest that increased ammonia levels can adversely affect various organ systems beyond the brain (Dasarathy et al., 2016). These effects highlight the importance of the effective management of renal impairment in order to avoid more comprehensive physiological disturbances. The recognition of the extensive consequences of high levels of ammonia compounds the need to include the KFTs in routine diagnostic procedures, particularly in patients who have underlying liver diseases. The tests help to generate important information on how renal failure interacts with the organ-wide implications, thereby allowing healthcare practitioners to assume a proactive role in treatment. Additionally, there is also an urgent need to manage patients with compromised renal function, and such a challenge mandates continuous changes in medical practices. The therapy of patients with kidney problems is still changing with the introduction of new therapeutic agents to treat concomitant diseases, especially diabetes. Conventional therapeutic strategies should also be reconsidered because the safety limits of drugs can vary considerably in the case of patients with renal dysfunction. Such a paradigm shift requires a corresponding change in the interaction of healthcare providers, as the KFTs should become the basis of developing treatment strategies that consider the unique needs of patients. As highlighted by the Italian Diabetes Society and the Italian Society of Nephrology, understanding the progression of diabetic kidney disease and its distinct phenotypes is crucial for implementing effective diabetes management strategies (Barutta et al., 2019). In this way, lifelong learning and investigation play a significant role in the maximization of care to patients with compromised renal functionality, which will eventually translate into better health outcomes in various organ systems (Figure 2.23).

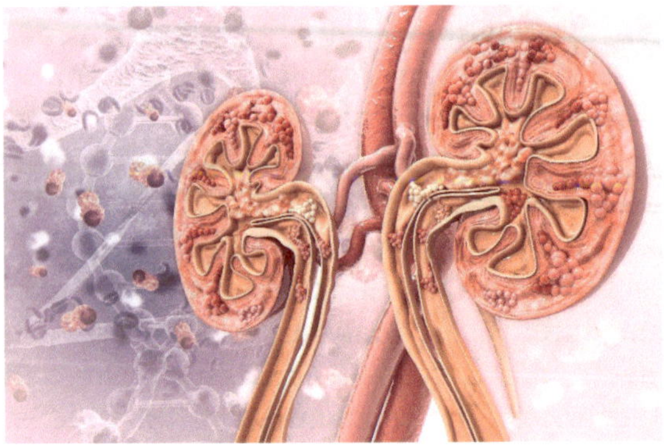

Figure 2.23. Medical illustration of human kidneys and associated structures.

Source: https://www.thecardiologyadvisor.com/wp-content/uploads/sites/17/2019/09/kidneysh1092756959_1502448-2.jpg.

2.6.3. Potential Diseases Indicated by Test Abnormalities

The lab interpretation of liver tests and KFTs gives significant information regarding potential diseases that may afflict the patients. Abnormal values obtained from the tests are suggestive of many health issues, particularly of CKD as well as liver disease. For example, high elevations of liver enzymes , such as AST and ALT, typically suggest inflammatory or injurious conditions of the liver. When coupled with altered renal function, this may suggest more severe underlying pathology like glomerulonephritis or hepatic cirrhosis. The interaction between liver and renal health is particularly relevant, as both organs are deeply engaged in metabolic activities and detoxification, showing how disease in one can influence the other, ultimately rendering patient prognosis and treatment choices increasingly more difficult, as seen in various studies (Dash et al., 2023). Liver and KFTs are not just employed as diagnostic procedures but also as follow-up procedures for chronic disease. Kidney impairment is reflected by abnormal values of glomerular filtration rate (eGFR) and is most typically suggestive of diseases , such as diabetic nephropathy or hypertensive kidney disease. The relationship between liver impairment and eGFR levels has been reported to show that dysfunctional kidney function can aggravate liver impairment by means , such as a shift in drug metabolism and accumulation of toxins (Kumar et al., 2022). Moreover, an evaluation of lipid profiles along with renal as well as LFTs provides the overall metabolic status of a patient. Elevated levels of lipids observed in patients with dysregulated eGFR establish an increased risk for CVD, highlighting organ system interdependence in the assessment of overall health status. Clinicians can use results obtained from liver and KFTs to develop particular disease prevention and control strategies. In populations with high CKD prevalence, such as, repeated monitoring of LFTs may help to identify underlying derangements of the liver co-existent with CKD that may complicate the process of care (Dash et al., 2023). Additionally, triaging of patients based on test results will enable prioritization of those who are at greater risk of adverse outcomes, particularly if SARS-CoV-2 infection is observed. The heightened liver enzyme elevation in the case of SARS-CoV-2-infected patients with CKD indicates the vulnerability of this group to multisystem disorders and careful and subtle medical management (Kumar et al., 2022). The awareness of potential diseases indicated by abnormal laboratory findings, therefore, promotes an anticipatory management of chronic diseases and improvement of patient care through early detection and intervention.

Test Your Knowledge

1. What are the implications of elevated liver enzymes?
2. What are the implications of impaired kidney function?

SUMMARY

Liver and kidney functional tests are important tests that are used to evaluate the health status of individuals, especially in determining whether there are any dysfunctions that might result in severe health conditions. By performing an extensive evaluation of these tests, medical professionals can successfully understand the level at which these organs are carrying out their vital functions, such as detoxification, metabolism, and excretion of waste. These tests are especially crucial in a population that is either environmentally exposed to toxins or a population that is on medical regimens that could affect the functioning of the organs. The importance of the continuous monitoring of these parameters has been recently emphasized, and it is necessary to continue the assessment to ensure the health of patients. For instance, research indicates that certain herbal supplements may not exhibit adverse effects on liver function, highlighting the importance of continued investigations into various treatments that could influence organ health and overall metabolic processes (Arsana et al., 2025). Liver and kidney function test implications are not only limited to the health examination of an individual; it is also a contributing factor to the wider scope of occupational health. Research studies on the occupational hazards of professionals, especially those working in high-risk areas like anesthesiology, can be used to explain how the body organs can be affected as a result of exposure to certain substances. For example, a longitudinal study indicated that exposure to anesthetic gases did not significantly alter liver and kidney marker levels over time, suggesting that careful monitoring and appropriate workplace safety measures can mitigate risks (Rahmani et al., 2024). The given finding supports the significance of routine health monitoring and the introduction of effective measures aimed at safeguarding the health of workers and simultaneously ensuring the optimal functioning of their organs. To conclude, liver and kidney functional tests are still very much critical in the assessment, both in clinical and occupational health settings. The tests offer crucial information about the physiologic functioning of these crucial organs, which informs the medical practitioners in their diagnosis and treatment plan. In addition, the incorporation of data obtained from research on occupational exposures helps to highlight the fact that research in the area of interaction between the environment and the health of organs should be continued. As the reviewed studies demonstrate, both herbal medicine and job protection can co-exist so that patients and employees can both enjoy the benefits of an informed decision-making process targeting the long-term health and wellness. Finally, promoting the understanding of the liver and kidney functioning will help achieve better results in diverse populations and environments.

The importance of liver and KFTs can hardly be overestimated, and these tests are of utmost importance in the diagnosis and treatment of a variety of health issues. The liver performs many vital roles, such as metabolism, detoxification, and the production of proteins that are important in blood clotting. LFTs measure various enzymes and proteins in the blood to assess liver health. LFT abnormalities may be a sign of liver disease or damage, which may not be accompanied by evident symptoms, particularly at the initial disease progression stages. As an example, liver dysfunction can be caused by fatty liver disease or hepatitis, and it might be revealed only during these tests. Early diagnosis with the help of LFTs makes it possible to actively manage the health of the liver, which is the key to avoiding more serious complications in the future. Equally important are KFTs, which evaluate the ability of the kidneys to filter waste products from the blood. Kidneys are extremely important organs that promote the maintenance of body fluid, electrolyte, and blood pressure balance, as well as acid-base homeostasis. KFTs often include measurements of serum creatinine and BUN, which serve as markers for kidney performance. An unusual outcome could indicate acute or chronic kidney damage, which may develop quite quickly unless sufficient attention is paid to it and appropriate measures are taken. Certain groups of people, including individuals with diabetes or hypertension, are more susceptible to kidney dysfunction, which is why regular tests are an important preventive health practice. With the early detection of kidney problems, medical professionals will be able to maximize the treatment protocols, which will ultimately result in the minimization of the chances of progressing to end-stage renal disease. Furthermore, the analysis of the liver and kidney functions cannot be reduced to the diagnosis alone, since the tests are also essential in terms of controlling the effectiveness of the current treatments and interventions. In patients receiving treatment for chronic illnesses, like diabetes, hypertension, or liver-related diseases, a routine check of the liver and kidney functions will provide valuable information on how the organs are managing within the treatment plans. As an illustration, some drugs might cause hepatotoxic or nephrotoxic outcomes in patients, and in this case, regular laboratory audits are necessary to prevent the development of additional issues. The use of biomarkers to monitor the health of the liver and kidneys underlines the importance of whole-of-care approaches. As outlined in recent studies, understanding these biomarkers is pivotal to improving health outcomes, since they guide personalized treatment approaches and enhance patient quality of life (Abdolrahim et al., 2017; Gutiérrez et al., 2019).

KEY TERMS FROM THIS CHAPTER

- Abdomen
- Acid-base balance
- Alanine aminotransferase
- Aspartate aminotransferase
- Bilirubin
- Blood coagulation
- Detoxification
- Fluid regulation
- Glycogen
- Lipid metabolism
- Loop of Henle
- Nephrons
- Renal dysfunction
- Serum protein electrophoresis
- Waste excretion

Critical Thinking Questions

1. What does a low albumin level indicate in liver function tests?
   a. Acute infection
   b. Chronic liver disease
   c. Dehydration
   d. Acute kidney injury

2. Prothrombin time (PT) is used to assess:
   a. Renal function
   b. Hepatic synthesis of clotting factors
   c. Electrolyte balance
   d. Bone health

3. Which of the following is the most commonly used test for kidney function?
   a. Bilirubin
   b. Serum creatinine
   c. ALT
   d. AST

4. An elevated blood urea nitrogen (BUN) level is indicative of:
   a. Kidney dysfunction
   b. Liver dysfunction
   c. Muscle damage
   d. Gallstones

5. Which test is used to estimate the glomerular filtration rate (GFR)?
   a. Urinalysis
   b. Creatinine clearance test
   c. Serum sodium
   d. Bilirubin

Short Answer Questions

1. What is the function of the liver in metabolism?
2. What is the anatomy of the kidney?
3. Name the 4 liver function tests.
4. What is alkaline phosphatase (ALP)?
5. How many types of kidney function tests are there?

Answers to Critical Thinking Questions

1. (b); 2. (b); 3. (b); 4. (a); 5. (b)

REFERENCES

1. Abdolrahim, M., Jazayeri, H. E., Rabiee, M., Rajab, A., et al. (2017). Evaluation of glycated albumin (GA) and GA/Hba1c ratio for diagnosis of diabetes and glycemic control: A comprehensive review. https://core.ac.uk/download/213086982.pdf (accessed on 12th June 2025).
2. Abo-Raia, G., El-Azab, G., Omar, M., Assem, M., & Abdel-Razek, W. (2015). Evaluation of serum cystatin C as a marker of early renal impairment in patients with liver cirrhosis. https://core.ac.uk/download/206132053.pdf (accessed on 12th June 2025).
3. Vilar-Gomez, E., Athinarayanan, S. J., Adams, R. N., Hallberg, S. J., Bhanpuri, N. H., McKenzie, A. L., Campbell, W. W., McCarter, J. P., Phinney, S. D., Volek, J. S., & Chalasani, N. (2019). Post hoc analyses of surrogate markers of non-alcoholic fatty liver disease (NAFLD) and liver fibrosis in patients with type 2 diabetes in a digitally supported continuous care intervention: an open-label, non-randomised controlled study. *BMJ open*, *9*(2), e023597. https://doi.org/10.1136/bmjopen-2018-023597 (accessed on 12th June 2025).
4. Ademi, B., Jaha, L., Haxhiu, I., Çuni, X., Tahiri, A., Gashi, J., Koshi, A., et al. (2024). Surgical management of renal cell carcinoma with subhepatic inferior vena cava tumor thrombus: A case report and review of the literature. *Journal of Medical Case Reports*, *18*. https://www.semanticscholar.org/paper/44d6fc93b3a073890ea73cffe10cd78a5cf205d2 (accessed on 12th June 2025).
5. Aguayo Calcena, A., Ariceta, G., Castaño González, L. A., García Castaño, A., et al. (2019). Variable phenotype in HNF1B mutations: Extrarenal manifestations distinguish affected individuals from the population with congenital anomalies of the kidney and urinary tract. https://core.ac.uk/download/211054684.pdf (accessed on 12th June 2025).
6. Alejandro, R., Carroll, P. B., Demetris, A. J., Fung, J., et al. (1992). Human islet isolation and allotransplantation in 22 consecutive cases. https://core.ac.uk/download/12204750.pdf (accessed on 12th June 2025).
7. Matar, Alaa; Al-Tamimi, Sarah; and Borjac, Jamilah (2024) "EVALUATION OF THE EFFECT OF VITAMIN D DEFICIENCY ON LIVER AND KIDNEY FUNCTIONS OF IRAQI TYPE II DIABETIC PATIENTS," *BAU Journal - Science and Technology*: Vol. 6: Iss. 1, Article 8. DOI: https://doi.org/10.54729/2959-331X.1139 (accessed on 12th June 2025).
8. Andant, T., Anderson, C., Andersson, L., Badawy, A., Balwani, M., Bissell, D. M., Bissell, M., et al. (2019). Acute hepatic porphyrias: Review and recent progress. https://core.ac.uk/download/323074395.pdf (accessed on 12th June 2025).
9. Arsana, I. N., Juliasih, N. K. A., Agung, A. A., Sauca, A., Widyantari, S., Widhiantara, I. G., et al. (2025). Subacute oral toxicity study of a new polyherbal formulation of Usadha on liver and kidney function of Wistar rats. *Biomedical and Pharmacology Journal*. https://www.semanticscholar.org/paper/9de50f46d66d28d597a1da383a31d89f0294bc46 (accessed on 12th June 2025).
10. Azab, A. E. (2022). An overview of oxytocin: Chemical structure, receptors, physiological functions, measurement techniques of oxytocin, and metabolism. *Journal of Clinical Research and Reports*. https://www.semanticscholar.org/paper/16eea2c132a587c9f09a31ae60d43cf7fb7304a8 (accessed on 12th June 2025).
11. Lockhart, P. B., Gibson, J., Pond, S. H., & Leitch, J. (2003). Dental management considerations

for the patient with an acquired coagulopathy. Part 1: Coagulopathies from systemic disease. *British dental journal*, *195*(8), 439–445. https://doi.org/10.1038/sj.bdj.4810593 (accessed on 12th June 2025).

12. Barutta, F., De Nicola, L., Di Paolo, S., Gesualdo, L., et al. (2019). Diabetic kidney disease. New clinical and therapeutic issues. Joint position statement of the Italian Diabetes Society and the Italian Society of Nephrology on "the natural history of diabetic kidney disease and treatment of hyperglycemia in patients with type 2 diabetes and impaired renal function". https://core.ac.uk/download/231749247.pdf (accessed on 12th June 2025).
13. Iwatsuki, S., Popovtzer, M. M., Corman, J. L., Ishikawa, M., Putnam, C. W., Katz, F. H., & Starzl, T. E. (1973). Recovery from "hepatorenal syndrome" after orthotopic liver transplantation. *The New England journal of medicine*, *289*(22), 1155–1159. https://doi.org/10.1056/NEJM197311292892201 (accessed on 12th June 2025).
14. Bhargava, R., Gao, M. H., Giamouridis, D., Guo, D., et al. (2020). Urocortin 2 gene transfer improves glycemic control and reduces retinopathy and mortality in murine insulin deficiency. https://core.ac.uk/download/323064390.pdf (accessed on 12th June 2025).
15. Biancofiore, G., Pucci, L., Cerutti, E., Penno, G., Pardini, E., Esposito, M., Bindi, L., Pelati, E., Romanelli, A., Triscornia, S., Salvadorini, M. P., Stratta, C., Lanfranco, G., Pellegrini, G., Del Prato, S., Salizzoni, M., Mosca, F., & Filipponi, F. (2006). Cystatin C as a marker of renal function immediately after liver transplantation. *Liver transplantation : official publication of the American Association for the Study of Liver Diseases and the International Liver Transplantation Society*, *12*(2), 285–291. https://doi.org/10.1002/lt.20657(accessed on 12th June 2025).
16. Biggins, S. W., Angeli, P., García-Tsao, G., Ginès, P., Ling, S. C., Nadim, M. K., Wong, F., et al. (2021). Diagnosis, evaluation, and management of ascites, spontaneous bacterial peritonitis and hepatorenal syndrome: 2021 practice guidance by the American Association for the Study of Liver Diseases. *Hepatology*, *74*, 1014–1048. https://doi.org/10.1002/hep.31884 (accessed on 12th June 2025).
17. Čolović, M. B., Krstić, D., Lazarević-Pašti, T., Bondžić, A. M., & Vasić, V. (2013). Acetylcholinesterase inhibitors: Pharmacology and toxicology. *Current Neuropharmacology*, *11*, 315–335. https://doi.org/10.2174/1570159x11311030006 (accessed on 12th June 2025).
18. Dasarathy, S., Mookerjee, R. P., Ott, P., Rackayova, V., et al. (2016). Ammonia toxicity: From head to toe? https://core.ac.uk/download/286115644.pdf (accessed on 12th June 2025).
19. Dash, P., Nayak, S. R., Sahoo, D., Rana, K., Nayak, S., Mohanty, K. C., Pati, S., et al. (2023). Serum biochemical changes among chronic kidney disease patients in a rural cohort of Odisha, India: A cross-sectional study. *Journal of Clinical and Diagnostic Research*. https://www.semanticscholar.org/paper/8ac7a4f0c605dc92f9e7bb864bdfd167198d553e (accessed on 12th June 2025).
20. De Rosa, S., Samoni, S., Villa, G., & Ronco, C. (2017). Management of chronic kidney disease patients in the intensive care unit: Mixing acute and chronic illness. *Blood Purification*, *43*, 151–162. https://doi.org/10.1159/000452650 (accessed on 12th June 2025).
21. Duswald, K. H., Jochum, M., Lenk, S., Nast-Kolb, D., et al. (1993). Increased serum levels of procollagen type III peptide in severely injured patients. https://core.ac.uk/download/12170584.pdf (accessed on 12th June 2025).
22. Elhady, M. M., Adly, S., Elshebiny, H. A., & Moselhy, S. S. (2023). Detection the severity

of organophosphate intoxication using sensitive serum biomarkers S100B and amyloid β (Aβ) in Egyptian subjects. *Environmental Science and Pollution Research International, 30,* 105194–105201. https://www.semanticscholar.org/paper/9898c37ffee6cfd5b59d803d4c7d557152eec31c (accessed on 12th June 2025).

23. Farahani, S., Kadivar, F., Khajeh, F., & Shojaeifard, M. B. (2025). Effect of non-ionizing radiations on liver and kidney function tests in an animal model. *Journal of Biomedical Physics & Engineering, 15,* 125–136. https://www.semanticscholar.org/paper/009c33738b695a7787905edfdadd6e71f521ccce (accessed on 12th June 2025).

24. Frączek, J., Sowa, A., Agopsowicz, P., Migacz, M., Dylińska-Kala, K., & Holecki, M. (2025). Non-invasive tests as a replacement for liver biopsy in the assessment of MASLD. *Medicina, 61.* https://www.semanticscholar.org/paper/285963a8e943e092ffafda0f54d67376a06ffaa8 (accessed on 12th June 2025).

25. Garshnek, V., Hooke, L. R., Radtke, M., Rowe, L., et al. (2025). *USSR Space Life Sciences Digest,* issue 3. https://core.ac.uk/download/pdf/42842161.pdf (accessed on 12th June 2025).

26. Gashaw, B., Dedefo, G., Abreham, A., Getaneh, A., Bayih, A., Abay, Y., Tsegaye, M., et al. (2025). Assessment of liver and renal function tests among patients with typhoid fever in Motta General Hospital, Northwest Ethiopia: A comparative cross-sectional study. *Pakistan Journal of Medical and Health Sciences.* https://www.semanticscholar.org/paper/bef82d6f08fd64c45709093521b55524d4b769e4 (accessed on 12th June 2025).

27. Goswami, S., & Kundra, P. (2019). Endothelial glycocalyx: Role in body fluid homeostasis and fluid management. https://core.ac.uk/download/212867445.pdf (accessed on 12th June 2025).

28. Gutiérrez Rodríguez, A. (2019). Diagnosis of some diseases through biomarkers. https://core.ac.uk/download/288157992.pdf (accessed on 12th June 2025).

29. Hilscher, M., Wells, M., Venkatesh, S. K., Cetta, F., & Kamath, P. S. (2022). Fontan-associated liver disease. *Hepatology, 75,* 1300–1321. https://doi.org/10.1002/hep.32406 (accessed on 12th June 2025).

30. Jalei, A. A., Omar, A. I., Hassan, S., Hassan, Y. S. A., & Ahmed, N. R. (2024). Establishment of reference intervals for common renal and liver function parameters in healthy adults in Mogadishu, Somalia: A cross-sectional study. *International Journal of General Medicine, 17,* 4163–4170. https://www.semanticscholar.org/paper/9ca5583476591e026f07663ea6a3809f95acb0b5 (accessed on 12th June 2025).

31. Kumar, R., Jana, P., Priyadarshini, I., Roy, S., Datta, P., & Das, S. (2022). An evaluation of liver function tests in severe acute respiratory syndrome–Corona virus 2 (SARS-CoV-2) infection in the backdrop of chronic kidney disease. *Journal of Family Medicine and Primary Care, 11,* 751–757. https://www.semanticscholar.org/paper/7e70dbf26d758e77c8dbd55f0881c320d1829c83 (accessed on 12th June 2025).

32. Kumar, S., Sagar, S., Subramanian, A., Albert, V., Pandey, R., & Kapoor, N. (2012). Evaluation of amylase and lipase levels in blunt trauma abdomen patients. *Journal of Emergencies, Trauma, and Shock, 5,* 135–142. https://www.semanticscholar.org/paper/214202af02ef564ca3810380cee9f35ffe104dc9 (accessed on 12th June 2025).

33. Levitsky, J. (2019). Does the liver provide immunosuppressive advantage? *Clinical Liver Disease, 13,* 180–183. https://doi.org/10.1002/cld.817 (accessed on 12th June 2025).

34. Liu, K., Chen, Y., Lin, R., & Han, K. (2020). Clinical features of COVID-19 in elderly patients: A comparison with young and middle-aged patients. *Journal of Infection*, *80*, e14–e18. https://doi.org/10.1016/j.jinf.2020.03.005 (accessed on 12th June 2025).

35. Lustosa do Carmo, T. L., de Siqueira, P. R., Azevedo, V. C., Tavares, D., Pesenti, E., Cestari, M. M., Martinez, C. B. R., et al. (2019). Overview of the toxic effects of titanium dioxide nanoparticles in blood, liver, muscles, and brain of a Neotropical detritivores fish. *Environmental Toxicology*, *34*, 457–468. https://doi.org/10.1002/tox.22699 (accessed on 12th June 2025).

36. Mach, F., Baigent, C., Catapano, A. L., Koskinas, K. C., Casula, M., Badimón, L., Chapman, M. J., et al. (2019). 2019 ESC/EAS guidelines for the management of dyslipidemias: Lipid modification to reduce cardiovascular risk. *European Heart Journal*, *41*, 111–188. https://doi.org/10.1093/eurheartj/ehz455 (accessed on 12th June 2025).

37. Martini, S., Muniroh, L., Nindya, T. S., Solfaine, N., et al. (2014). Effect of *Plectranthus amboinicus* extract on BUN and creatinine levels and cellular response proinflammatory factors TNF-α and IL-1β on gout arthritis patients. https://media.neliti.com/media/publications/150596-EN-effect-of-plectranthus-amboinicus-extrac.pdf (accessed on 12th June 2025).

38. Mauvais-Jarvis, F., Bairey Merz, C. N., Barnes, P. J., Díaz Brinton, R., Carrero, J. J., DeMeo, D. L., De Vries, G. J., et al. (2020). Sex and gender: Modifiers of health, disease, and medicine. *The Lancet*, *396*, 565–582. https://doi.org/10.1016/s0140-6736(20)31561-0 (accessed on 12th June 2025).

39. Mo, J., Liu, J., Wu, S., Lü, A., Xiao, L., Chen, D., Zhou, Y., et al. (2020). Predictive role of clinical features in patients with coronavirus disease 2019 for severe disease. *Zhong nan da xue xue bao. Yi xue ban = Journal of Central South University. Medical sciences*, *45*(5), 536–541. https://www.semanticscholar.org/paper/74eadf9e0cee07f25d5f7b5aebc9c89bca3a1bf7 (accessed on 12th June 2025).

40. Mukhtar, S., Shahid, Z. B., Hussain, I., Ullah, N., Ather, M. M., & Rasheeq, T. (2023). Assessment of mortality in liver cirrhosis and acute kidney injury cases. *Biological and Clinical Sciences Research Journal*. https://www.semanticscholar.org/paper/6f5729d3fd53d28fd4ee029ef3c2ec7407f79e09 (accessed on 12th June 2025).

41. Muluye, D., Getachew, P., Tekalign, T., Woldekidan, S., & Biftu, T. (2024). Evaluation of the antihyperglycemic and antihyperlipidemic effects of *Trigonella foenum-graecum* L. and *Coffea arabica* L. seeds in STZ-induced diabetic mice: Impact on kidney and liver functions. *The Pan African Medical Journal*, *49*. https://www.semanticscholar.org/paper/42ccddd893d0b3301197c12a95c5b7f4ae14ade8 (accessed on 12th June 2025).

42. Obaid, R. M. (2024). Estimation of some physiological biomarkers associated with kidney failure and liver damage in COVID patients. *Full Text Book of Minar Congress12*. https://www.semanticscholar.org/paper/955c88f184a60666608bda6b6ed7f3d08ae4441b (accessed on 12th June 2025).

43. Patra, J. K., Das, G., Fraceto, L. F., Ramos Campos, E. V., Rodriguez-Torres, M. del P., Acosta-Torres, L. S., Díaz-Torres, L. A., et al. (2018). Nano based drug delivery systems: Recent developments and future prospects. *Journal of Nanobiotechnology*, *16*. https://doi.org/10.1186/s12951-018-0392-8 (accessed on 12th June 2025).

44. Rahmani, A., Dini, G., Montecucco, A., Priano, L., Leonetti, M., Manca, A., Kusznir Vitturi, B., et al. (2024). Monitoring of liver and kidney profiles in anesthesiologists working in a regional

reference teaching hospital in Northern Italy: Analysis of health surveillance data using a linear mixed model. *International Journal of Occupational Medicine and Environmental Health*, *37*, 557–568. https://www.semanticscholar.org/paper/00aa8fe66fdcdf0787585c309bb4c3ff3d0a9adf (accessed on 12th June 2025).

45. Rinella, M. E., Neuschwander-Tetri, B. A., Siddiqui, M. S., Abdelmalek, M. F., Caldwell, S. H., Barb, D., Kleiner, D. E., et al. (2023). AASLD practice guidance on the clinical assessment and management of nonalcoholic fatty liver disease. *Hepatology*, *77*, 1797–1835. https://doi.org/10.1097/hep.0000000000000323 (accessed on 12th June 2025).
46. Schröder, A., Majumder, A. A. S., Butterworth, A. S., Reiner, A. P., Malarstig, A., Johnson, A. D., Justice, A., et al. (2017). Fifteen new risk loci for coronary artery disease highlight arterial-wall-specific mechanisms. https://core.ac.uk/download/82958631.pdf (accessed on 12th June 2025).
47. Singh, G., Phadke, C., Dighe, T., Sajgure, A., Bale, C., Shinde, N., Wakhare, P., et al. (2024). #2418 Effects of correction of acidosis on body composition and biochemical parameters in CKD patients on maintenance hemodialysis. *Nephrology Dialysis Transplantation*. https://www.semanticscholar.org/paper/244c35e7ca50153bd2dda7979adf74e4cbfe6606 (accessed on 12th June 2025).
48. Singh, S., & Singh, S. (2024). Exploring the role of peroxisome proliferator-activated receptors α and peroxisome proliferator-activated receptors δ in stress adaptation and metabolic regulation in liver and kidney of freshwater fish *Channa punctatus* (Bloch, 1793). *Journal of Environment and Bio-Science*. https://www.semanticscholar.org/paper/852733fc1002cb42eb8e113a4f6b3ab8bd6eb3e4 (accessed on 12th June 2025).
49. Tzakis, A., Zeevi, A., Zeevi, A., Demetris, A. J., Demetris, A. J., Alper, M., Asonuma, K., et al. (1993). Baboon-to-human liver transplantation. https://core.ac.uk/download/12204908.pdf (accessed on 12th June 2025).
50. Zhang, X., Xiao, X., Luo, Y., Xiao, W., Cao, Y., Chang, Y., Wu, D., et al. (2025). Machine learning based early diagnosis of ADHD with SHAP value interpretation: A retrospective observational study. *Neuropsychiatric Disease and Treatment*, *21*, 1075–1090. https://www.semanticscholar.org/paper/8b4dc6793ac4b0c3164e3ea0bcddd482b467c184 (accessed on 12th June 2025).
51. Zhao, T. (2024). Comparison of hepatic and renal functions during intraoperative sedation with remimazolam in elderly patients under intrathecal anesthesia. *Asploro Journal of Biomedical and Clinical Case Reports*. https://www.semanticscholar.org/paper/1405a4d79f7ea03363b6164e428935c2bb9774a8 (accessed on 12th June 2025).

BLOOD BIOCHEMISTRY

3

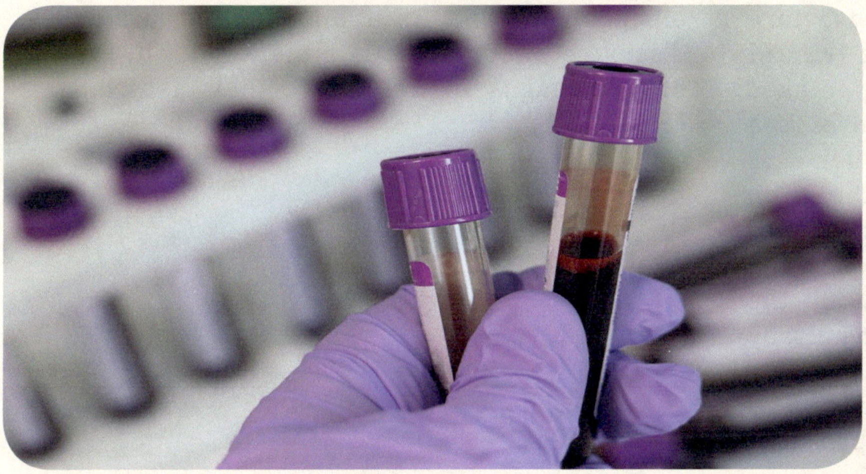

LEARNING OBJECTIVES

After studying this chapter, you will be able to:

1. Understand the composition of blood;
2. Know the metabolic pathways in blood;
3. Describe the blood proteins and their functions;
4. Understand the hormonal regulation in blood biochemistry;
5. Describe the blood disorders and biochemical implications;
6. Know the diagnostic techniques in blood biochemistry.

Introduction

Blood biochemistry knowledge is essential as it entails the study of the chemical substances and processes in blood, a critical component of biological systems. Blood serves numerous roles, including supplying oxygen and nutrients to cells, eliminating metabolic wastes, and regulating body temperature and pH levels. Basically, blood is made up of plasma, RBCs, white blood cells (WBCs), and platelets, each with a function in its diverse roles. Plasma, which constitutes about 55% of blood volume, contains water, electrolytes, proteins, hormones, and waste products, thereby acting as a medium for a number of biochemical reactions. Furthermore, metabolic parameters derived from blood could provide insight into the health and functioning of organs. For example, studies have recognized distinctive metabolic rates of the canine and human livers, showing the effect of size and evolutionary requirements on nutrient processing in blood biochemistry

(Shestopaloff et al., 2014). Metabolic patterns derived from blood testing not only enable one to diagnose diseases but also underscore the significance of biochemistry in medicine. Blood chemistry is the foundation in clinics to measure organ function, detect infection, and monitor conditions like diabetes and anemia. Another impressive aspect of blood biochemistry is its association with lifestyle factors that potentially influence health outcomes. Research shows that certain metabolic changes in a subject can be attributed to external factors, including dietary intake and environmental exposures (Hamid et al., 2015). For example, varying intakes of essential nutrients in humans can have a profound impact on blood composition and consequently, impact overall well-being. Such an interrelation between lifestyle and blood composition illustrates the complex association that exists within biological systems and the necessity of understanding such biochemically mediated interactions. Secondly, advancements in blood biochemistry have provided new approaches in diagnostics and therapies that enhance our ability to manage diseases. As more research is conducted, researchers are finding out how some biochemical indicators in the blood can be excellent predictors for the early diagnosis of disease. Beyond diagnosis, blood biochemistry now has its implications extend to such treatment and management decisions as well. With biochemical data obtained from blood, medical practitioners are able to tailor therapy to suit an individual's requirements, thereby maximizing patient outcomes. These developments highlight the potency of blood biochemistry to unveil the benefits of personalized medicine in defining the intricate relationship between biochemical pathways, lifestyle, and health outcomes. With further research progressing, it is important to investigate the interrelated dynamics of blood biochemistry and its application in various disciplines, in order to pave the way for future breakthroughs in healthcare and medicine (Figure 3.1).

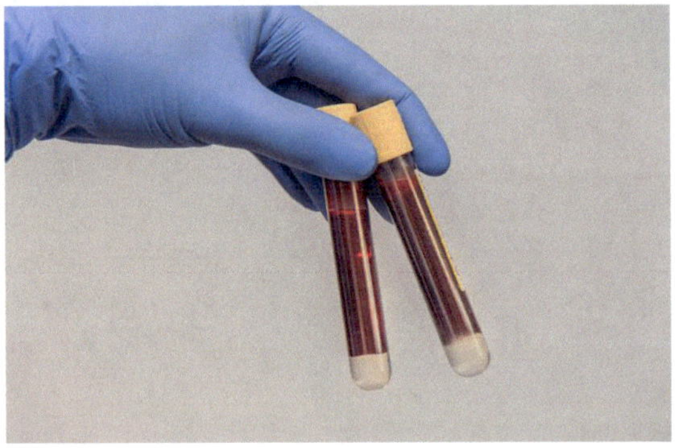

Figure 3.1. Blood biochemistry.

Source: https://en.seamaty.com/Uploads/2022-09-14/63218fa7b3d1b.jpg.

3.1. Composition of Blood

Learning Outcome

1. Understand the plasma and its functions;
2. Describe the cellular components of blood;
3. Describe the role of electrolytes in homeostasis.

Blood composition is a complex topic that involves a number of cellular and plasma constituents, which have their own individual role in the process of homeostasis in the body. Blood primarily consists of RBCs (erythrocytes), WBCs (leukocytes), platelets, and plasma. Erythrocytes play an important role in the transportation of oxygen, whereby they use hemoglobin to combine with oxygen in the lungs and deliver it to tissues. Leukocytes, on the contrary, are part of the immune system, and they promote the defense mechanism of the body against disease-causing organisms. Platelets are small fragments of cells that play a significant role in blood clotting to ensure that excessive bleeding does not occur when one is injured. The intricate combination of these elements makes blood not only the substance that performs its transporting responsibilities but also takes an active part in the regulation processes. Knowledge of this complex composition forms the basis of the analysis of the possibility of changes in these components to influence the state of health in general, which is one of the main problems in blood biochemistry. Plasma is the liquid component in which the cellular components are suspended and it comprises about 55% of the blood volume. Blood is mostly made up of water, proteins, electrolytes, hormones, and waste products, all of which serve the different physiological functions of blood. The proteins present in plasma are albumin, which is significant in the maintenance of oncotic pressure, and globulins, which are vital in immune functioning. Another significant protein is fibrinogen, which plays a vital role during the process of clotting. Electrolytes include sodium and potassium, which play a crucial role in balancing acid-base and passing electrical signals in nerve cells and muscle cells. The metabolic and physiological importance of the plasma constituents could not be overestimated, and all of them contribute to the maintenance of the crucial processes of transporting nutrients, removing wastes, and maintaining body temperature, which emphasizes the value of the blood composition analysis in the scope of biochemistry. The biochemical profiles linked to the blood of different species have been studied recently, and the importance of blood composition in health conditions and disease diagnosis has been revealed.

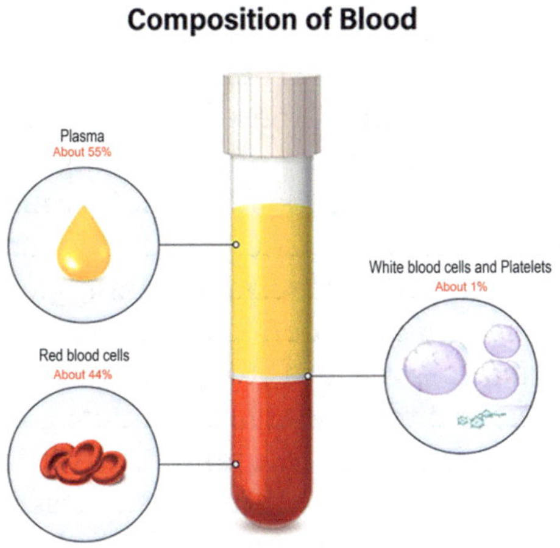

Figure 3.2. The composition of blood.

Source: https://www.hematology.org/-/media/hematology/images/patients/blood-composition.png?la=en&h=501&w=872&hash=04A91A7CB1617CEB0595141AA9C10955.

For instance, variations in biochemical parameters , such as total protein and alkaline phosphatase (ALP) have been linked to physiological status in wild bird populations, showcasing how external factors can influence blood chemistry (Gallo et al., 2017). Similarly, breed-specific differences in serum biochemical traits have been documented in domestic dogs, indicating that genetic predispositions can influence biochemical variations (Chang et al., 2016). The importance of this kind of discovery is in the need to consider the blood composition in the context of a health assessment. Such discoveries not only enrich our knowledge about blood biochemistry but also lead to the personalization of veterinary and medical practice, which shows how the study of blood composition can be applied in practice (Figure 3.2).

3.1.1. Plasma and Its Functions

The knowledge about plasma and its different roles is essential in the framework of blood biochemistry because this yellowish liquid constituent takes up approximately 55% of the entire blood volume. Plasma is mostly composed of water, electrolytes, proteins, hormones, and waste products and is therefore very crucial in the maintenance of homeostasis. Among its many essential functions is the fact that it transports nutrients, gases, and waste products around the body. Plasma proteins, e.g., albumin, globulins and fibrinogen, have defined functions, e.g., to exert oncotic pressure, to promote immune responses, and to play key roles in coagulation. These proteins make the difference in terms of the physiological stability of the tissues and organs since they can successfully deal with the dynamics of fluids and immune reactions and, therefore, the crucial importance of the plasma in health and biological functioning in general. Also, the plasma plays a significant role in the maintenance of pH and electrolyte levels, providing that the internal environment is favorable to the activities of cells. Plasma proteins, bicarbonate and other electrolytes provide buffering capacity to stabilize the blood pH to a narrow range that is vital to physiological processes. In addition, the plasma carries vital ions, including sodium, potassium, and calcium, which are imperative in cellular homeostasis and signal transduction. Such ionic balances affect the contraction of the muscle, the transmission of nerve impulses and the general functioning of the cell. It has been demonstrated that disturbances of plasma chemistry may cause serious pathophysiological states, e.g., acidosis or alkalosis, and thus the role of plasma is rather important in the context of homeostasis and stimulation of adaptive processes of the body to varying internal and external conditions. This role is not just a transportation and chemical equilibrium, but it is also a storage of several bioactive molecules that help in physiological activities. For instance, sphingosine 1-phosphate (S1P), a significant bioactive lipid present in plasma, is implicated in multiple regulatory pathways within different organs, including the kidney. Research shows that S1P modulates various signaling mechanisms that influence renal function, impacting conditions like diabetic nephropathy and glomerulonephritis (Huwiler et al., 2013).

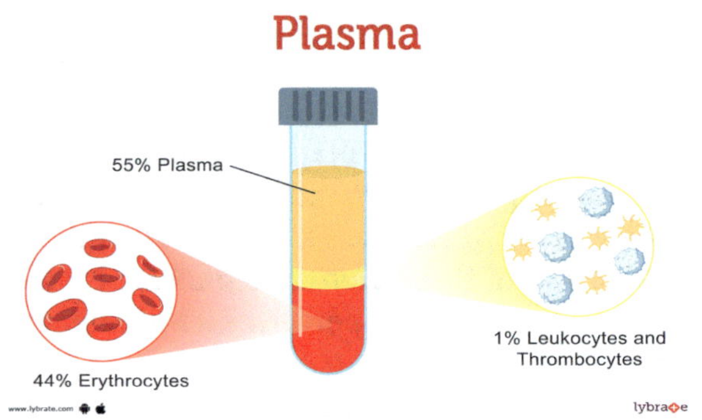

Figure 3.3. Plasma.

Source: https://assets.lybrate.com/imgs/tic/enadp/image-of-the-plasma.jpg.

Furthermore, specific oxysterols present in the plasma have been linked to the regulation of RBC lifespan and erythrocyte function, showcasing the intricate biochemistry of plasma components. The interactions between plasma constituents and cellular pathways stress the importance of plasma in both normal physiology and the pathogenesis of various diseases (Allegra et al., 2019). Therefore, plasma can be considered an active constituent of blood, the element that is closely connected to various biological processes and health conditions (Figure 3.3).

3.1.2. Cellular Components: Red Blood Cells, White Blood Cells, and Platelets

Red blood cells (RBCs) or erythrocytes are simple cellular components of blood primarily responsible for the oxygen delivery from the lungs to various tissues and carrying carbon dioxide back to the lungs for excretion. They are biconcave, anucleate cells with a high hemoglobin concentration, a protein molecule that facilitates gas exchange by binding oxygen and carbon dioxide. Their unique structure not only enhances surface area for gas diffusion but also adds to flexibility such that they can pass through microcapillaries with ease.

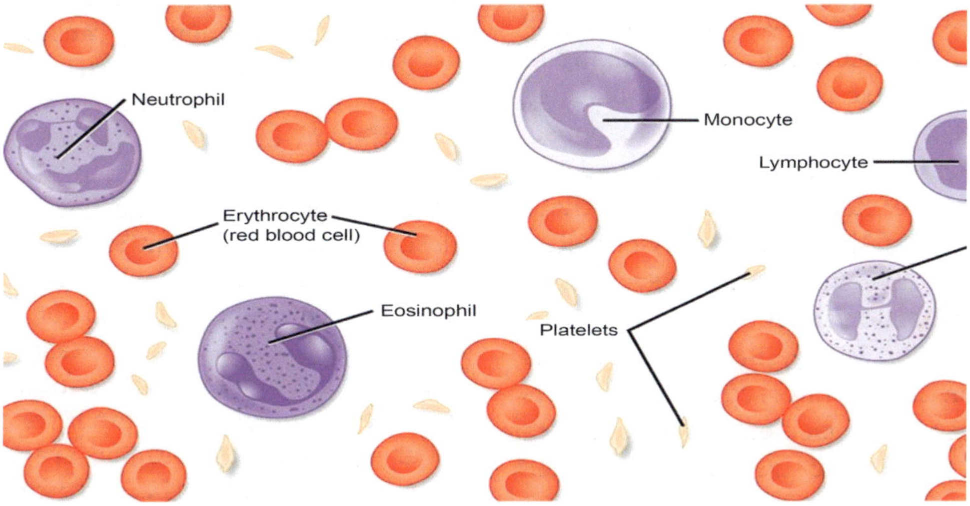

Figure 3.4. The cells and cellular components of human blood are shown. Red blood cells deliver oxygen to the cells and remove carbon dioxide. White blood cells—including neutrophils, monocytes, lymphocytes, eosinophils, and basophils—are involved in the immune response. Platelets form clots that prevent blood loss after injury.

Source: https://open.lib.umn.edu/app/uploads/sites/272/2019/07/Figure_40_02_01.jpg.

RBCs have a lifespan of approximately 120 days in the bloodstream before they are taken out of circulation by splenic and hepatic macrophages. This is a continuous process that highlights the importance of erythropoiesis, the creation of new RBCs, and is tightly regulated by processes , such as erythropoietin and iron availability. WBCs, or leukocytes, are the pillars of the immune system, shielding the body from infection and invasion. Unlike RBCs, WBCs are nucleated and highly diverse in structure and function, with several subtypes consisting of neutrophils, lymphocytes, monocytes, eosinophils, and basophils. They each specialize, with neutrophils having a key role during the acute inflammatory response and lymphocytes having a key role in adaptive immunity. Their ability to proliferate in numbers during infections highlights their important contribution to health promotion. Current studies emphasize the point that leukoreduction, or the removal of WBCs from blood products, can prevent transfusion-related adverse effects, such as febrile non-hemolytic transfusion reactions. This practice is evidence-based and guided by recommendations that consider the clinical efficacy of leukoreduction in preventing immune-related adverse effects for recipients (Bianchi et al., 2015). Platelets, or thrombocytes, are pivotal in the process of hemostasis, the body's system of avoiding bleeding. These small, disc-shaped cell fragments, which are produced by megakaryocytes in the bone marrow, coagulate upon vascular trauma and play a key role in the formation of a solid blood clot. Several factors induce activation, including contact with von Willebrand factor and collagen when the endothelial covering is disrupted. While performing predominantly in clotting, platelets also release signal molecules that promote healing and immune response. Furthermore, recent work has validated the role of oxidative stress in platelet activity and, therefore, an imbalance between ROS and antioxidant substances was revealed to regulate their function and lifespan significantly (Marrocco et al., 2017). Such biochemical sophistication in the interaction of platelets with the other blood elements is essential in the design of therapeutic strategies towards the management of thrombotic as well as bleeding disorders (Figure 3.4).

3.1.3. Electrolytes and Their Role in Homeostasis

Electrolytes are important in homeostasis, the condition of internal stability and balance in the body especially in the physiological environment of blood. Major electrolytes like sodium, potassium, calcium, and magnesium play a vital role in different functions in the cell, like nerve impulse, muscle contraction, and acid-base regulation. These ions are present in the blood plasma in certain concentrations and any deviation may cause dysfunction. To take an example, sodium is the main element that balances the fluids and has a direct effect on the regulation of blood pressure. A disproportion, either hypernatremia or hyponatremia, may disturb the stability of the cardiovascular system and affect the general condition. Homeostatic processes of the body, such as hormonal control through aldosterone and ADH, are responsible for maintaining these electrolyte concentrations in a careful range, which are conducive to proper physiological functioning. Electrolytes are also involved in metabolism and enzyme activities in the blood, besides their known functions in body fluid balance and nerve activity. As an example, calcium ions play an essential role not just in bone health but also in blood clotting and in the secretion of neurotransmitters. The calcium homeostasis disruption may cause diverse clinical conditions, ranging from muscle spasms and the serious health-related issues, such as cardiac arrhythmias. In addition, potassium is central to the resting membrane potential and the action potential in cardiac and skeletal muscle tissues. This intricate interplay of electrolytes underscores the importance of electrolyte balance in preventing metabolic disorders and maintaining cellular homeostasis, highlighting the connections between nutrition, metabolism, and health outcomes as emphasized by Sarmidi et al. (2012). New studies are beginning to illuminate the genetic basis which is associated with electrolyte homeostasis and its role in the regulation of blood pressure. One good example is the WNK1 gene, which was linked to the changes in blood pressure as well as urinary potassium excretion. The translational potential of this study is enormous because the knowledge of the genetic factors in the electrolyte balance can be used to customize clinical responses to hypertension and other metabolic diseases. Variants in the genes responsible for electrolyte transport can affect blood pressure significantly, with specific genotypes impacting the efficacy of dietary potassium in regulating blood pressure, as noted by Brown et al. (2009). In this way, the complexity of the connection among electrolyte concentrations, genetic predisposition, and environmental determinants highlights the complexity of the homeostasis of blood biochemistry, advocating the need for integrative health and nutrition (Figure 3.5).

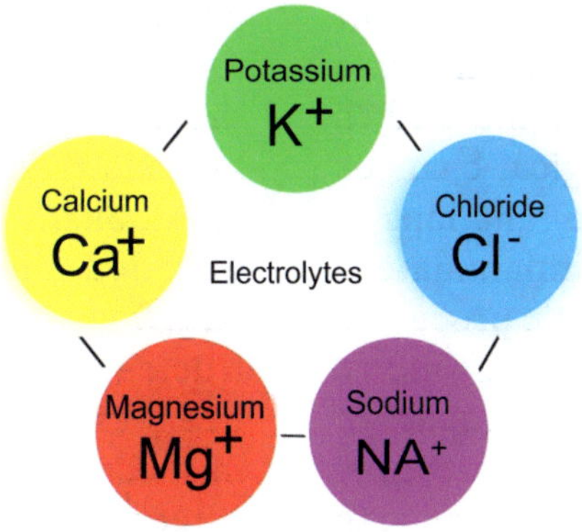

Figure 3.5. Electrolytes.

Source: https://cdn.shopify.com/s/files/1/0068/3815/7410/files/ViDrate_Electrolytes4.jpg?v=1590649555.

Test Your Knowledge

1. What is plasma and its function?
2. What is the role of electrolytes in homeostasis?

3.2. Metabolic Pathways in Blood

Learning Outcome

1. Understand glycolysis and its significance;
2. Describe the citric acid cycle (CAC) in energy production;
3. Understand the urea cycle for comprehending nitrogen metabolism.

Metabolic pathways in blood play a major role in homeostasis and general physiological activity. Metabolite (, such as glucose, fatty acids, and amino acids) regulation is achieved by complex sets of enzymatic reactions that guarantee the provision of energy to cellular processes and metabolic balance. Specifically, glycolysis, CAC, and oxidative phosphorylation are more basic pathways, which break down substrates to produce usable energy. The interruption of these routes may cause metabolic disorders like diabetes and CVDs. With this knowledge of the complexities of these pathways, it will be possible to design specific interventions to correct metabolic health, highlighting the importance of the relationship between blood composition and metabolic activity. The transport proteins, especially those that take part in the transport of organic anions, play a central role in the mediation of metabolic exchanges in blood. As an example, the URAT1 transporter is mainly known to mediate renal reabsorption of uric acid, but studies also suggest that it can transport numerous other organic molecules, which influence metabolism. The results of the studies with the help of knockout mice models demonstrated that the changes in the expression of URAT1 result in considerable alterations of the plasma and urinary levels of a variety of metabolites, involving broader changes in metabolic pathways. These alterations spread to those that control the metabolism of nucleotides, carbohydrates, and steroids, which underscores the interdependence of blood biochemistry and metabolic control. The implications of these investigations shed light on the intricate biochemical networks that govern the body's metabolic adaptation to physiological changes (Eraly et al., 2015). Along with the functions of different transport proteins, the inflammatory processes also regulate the metabolic processes in the blood, especially in reaction to infections. A study of bovine mastitis shows the impact of systemic inflammation on monocyte functionality and the overall metabolic picture. In response to infection, the differentially expressed genes in monocytes isolated in blood indicate profound interaction with immune signaling and changes in metabolic regulation. It is interesting to note that up-regulated genes in an inflammatory response are enriched in pathways related to interferon activity, whereas down-regulated genes are enriched in metabolic pathways. Moreover, the fact that these responses are modulated by miRNAs highlights the sophistication of inflammatory signaling and metabolism in blood. As such, unraveling these interactions expands our understanding of how blood biochemistry can be responsive to both metabolic and immune demands (Baker et al., 2014).

3.2.1. Glycolysis and Its Significance

Glycolysis, the biochemical process that breaks down glucose to give pyruvate, is a vital cellular process in energy generation. It is an anaerobic process that is important in that it generates ATP, which is one of the most important energy currencies in cells. Interestingly, glycolysis is not only important in aerobic conditions but is also significant in hypoxia, which is when the available oxygen is low. In such situations, cells are more reliant on glycolysis for cellular needs, highlighting the importance of its role in cellular maintenance under duress. Its importance in the blood biochemistry is also highlighted by the ischemia process, where oxygen deprivation can drastically impair cellular metabolism. Glycolysis offers a quick response pathway that preserves ATP levels irrespective of damage to mitochondrial oxidative phosphorylation, thereby guaranteeing cellular survival under hypoxia (Dyson et al., 2013). As concerns bone metabolism and health, current studies have unveiled the intricate function of glycolytic pathways in osteogenesis. Transcription factor Nuclear Matrix Protein 4 (Nmp4) has also been established to play an important role in mesenchymal stem/progenitor cells during osteogenic differentiation, in terms of glycolysis. Mice with no transcription factor for Nmp4 exhibit an increased process of mineralization, with consequent increases in bone density and structural quality. This provides proof that higher glycolysis in $Nmp4^{-}/^{-}$ cells stimulates greater collagen synthesis and secretion, which are vital for creating the bone matrix. These findings identify glycolysis not only as a major player in energy production but also as a most critical factor in bone anabolism, and thus overall skeletal well-being (Adaway et al., 2019). This is an even larger implication of glycolysis than is known in the classical metabolic pathways, pushing its reach into physiological processes. The study of glycolysis in blood biochemistry also identifies it as central to the pathogenesis of varied metabolic diseases, including diabetes and CVD. In diabetes, alteration of glycolytic flux can lead to hyperglycemia and long-term complications due to the inability to properly utilize glucose. Understanding the regulatory mechanisms of glycolysis would thus be useful in proposing therapeutic schemes that enhance glycemic control and alleviate complications. Similarly, in CVD, impaired glycolytic metabolism can trigger myocardial ischemia, and additional research on metabolic adaptation in response to hypoxia is warranted. Therefore, glycolysis continues as a staple in blood biochemistry, not only demonstrating its pivotal role in energy metabolism but also emphasizing its vulnerability to therapeutic intervention in a number of diseases (Dyson et al., 2013) (Figure 3.6).

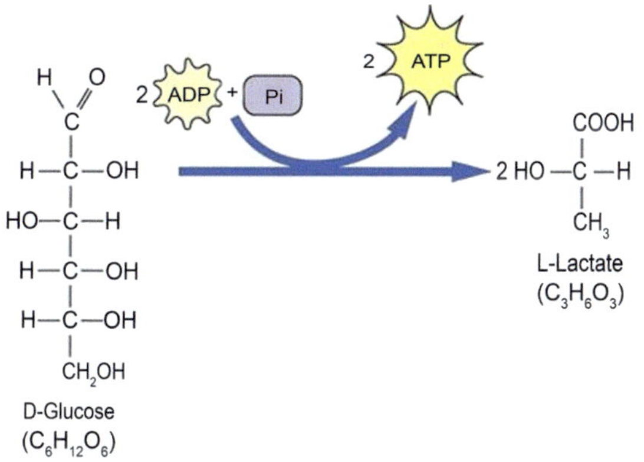

Figure 3.6. Conversion of glucose to lactate during anaerobic glycolysis.

Source: https://doctorlib.org/medical/biochemistry/biochemistry.files/image192.jpg.

3.2.2. The Citric Acid Cycle and Energy Production

The citric acid cycle (CAC), also known as the Krebs cycle, plays a pivotal role in cellular respiration, serving as a central hub for energy production within metabolic pathways. The cycle allows the cell to utilize energy efficiently by converting the carbohydrates, fats, and proteins breakdown products acetyl-CoA, into electron carriers NADH and FADH2. This is done in the matrix of mitochondria, where a set of chemical reactions occurring under the facilitation of enzymes oxidize acetate to carbon dioxide. The significance of the CAC does not only stop at energy production since it also plays a role in the synthesis of important metabolites and intermediates that are important in several biosynthetic pathways. As an example, one of the intermediates of the cycle, alpha-ketoglutarate, plays a central role in amino acid synthesis, therefore, connecting energy metabolism to biosynthetic needs that are important to sustain cellular functions. These interactions of the CAC are highly regulated and capable of adjusting to shifting metabolic circumstances, like hypoxia, in which oxygen is restricted. In this case, the CAC might not operate as it normally does through oxidative pathway but some of its parts are still active. The ability to operate in oppositional directionalities to maintain energy production by substrate-level phosphorylation in spite of the inhibited electron transport chain activity testifies to this adaptability. This phenomenon underscores the metabolic flexibility of the CAC. The alpha-ketoglutarate dehydrogenase complex emerges as a crucial player, influencing the directional flow of metabolic intermediates based on the cellular energy demands, thereby demonstrating how the CAC can dynamically support cellular processes even in conditions of energetic imbalance (Christos, 2013).

Consequences of perturbed energy production through the CAC may be severe, especially in pathological situations. There are considerable biochemical changes in tissues as demonstrated in post-mortem research, affecting metabolic markers, which demonstrate cellular energetics. As an illustration, the build-up of lactic acid, a metabolite of anaerobic glycolysis, is characteristic of a transition to anaerobic metabolism in limited oxygen conditions. This results in an increase of metabolites like hypoxanthine and ammonia, which are products of cellular breakdown after death. These are the changes that can be detected by blood biochemistry and which could become important indicators in forensic science to determine the post-mortem interval. Furthermore, understanding the alterations in blood biochemistry in relation to the CAC provides insights into the broader implications of energy metabolism in essential physiological and pathological processes (Donaldson, 2013) (Figure 3.7).

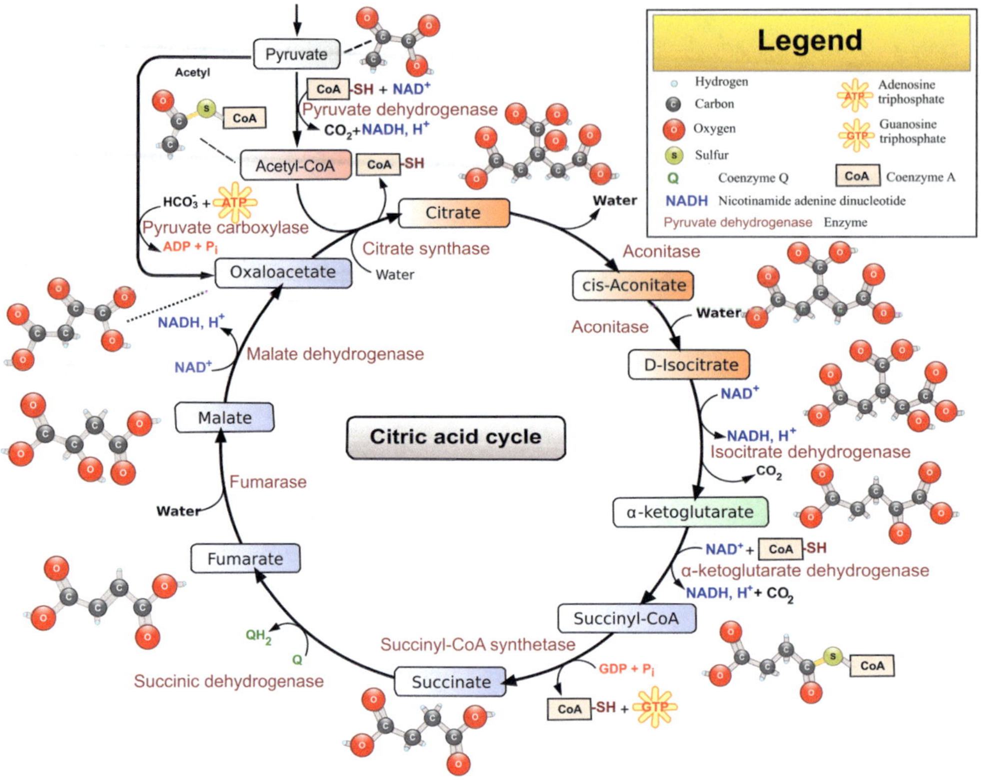

Figure 3.7. Overview of the citric acid cycle.

Source: https://upload.wikimedia.org/wikipedia/commons/0/0b/Citric_acid_cycle_with_aconitate_2.svg.

3.2.3. The Urea Cycle and Nitrogen Metabolism

The study of the urea cycle is an essential part of the nitrogen metabolism and its influence on blood biochemistry. The urea cycle takes place mainly in the liver and its purpose is to transform ammonia, a highly toxic product of amino acids decomposition, into urea, which could be easily excreted in the urine. The process is also interconnected with other metabolic pathways , such as those of amino acid synthesis and degradation. The urea cycle is a series of enzyme reactions that produce urea out of ammonia and bicarbonate. A deficiency of any of these enzymes may cause the build-up of toxic intermediates and disorders, including hyperammonemia, which is the excess amount of ammonia in the blood. Thus, the urea cycle is not just important in detoxification, but it is also a crucial marker of metabolic health, requiring further insight into its working and regulation. A major effect of perturbed nitrogen metabolism is the presence of orotic aciduria, which is a disorder connected with the perturbed pathway of pyrimidine synthesis. Since the production of orotic acid occurs in the course of nucleotide synthesis, the disruption of the urea cycle can provoke the elevated concentration of orotic acid in the urine. This condition may arise from inborn errors of metabolism, specifically genetic defects affecting the bifunctional enzyme uridine monophosphate synthase (UMPS). The symptoms usually appear in neonatal patients in the form of lethargy and feeding problems, as well as serious metabolic disorders, such as megaloblastic anemia and problems with neural development. As noted, prompt diagnosis and treatment are very important, since they will reduce the chances of getting severe outcomes like mental retardation or coma. Effective management of orotic aciduria emphasizes the intricate links between nitrogen metabolism, the urea cycle, and overall metabolic health in humans (Fonteh, 2018). New research developments provide novel platforms to investigate metabolic heterogeneity, especially in the liver, which plays a central role in nitrogen metabolism. The metabolic patterning on a chip (MPOC) technology has been developed to create dynamic metabolic patterns highlighting the liver's zonal differences. This platform has been shown to accurately predict the differences in nitrogen and carbohydrate metabolism between liver tissues recapitulates the complex metabolic activities that define the efficiency of the urea cycle. By emulating *in vivo* conditions, researchers have been able to get insights into the interaction of different metabolic processes within the liver that lead to the development of knowledge on the cause of diseases associated with nitrogen imbalance. This technological advancement not only elucidates the pathophysiology of conditions associated with urea cycle dysfunction but also informs therapeutic strategies for improving metabolic health, underscoring the profound relevance of the urea cycle in blood biochemistry (Eo et al., 2018) (Figure 3.8).

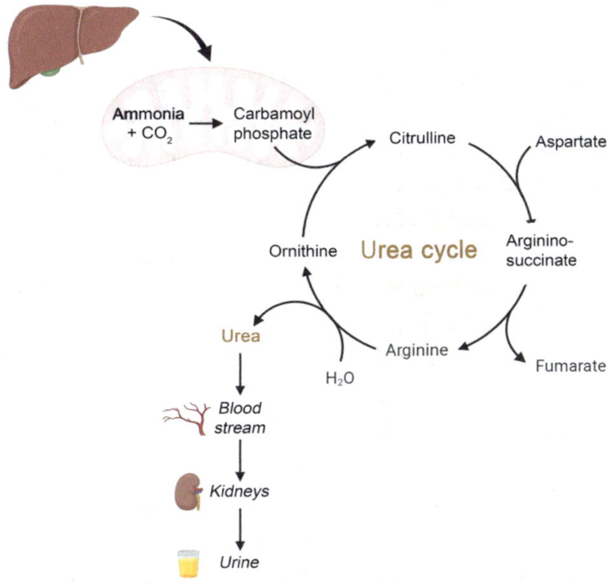

Figure 3.8. Urea cycle steps and reactions.

Source: https://microbenotes.com/wp-content/uploads/2023/10/Urea-Cycle-Steps-and-Reactions.jpeg.

Test Your Knowledge

1. What is the significance of glycolysis?
2. What is the role of the citric acid cycle in energy production?

3.3. Blood Proteins and Their Functions

Learning Outcome

1. Describe the types of blood proteins;
2. Understand the role of antibodies in immune response;
3. Know the enzymatic functions of blood proteins.

Proteins in the blood are crucial in maintaining homeostasis and the functioning of a number of physiological processes in the body. Among the proteins, albumin is the most common, responsible for maintaining osmotic pressure and serving as a transport molecule for hormones, fatty acids, and drugs. Apart from albumin, globulins are an equally significant category of proteins that include immunoglobulins that form the foundation of the immune response. The multifunctionality of blood protein functions highlights their importance in transport, pathogen defense, and fluid balance. In addition, the dynamic nature of the proteins supports the ability to respond quickly to alterations in physiological states, particularly required in stress or injury. Multifunctionality thus asserts the pivotal role of blood proteins in general health and metabolism, affirming their foundational status in blood biochemistry. The effect of blood proteins also extends to the complicated processes of the immune response, where they play a vital mediating role. Immunoglobulins or antibodies not only recognize and bind to foreign antigens but also mark pathogens for destruction by other immune cells, thus playing an important role in immunological defense. In addition, acute-phase proteins like the C-reactive protein are rapidly synthesized after inflammation, making their role important in the human body's reaction to trauma or infection. Their regulation and synthesis are a multi-dimensional one between the immune system and other physiological processes, which are vital adaptive mechanisms. This multianalytical nature of blood proteins is a condition for the neutralization of diseases and healing, underlying their significance in the context of more general blood biochemistry. Under disease conditions, modification of blood proteins can provide a great deal of information concerning disease mechanisms and health in general.

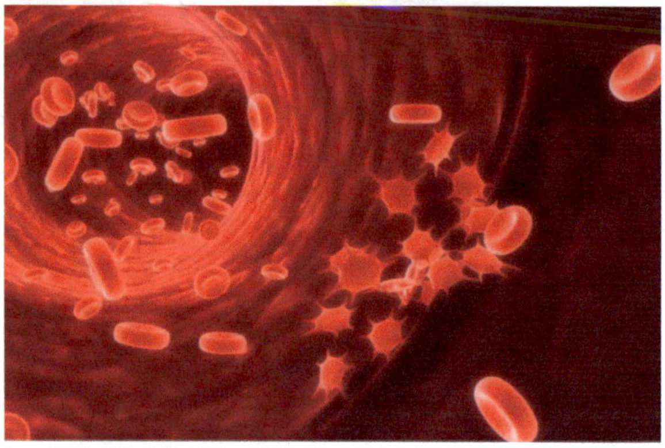

Figure 3.9. Illustration of red blood cells and platelets flowing through a blood vessel.

Source: https://news.liverpool.ac.uk/wp-content/uploads/2016/02/blood-n.jpg.

For example, disease states causing oxidative stress may influence the amount and activity of various blood proteins, including transport proteins and proteins involved in the immune response. Elevated levels of oxidative stress markers have been associated with numerous diseases, such as cardiovascular events and metabolic syndromes. Furthermore, the concordance between blood protein profiles and biomarkers for oxidative stress reflects the interrelationship between biochemical pathways in promoting health. The complexity of such interactions warrants further investigation, as understanding the dynamics between blood proteins and their functioning can open doors to medical interventions and therapy to correct imbalances in the body, ultimately furthering blood biochemistry knowledge (Figure 3.9).

3.3.1. Types of Blood Proteins: Albumin, Globulins, and Fibrinogen

Blood proteins play an essential role in homeostasis and the execution of other physiological processes, and three main types of them are albumin, globulins, and fibrinogen. Albumin is the most prominent protein in human plasma and makes up about 60% of the total serum protein concentration. Its major functions are to provide oncotic pressure that aids in regulating fluid balance between blood vessels and tissues and to carry different substances, including hormones, fatty acids, and drugs. As the key player in the edema prevention and adequate hydration of tissues, the albumin levels are frequently checked in medical practice to determine the nutritional status of a patient or his/her liver functions. Due to the dynamic character of the albumin level, it can also give information about inflammatory processes and other systemic diseases, which makes it significant in the blood biochemistry. Globulins are a heterogeneous group of proteins that are further divided into alpha, beta and gamma globulins that have different roles in immune response and transportation. Alpha globulins are mostly made up of transport proteins, whereas beta globulins comprise transferrin that binds and carries iron, which is vital in erythropoiesis. Immunoglobulins, also known as gamma globulins, are essential elements of the immune system that are synthesized by B cells as a reaction to pathogens. An increase or decrease in the globulins may be significant of various health conditions; specifically, elevated gamma globulins are significant of chronic inflammatory disease or immune system malfunction. Serum protein electrophoresis aids in the diagnosis of diseases by analyzing these protein fractions and thereby allowing a clinician to identify abnormalities in immune responses. Consequently, understanding the roles and variations of globulins enhances the diagnostic potential of blood protein analysis (Mihajlovičová et al., 2017). The last large group of blood proteins is fibrinogen, which is central to the coagulation cascade and thus part of hemostasis and wound healing. Fibrinogen is synthesized in the liver and transformed into fibrin as part of the clotting process; fibrin provides a mesh-like structure that stabilizes blood clots and helps to prevent excessive bleeding. An increase in fibrinogen may signify inflammation or tissue injury, whereas low fibrinogen may cause a bleeding disorder or delayed wound healing.

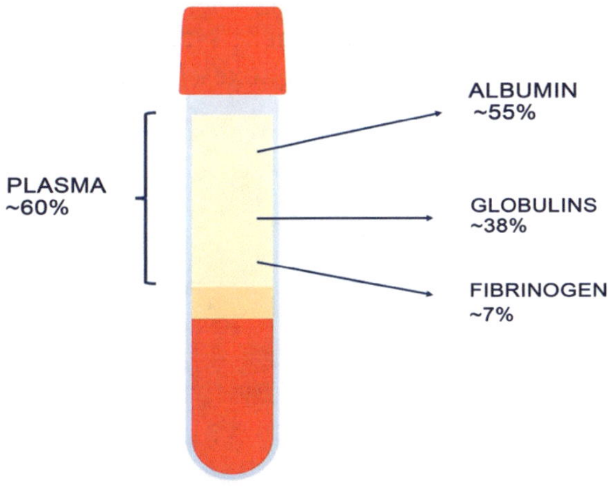

Figure 3.10. Top three proteins found in plasma are: Albumin, globulins, and fibrinogen.

Source: https://interactivebiology.com/wp-content/uploads/2022/01/Plasma-components.jpg.

In clinical practice, measuring fibrinogen levels is essential for evaluating coagulation pathways and diagnosing conditions like disseminated intravascular coagulation (DIC) or thrombosis. Furthermore, shifts in fibrinogen concentrations may provide insights into an individual's inflammatory status or risk for cardiovascular events, highlighting the importance of this protein in both coagulation and broader health assessments (Bonde et al., 2018) (Figure 3.10).

3.3.2. Role of Antibodies in Immune Response

Antibodies are important elements of a complex system, the immune response of the body, which plays the key role in homeostasis maintenance. Immunoglobulins or antibodies are glycoproteins that are synthesized by B cells in response to antigens that are foreign substances like pathogens or toxins. When an antigen is encountered, the B cells undergo clonal selection and clonal expansion to produce both memory cells and plasma cells, which produce large amounts of antibodies. These antibodies are very specific; they have special variable regions that enable them to combine with specific antigens with high affinity. This interaction not only inactivates the pathogen but also tags it to be destroyed by other immune cells, making the immune response as a whole more effective. The intricate interaction between antibodies and antigens is illustrative of the important adaptive processes by which the immune system protects against disease. Antibodies do more than just neutralize pathogens; they can also initiate several immune pathways, which then allow a complex assault to be carried out against invading organisms. As an example, antibody binding to antigens may activate the complement system, which leads to the direct lysis of target cells by the formation of membrane attack complexes (MACs).

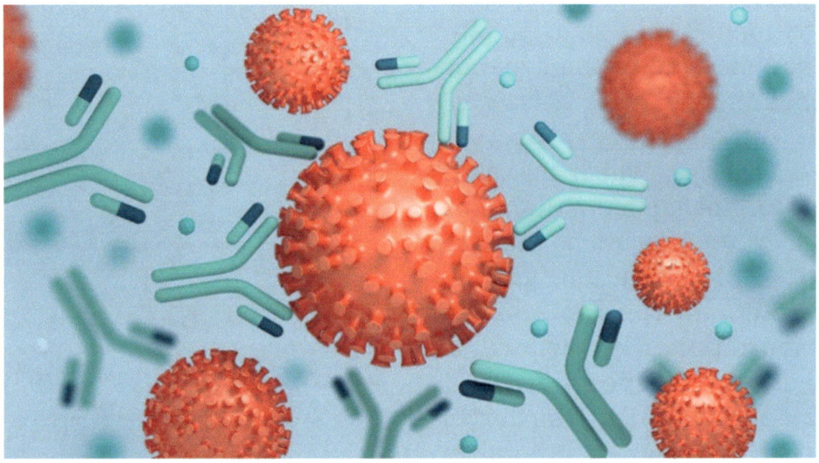

Figure 3.11. An artist's illustration of antibodies (blue-green structures) attempting to latch onto the antigens on the outer surface of a coronavirus (red). Antibodies are one of the major players in the immune system's attack against viruses.

Source: https://www.snexplores.org/wp-content/uploads/2020/07/1030_antibodies_explainer.jpg.

In addition, the antibodies can opsonize pathogens, which increases their phagocytosis by the immune cells, including macrophages and neutrophils. This opsonization is especially important in the early stages of infection when the adaptive immune response has not yet developed fully. Moreover, some classes of antibodies, e.g., IgG, are able to pass through the placenta, thus passively immunizing the fetus and the newborn, which underlines the great importance of antibodies in ensuring the continuity of immunity between generations. Antibodies are important in the innate and adaptive immune responses because of their versatility and functionality. Moreover, antibody biochemistry demonstrates the structural complexity and flexibility to different immunogenic challenges. The heavy and light chains form the antibodies and are responsible for giving the antibodies a characteristic Y-shape that allows them to bind flexibly with antigens as well as conferring stability and solubility in blood. The genetic processes that result in antibody diversity are illustrative of the rapid adaptation to novel threats which the immune system is capable of achieving. The final steps of antibody specificity and function refinement, which further increase immune protection, are somatic hypermutation and class switching. As they have such important functions, the dynamics of antibodies are crucial to the creation of therapeutic interventions, such as mAbs, which are applied during the treatment of infections, cancers, and autoimmune diseases. The current studies of the antibody functioning and optimization are going to further develop the knowledge of the blood biochemistry and its use in the medical practice (Figure 3.11).

3.3.3. Enzymatic Functions of Blood Proteins

The enzymatic function of blood proteins is what guarantees homeostasis and facilitates various physiological processes. Enzymes, which are mostly protein in composition, act as catalysts, accelerating biochemical reactions but not being consumed in the process. Such important enzymes in the blood are those that catalyze the coagulation cascade, such as thrombin and clotting factors, which facilitate hemostasis. These enzymes can influence the velocity and effectiveness of blood clotting and hence inhibit excessive bleeding into the body. Blood proteins , such as metabolic enzymes for glucose, hexokinase, and glucokinase (GK), regulate energy production necessary for cellular function.

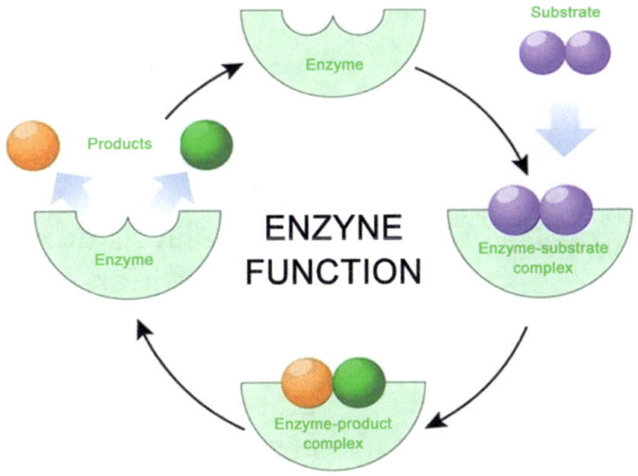

Figure 3.12. Enzyme function.

Source: https://www.news-medical.net/image-handler/ts/20180813125340/ri/673/picture/2018/8/shutterstock_760624435.jpg.

This intricate interdependence of enzymatic activity highlights the pivotal position of blood proteins in the homeostatic regulation of metabolism and the entire body, a tribute to their ancient significance in blood biochemistry. Besides, blood enzymes are also involved in the detoxification of metabolic end products and toxic agents. For example, enzymes like ALP and AST play significant roles in the function of the liver, facilitating the breakdown of various compounds and facilitating the excretion of the same. Such detoxification is essential to remove excess nitrogenous waste from the system so that it doesn't accumulate and become toxic. Blood proteins involved in oxidative stress response, such as SOD and catalase, also exhibit enzymatic activity that protects cellular structures from damage by ROS. Efficient enzymatic activity in the blood not only detoxifies but also aids tissue repair processes and the promotion of overall well-being, illustrating the complex biochemical interdependencies of blood dynamics. In addition, the versatility of blood proteins is also their ability to act as enzymes in the course of the immune response. Immunoglobulins, or antibodies, not only respond to pathogens but can have enzymatic activity under certain conditions and thus enhance immune defense mechanisms. Enzymic activities of blood proteins can modulate inflammation and facilitate the identification of foreign antigens, thus accelerating the immune response. For instance, proteolytic enzymes, which are secreted during the inflammatory response, can be helpful in antigen processing into more recognizable diminutive peptides for proper antigen-presenting cell presentation. This multi-functional ability addresses the essential role these proteins play both in enzymatic and non-enzymatic activities, demonstrating their central position within the overall blood biochemistry domain. These proteinase activities of blood proteins encapsulate the critical, dynamic functions they perform in maintaining physiological homeostasis, responding to stressors, and clearing deleterious agents from the circulation, thereby more strongly highlighting their overall significance in human health (Figure 3.12).

Test Your Knowledge

1. Name the 3 main blood proteins.
2. What is the role of antibodies in the immune response?

3.4. Hormonal Regulation in Blood Biochemistry

Learning Outcome

1. Understand the role of insulin and glucagon in blood sugar regulation;
2. Describe the impact of cortisol on metabolism;
3. Know the thyroid hormones and their influence on blood chemistry.

This is because of the complex interaction of the hormones, which largely affect the biochemistry of the blood, controlling different metabolic pathways that help in the maintenance of homeostasis. Insulin is one of these hormones, and it is central in glucose metabolism, as it promotes the intake of glucose by tissues, thus maintaining the blood sugar levels. When one eats, the pancreas releases insulin, which tells the cells to take up glucose to use as energy or store as glycogen. At the same time, another pancreatic hormone, glucagon, has an effect opposite to insulin, i.e., it raises the blood glucose levels during fasting by stimulating the decomposition of glycogen. This feedback loop is an example of how hormonal communication coordinates metabolic networks to make sure that the concentration of glucose stays within a small range, which is essential to cellular functioning. As a result, a violation in the hormonal pathways can cause a metabolic disorder in the form of diabetes, which is why hormonal control is significant in the blood biochemistry. Thyroid hormones, particularly thyroxine (T4) and triiodothyronine (T3), further illustrate the profound impact of hormonal regulation on blood biochemistry through their role in metabolic rate modulation. The hormones play a central role in the control of basal metabolism, affecting oxygen intake and macronutrient metabolism speed. As an example, the rise of T3 may stimulate the metabolic rate, which will promote the further generation of glucose and fatty acids out of the stored energy, thereby directly influencing the blood biochemistry. Moreover, the connection between thyroid hormones and energy expenditure is well-reported in the literature, as the changes in the levels of thyroid hormones are associated with alterations in metabolic efficiency and adaptation to fasting. This kind of hormonal interaction supports the existence of complex regulatory networks that control energy metabolism and points to how thyroid dysregulation can have such an enormous impact on metabolic health, as seen in the case of hypothyroidism and hyperthyroidism. Moreover, the effects of hormones reach the regulatory functions of leptin and ghrelin, the main task of which is to regulate appetite and energy balance. Leptin is a hormone produced by adipose tissue and Leptin signals satiety and appetite suppression, whereas ghrelin is a hormone produced in the stomach that stimulates hunger. The interaction of these hormones also influences the biochemistry of blood in terms of lipid metabolism and glucose homeostasis. Notably, during periods of prolonged fasting, such as seen in northern elephant seals, hormonal adaptations occur, including altered levels of leptin and ghrelin, which help manage energy utilization effectively (Costa et al., 2012). Such flexibility is essential to survive in periods of nutrient shortage, and it demonstrates that physiological needs determine hormonal reactions and, thereby, blood biochemistry. Moreover, the consideration of the roles of these hormones in the framework of energy expenditure helps to clarify the difficulties of metabolic regulation, indicating the significance of the hormonal balance in the maintenance of overall metabolic health and the prevention of metabolic disorders.

3.4.1. Role of Insulin and Glucagon in Blood Sugar Regulation

Blood sugar regulation is a vital mechanism that occurs in the body in the process of homeostasis, which is mainly facilitated by the insulin and glucagon hormones. Insulin is a hormone that is responsible for the reduction of blood glucose levels after a meal. This is achieved through the stimulation of glucose uptake into cells, especially those in the muscle and adipose tissues, which is produced by the beta cells of the pancreas. The process not only results in the reduction of blood glucose level but also provokes the process of glycogenesis, the formation of glycogen in which glucose is stored, which prevents hyperglycemia. On the other hand, glucagon is a counter-regulatory hormone secreted by the alpha cells of the pancreas to raise the level of blood sugar between meals or during fasting. By stimulating glycogenolysis and gluconeogenesis in the liver, glucagon ensures that the body maintains adequate glucose levels to meet its metabolic demands, especially during periods of stress or energy deficit (Mujtahid et al., 2020). The insulin-glucagon balance is critical; its disruption may result in pathological conditions, including diabetes mellitus. In type 1 diabetes, the body's immune system attacks and destroys the insulin-producing beta cells in the pancreas, leading to low production of insulin and hence, high levels of glucose in the blood. In type 2 diabetes, the body cells develop insulin resistance, once more resulting in a high concentration of glucose in the blood. A failure of insulin to carry out its duty may lead to severe long-term complications, including CVD and neuropathy. As noted in studies, the tight regulation of blood glucose is a complex interplay involving not only insulin and glucagon but also other hormones , such as cortisol and adrenaline, which further signifies the importance of these hormonal pathways in metabolic health and disease (Ambrosio et al., 2016). Moreover, one cannot overestimate the importance of lifestyle factors in terms of their ability to adjust the impact of insulin and glucagon. Examples of such activities include regular exercise, which has been demonstrated to result in insulin sensitivity, or the ability of the body to utilize glucose more effectively.

Exercise induces positive metabolic changes, including enhancement of beta cell mass and pancreatic functioning, especially in people at risk of diabetes. This relationship underscores the potential benefits of incorporating exercise into daily routines to counteract the adverse effects of dietary choices, such as excessive cola consumption, which might impair pancreatic morphology and function (Ambrosio et al., 2016). Therefore, the complicated process of blood sugar control via insulin and glucagon not only indicates the physiological process but also shows the significant influence of lifestyle habits on metabolic health (Figure 3.13).

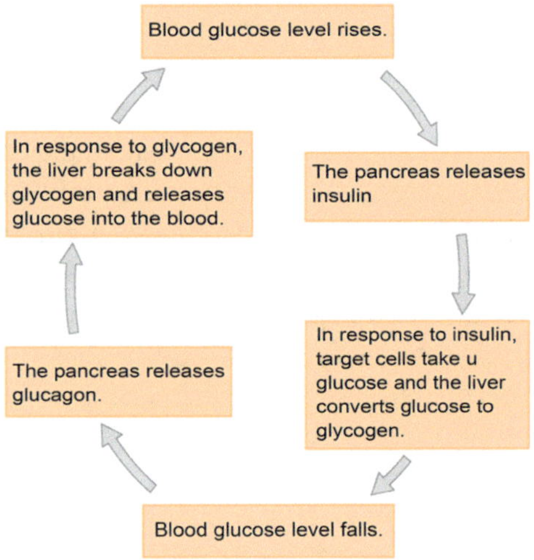

Figure 3.13. Insulin and glucagon regulate blood glucose levels.

Source: https://s3-us-west-2.amazonaws.com/courses-images/wp-content/uploads/sites/1223/2017/02/07230445/Figure_37_03_05.png.

3.4.2. The Impact of Cortisol on Metabolism

The role of cortisol metabolism is multifaceted, with widespread action on both energy expenditure and homeostasis. The glucocorticoid hormone secreted by the adrenal cortex is responsible for regulating glucose during stress, primarily by enhancing gluconeogenesis within the liver. The rise in blood glucose produces a reserve pool of energy that the body can use to deal with the stressors. However, sustained cortisol elevations have the potential for adverse metabolic effects. Elevated and continuous exposure to cortisol has been found to correspond with insulin resistance, a pretype 2 diabetes syndrome, which compromises the body's capacity to regulate glucose balance. It has also been shown in certain investigations that the adrenal gland exhibits circadian and seasonal variability of cortisol secretion, which affects metabolic control throughout the year. For instance, increased plasma cortisol levels have been noted in November during peak weight gain and metabolic readiness in red deer stags (Crockford et al., 1999). The influence of cortisol on protein metabolism is also illustrative of its role in the control of metabolism. With chronic stress or low dietary energy, cortisol will cause catabolism of protein to enable the release of amino acids into the circulation. This response serves to preserve glucose reserves for essential physiological functions, particularly in the brain. Nevertheless, such catabolic effects can cause muscle wasting and weakening in the event that cortisol generation continues to be elevated for prolonged durations. This disease affects muscle cells and is a common condition across most populations that can experience chronic stress, including athletes undergoing strenuous training regimens and persons experiencing emotional stress. Furthermore, cortisol also impacts lipid metabolism, causing the mobilization of fatty acids from adipose tissue, which may result in the abnormal distribution of fat; a condition commonly experienced by individuals with obesity related to metabolic syndrome (Ackerman et al., 2019). While cortisol is crucial for the body's acute metabolic response, acute elevation of cortisol could be detrimental to one's health. Chronic stress, by inducing sustained high levels of cortisol secretion, has been implicated in obesity, CVD, and other metabolic disorders. This implies the necessity of understanding cortisol regulation not only with reference to short-term survival requirements, but also in the context of long-term metabolic health. Furthermore, variability in cortisol secretion may influence variability in stress responses and hence control metabolic outcomes. The complex interaction among cortisol, metabolism, and health illustrates the necessity of additional research into blood biochemistry, specifically the determination of how to avoid the harmful effects of chronic stress and cortisol disturbances. A comprehension of these dynamics can optimize preventive techniques and treatment plans for metabolic diseases associated with stress and hormonal imbalance (Figure 3.14).

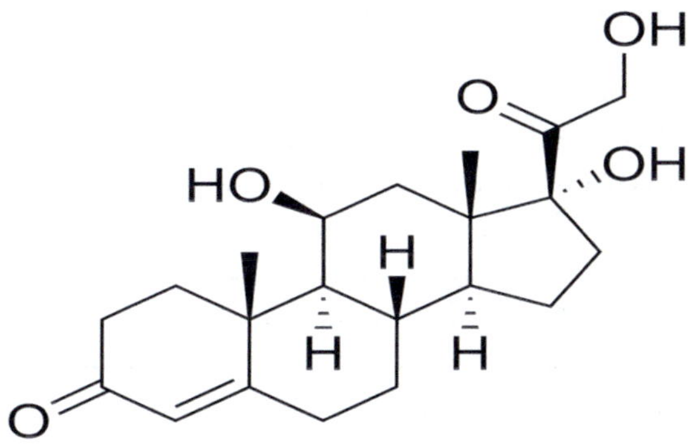

Figure 3.14. Structure of cortisol.

Source: https://upload.wikimedia.org/wikipedia/commons/9/96/Cortisol3.svg.

3.4.3. Thyroid Hormones and Their Influence on Blood Chemistry

Thyroid hormones, primarily thyroxine (T4) and triiodothyronine (T3), play a pivotal role in regulating various metabolic processes within the body, significantly influencing blood chemistry. They are critical hormones in metabolic homeostasis, and they influence carbohydrate metabolism, protein metabolism, and lipid metabolism. On release of thyroid hormones into the blood, a series of biochemical reactions are promoted which permit growth of tissues, production of energy and general metabolic efficiency. In hypothyroidism states, when the hormone levels are low, the reduction of metabolic rates may result in disorganized blood chemistry, such as increased cholesterol levels and altered glucose metabolism. Conversely, hyperthyroidism often results in increased metabolic rates, which can manifest as lower cholesterol levels, rapid weight loss, and altered glucose homeostasis, illustrating the intricate balance that thyroid hormones maintain in blood chemistry (Gross et al., 2001). The thyroid hormone connection with blood chemistry is also applicable to other biochemical parameters that indicate metabolic well-being. As an example, thyroid hormones have a great impact on the serum lipid levels, and this triggers alterations in the way the body metabolizes fats. An increase in T3 has been linked to decreased serum lipid levels by increasing lipolysis and stimulating lipid oxidation. Moreover, thyroid hormones have the ability to influence blood glucose levels through increasing insulin sensitivity, and hence they are important in glucose metabolism. These processes may be impaired by abnormal levels of thyroid hormones, resulting in hyperlipidemia or glucose intolerance. As such, monitoring thyroid function is imperative in assessing overall metabolic health and can provide valuable insights into the underlying causes of dyslipidemia and altered glucose metabolism in patients (Herndl et al., 1980). Also, the effect of thyroid hormones on blood chemistry includes the fact that they affect the electrolyte balance, which is essential to many physiological processes. Thyroid hormones have the ability to increase renal excretion of sodium and potassium and other electrolytes, which affect cardiovascular stability. Such control of electrolytes is necessary to sustain the fluid balance and avoid complications in the form of hypertension or arrhythmias. Moreover, thyroid malfunction may cause electrolyte imbalance, worsen the initially presented health issues, or develop new metabolic disorders. Understanding the influence of thyroid hormones on these biochemical markers aids in the diagnosis and management of disorders associated with both hypo- and hyperthyroidism, thereby highlighting the importance of thyroid hormone assessment in clinical practice and its broader implications within blood biochemistry (Gross et al., 2001).

Test Your Knowledge

1. What is the role of insulin and glucagon in blood sugar regulation?
2. What is the role of cortisol in metabolism?

3.5. Blood Disorders and Biochemical Implications

Learning Outcome

1. Describe the types and biochemical causes of anemia;
2. Understand the hemophilia and coagulation pathways;
3. Know diabetes mellitus and its biochemical markers.

The complexity of the connection between blood disorders and biochemical implications of such disorders introduces a substantial field of interest in the sphere of blood biochemistry. The significance of the influence of different blood disorders on the biochemical processes may shed light on the possible channels of diagnostics and therapy. As an example, diseases , such as anemia greatly change the level of hemoglobin and the functioning of RBCs, which consequently influences the transportation of oxygen within the body. These disruptions are not only localized but also affect systemic health, which can result in complications in various organ systems due to the initiation of biochemical cascades. Such complexity warrants further sophisticated investigative techniques that explore the interaction between blood composition and biochemical markers to improve clinical outcomes and management strategies of the patients. In addition, liver enzyme values are important parameters when it comes to the study of blood disorders, especially with reference to the biochemical basis of the same. An evaluation of the activities of liver enzymes in healthy blood donors indicated that there were variations according to the ethnic backgrounds and this demonstrated that there might be metabolic differences that would influence the safety and effectiveness of blood donation. Specifically, alterations in serum γ-Glutamyl transferase (GGT), ALT, and AST levels offer insights into liver function and its intricate relationship with blood quality. The findings underscore the importance of identifying individuals at risk for hepatic dysfunction, emphasizing the need for routine screenings within populations with a high prevalence of liver disease, as indicated in the research (Marjani et al., 2016). Lastly, nutrition and biochemical homeostasis are complexly balanced and have a central role in the health of blood. Blood-related disorders can be worsened or improved through proper dietary intake, and this is a critical area of handling conditions like thrombocytopenia or hemophilia. The relations among food, metabolism, and the biochemical reactions in the body explain how dietary approaches can be used to promote cellular health and counter the consequences of metabolic disorders. With the emphasis on the collaboration between biochemistry and nutrition, researchers will be able to design interventions aimed at achieving the optimal blood composition and functioning, which will eventually translate into better patient outcomes and an increased quality of life. Emphasizing this connection equips healthcare providers with a broader toolkit for addressing blood disorders and demonstrates the necessity for an integrated approach to health management (Sarmidi, 2012) (Figure 3.15).

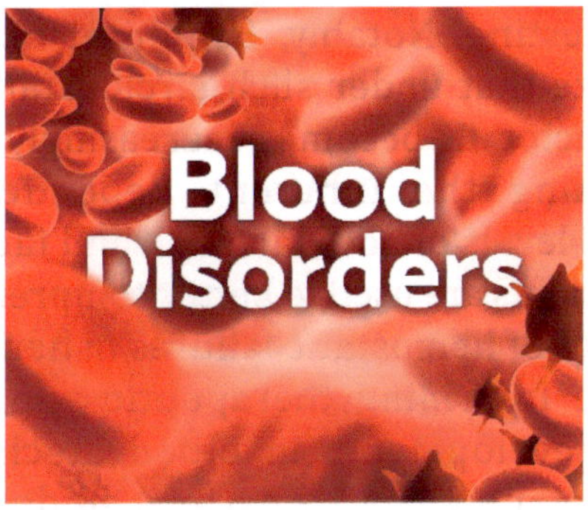

Figure 3.15. Blood disorders.

Source: https://www.dlshsi.edu.ph/dlsumc/wp-content/uploads/sites/3/2021/02/Blood-disease-1.jpg.

3.5.1. Anemia: Types and Biochemical Causes

Anemia is a multivalent medical condition where there is a decrease or dysfunction of the number or quality of RBCs, which results in compromised oxygen delivery to the body. Anemia exists in a number of types, and each has varying biochemical etiologies. For instance, iron-deficiency anemia, the most common type, is when there is a lack of sufficient iron for hemoglobin production, resulting in microcytic and hypochromic RBCs. Additionally, megaloblastic anemia is produced by impaired DNA synthesis, typically due to vitamin B12 or folate deficiency, to produce unusually large erythrocytes. Such pathophysiologic distinctions necessitate special diagnostic techniques and therapeutic regimens, highlighting the importance of understanding the biochemistry producing each anemia in the context of blood biochemistry. The biochemical pathogenesis of anemia can also be linked with derangements of metabolic pathways crucial to normal erythropoiesis. For instance, orotic aciduria, an extremely rare metabolic disorder, is caused by defects in the enzyme UMPS, part of pyrimidine synthesis. The consequent increase in orotic acid may further exacerbate megaloblastic anemia and other manifestations, such as developmental retardation and lethargy. When evaluating anemic patients, it is crucial to examine not only iron content but also the integrity of metabolic pathways involved in nucleic acid synthesis, which is indicative of broader implication for cellular proliferation and differentiation.

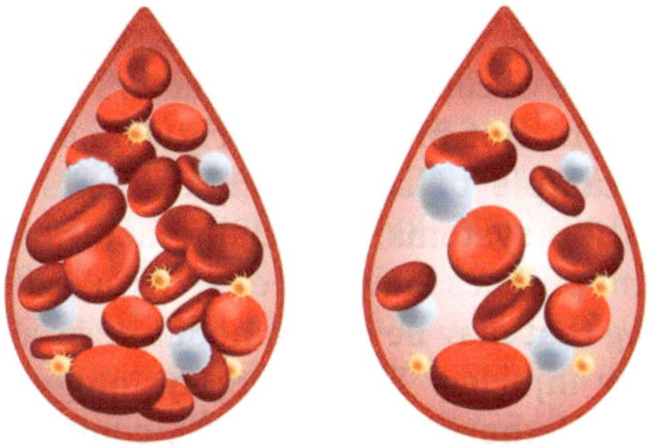

Figure 3.16. Anemia.

Source: https://www.diagnopein.com/img/BlogImages/Common%20symptoms%20of%20anemia,%20causes%20anemia,%20anemia%20diagnosed.jpg.

Biochemical derangement of these biochemical pathways provides insight into potential therapeutic targets that are likely to enhance anemia's impact on overall well-being and health. Moreover, immunological and hematological systems makes the clinical presentation of anemia even more complex. Research on disease conditions like protein-losing nephropathy (PLN) in dogs clearly shows the way an infection, in this instance by Borrelia burgdorferi, can lead to anemia along with renal dysfunction. This correlation serves to underscore the importance of recognizing individuals at risk of unfavorable cardiovascular incidents even before the occurrence of diabetes. Thus, integrating these biomarkers into routine clinical practice can enhance the stratification of cardiovascular risk in diabetic patients, leading to more tailored and preventive care strategies (Pasupathi et al., 2011) (Figure 3.18).

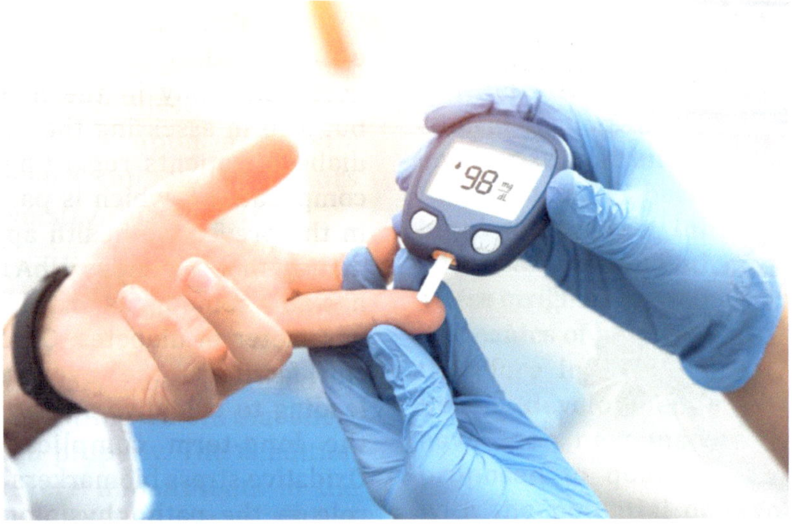

Figure 3.18. Diabetes mellitus.

Source: https://drraghu.com/wp-content/uploads/2023/01/Diabetes-mellitus.jpg.

Test Your Knowledge

1. What are the biochemical causes of anemia?
2. What is hemophilia?

3.6. Diagnostic Techniques in Blood Biochemistry

Learning Outcome

1. Understand the types and their significance of blood tests;
2. Describe the biochemical markers for disease detection;
3. Describe the advances in blood analysis technology.

Advances in the diagnostic techniques of blood biochemistry have totally revolutionized the area of medical diagnostics, so that numerous health disorders can be diagnosed at the early stage and controlled. Modern techniques currently utilize a range of instruments , such as immunoassays and mass spectrometry to analyze biomolecules in high specificity and sensitivity. Immunoassays, which are based on the application of antigen-antibody interaction, are essential in the detection of specific proteins and hormones from blood samples. This technique is highly useful in clinical diagnosis, whereby the disease biomarkers of conditions , such as diabetes and cancers may be determined. Furthermore, automation and robot integration into these processes enhance throughput and reduce human errors, thereby simplifying lab procedures. The integration of new technologies and traditional methods is transforming blood biochemistry and leads to increased accuracy and speed of diagnoses, which are the backbone of improved patient care. Mass spectrometry is now a cornerstone in blood biochemistry diagnosis because of its ability to provide precise molecular characterization of analytes at trace levels. The technique is especially desirable in the analysis of metabolites, drugs, and disease markers that require precise quantitation for clinical relevance. For instance, its application in the quantitation of cardiac biomarkers has taken center stage in the diagnosis of conditions like acute MI, where prompt identification is crucial. The highly sensitive nature of mass spectrometry makes it capable of detecting cardiac troponin, a critical biomarker of myocardial damage, which remains elevated for a couple of days after the incident, thus a critical tool in clinical decision-making (Goodson et al., 2015). Besides, the ability to examine complex biological blends with minimal preparation continues to expand mass spectrometry's use in clinical laboratories, making it a mainstay technique in blood biochemistry diagnosis. As diagnostic techniques in blood biochemistry continue to evolve, focus increasingly falls on tailored medicine and the utilization of biomarkers. With the development of omics sciences, such as proteomics and genomics, researchers are now capable of identifying disease-specific biomarkers that can translate to individualized treatment strategies. For example, the potential to utilize specific protein signatures from blood samples can help oncologists determine the most effective treatment strategy for cancer patients. Application of such specific strategies not only maximizes intervention effectiveness but also minimizes the side effects of less specific interventions. In this regard, attempts to foster collaboration between industry and academia are crucial to advance research and translate results into clinical practice (Seaman & Whitehouse, 2001). Ultimately, the continuous advancement and utilization of methods of blood biochemistry diagnosis have the ability to transform the future of health, striving for improved patient results and precision in medical care.

3.6.1. Blood Tests: Types and Their Significance

Blood tests constitute a milestone in the area of blood biochemistry as they help to obtain important information about the health state of a person and help to diagnose countless numbers of health issues. There are numerous kinds of blood tests that are used, each with a specific purpose. For instance, complete blood counts (CBC) are instrumental in evaluating red and white blood cell levels, enabling healthcare providers to detect anemia, infection, and other hematological disorders. Likewise, metabolic panels are used to measure various blood substances, including glucose, electrolytes, and proteins, and provide an overall picture of metabolism and organ functioning. These tests are important not only in their diagnostic value but also in the continuous monitoring of the patient, thus providing timely interventions in case of any abnormality, which will improve patient outcomes and personalized health approaches. The results of blood tests interpreted in clinical conditions should be viewed with a sophisticated perception of pre-analytical, analytical, and post-analytical factors that may affect the results. As a case in point, pre-analytic factors like sample collection time and storage temperature could significantly affect the concentration of analytes and the overall test precision. Even though the analytical part of blood tests is usually very regulated, inconsistencies in sample treatment may provide inappropriate results. Moreover, as noted in the literature on the subject of clinical biochemistry, the interpretation can only be efficiently performed with the establishment of reference ranges. These systems help clinicians to evaluate the abnormalities of the normal values, which eventually support crucial decision-making during diagnosis and treatment. The emphasis on standardized protocols ensures that blood tests, such as those used in aquatic veterinary medicine, can be effectively translated into practice, thus extending the utility of biochemistry beyond traditional applications (Ashby et al., 2016). There are also implications of blood tests in the area of environmental health and toxicological studies. As an example, the research on the impact of environmental stressors on the organism has led to the emphasis on the blood biochemistry as an indicator of the physiological alterations when an organism is exposed to toxins. In particular, research on the acute effects of substances like Malathion demonstrates how biochemical markers can indicate disruptions in glucose homeostasis and insulin resistance (Ekremoğlu et al., 2020). The findings of this kind underline the significance of blood tests in not only clinical diagnosis, but also the need to understand the larger picture of how the environmental health is reflected in biological systems. In such a way, blood tests can be used both in clinical diagnostics, which is their essential application, and in environmental science, which is their rapidly developing application area, showing the complex nature of interactions between biochemistry and health outcomes in different settings (Figure 3.19).

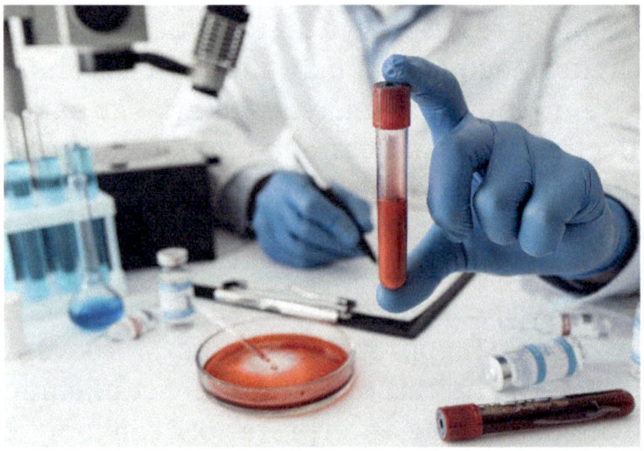

Figure 3.19. Blood tests.

Source: https://abiscans.com/wp-content/uploads/2023/09/coronavirus-vaccine-composition-lab-1-scaled.jpg.

3.6.2. Biochemical Markers for Disease Detection

Discovery and application of biochemical markers are invaluable instruments in detection of a variety of diseases in the context of blood biochemistry. These markers are usually proteins, enzymes or metabolites that may reflect pathological changes in the body. As an example, an increase in certain enzymes can indicate liver dysfunction or heart attacks, and an abnormality in metabolic products can indicate a hormonal disorder. Clinical utility of such markers is not only in their power to confirm the diagnosis, but also, they may be used to monitor the evolution of the disease and its sensitivity to therapy. The introduction of biochemical markers in everyday clinical practice indicates that there is a necessity for continuous research to prove the accuracy and reliability of such tests in order to ensure that they will really help in providing useful information about the health of the patients. The area of biochemical markers is however, dogged by difficulties which pertain to standardization and methodology. The absence of an agreement on the method of measuring oxidative stress and other markers raises serious concerns that may hamper their applicability in clinical practices. According to recent sources, the difference in the measurement methods may cause a difference in the outcomes, and the redox status of a patient may be challenging to interpret. Marrocco et al. (2017) offer insights into these methodological biases, emphasizing that a unified approach to defining and measuring oxidative stress is crucial for the development of reliable diagnostic tools. Therefore, scientists recommend the implementation of composite indices including several oxidative stress markers, depending on particular clinical conditions, that would improve the specificity and relevance of diagnosis. In addition, there is an ever-growing necessity for rationalization of laboratory tests in healthcare as medical services are getting more and more demand. The need to continue practicing cost-effectively and the pressure to increase the number of available tests may lead to overusing some of the biochemical markers. Buhagiar et al. (2005) underscore the tendency to request tests based merely on their availability rather than their clinical significance. Besides straining the resources of the laboratory, this trend can also cause undue stress to both the patients and the health practitioners. The careful consideration of the clinical utility of current and new tests is needed to rationalize laboratory services and provide patients with reasonable and justified diagnostic assessment. Such a negative attitude towards the application of biochemical markers is essential in developing the area of blood biochemistry and enhancing the outcomes of patients in general.

3.6.3. Advances in Blood Analysis Technology

New technology in the analysis of blood has changed the science of blood biochemistry and allowed for a more advanced understanding of human health. Such new technology includes making microfluidics, which allows for rapid analysis of small volumes of blood. Microfluidic devices reduce laboratory operations down to miniaturization and not only reduce the level of blood needed but also enhance the speed and accuracy of biochemical assays. This effectiveness is most critical in point-of-care diagnostics, where prompt results are critical to timely medical treatment. Further, such technologies may facilitate more cost-effective diagnostics, thus expanding access to valuable health screening in resource-limited settings.

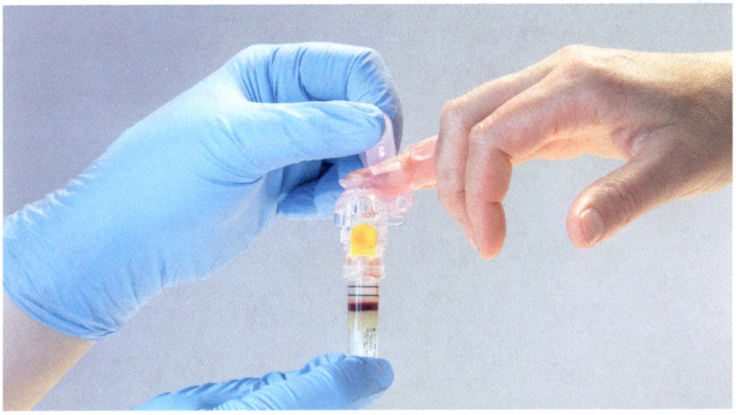

Figure 3.20. Gloved hands collecting a small-volume blood sample using a microcollection device.

Source: https://images.fastcompany.com/image/upload/f_webp,c_fit,w_1920,q_auto/wp-cms/uploads/2023/12/p-1-91002941-bd-launches-mini-draw-a-version-of-theranos-that-actually-works.jpg.

The integration of microfluidics into routine clinical use is a paradigm shift toward more individualized and efficient healthcare delivery. In addition to microfluidic technology, the advent of genomic and proteomic analysis instruments has changed blood analysis. High-throughput sequencing and advanced mass spectrometry approaches enable researchers to probe the genetic and protein content in blood specimens. This makes it possible to identify biomarkers for diseases like cancer and metabolic disorders and thus initiate a new era of precision medicine. For instance, the potential for analyzing circulating tumor DNA in the blood has presented opportunities for early cancer detection and tracking of cancer development. Such sophisticated techniques not only improve the accuracy of diagnosis but also provide insight into the biological mechanisms of diseases, thereby enabling improved treatment approaches. As technological abilities improve, the combination of genomic and proteomic analysis into routine blood testing has great potential for improving patient results. Moreover, the epigenetic revolution highlights the need for continued research in blood analysis technology. Epigenetic biomarkers hold the potential to yield valuable information about the biological age of a subject, distinguish between genetic profiles , such as monozygotic twins, and identify specific body fluid sources in admixed samples. These advances have immense potential to make significant contributions to forensic science and other diagnostic applications, as they enable enhanced understanding of biological samples beyond what has been achieved with traditional DNA profiling strategies. Research has shown that proteomics methods, particularly mass spectrometry, can be incorporated into existing DNA research without compromising the integrity of genetic material (Eilerts, 2016). This crosspoint between proteomics and epigenetics is crucial for the development of improved strategies that can guide clinical and forensic applications, whereby blood analysis remains at the pinnacle of biomedical science and practice (Capiau et al., 2016) (Figure 3.20).

Test Your Knowledge

1. What is the significance of a blood test?
2. What are biochemical markers for disease detection?

SUMMARY

The conclusion of a chapter about blood biochemistry represents the complexity of connections between biochemical markers and their health-related consequences. As has been revealed in the discussion, blood biochemistry is an important instrument for interpreting a number of pathological conditions , such as hematological malignancies and metabolic disorders. For instance, studies of non-Hodgkin Lymphomas (NHL) reveal a notable association between elevated Epstein-Barr Virus (EBV) loads and the incidence of different lymphoma subtypes in children. The identified odds ratio indicates a significant risk factor, emphasizing the necessity for effective screening and early diagnosis in at-risk populations (Filipovich et al., 2013). It highlights the role that biochemistry can play in highlighting disease progression pathways and provides insights into targeted therapeutics. Moreover, the discussion of circulating oxysterols with regard to obesity and metabolic syndrome indicates the biochemical changes that happen in accordance with the pathophysiological alterations. Evidence suggests that alterations in oxysterol profiles correlate with changes in fatty acid levels, thereby establishing a metabolic interplay that may contribute to CVDs and increased cancer risks (Tremblay-Franco et al., 2015). The discovery of these biochemical signatures not only adds value to our knowledge of the involved biological processes but also helps to design the possible therapeutic interventions that could help to reduce the health risks associated with obesity. Finally, the comprehensive approach incorporating the results of the research on blood biochemistry opens the door to new methods of diagnosing and treating the diseases that have a serious implication on the population's health. The inferences made on the basis of the correlations between the biochemical markers and the disease conditions demonstrate the significance of continued research in the given sphere. Disentangling these complicated biochemical interactions will lead to personalized medicine and better health outcomes, and this is just how relevant blood biochemistry is in clinical and research environments. This conclusion restates the importance of biochemistry in the transition between laboratory-based science and patient-based care, which will eventually lead to an improved health management approach.

The complex interactions of different biochemical constituents of blood are central to normal physiology as well as pathological states. Biochemistry of blood involves a huge number of substances, such as proteins, enzymes, hormones, electrolytes, and metabolites, which all have a combined effect on metabolic processes. The involvement of inflammatory mediators in diseases like severe malaria is one of the important factors that have been pointed out by present research. For instance, recent research indicates that orally administered activated charcoal can significantly enhance survival rates in experimental cerebral malaria by modulating immune responses associated with inflammation, suggesting its potential as an adjunct therapy (Alexander et al., 2010). The elucidation of biochemical pathways underlying the process of inflammation not only adds to the knowledge on the disease processes but also creates the possibility of designing specific therapeutic interventions. Besides, the profile and control of blood components are extremely important in the determination of health conditions and disease diagnosis. The profile of the expression of different genes and miRNAs in immune cells has become of interest, especially with regard to inflammation-associated diseases , such as mastitis. Sensitive sequencing methods show deep changes in gene expression related to immune reactions. For example, genes up-regulated in monocytes exposed to infection show significant enrichment in inflammation-related pathways, emphasizing the role of innate immunity (Baker et al., 2014). The significance of this kind of finding is in the need to combine molecular biology with the established blood biochemistry to come up with a comprehensive perspective of the disease evolution and reaction to therapy. Moreover, blood chemistry regarding the pharmacokinetics of therapeutic agents is also vital when it comes to the optimization of treatment courses. The interplay between exaggerated inflammatory reactions and various pharmacological interventions is a subject of active investigation. For instance, the co-administration of adjunct therapies that do not interfere with primary treatments, like how oral activated charcoal did not affect the pharmacokinetics of artesunate, is essential for patient safety and therapeutic efficacy (Alexander et al., 2010). This collaboration of different biochemical modalities opens up thrilling prospects for researchers and health practitioners in general, as it will help in the enhancement of clinical outcomes due to the application of customized therapeutic approaches. In general, molecular, biochemical, and pharmacological points of view on the problem demand synthesis of data to develop our knowledge on blood biochemistry in health and disease.

KEY TERMS FROM THIS CHAPTER

- Acidosis
- Adaptive immunity
- Alkalosis
- Blood analysis
- Blood biochemistry
- Blood cells
- Blood tests
- Blood volume
- Electrolytes
- Erythrocytes
- Glomerulonephritis
- Hormones
- Hypernatremia
- Hyponatremia
- Leukocytes
- Plasma

CRITICAL THINKING QUESTIONS

1. **What is the primary component of blood plasma?**
   a. Proteins
   b. Glucose
   c. Water
   d. Electrolytes
2. **Which protein is the most abundant in plasma?**
   a. Fibrinogen
   b. Hemoglobin
   c. Albumin
   d. Globulin
3. **What is the primary function of hemoglobin in red blood cells?**
   a. Transport carbon dioxide
   b. Transport oxygen
   c. Regulate blood pH
   d. Fight infections
4. **Hypernatremia refers to:**
   a. Low sodium levels in the blood
   b. High sodium levels in the blood
   c. Low potassium levels in the blood
   d. High potassium levels in the blood
5. **What is the most abundant type of white blood cell in healthy individuals?**
   a. Lymphocytes
   b. Neutrophils
   c. Monocytes
   d. Eosinophils

Short Answer Questions

1. What is blood biochemistry?
2. What are the 3 cellular components of blood?
3. What are the 4 metabolic pathways?
4. What types of protein are in the blood?
5. What is hormonal regulation in the blood?

Answers to Critical Thinking Questions

1. (c); 2. (c); 3. (b); 4. (b); 5. (b)

REFERENCES

1. Goodson, W. H., 3rd, Lowe, L., Carpenter, D. O., Gilbertson, M., Manaf Ali, A., Lopez de Cerain Salsamendi, A., Lasfar, A., Carnero, A., Azqueta, A., Amedei, A., Charles, A. K., Collins, A. R., Ward, A., Salzberg, A. C., Colacci, A., Olsen, A. K., Berg, A., Barclay, B. J., Zhou, B. P., Blanco-Aparicio, C., ... Hu, Z. (2015). Assessing the carcinogenic potential of low-dose exposures to chemical mixtures in the environment: the challenge ahead. *Carcinogenesis*, *36 Suppl 1*(Suppl 1), S254–S296. https://doi.org/10.1093/carcin/bgv039(accessed on 12th June 2025).

2. Abdolrahim, M., Alhosseini, S. N., Rabiee, M., Tahriri, M., et al. (2015). Development of optical biosensor technologies for cardiac troponin recognition. https://core.ac.uk/download/213059311.pdf (accessed on 12th June 2025).

3. Abreu, I., Adlard, R., Alvarez-Pellitero, P., Alves, A., Aravindan, V., Bayne, C., Becker, T., et al. (2017). Physiological responses of reared sea bream (*Sparus aurata* Linnaeus, 1758) to an *Amyloodinium ocellatum* outbreak. https://core.ac.uk/download/322918622.pdf (accessed on 12th June 2025).

4. Ackerman, M., Alfaro, M., Almeida, L., Araújo-Luna, A., Arends, J., Ashley, M., Auer, H., et al. (2019). Tissue-specific orchestration of gilthead sea bream resilience to hypoxia and high stocking density. https://core.ac.uk/download/228073311.pdf (accessed on 12th June 2025).

5. Adaway, M., Allen, M. R., Bidwell, J. P., Brustovetsky, T., et al. (2019). Loss of Nmp4 optimizes osteogenic metabolism and secretion to enhance bone quality. https://core.ac.uk/download/187423805.pdf (accessed on 12th June 2025).

6. Alexander, N. D., Aziz, N., Conway, D. J., de Souza, J. B., et al. (2010). Oral activated charcoal prevents experimental cerebral malaria in mice and in a randomized controlled clinical trial in man did not interfere with the pharmacokinetics of parenteral artesunate. https://core.ac.uk/download/13096831.pdf (accessed on 12th June 2025).

7. Allegra, M., Attanzio, A., Cilla, A., Frazzitta, A., Livrea, M. A., & Tesoriere, L. (2019). 7-Keto-cholesterol and cholestan-3β, 5α, 6β-triol induce eryptosis through distinct pathways leading to NADPH oxidase and nitric oxide synthase activation. https://core.ac.uk/download/275693511.pdf (accessed on 12th June 2025).

8. Marrocco, I., Altieri, F., & Peluso, I. (2017). Measurement and Clinical Significance of Biomarkers of Oxidative Stress in Humans. *Oxidative medicine and cellular longevity*, *2017*, 6501046. https://doi.org/10.1155/2017/6501046(accessed on 12th June 2025).

9. Ambrosio, G., Azzato, F., Cao, G. F., Gonzalez, A., et al. (2016). Exercise ameliorates endocrine pancreas damage induced by chronic cola drinking in rats. https://core.ac.uk/download/159294453.pdf (accessed on 12th June 2025).

10. Timothy S. Gross, Beverly S. Arnold, Maria S. Sepulveda, and Kelly McDonald (2001). Relations of environmental contaminants, algal toxins, and diet with the reproductive success of American alligators on Florida lakes. USGS-Florida Caribbean Science Center and The Department of Physiological Sciences, College of Veterinary Medicine, University of Florida, Gainesville, Florida. (accessed on 12th June 2025).

11. Ashby, A., Braceland, M., Eckersall, P. D., Haining, H., et al. (2016). Technical pre-analytical effects on the clinical biochemistry of Atlantic salmon (*Salmo salar* L.). https://core.ac.uk/download/42370197.pdf (accessed on 12th June 2025).

12. Baarendse, P. J. J., Brand, H., van den Bruggeman, V., et al. (2008). Involvement of the hypothalamic-pituitary-thyroid axis and its interaction with the hypothalamic-pituitary-adrenal axis in the ontogeny of avian thermoregulation: A review. https://core.ac.uk/download/pdf/29259797.pdf (accessed on 12th June 2025).
13. Baker, M., Bryan, K., Lawless, N., Lippolis, J., et al. (2014). MicroRNA regulation of bovine monocyte inflammatory and metabolic networks in an *in vivo* infection model. https://core.ac.uk/download/45656557.pdf (accessed on 12th June 2025).
14. Beguin, S., Hemker, H. C., & Xi, M. (1989). Importance of factor-IX-dependent prothrombinase formation–the Josso pathway–in clotting plasma. https://core.ac.uk/download/323361379.pdf (accessed on 12th June 2025).
15. Bianchi, M., Vaglio, S., Pupella, S., Marano, G., Facco, G., Liumbruno, G. M., & Grazzini, G. (2016). Leucoreduction of blood components: an effective way to increase blood safety?. *Blood transfusion = Trasfusione del sangue, 14*(2), 214–227. https://doi.org/10.2450/2015.0154-15(accessed on 12th June 2025).
16. Bonde, R. K., de Wit, M., Harr, K. E., et al. (2018). Serum proteins in healthy and diseased Florida manatees (*Trichechus manatus latirostris*). https://core.ac.uk/download/188135031.pdf (accessed on 12th June 2025).
17. Brown, M., Brunner, E., Burke, B., et al. (2009). Polymorphisms in the WNK1 gene are associated with blood pressure variation and urinary potassium excretion. https://core.ac.uk/download/1730056.pdf (accessed on 12th June 2025).
18. Buhagiar, G. (2005). *Rationalization of the Biochemistry Laboratory: Which Way Forwards?* https://core.ac.uk/download/46602008.pdf (accessed on 12th June 2025).
19. Capiau, S., Stove, C., & Velghe, S. (2016). Opening the toolbox of alternative sampling strategies in clinical routine: A key-role for (LC-)MS/MS. https://core.ac.uk/download/84043363.pdf (accessed on 12th June 2025).
20. Chang, Y. M., Garden, O. A., Hadox, E., et al. (2016). Serum biochemical phenotypes in the domestic dog. https://core.ac.uk/download/36779275.pdf (accessed on 12th June 2025).
21. Chinopoulos, C. (2013). Which way does the citric acid cycle turn during hypoxia? The critical role of alpha-ketoglutarate dehydrogenase complex. https://core.ac.uk/download/50566105.pdf (accessed on 12th June 2025).
22. Costa, D. P., Crocker, D. E., Houser, D. S., et al. (2012). Hormone and metabolite changes associated with extended breeding fasts in male northern elephant seals (*Mirounga angustirostris*). https://core.ac.uk/download/56705017.pdf (accessed on 12th June 2025).
23. Crockford, J. N., Ingram, J. R., & Matthews, L. R. (1999). Ultradian, circadian and seasonal rhythms in cortisol secretion and adrenal responsiveness to ACTH and yarding in unrestrained red deer (*Cervus elaphus*) stags. https://core.ac.uk/download/29195391.pdf (accessed on 12th June 2025).
24. Donaldson, A. (2013). Biochemistry changes that occur after death: Potential markers for determining post-mortem interval. https://core.ac.uk/download/322841937.pdf (accessed on 12th June 2025).
25. Dyson, A., Audibert, G., Berne, R. M., Blitzer, M. L., Boutilier, R. G., Brown, I. P., Devlin, C., et al. (2013). The key role of nitric oxide in hypoxia: Hypoxic vasodilation and energy

supply-demand matching. *Antioxidants & Redox Signaling*, *19*(14), 1690–1710. https://doi.org/10.1089/ars.2012.4979 (accessed on 12th June 2025).

26. Eilerts, Diane F. (2016) "Beyond DNA: Epigenetics and Proteomics in Forensic Science," *Themis: Research Journal of Justice Studies and Forensic Science*: Vol. 4 : Iss. 1 , Article 10. DOI: https://doi.org/10.31979/THEMIS.2016.0410 https://scholarworks.sjsu.edu/themis/vol4/iss1/10(accessed on 12th June 2025).
27. Ekremoğlu, M., Pasaoğlu, H., Pasaoğlu, Ö. T., et al. (2020). An investigation of acute effects at various doses of malathion on glucose homeostasis and insulin resistance in rat liver, pancreas and serum. https://core.ac.uk/download/304672915.pdf (accessed on 12th June 2025).
28. Eo, J., & Kang, Y. B. (Abraham), Mert, S., et al. (2018). Metabolic patterning on a chip: Towards *in vitro* liver zonation of primary rat and human hepatocytes. https://digitalcommons.georgefox.edu/cgi/viewcontent.cgi?article=1056&context=mece_fac (accessed on 12th June 2025).
29. Eraly, S. A., Jamshidi, N., Liu, H. C., et al. (2015). Transcriptome-based reconstructions from the murine knockout suggest involvement of the urate transporter, URAT1 (*SLC22A12*), in novel metabolic pathways. https://core.ac.uk/download/323080180.pdf (accessed on 12th June 2025).
30. Ferru, E., Pantaleo, A., & Turrini, F. M. (2012). A new method for the capture of surface proteins in *Plasmodium falciparum* parasitized erythrocytes. https://core.ac.uk/download/11693500.pdf (accessed on 12th June 2025).
31. Filipovich, A. H., De Rossi, A., Cavdar, A. O., Kidenya, B., Klumb, C. E., Kim, D., Mwizamuholya, D., et al. (2013). Relationship between non-Hodgkin's lymphoma and blood levels of Epstein-Barr virus in children in north-western Tanzania: A case control study. https://core.ac.uk/download/pdf/11307798.pdf (accessed on 12th June 2025).
32. Fonteh, A. L. (2018). *Erotic Aciduria.* https://core.ac.uk/download/213462592.pdf (accessed on 12th June 2025).
33. Gallo, L., Quintana, F. R., Svagelj, W. S., et al. (2017). Plasma biochemistries and morphometric indices of body condition in imperial cormorant (*Phalacrocorax atriceps*) chicks. https://core.ac.uk/download/159291883.pdf (accessed on 12th June 2025).
34. Goldstein, R. E., Grauer, G. F., Kalish, R. A., Levy, S., Levy, S. A., Rolla, D., & Scorpio, D. G. (2019). Differences in clinicopathologic variables between Borrelia C6 antigen seroreactive and Borrelia C6 seronegative glomerulopathy in dogs. https://core.ac.uk/download/323071861.pdf (accessed on 12th June 2025).
35. Tremblay-Franco, M., Zerbinati, C., Pacelli, A., Palmaccio, G., Lubrano, C., Ducheix, S., Guillou, H., & Iuliano, L. (2015). Effect of obesity and metabolic syndrome on plasma oxysterols and fatty acids in human. *Steroids*, *99*(Pt B), 287–292. https://doi.org/10.1016/j.steroids.2015.03.019 (accessed on 12th June 2025).
36. Herndl, R., Marschner, I., & Scriba, P. C. (1980). Comparison of four different algorithms for the calculation of radioimmunoassay standard curves. https://core.ac.uk/download/12169087.pdf (accessed on 12th June 2025).

37. Huwiler, A., Koch, A., & Pfeilschifter, J. M. (2013). Sphingosine 1-phosphate in renal diseases. https://core.ac.uk/download/16515935.pdf (accessed on 12th June 2025).

38. Kalachniuk, L. (Liliia), Luhova, Y. (Yeseniia), & Maliuk, I. (Inna). (2016). The protein metabolism in small animals with chronic renal failure and its correction. https://media.neliti.com/media/publications/297166-the-protein-metabolism-in-small-animals-307fcaf7.pdf (accessed on 12th June 2025).

39. Majidi, F., Marjani, A., Naseri, F., et al. (2015). Prevalence of metabolic syndrome in Baluch women in Chabahar. https://core.ac.uk/download/52205795.pdf (accessed on 12th June 2025).

40. Marjani, A., Mehrpouya, M., & Pourhashem, Z. (2016). Serum γ-glutamyl transferase, alanine aminotransferase and aspartate aminotransferase activity in healthy blood donors of different ethnic groups in Gorgan. https://core.ac.uk/download/52205537.pdf (accessed on 12th June 2025).

41. Mihajlovičová, X., Nagy, O., & Tóthová, C. (2017). The use of serum proteins in the laboratory diagnosis of health disorders in ruminants. https://core.ac.uk/download/322433768.pdf (accessed on 12th June 2025).

42. Mujtahid, M. (2020). Blood glucose regulating hormones and their physiological and biochemical roles. https://core.ac.uk/download/356679375.pdf (accessed on 12th June 2025).

43. Palanisamy, P., Rao, Y. Y., Farook, J., Subramaniyam, S., Ponnusha, B. S., & Ambika, A. (2011). The combinational effect of cardiac and biochemical markers in diabetic patients with cardiovascular disease. *International Journal of Current Biomedical Sciences.* https://core.ac.uk/download/pdf/14681.pdf (accessed on 12th June 2025).

44. Perdomo, J. L. (2016). *Mathematical Modeling of Blood Coagulation.* https://core.ac.uk/download/80535721.pdf (accessed on 12th June 2025).

45. Sarmidi, M. R. (2012). *Food is Our Medicine.* https://core.ac.uk/download/11801185.pdf (accessed on 12th June 2025).

46. Seaman, W., & Whitehouse, J. H. (2001). *Florida Marine Biotechnology: Research, Development and Training Capabilities to Advance Science and Commerce.* Sea Grant Technical Paper Number 110 March 2001. https://core.ac.uk/download/11016354.pdf (accessed on 12th June 2025).

47. Shestopaloff, Y. K. (2014). Method for finding metabolic properties based on the general growth law. Liver examples. *A General Framework for Biological Modeling.* http://arxiv.org/abs/1509.03516 (accessed on 12th June 2025).

FREE RADICALS AND ANTIOXIDANTS

4

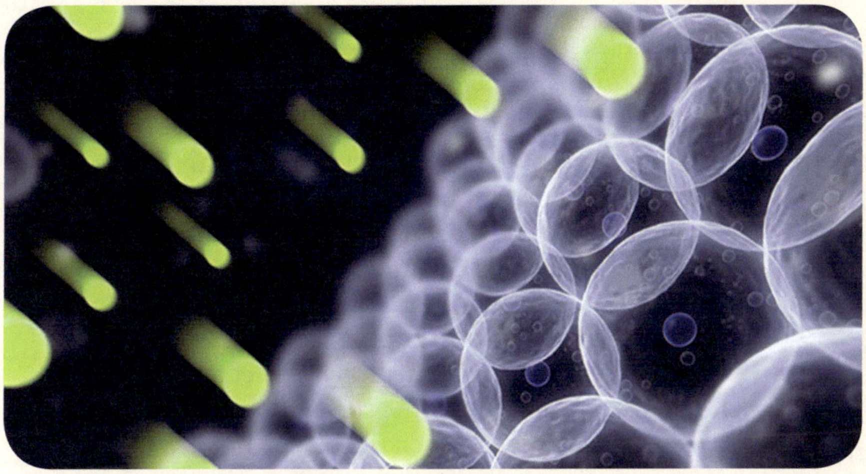

LEARNING OBJECTIVES

After studying this chapter, you will be able to:

1. Understand the science of free radicals;
2. Describe the role of free radicals in the human body;
3. Describe the antioxidants in nature's defense;
4. Understand the role of antioxidants in disease prevention.

Introduction

The intricate dance between free radicals and antioxidants illustrates a fundamental principle of biological chemistry and pathology. Free radicals, which are most often generated by metabolic processes and environmental stress, play a dual role in the body; while they are necessary for certain cellular functions, their excessive production leads to oxidative stress. This stress is a condition that entails a lack of balance between ROS and the body's ability to detoxify toxic intermediates or to repair the resulting damage. For instance, smoking cigarettes has been revealed as a significant causative factor of oxidative stress since it accelerates the production of free radicals, and these can lead to cellular damage and a host of diseases like cancer and CVDs, as per Kakako et al. (2025). Therefore, it is important to understand the dynamics of free radicals to develop effective therapeutic interventions against oxidative stress. Antioxidants serve the function of a vital countermeasure to the deleterious actions of free radicals as they strive to neutralize the same reactive species and restore oxidative balance. The body's internal antioxidant defense systems, including enzymes , such as SOD and glutathione (GSH) peroxidase, play a significant role in protecting against oxidative damage. Antioxidants in foods, like vitamins C and E, can be consumed through normal foods and supplements as an external protective mechanism.

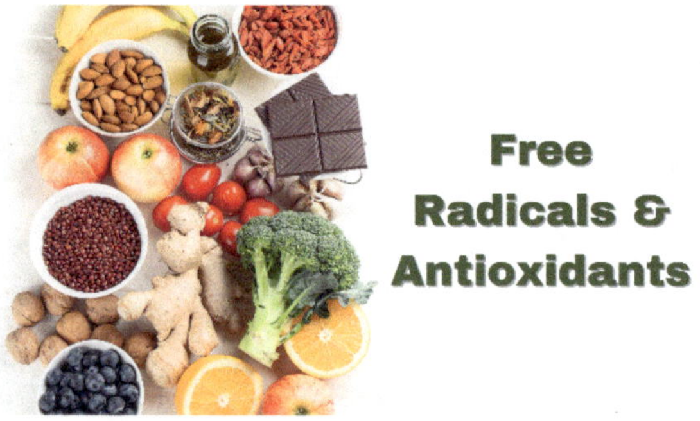

Figure 4.1. Free radicals and antioxidants.

Source: https://molecularhydrogeninstitute.org/wp-content/uploads/2023/02/free-radicals-and-antioxidants-1.png.

The function of such antioxidants is evidently seen in individuals who are exposed to excessive oxidative stress, such as smokers or individuals exposed to environmental pollutants. Evidence presented by Shuja (2025) points to the way oxidative stress is also manifested through cellular architectures, leading to electrical changes, thus making the function of antioxidants important to physiological and public health significance. In the future, the search for antioxidants is both a therapeutic intervention and a lifestyle modification that enhances endogenous protective mechanisms. Clinical studies demonstrate that antioxidant supplementation may reduce the incidence of oxidative stress-related disease and health effects overall. As continued advances in research reveal the complex interaction between free radicals and antioxidants, there is growing interest in establishing a paradigm of surveillance that identifies at-risk groups, particularly with genetic predisposition or environmental risk. Integration of public health interventions with emphasis on dietary modification will be essential in raising awareness about antioxidant activities and encouraging an active response to thwart the pervasive reach of oxidative stress and enhance community health programs using the most current scientific data (Figure 4.1).

Definition of Free Radicals

Free radicals are very reactive molecules that have unpaired electrons in their outermost shell. This peculiar structure not only causes their instability but also motivates them to achieve stability through chemical reaction with other molecules around. The outcome can be harmful, causing oxidative stress, a condition where there is an imbalance of free radicals and antioxidants in the body. The consequences of free radical action are far-reaching in that they may trigger a chain of events leading to the destruction of lipids, proteins and even DNA. This damage has been implicated in numerous pathophysiological states , such as CVDs, cancers, and neurodegenerative disorders. It is important to understand the nature of free radicals due to the fact that they are not only byproducts of normal metabolic processes but are also produced by external environmental factors, including pollution and radiation, hence the dualistic nature of their involvement in biological systems. Under pathological conditions, the formation of free radicals may be greatly enhanced, e.g., during ischemia/reperfusion when the abrupt reestablishment of blood flow results in oxidative tissue damage. This happens when there is overproduction or accumulation of free radicals, which may stimulate the peroxidation of lipids and oxidation of proteins, making them inactive. These molecular changes can induce inflammation, which further promotes the cellular damage. As an example, oxidative stress commonly leads to the formation of pro-inflammatory cytokines, which have been determined as contributing factors in the case of several types of MI. The interplay between free radicals and inflammatory mediators demonstrates how these reactive species not only contribute to cellular injury but also drive broader inflammatory pathways, complicating the body's response and recovery processes (Cerretani et al., 2015). Besides the harmful effects, free radicals also have a paradoxical role in physiology, as they are signaling molecules, able to regulate several biological functions. Although usually linked with degeneration and pathology, some amounts of free radicals are required for normal cellular physiology, especially immune responses and cellular signaling. Such a subtle role has a curious dichotomy, in that low doses can promote protective processes, but excessive accumulation leads to oxidative stress, which is harmful to cellular integrity. Furthermore, the application of synthetic antioxidants like synthetic phenolic antioxidants (SPAs) has been shown to help mitigate the adverse effects of free radicals by extending the shelf life of food products, showcasing their utility in both health and industry. This balance between free radicals and antioxidants underscores the importance of maintaining homeostasis within biological systems (Yong et al., 2007) (Figure 4.2).

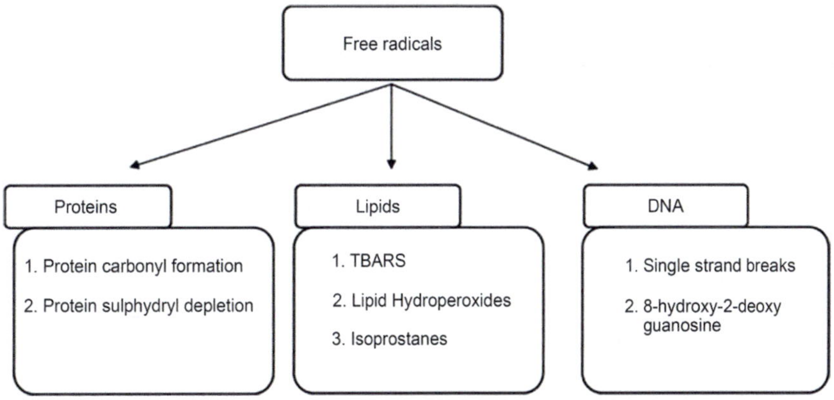

Figure 4.2. Impact of free radicals on biomolecules present in cells leads to the formation of adducts, markers of various diseases.

Source: https://cdnintech.com/media/chapter/65067/1512345123/media/F1.png.

Importance of Antioxidants

The role of antioxidants in checking the destructiveness of free radicals cannot be overestimated. Highly reactive molecules known as free radicals, produced as a result of different metabolic reactions, environmental stress, or pollution, present a significant danger to cellular integrity. The disturbance generated by these radicals is known to result in a situation called oxidative stress, which has been attributed to a host of chronic diseases like cancer and cardiovascular disorders. Antioxidants checkmate this harm by neutralizing free radicals in different ways, hence protecting cellular components like lipids, proteins, and DNA. Research has helped us to understand how dietary antioxidants can support the innate immunity of the body, thus promoting good health and prevention of disease. Dietary intake of antioxidants, as one of the most significant elements of health maintenance, is of paramount importance in terms of longevity and the reduction of the harmful impacts of oxidative stress. In addition, it is not true that antioxidants are only obtained through the diet since they can also be synthesized endogenously following an exercise. Studies have pointed out the significant effect of exercise in boosting antioxidant defense in the body.

Engaging in regular exercise can stimulate the production of endogenous antioxidants, such as SOD, which helps mitigate oxidative damage during stress exposure. For instance, a study on sled dogs revealed a significant increase in SOD levels during environmental stress events, a response indicative of the body's adaptive mechanisms to counteract oxidative stress (Witkop, 2019). Additionally, sustained exercise has been shown to elevate total antioxidant power (TAP), indicating an increased cytoprotective effect following repeated physical activity. This reiterates the need to ensure that foods rich in antioxidants are incorporated into the diet and that an individual leads an active lifestyle in order to ensure that the body is as resistant as possible to oxidative stress. Lastly, the clinical significance of antioxidants is that the assessment of oxidative stress biomarkers requires a more subtle approach. As recent debates have indicated, current approaches to the measurement of oxidative stress are usually inconsistent and biased, which makes it particularly important to employ a multi-faceted approach to assessment. Any thoroughgoing index of oxidative stress ought to incorporate a number of biomarkers so that it may mirror the redox status in the human body. This can be used to give crucial information on health health-promoting properties of antioxidants. Researchers can further clarify the possible therapeutic effects of antioxidants in the prevention of diseases and promotion of health by determining and overcoming methodological shortcomings. The integration of robust analytical methods will ensure a clearer understanding of antioxidant efficacy, further highlighting their critical role in combating oxidative stress and improving health outcomes in diverse populations (Marrocco et al., 2017) (Figure 4.3).

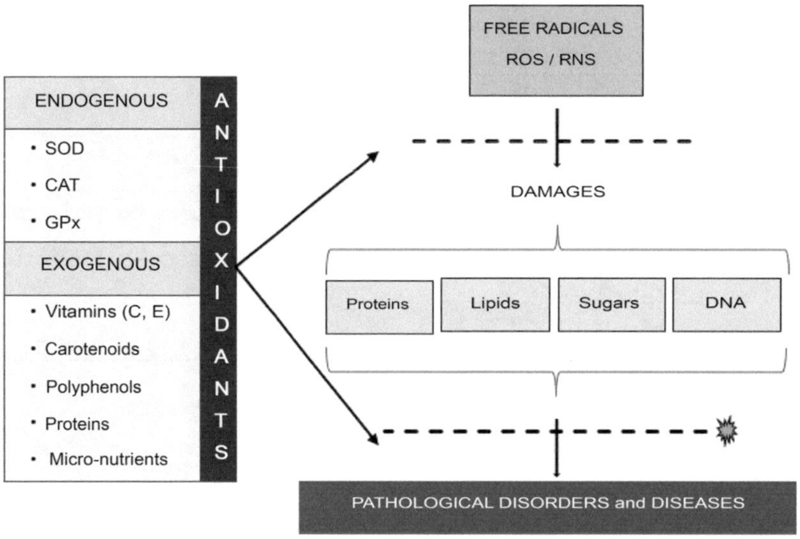

Figure 4.3. Antioxidant defense against free radicals.

Source: https://www.mdpi.com/oxygen/oxygen-02-00006/article_deploy/html/images/oxygen-02-00006-g004.png.

4.1. The Science of Free Radicals

Learning Outcome

1. Know the formation of free radicals;
2. Describe the types of free radicals;
3. Understand the role of free radicals in biological processes.

The sensitive balance between free radicals and antioxidants is crucial to the health of cells. Free radicals are highly reactive molecules with loose electrons, which make them chase stability by targeting molecules, resulting in cell damage. Oxidative stress is also linked to various diseases like CVDs, cancer, and neurodegenerative disorders. Free radical chemistry highlights both the harm that free radicals have the capacity to do and their important physiological roles, such as enhancement of immune response and cellular signaling. Understanding the fundamental mechanisms by which free radicals interact with biological systems is essential in the development of preventive interventions against oxidative damage, underscoring the necessity of ongoing research on this complex field. Antioxidants are either synthetic or natural compounds that cancel out the damaging effects of free radicals. They do this by donating electrons to neutralize free radicals without themselves becoming harmful. The body generates some antioxidants endogenously, such as GSH, while others need to be ingested through food, such as vitamins C and E. New studies show that an interactive increase in the action of a number of antioxidants is with their synergistic interaction. For instance, natural pomegranate-derived antioxidants, such as pomegranate peel extracts (PPE) and seed extracts (PSE), have been reported to be promising in lipid peroxidation inhibition, a process that is highly stimulated by free radicals. The blending of these extracts with other antioxidants like tocopherol and quercetin has been reported to have an increased lag phase of lipid degradation, which indicates their combined capacity to protect cell membranes against oxidative deterioration (Altunkaya, 2014). Current development in research has also explored the use of waste materials from industries, like those from pomegranate juice, as a source of valuable antioxidants. The approach is not only focused on the dual challenge of waste management and promoting health, but also responds to opportunities for green solutions to combat oxidative stress. By pursuing the antioxidative capacity of natural products, scientists aim to develop new means to enhance the body's ability to combat free radicals. The mounting evidence for the effectiveness of natural antioxidants underscores the importance of including such substances in a prevention strategy for health. As such, insight into the mechanistic pathways relating free radicals, antioxidants, and cell health may lay the groundwork for novel therapeutic strategies aimed at neutralizing oxidative stress cytotoxicity and promoting overall well-being (Gray et al., 2014) (Figure 4.4).

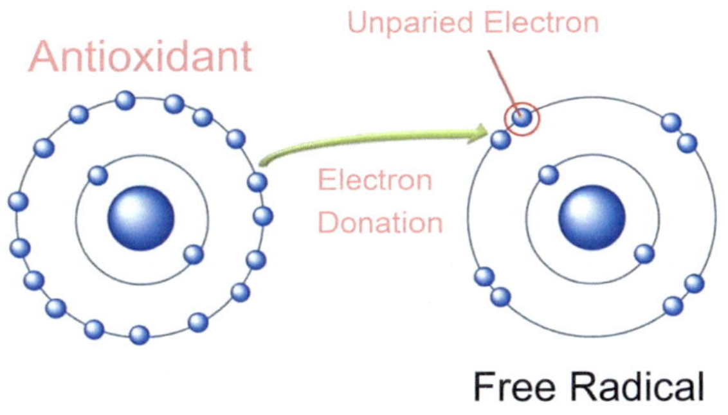

Figure 4.4. When an electron loses its partner, it creates a free radical, which is usually unstable and highly reactive.

Source: https://media.hswstatic.com/eyJidWNrZXQiOiJjb250ZW50LmhzdzN0YXRpYy5jb20iLCJrZXkiOiJnaWZcL2ZyZWUtcmFkaWNhbHMuanBnIiwiZWRpdHMiOnsicmVzaXplIjp7IndpZHRoIjo4Mjh9LCJ0b0Zvcm1hdCI6ImF2aWYifX0=.

4.1.1. Formation of Free Radicals

The generation of free radicals is a complicated biochemical process which has decisive roles in normal bodily capabilities as well as pathophysiological states. Free radicals are unstable chemicals that have unpaired electrons, which make them very reactive and they can cause chain reactions that may harm the cell components. These radicals can be produced through various endogenous pathways, such as mitochondrial respiration, where oxygen is incompletely reduced, generating ROS like superoxide anion. Moreover, exogenous sources of free radicals include UV radiation, pollution, tobacco smoke, etc., which can further increase the level of oxidative stress in the body. The intricacies of these processes underscore the necessity for a balanced redox state to maintain cellular integrity and function, highlighting the dual nature of free radicals as both participants in essential biological pathways and potential agents of harm, particularly when their levels exceed the body's antioxidant defenses (Chandimali et al., 2025). In addition, the creation and effects of free radicals also apply to the metabolism process, especially in terms of digesting nutrients in the body. The metabolic activities help to convert food into energy, yet they also result in generating free radicals as byproducts unintentionally. Remarkably, dietary antioxidants can affect the efficient digestion and utilization of feed nutrients, as they can be used to alleviate oxidative stress. Studies indicate that some natural products like carotenoids have a high antioxidant capacity, hence they check the generation of free radicals in metabolism.

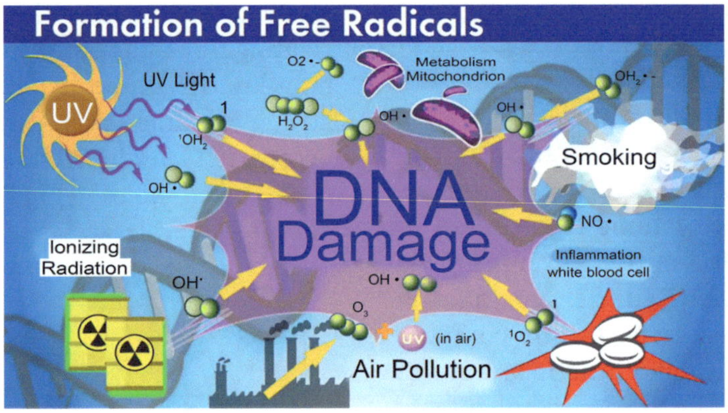

Figure 4.5. Free radicals form because of many things in modern life, including UV light, pollution, smoking and even our diet.

Source: https://media.hswstatic.com/eyJidWNrZXQiOiJjb250ZW50Lmhzd3N0YXRpYy5jb20iLCJrZXkiOiJnaWZcL2ZyZWUtcmFkaWNhbC1jYXVzZXMuanBnIiwiZWRpdHMiOnsicmVzaXplIjp7IndpZHRoIjo4Mjh9LCJ0b0Zvcm1hdCI6ImF2aWYifX0=.

As an example, astaxanthin, a carotenoid possessing strong antioxidative potential, has been revealed to promise the improvement of the physiological health of diverse organisms. The intricate relationship between metabolism, free radical formation, and antioxidant presence emphasizes the importance of understanding these mechanisms for developing effective dietary strategies to combat oxidative damage (Akhmedzhanova et al., 2023). The consequences of the formation of free radicals are far-reaching, especially when chronic diseases are considered. High levels of free radicals are linked to extensive damage to cells, which leads to the development of several disorders, such as cancer, cardiovascular and neurodegenerative diseases. This property of free radicals to react and destroy important biomolecules, including DNA, proteins, and lipids, may result in the changed functioning of cells and accelerated inflammation. Therefore, elucidation of the processes involved in the generation of free radicals and their effects on health are imperative in the design of therapeutic interventions. In addition, increasing the antioxidant defenses of the body with the help of the diet can be a strategic way of dealing with oxidative stress and the health risks related to it. Future research into the nuances of free radical biology and antioxidant utilization will be vital in elucidating effective preventive and therapeutic strategies against oxidative stress-related diseases (Chandimali et al., 2025) (Figure 4.5).

4.1.2. Types of Free Radicals

Free radicals' classification is wide and can be divided into several types, which vary in their structure and reactivity. At the forefront are ROS, which include superoxide anions, hydrogen peroxide, and hydroxyl radicals. Such species have been known to occur as a result of normal metabolism, especially during cellular respiration. Although ROS are essential in cell signaling and homeostasis, their over-accumulation may cause oxidative stress, which harms proteins, lipids, and DNA. This oxidative injury has been linked to many health disorders, such as neurodegenerative diseases and cancer, so the balance between ROS generation and antioxidant defense is a key research area. Knowledge of the different kinds of free radicals and their causes enables scientists to come up with specific antioxidant treatments to counter the harmful effects of oxidative stress on human health observed in numerous studies and health-related interventions that attempt to redress this balance. Another significant category is reactive nitrogen species (RNS), which includes radicals , such as nitric oxide and peroxynitrite. Such radicals may be generated during the metabolism of compounds that contain nitrogen and may combine with ROS to create more complex species that are harmful to cellular integrity. RNS plays a central role in several physiological functions, such as vasodilation and immune reactions. Nevertheless, in pathological conditions, RNS may also participate in inflammation and tissue damage, especially in such diseases as diabetes and cardiovascular disorders. For instance, oxidative damage caused by free radicals has been shown to play a role in the progression of type II diabetes mellitus (TIIDM), further complicating patient outcomes and management strategies. An elucidation of the pathways through which RNS mediate cellular damage and aging sheds light on possible therapeutic avenues , such as dietary antioxidants, which could protect these damaging species. Also, alkoxy and peroxy radicals formed upon the peroxidation of lipids deserve much attention because of their reactivity and role in lipid metabolism. These radicals can cause chain reactions that result in massive damage to the cellular level, further increasing oxidative stress in the body. The connection between chronic diseases and lipid peroxidation supports the significance of dietary antioxidants, especially those contained in fruits. According to recent studies, these bioactive compounds counteract free-radical development and reduce oxidative stress, thus mitigating risks associated with aging and degenerative diseases like cancer and diabetes (Dhalaria et al., 2020). Consequently, understanding the various types of free radicals, their sources, and their effects enhances the potential for antioxidant strategies that can promote health and longevity in populations prone to oxidative stress-related disorders (Joshua et al., 2017) (Figure 4.6).

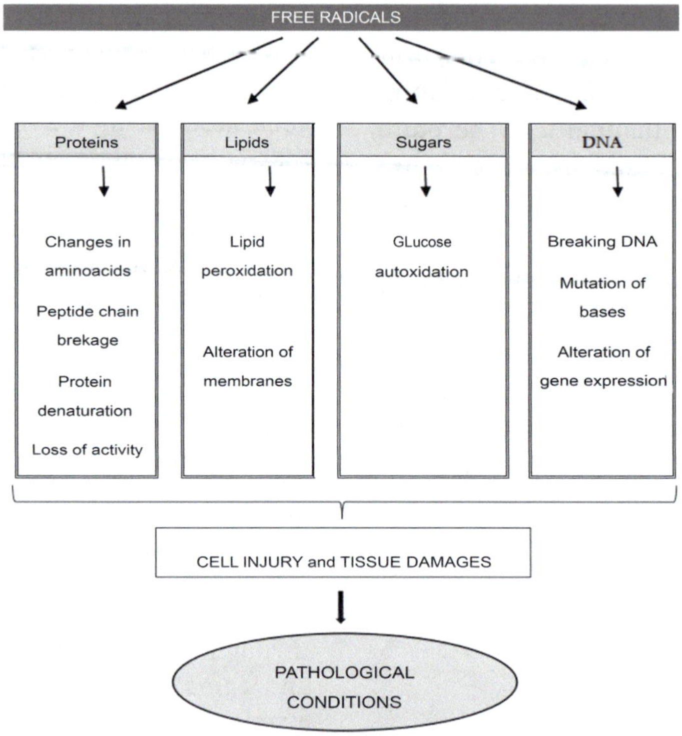

Figure 4.6. The molecular target of free radicals and oxidative damage.

Source: https://www.mdpi.com/oxygen/oxygen-02-00006/article_deploy/html/images/oxygen-02-00006-g002.png.

4.1.3. Role of Free Radicals in Biological Processes

Free radicals are very reactive molecules with multidimensional functions in biological systems, with huge impacts on cellular activities and general health. Their presence is a natural consequence of metabolic processes, especially during aerobic respiration when oxygen is broken down to release energy. However, while free radicals , such as ROS and RNS are required for normal physiological function, they also pose the risk of destabilizing cellular integrity when produced in excess. Curiously, free radicals have a role in immune reactions, with important functions as powerful signaling molecules in aiding the killing of pathogens during the inflammatory response. This duality indicates the delicate equilibrium that must be found by organisms between the beneficial and deleterious actions of free radicals, underscoring their important but complex function in biological processes. A balance between free radicals and antioxidants is lost; however, a situation known as oxidative stress, characterized by an overabundance of free radicals capable of leading to intense cellular damage. Oxidative stress is associated with protein, lipid, and DNA deterioration, which is capable of triggering unwanted processes linked with various illnesses, for example, cancer. Of special note, excessive ROS build-up could lead to damage in DNA, a key element in the establishment and development of oncogenesis. There are proofs that oxidative stress participates in the activation of signaling pathways towards tumor development and growth. Furthermore, the abnormal cellular microenvironment in oxidative stress provides a fertile ground for malignant transformation, proposing that one should value the mechanisms of free radical-mediated alterations in cellular processes as a framework for directing therapeutic interventions into cancer management (Zahra et al., 2021). Importantly, the coordination between free radicals and biological processes goes beyond disease pathology to therapeutic interventions. Increased attention has been devoted to utilizing antioxidants in a strategy to combat oxidative stress and associated cellular damage. Antioxidants' enzymatic and non-enzymatic functions include detoxification of free radicals and the restoration of oxidative balance and therefore protection against cellular damage. Antioxidant therapy was revealed by recent studies to improve the outcome of the treatment of various forms of cancer by efficiently modulating oxidative stress pathways. Nonetheless, the use of antioxidant supplements remains controversial, particularly their excessive use, as it can sometimes cause adverse effects, like enhanced cancer risk (Che et al., 2021). Lastly, with the understanding of free radicals' dual role in health and disease, efficient therapeutic strategies could be developed in managing oxidative stress disorders.

Test Your Knowledge

1. What are free radicals?
2. What is the role of free radicals in biological processes?

4.2. The Impact of Free Radicals on Health

Learning Outcome

1. Know the oxidative stress and its consequences;
2. Understand the relationship between free radicals and chronic diseases;
3. Describe the aging and free radical damage.

The importance of free radicals in the human body has attracted a lot of interest, especially because they are considered as potentially dangerous and at the same time useful molecules. Free radicals are highly reactive species that are usually produced during metabolism and may react with cell components, resulting in oxidative stress. This occurs when the free radicals are more than the antioxidant defenses in the body, leading to damage to proteins, lipids as well as DNA. This type of oxidative damage has been linked to the pathogenesis of many chronic diseases , such as cancer, CVDs, and neurodegenerative diseases. Thus, the relationship between free radicals and antioxidants is very important in the determination of health and disease prevention. The quest for effective strategies to mitigate oxidative stress has led researchers to explore natural antioxidants as a preferable alternative to synthetic options, which may pose health risks (Zahid et al., 2024). Among the potential opportunities in the fight against oxidative stress is the use of natural plant-based antioxidants. Flavonoids, a class of antioxidants abundant in fruits, vegetables, and herbs, exhibit remarkable capabilities to scavenge ROS and protect cells from oxidative damage. The compounds not only play a vital role in plant tolerance to abiotic stresses but also have great importance in human health, as they may have anti-inflammatory and antimicrobial activity. Current research indicates that by including flavonoid-rich foods in the diet, total antioxidant capacity may be increased, which may reduce the risk of developing chronic diseases linked to oxidative stress. Moreover, with growing consumer awareness regarding dietary choices, there is an increasing shift towards natural sources of antioxidants, as these are perceived to be safer and more beneficial than synthetic alternatives (Dias et al., 2021). The inclusion of natural antioxidants in dietary habits is also justified by the developments in extraction technologies, which are directed at the maximization of their activity and, at the same time, environmental friendliness. It has also been shown that extracted antioxidants from fruits and vegetable waste can be effectively used to extend the oxidative stability of edible oils, hence making them safer and more nutritionally balanced. These methods can prolong the shelf life of food products, making them ecologically sustainable as they make use of waste materials to add value to the waste. With the growing concern for health conscious and eco-friendly products among consumers, the need to have natural sources of antioxidants in food is on the increase. This trend underscores the critical importance of antioxidants in combating the effects of free radicals and reflects a broader movement towards healthier dietary practices in contemporary society (Zahid et al., 2024) (Figure 4.7).

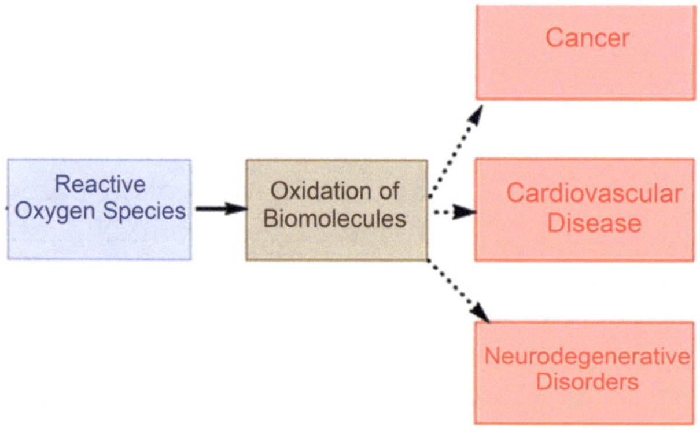

Figure 4.7. Reactive oxygen species are involved in the development of various pathological disorders.

Source: https://cdnintech.com/media/chapter/65067/1512345123/media/F3.png.

4.2.1. Oxidative Stress and Its Consequences

Oxidative stress is an extremely vital notion in the biological effects of free radicals. Oxidative stress occurs when there is an imbalance between the production of ROS and the body's ability to neutralize these potentially harmful agents. This imbalance may cause huge harm to biomolecules like proteins, lipids, and DNA. To keep the redox balance organisms have several mechanisms that prevent the occurrence of oxidative stress, intercept it when it happens, and repair the damage it produces. Paradoxically, although an extreme oxidant challenge may be harmful, a degree of oxidative signaling, termed oxidative eustress, does play critical regulatory roles in cellular responses. This nuanced understanding blurs the lines between oxidative damage and physiological signaling, prompting researchers to explore how redox balance might be manipulated for therapeutic purposes (Sies et al., 2017). Oxidative stress has implications in many areas of health-related issues, especially chronic diseases. High levels of oxidative stress have been associated with diseases including CVD, neurodegenerative diseases, and cancer. As in the example of cardiovascular health, oxidative stress plays a role in endothelial dysfunction and atherosclerosis development. Oxidative stress is frequently worsened by chronic inflammation, which further complicates the disease courses. It is important to note that antioxidants are significant in the reduction of the impact of oxidative stress, hence providing protective functions against oxidative damage, which is caused by ROS. Consequently, antioxidants can alleviate the development or exacerbation of multiple disorders, which underlines the significance of dietary elements, including flavonoids, which possess strong antioxidative abilities. These connections underscore the need for continued investigation into the duality of oxidative stress and its relationship with disease (Archana et al., 2016). Besides, the knowledge of the outcomes of oxidative stress leads to the innovation of therapeutic approaches. This interaction between ROS and antioxidant defenses forms a rich area of research in nutraceuticals and pharmaceutical agents capable of modulating oxidative pathways. As an example, flavonoids, a family of natural products with diverse phenolic structures, have been reported as potent antioxidants that can regulate cellular activities and present anti-inflammatory effects. Modern research is confirming their historical use in traditional medicine and is ongoing to discover their mechanisms of action and possible health benefits. This ongoing investigation highlights the critical role that antioxidants can play in countering oxidative stress and addressing chronic health conditions, reflecting a broader trend toward integrative approaches in healthcare that recognize the significance of redox biology in human health (Archana et al., 2016) (Figure 4.8).

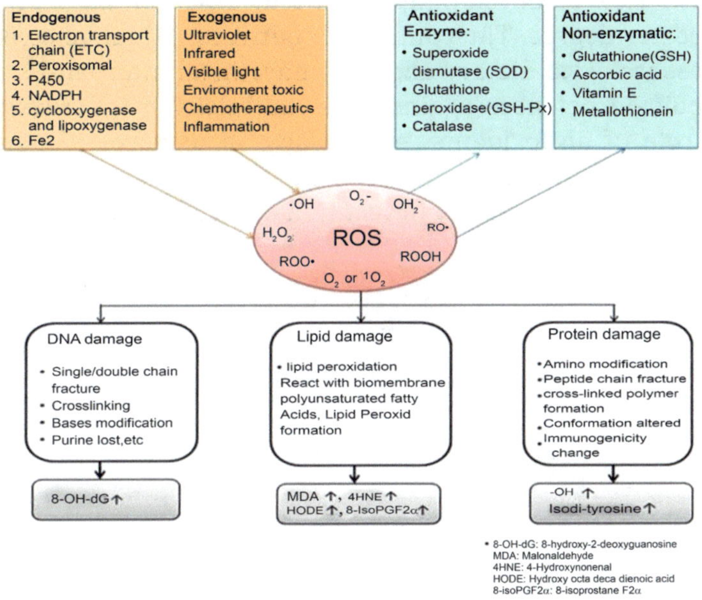

Figure 4.8. The functions of free radicals on biomolecules and its consequences.

Source: https://cdnintech.com/media/chapter/65067/1512345123/media/F2.png.

4.2.2. Connection to Chronic Diseases

The relationship between free radicals and chronic conditions is a significant field of research, particularly in light of the involvement of oxidative stress in pathophysiological conditions. Chronic conditions , such as neurodegenerative diseases are increasingly accounted for by considering oxidative damage caused by free radicals. For instance, a diet intervention rich in bioactive compounds is said to reverse oxidative stress, a pathogenic causation of neurodegeneration, according to some research. Among these compounds are ghee and curcuminoids, chlorogenic acid, and conjugated linoleic acid, which possess anti-inflammatory, free radical scavenging, and antioxidant properties. Toward this end, the interconnection between free radicals and chronic disease underscores nutrition's role in therapy for the prevention or treatment of diseases like Alzheimer's disease, where oxidative stress is a prime cause of disease pathogenesis (Amato et al., 2019). CVDs represent another high-profile category of chronic disease that is intensely impacted by free radical activity and oxidative stress. End-stage heart failure pathogenesis, a CVD complication, consists of complex interactions between cellular injury and metabolic disturbance evoked by free radicals. Research has established that certain pharmaceutical agents employed in the treatment of chronic disease, including doxorubicin, can potentially augment mitochondrial dysfunction, leading to cardiomyocyte oxidative damage. This highlights a critical intersection where both drug therapy and free radicals contribute to the development of the disease. Melatonin, a natural antioxidant, has protective actions against such oxidative damage, and it is suggested that antioxidants may be beneficial adjunct therapies for improving patient outcomes in heart failure and other drug-induced cardiac dysfunction (Ganeshan et al., 2019). Understanding the role of antioxidants in the suppression of the impact of free radicals on chronic diseases reflects the tremendous therapeutic potential. By taking more antioxidants through food or supplements, patients can reduce their risk of developing chronic diseases or manage those with prevailing chronic diseases to a greater degree. The connection between oxidative stress and disease state is the basis for ongoing research into dietary and pharmaceutical interventions aimed at modulating the use of the body's built-in defenses against free radicals. With increasing evidence regarding the disease-protective role of antioxidants, particularly in diseases like neurodegeneration and heart failure, it is increasingly critical to integrate such information into public health programs and individualized health care plans for the prevention and control of diseases (Amato et al., 2019; Ganeshan et al., 2019) (Figure 4.9).

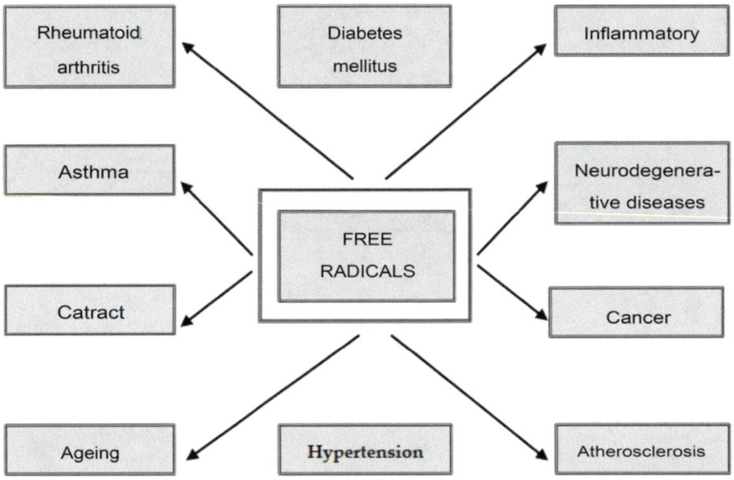

Figure 4.9. Free radicals and diseases.

Source: https://www.mdpi.com/oxygen/oxygen-02-00006/article_deploy/html/images/oxygen-02-00006-g003.png.

4.2.3. Aging and Free Radical Damage

Aging is closely connected with the active process of the fight between free radicals and antioxidants in the body. Free radicals are very reactive molecules produced as byproducts of cellular metabolism that can produce widespread damage to cells by attacking a variety of biomolecules, such as lipids, proteins, and DNA. With aging, the effectiveness of the antioxidant defense systems of the body is likely to decline and this leads to a high occurrence of oxidative stress. This is one of the causes of degenerative processes in aging, because the free radicals cause damage that accumulates with time. Various studies suggest that the accumulation of such oxidative damage is implicated in age-related diseases , such as Alzheimer's and cardiovascular ailments, highlighting the critical role of free radicals in the aging continuum (Akbari et al., 2022). In addition, interactions between the environment and the generation of free radicals enhance the process of aging. UV radiation and pollutants are exogenous factors that may increase the levels of free radicals and worsen the situation with oxidative stress. For instance, research has indicated that exposure to carbon tetrachloride, a known hepatotoxic agent, can lead to extensive oxidative damage through the generation of toxic free radicals, resulting in conditions like liver cirrhosis and other systemic complications (Velid et al., 2020). The subsequent oxidative stress catalyzes cellular senescence, inflammation, and apoptosis and thus facilitates the deterioration of physiological functions with age. Therefore, a strong perception of the role of environmental factors in the formation of free radicals is critical in the establishment of ways of reducing their adverse effects on aging. As a follow-up to the challenges of free radicals, the increase in antioxidant intake can be considered a proactive strategy to counteract the oxidative damage and even extend healthy lifespan. Antioxidants are important in counteracting the free radicals and hence preventing the damage of cells and the homeostasis. Fruits and vegetables contain natural antioxidants that have shown a great deal of anti-aging effects due to their capability of counteracting oxidative stress. In addition, inclusion of these natural compounds in the diet is linked with decreased incidence of chronic diseases that are prevalent among elderly people. As aging individuals are advised to enhance their antioxidant-rich food consumption, they may experience a slowdown in the progression of age-related diseases and an improvement in overall well-being, underscoring the importance of adopting dietary measures as part of aging management strategies (Akbari et al., 2022) (Figure 4.10).

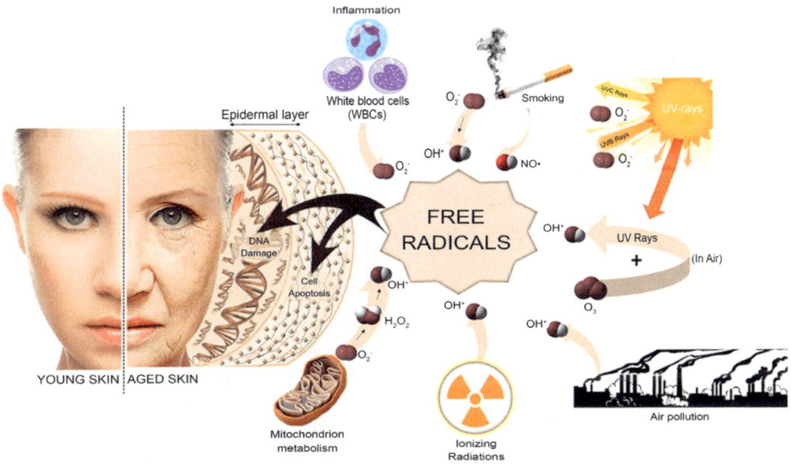

Figure 4.10. Illustration of different factors responsible for free radical generation resulting in aging.

Source: https://www.researchgate.net/publication/361734785/figure/fig1/AS:1143128109739 1457@1668567035522/Illustration-of-different-factors-responsible-for-free-radical-generation-resulting-in.png.

Test Your Knowledge

1. What is oxidative stress?
2. What is the relationship between free radicals and chronic diseases?

4.3. Antioxidants: Nature's Defense

Learning Outcome

1. Define the antioxidants;
2. Describe the sources of antioxidants in diet;
3. Know the mechanisms of action of antioxidants.

Antioxidants form a vital part of the intricate relationship between oxidative stress and cellular health as the defense mechanism provided by nature. Free radicals, particularly ROS and RNS, are generated as by-products of various metabolic processes, including mitochondrial respiration. When the production of free radicals and antioxidant defense systems is not in balance, as occurs under oxidative stress conditions like heat stress in animals, cellular damage can result. It has been shown that the buildup of free radicals is a major factor that causes several pathologies through the oxidation of vital macromolecules , such as DNA, lipids and proteins, thereby affecting the functioning of the cells. Understanding the mechanisms through which antioxidants mitigate these effects is crucial for developing interventions that support cellular integrity and health, an area that warrants further scientific exploration (Aryal et al., 2025). There are several major categories of antioxidants: enzymatic and non-enzymatic. Enzymatic antioxidants include SOD and catalase, which catalyze reactions to neutralize free radicals and thereby minimize oxidative damage. Conversely, non-enzymatic antioxidants, including vitamins C and E, phytochemicals, e.g., polyphenols and flavonoids, and other dietary constituents, also help in the defense of the body by directly scavenging free radicals. These compounds are increasingly recognized for their therapeutic potential in preventing chronic diseases linked to oxidative stress, including CVDs and diabetes (Allison et al., 2025). The emerging popularity of herbal medicine signifies the need to introduce antioxidant-rich herbs into the dietary routine as a natural means of health promotion and prevention of various diseases. The importance of antioxidants is not limited to personal health only, as they could also contribute to longevity and wellness. Modern scientific literature on this topic underlines the necessity of more detailed studies in order to assess the synergistic action of different foods and herbs rich in antioxidants to develop effective preventive measures in the development of oxidative stress-related diseases. These studies not only concentrate on the molecular action of antioxidants but also find out how eating habits that involve the use of these defensive compounds can lead to better health prospects. Through the incorporation of antioxidants as a basic element of preventive healthcare, society can harness the natural potential of counteracting oxidative stress and reduce the threat of developing chronic illnesses. Emphasizing a holistic approach that includes a diverse range of antioxidant sources will not only enhance individual health but also promote a sustainable lifestyle aligned with natural defense mechanisms (Allison et al., 2025) (Figure 4.11).

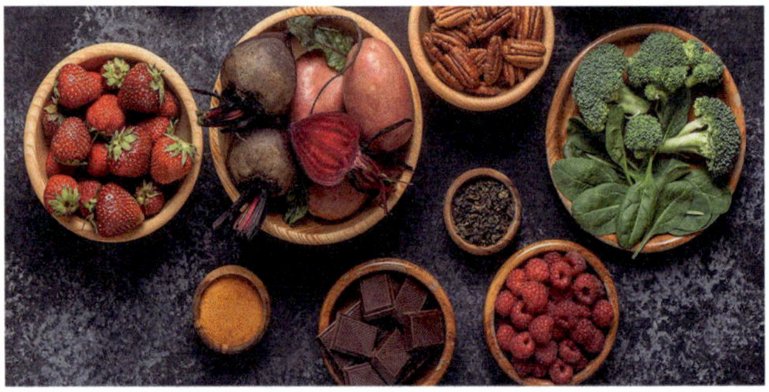

Figure 4.11. Antioxidant foods: The power of nature's defense.

Source: https://skinjournal.co.uk/wp-content/uploads/2023/05/Antioxidant-Foods-The-Power-of-Natures-Defence.jpg.

4.3.1. Definition and Types of Antioxidants

Antioxidants are compounds that play a critical role in countering the destructive effects of free radicals in the body. Free radicals are reactive molecules with loose electrons that are capable of causing oxidative stress, resulting in cell, protein, and DNA destruction. Oxidative damage has been associated with chronic diseases like cancer, CVDs, and neurodegenerative disorders. Antioxidants neutralize free radicals by donating electrons, hence stabilizing the reactive species and preventing cell damage. Some of the numerous categories of antioxidants are produced endogenously in the body, such as GSH and SOD enzymes. Others, however, must be obtained from diet, and this highlights the influence lifestyle has on promoting health and preventing disease. Among dietary antioxidants, the polyphenols are a significant class, which, with their antioxidant activity, exhibit a broad array of health benefits. Fruits, vegetables, tea, and wine are typical sources of polyphenols, and specific fruits like *Aronia melanocarpa* are noted for their tremendously high antioxidant activity. Research shows that the dietary content of antioxidants can effectively neutralize oxidative stress to a great extent. For instance, studies have found that Aronia juice reduces bladder cancer cell viability due to its high content of total polyphenols, thereby demonstrating the potential of dietary antioxidants in cancer prevention (Nowak et al., 2025). Similarly, other polyphenol sources contribute to overall well-being by their potential to defend against free radicals, which emphasizes the importance of an evenly balanced diet with the same bioactive components. Another antioxidant class that is widely recognized is vitamins and minerals, which function as enzyme reaction co-factors in combating oxidative stress. Vitamins A, C, and E are classic antioxidants that, in addition to stabilizing free radicals, also regenerate antioxidants, giving a chain of protection against oxidative stress. An example is vitamin C being vital in killing ROS, while vitamin E protects cell membranes from lipid peroxidation. For this purpose, mineral antioxidants , such as zinc and selenium aid in the operation of antioxidant enzymes. Therefore, their inclusion in food is vital to provide strong antioxidant defense (Djabali et al., 2024). Overall, the various types of antioxidants highlight the multifaceted approach required to reverse oxidative damage and help one stay healthy (Figure 4.12).

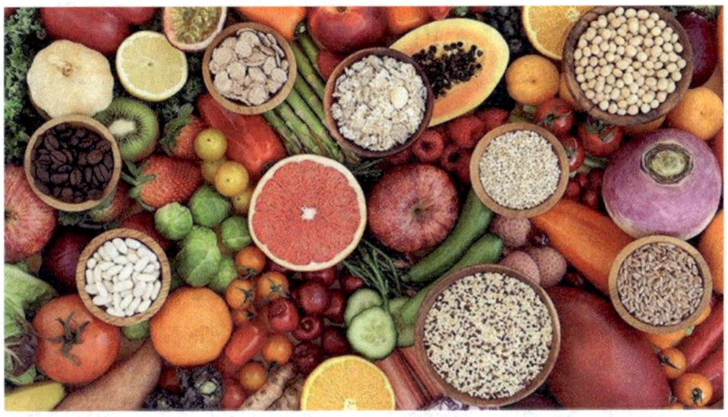

Figure 4.12. Antioxidants, which can be found in some foods, can fight damage caused by some free radicals.

Source: https://www.mdanderson.org/content/mda/en/cancerwise/2024/08/what-are-free-radicals-a-dietitian-explains/jcr:content/blog/adaptiveimage.resize.jpg.

4.3.2. Sources of Antioxidants in Diet

These important elements of a balanced diet are abundantly present in different food sources that may have a great effect on the human body. These compounds are especially abundant in fruits and vegetables, and they are essential in counteracting free radicals and reducing oxidative stress. Of these, berries, including blueberries and strawberries, have been of interest because of their anthocyanin content, a flavonoid with strong antioxidant activity. Moreover, green leafy vegetables, such as spinach and kale, have a strong antioxidant capacity, as it is confirmed by the studies that have used the DPPH assay to test the free radical scavenging activity of these vegetables. The incorporation of such nutrient-dense foods into one's diet can provide essential protection against chronic diseases, emphasizing the importance of dietary choices in promoting overall health and well-being as stated in the exploration of vegetable antioxidant activity in previous studies (Jahan et al., 2024). Other foods that contain antioxidants besides fruits and vegetables have a great potential to improve health. Walnuts and sunflower seeds are good examples of nuts and seeds that contain vitamin E and selenium, which add to the antioxidant capacity of nuts and seeds. Moreover, phenolic compounds with a great antioxidant capacity are found in whole grains , such as oats and barley. Herbs and spices, such as turmeric and cinnamon, also stand out due to the high content of antioxidants, which in many cases exceed the content in the traditional food products. Such varied sources of antioxidants not only contribute to the flavor but also have protective value against free radicals' harmful effects. As the research continues to unveil the connections between dietary antioxidants and health outcomes, it becomes increasingly essential to recognize and incorporate these foods into daily diets to harness their health-promoting properties (Cîrțînă et al., 2024). The relationship between foods with high antioxidant content and health effects is supported by the possibility that these substances to affect the prevention of chronic diseases and increase life span. Dietary antioxidants are important in the body because their regular intake could help in the enhancement of immune activity and lowering of inflammation, which are essential in countering several chronic diseases. Scientific investigations, such as those utilizing the DPPH assay, have illustrated the profound capacity of certain vegetables to protect against oxidative stress, thereby supporting the notion that a diet rich in antioxidants can confer health benefits (Jahan et al., 2024). Additionally, the synergistic action of diverse sources of antioxidants can improve the overall quality and resistance of the diet, which is essential under the conditions of the contemporary lifestyle. As research progresses, identifying and optimizing the inclusion of diverse antioxidant-rich foods in dietary patterns can foster a more comprehensive understanding of their role in enhancing health and combating degenerative diseases (Cîrțînă et al., 2024) (Figure 4.13).

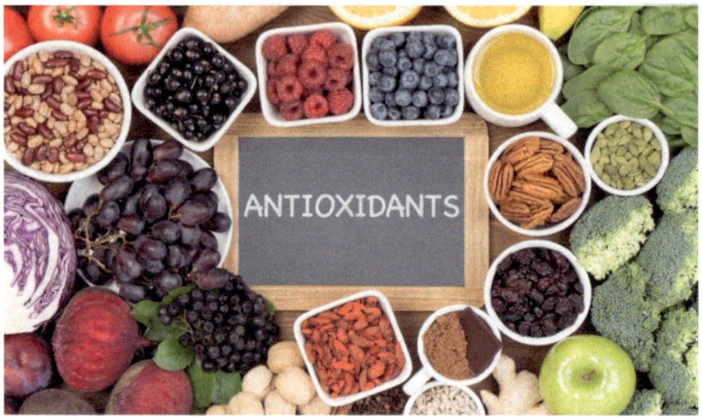

Figure 4.13. Sources of antioxidants.

Source: https://www.fitpaa.com/wp-content/uploads/2023/06/Untitled-design-2023-06-28T182737.452.jpg.

4.3.3. Mechanisms of Action of Antioxidants

Antioxidants are important in countering oxidative stress in biological systems, mainly because of their mechanisms of action, which entail neutralization of free radicals. Antioxidants can donate electrons to free radicals and make them stable, eventually stopping the chain of cell destruction that occurs due to oxidative reactions. Such stabilization results in fewer reactive species, which reduces further oxidative damage to lipids, proteins, and DNA. Natural antioxidants like vitamins C and E and other phytochemicals act by intercepting the free radicals and neutralizing them, thus making them harmless. Moreover, the flavonoids are representatives of a class of antioxidants that actively scavenge free radicals, which implies their possible therapeutic applications in a variety of diseases with oxidative stress. This kind of efficacy highlights the need to incorporate these bioactive compounds in nutritional thinking and treatment plans, in order to boost antioxidant defenses in the body. The protective mechanisms by which antioxidants exert their action are not only restricted to scavenging of the reactive species, but also by regulating the oxidative stress-related signaling pathways. There are a number of antioxidants that have been found to regulate the expression and activity of endogenous antioxidant enzymes, e.g., SOD and GSH peroxidase. This enzymatic regulation increases the inherent capability of the body to oppose oxidative stress. The best example of such dual action is natural polyphenols, which are abundant in fruits and vegetables, and which not only neutralize free radicals but also stimulate the defense systems of the cell. Here, the antioxidant ability of polyphenols is important, since these may regulate the expression of genes involved in response to oxidative stress. Therefore, it is clear that the numerous actions of antioxidants, both direct scavenging and indirect regulation of oxidative stress signaling, provide insight into their important contribution to cellular homeostasis and health. The discussion of the mechanisms of antioxidant action requires a concentration on certain groups of compounds, especially polyphenols, which have various bioactive properties. Polyphenols (flavonoids and phenolic acids) have been of interest due to their remarkable antioxidant activity, defined by free radical scavenging activity and induction of endogenous defenses. The biochemical details behind these activities are complex molecular interactions, in which polyphenols may serve as hydrogen atoms or electron donors to free radicals, generating stable final products and inhibiting cell damage. Current studies have conducted a systematic review of the antioxidant action of different polyphenolic compounds, which have shown a possibility of reducing the consequences of oxidative stress. Such insights contribute to the ongoing exploration of natural antioxidants as favorable alternatives to synthetic options, reinforcing the role of plant-derived compounds in health promotion and disease prevention, as emphasized in recent literature (Qi-Zhuang et al., 2021; Tumilaar et al., 2024).

Test Your Knowledge

1. What are the three types of antioxidants?
2. What is the main source of antioxidants in the diet?

4.4. The Role of Antioxidants in Disease Prevention

Learning Outcome

1. Describe the antioxidants in cardiovascular health;
2. Understand the role of antioxidants in cancer prevention;
3. Know the antioxidants and neurodegenerative diseases.

Prevention of chronic diseases through the application of antioxidants has been an area of interest in the scientific community. Antioxidants, due to their ability to scavenge free radicals, are essential in preventing oxidative stress that contributes to the onset of most diseases. These substances are derived from a variety of sources of food sources, from fruits and vegetables to nuts and whole foods, highlighting the importance of healthy eating in maintaining health. For instance, studies illustrate how antioxidants not only protect cell integrity but also ensure the body's immune system, thereby strengthening the body against disease. In addition, the summative health benefit of these substances extends beyond protection of the cell, indeed even slowing the aging process itself, and this underscores the need for adequate antioxidant intake in the everyday diet, as indicated by extensive literature evidence (Daniela et al., 2024). The relationship between free radicals, chronic inflammation, and disease worsening is well documented. Especially, the role of ROS in inducing inflammatory cascades can lead to the development of conditions , such as CVD and metabolic syndrome. It is crucial that this correlation be identified because oxidative damage induced by free radicals leads to cell malfunction and tissue injury. High antioxidant availability would be required to reverse these harmful effects. For example, recent research on periodontal health has shown that antioxidants can enhance tissue damage induced by ROS of disease-promoting bacteria in dental plaque. The findings suggest the therapeutic potential of antioxidants not just in systemic illness but also for localized diseases, such as periodontitis, suggesting the importance of further exploring their application in the clinic to enhance patient success (Seth, 2021). Furthermore, the use of diet strategies high in antioxidants could also be a preventive method for long-term diseases. Encouraging the consumption of various antioxidant foods has the potential to enable people to take active steps toward strengthening their overall health status. Apart from motivating antioxidant use, these modifications can also enhance overall gains in health, such as improved nutrient absorption and metabolism. Public health initiatives directed towards enlightening individuals about the importance of antioxidants are particularly significant, as they can directly function to reduce the prevalence of diseases caused by oxidative stress. Additionally, the application of antioxidants in disease therapy regimens is a promising area for enhancing therapeutic efficiency. The ongoing research on the mechanisms of action of dietary antioxidants reaffirms their vital role in disease prevention and underscores the importance of recognition of the advantages of their health benefits (Daniela et al., 2024) (Figure 4.14).

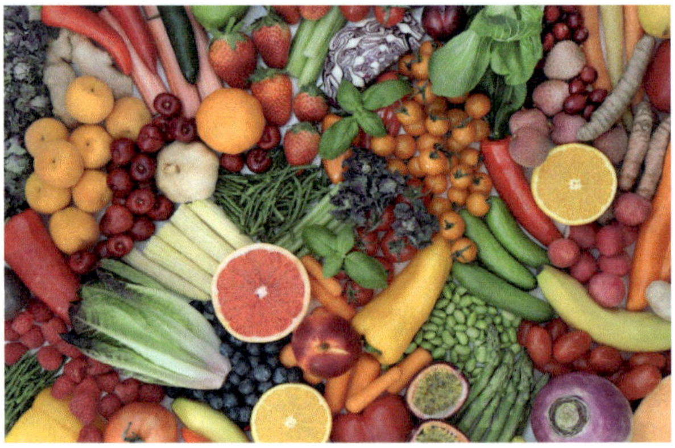

Figure 4.14. The role of antioxidants in disease prevention.

Source: https://umedoc.com/wp-content/uploads/2024/07/AdobeStock_404223776.jpeg.

4.4.1. Antioxidants and Cardiovascular Health

Interactions between antioxidants and CVD are a vital field of research considering the toxic effects of free radicals on the cardiovascular system. Free radicals, a group of highly reactive ROS, are the culprits behind oxidative stress that causes the endothelial cell lining of blood vessels to degenerate, culminating in atherosclerosis and heart disease. Antioxidants serve as a defense mechanism against oxidative stress by removing free radicals. The capacity of dietary antioxidants , such as vitamins C and E, flavonoids, and carotenoids, to lower cardiovascular risk has prompted widespread investigation of their mechanisms of action and efficacy *in vivo*. Nevertheless, it is crucial to appreciate that the availability of antioxidants in the diet does not necessarily equate to their presence in tissues at concentrations that are adequate to provide protective effects, since absorption and metabolism have considerable bearing on their effectiveness (Gordon, 2011). The contribution of dietary sources of antioxidants cannot be overemphasized, especially when considering cardiovascular outcomes of health. Fruits and vegetables, being rich in vitamins, minerals, and phytochemicals, abound with high antioxidant power. For example, the carotenoids found in colored vegetables like kale have shown strong antioxidative activity, which supports cardiovascular well-being through an anti-oxidant potential to oxidants. However, the daily consumption of fruits and vegetables is typically not achieved; thus, dietary supplements become a likely option. These supplements can enhance the uptake of beneficial antioxidants, making it convenient for individuals to meet their dietary needs within a controlled setting. Research has indicated that carotenoid-type supplements can enhance skin and possibly heart health, highlighting the importance of incorporating antioxidants in diets to promote overall well-being (GrayElpelt et al., 2019). Despite the promising links between antioxidants and cardiovascular health, there are some factors that complicate comprehending their effectiveness. An essential area of consideration is the bioavailability of antioxidants, which may vary greatly between individuals due to differences in metabolism as well as nutrient absorption. Also, the mode of action of antioxidants may extend beyond such rudimentary free radical scavenging as might be quantified using laboratory analysis, to involve modifications of cell signaling pathways and alterations of gene expression. This is why additional studies are required to assist with elucidation of the optimal type and amount of antioxidants for cardiac health. While consumption of a wide range of foods with antioxidants is definitely desirable, there are more studies to be done in order to develop precise guidelines that would realistically utilize dietary antioxidants' potential for the upkeep of cardiovascular health (Gordon, 2011) (Figure 4.15).

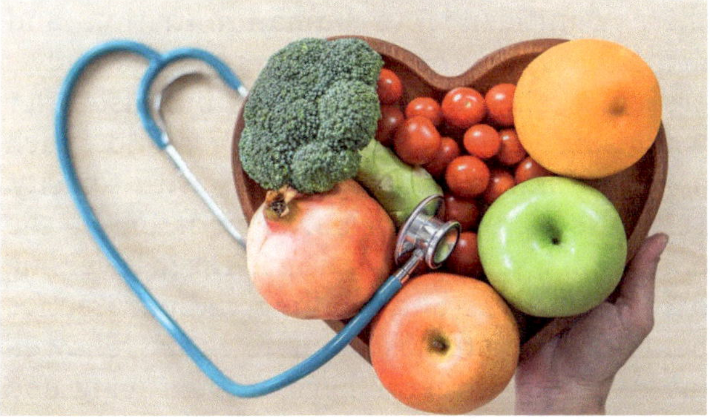

Figure 4.15. Antioxidants may help cardiovascular health.

Source: https://www.wholehealthweb.com/wp-content/uploads/2017/10/heart-2-1080x640.jpg.

4.4.2. Antioxidants in Cancer Prevention

The antioxidant function in cancer prevention becomes increasingly appreciated as being the top priority, particularly in the context of free radical-induced damage involved in cancer initiation and growth. Antioxidants remove such toxic compounds, thus lowering oxidative stress that may result in cell damage and cancer formation. Among the many natural antioxidants, certain polyphenols have emerged as being among the most significant in this context. Research has shown that these compounds, like mangiferin, found in *Mangifera indica*, exhibit robust antioxidant activity that reduces oxygen-free radical levels. Not only does this reduce DNA damage, but it also regulates key inflammatory pathways commonly overexpressed in cancer cells, thus halting the disease process. The study of such compounds highlights the importance of ongoing research into their chemopreventive activity in human health (Khurana et al., 2016). In addition to polyphenols, many herbs and plants have also been tested for antioxidant activity and for cancer preventive potential. Traditional medicine illustrates the utilization of such natural compounds over time, highlighting their significance to human nutrition and health. They not only contribute to the body's arsenal against oxidative stress but also offer wholesome benefits that drugs may not, such as fewer side effects and issues with toxicity. Scientific literature has borne testimony to the efficacy of a variety of natural herbs in reversing oxidative stress and yielding radioprotective benefits. The studies point towards renewed interest among researchers in identifying and verifying the mechanisms by which these plant sources can yield cancer-preventive benefits. The multidisciplinary research involving botanists, pharmacologists, and molecular biologists optimizes the scientific knowledge of the natural products and opens the way to their use for cancer prevention (Choong et al., 2014). Nevertheless, although the effectiveness of antioxidants for cancer prevention is suggested by a variety of studies, more research is still needed in order to gain a full understanding of their mechanisms and the optimal use in clinical trials. The sophistication of the biology of cancer and various reactions to antioxidant treatment across populations requires a more advanced approach. Researchers must strive to comprehend the various molecular pathways through which antioxidants exert their effects and engage with other therapeutic modes. Comparative clinical trials of the effectiveness of various antioxidants should be a high priority, as well as research into optimal dosing and interactive effects with other food components. These efforts will be crucial in closing the gap between theoretical concepts and actual implementation of such natural compounds in oncology, eventually in the advancement of preventive interventions and in patient outcomes with an increased value for antioxidants in cancer prevention (Khurana et al., 2016) (Figure 4.16).

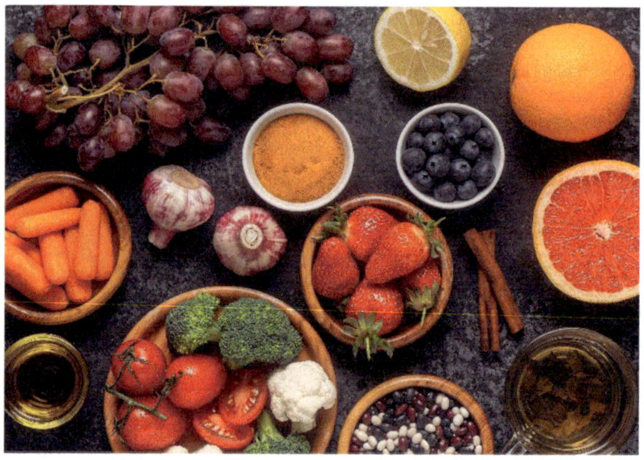

Figure 4.16. The role of antioxidants in cancer prevention.

Source: https://images.squarespace-cdn.com/content/v1/59f0e6beace8641044d76e9c/1697214925327-8727YAV278M7P8SHU4U5/Social+Antioxidants.jpg.

4.4.3. Antioxidants and Neurodegenerative Diseases

The relationship between free radicals and neurodegenerative disorders, and particularly that of antioxidants, has drawn special scientific interest due to its public health relevance. Neurodegenerative disorders , such as Alzheimer's disease, have been characterized by progressive neuronal impairment and loss of integrity, leading to extreme cognitive and functional impairments. Oxidative stress due to a discrepancy between the production of free radicals and antioxidant defenses is the pathophysiology of these diseases. Research has found that heightened oxidative stress can hasten the damage to neurons, causing the escalation of neurodegenerative diseases. As a natural defense strategy, antioxidants can neutralize free radicals, thereby preventing cellular damage and slowing down the disease process. Understanding the mechanisms of antioxidants in combat against oxidative stress is crucial for designing prevention measures and therapies for neurodegenerative illnesses. Gallic acid is a related antioxidant that shows much potential for therapy against neurodegenerative diseases like Alzheimer's. The phenolic acid, contained in numerous plant food sources, possesses potent antioxidant activities that can reverse oxidative stress as well as its deleterious effects on neuronal cells. Studies have demonstrated the potential for gallic acid to prevent Alzheimer's disease progression through the inhibition or suppression of free radical-induced damage. The study emphasizes the need for further research into the specific interactions of gallic acid and neurodegenerative pathways, with current literature reflecting scant understanding of its mechanism, given favorable outcomes. Through additional research in this area, researchers might find new means of tapping into the beneficial effects of gallic acid, ultimately creating new avenues of therapy for Alzheimer's disease treatment. The complex interaction between oxidative stress and neurodegenerative diseases also indicates the multifaceted role of antioxidants in promoting neurological health. As discussed in the literature, there are multiple causes of oxidative stress, including unhealthy lifestyles and environmental causes, which lead to the degradation of cognitive abilities and the development of chronic diseases, including neurodegenerative diseases (Kumari, 2023). Antioxidants from a rich diversity of natural products, particularly medicinal plants, play a vital role in reversing the effects of oxidative damage. These molecules, such as flavonoids and phenolics, are instrumental in maintaining cellular integrity and enhancing resistance of the body to stress-related damage. Thus, they not only contribute to the treatment of neurodegenerative disorders but are also supportive in treating an abundance of other chronic conditions. As the demand for effective treatments grows, ongoing studies on natural antioxidants can lead to spectacular advances in understanding and treating neurodegenerative disorders (Figure 4.17).

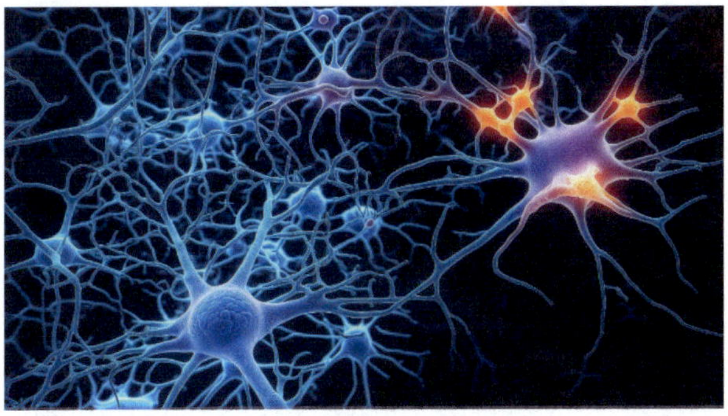

Figure 4.17. Illustration of neural networks with activated neurons, representing neurodegenerative processes.

Source: https://taurx.com/images/Neurodegenerative-disorders.jpg.

Test Your Knowledge

1. What is the role of antioxidants in cardiovascular disease?
2. What is the role of antioxidants in cancer prevention?

SUMMARY

Briefly, the intricate interaction between free radicals and antioxidants has far-reaching consequences for disease and the management of health. Free radicals, which are reactive molecules found naturally, have the capacity to cause oxidative stress and play a significant role in the etiopathogenesis of several diseases, including cancer, CVDs, and neurodegenerative diseases. The continuous formation and accumulation of these free radicals overwhelm the body's natural defense mechanisms, leading to cell damage. This highlights the need for antioxidant consumption, which can offset free radicals, achieve equilibrium, and diminish oxidative stress. Antioxidants are naturally found as phenolic compounds in other therapeutic plants and perform vital protective roles at the molecular level, highlighting the role of these agents in prevention protocols. Research on various plant antioxidants has provided insight into the effectiveness of these plant antioxidants in oxidative stress prevention. A prominent example is Moringa oleifera, a plant that has been studied in-depth for the high levels of phenolics and flavonoids it contains, and which are renowned for their antioxidant activity. Research has shown that Moringa oleifera extracts exhibit high antioxidant activity, as shown by their efficiency in scavenging free radicals. Such research supports the efficacy of incorporating such natural sources into diets in order to promote health and fight diseases related to oxidative stress. These findings reinforce the proposal that the use of plant-based antioxidants may represent a key strategy towards the promotion of general health and the prevention of chronic diseases and hence public health initiatives. Moreover, the role of dietary habits in the context of oxidative stress cannot be overstated. The consumption of high-lipid diets has been linked to the generation of free radicals, leading to a cascade of adverse health effects, including hyperlipidemia and tissue damage. The results of current studies on the effects of the impact of these diets highlight a key trend in which detrimental food intake drives chronic inflammation and oxidative damage. Through approaches in the diet and promoting the intake of more healthful foods, these dangers can be reduced and the antioxidant effects used against free radical harm. With this in mind, existing research and public health efforts should remain focused on efforts to learn about and promote antioxidant-rich diets as a fundamental approach to health improvement and disease prevention.

Free radicals are highly reactive molecules with one or more free electrons and are a part of many biochemical reactions in the body. Free radicals are generated as a natural consequence of metabolic processes, interaction with the environment, and even exercise. Free radicals do, however, induce oxidative stress if produced in large numbers, and this would irreversibly harm cells, proteins, and DNA. This oxidative free radical damage is implicated in many diseases, including cancer, CVDs, and neurodegenerative diseases. Shedding light on the balance between free radical production and the body's reactions becomes essential for formulating therapeutic strategies to overcome oxidative stress. In addition, free radical regulation offers avenues for the creation of new treatments as researchers discover new ways to right this balance and uphold cellular integrity. Antioxidants, compounds that eliminate free radicals, play an essential role in maintaining cellular health and preventing oxidative stress. They act by donating electrons to free radicals and thus stabilizing them, preventing biological structures from damage. Antioxidants can be either endogenous, which are body-synthesized naturally, or exogenous, which are obtained from foods , such as fruits, vegetables, and other supplements. Polyphenols, for example, are important antioxidants that are widely recognized to have the capability of modulating inflammatory pathways and enhancing the immune system. Recent research identifies their multi-faceted modes of action, which include inhibiting pro-inflammatory cytokines as well as modulation of gene expression pathways against oxidative stress (Yahfoufi et al., 2018). Their interactions demonstrate the importance of a nutrient-rich diet with high levels of antioxidants as a protective measure against chronic diseases related to oxidative injury. The equilibrium between antioxidants and free radicals is increasingly recognized to be at the heart of health and disease considerations. The novel concept of ferroptosis, a unique iron-dependent form of programmed cell death that is connected to lipid peroxidation, is emblematic of the complex chemistry involved in oxidative processes (Li et al., 2020). This process not only underscores the pathogenicity of uncontrolled free radical activity but also the potential therapeutic benefit of ferroptosis inhibition in disease management. As the investigation further pursues the distinctive molecular events underlying ferroptosis and how this is related to pathologies, it can be seen that manipulation of this process holds the promise to bring about novel therapeutic avenues. In this context, it is important to differentiate the roles of both free radicals and antioxidants to devise comprehensive methods to prevent and treat oxidative stress-induced and inflammation-related diseases.

KEY TERMS FROM THIS CHAPTER

- Antioxidants
- Cancer
- Chronic diseases
- Free radicals
- Hydrogen peroxide
- Neurodegenerative disorders
- Stress exposure
- Superoxide dismutase
- Biological systems
- Cardiovascular disorders
- Environmental stressors
- Glutathione peroxidase
- Hydroxyl radicals
- Pollution
- Superoxide anions

CRITICAL THINKING QUESTIONS

1. **What are free radicals?**
   a. Molecules that contain oxygen
   b. Molecules with an unpaired electron
   c. Antioxidant molecules
   d. Molecules rich in hydrogen
2. **Which of the following is an example of a reactive oxygen species (ROS)?**
   a. Superoxide anion (O_2^-)
   b. Carbon dioxide (CO_2)
   c. Nitric oxide (NO)
   d. Oxygen (O_2)
3. **What is the primary function of antioxidants in the body?**
   a. To repair DNA damage
   b. To neutralize free radicals
   c. To produce ATP
   d. To act as enzymes
4. **Which of the following vitamins acts as a major antioxidant?**
   a. Vitamin B12
   b. Vitamin C
   c. Vitamin D
   d. Vitamin K
5. **Which enzyme is responsible for converting superoxide radicals into hydrogen peroxide?**
   a. Catalase
   b. Superoxide dismutase (SOD)
   c. Glutathione peroxidase
   d. Peroxidase

Short Answer Questions

1. Define the free radicals.
2. How many types of free radicals are there?
3. What is the role of free radicals in the human body?
4. What are antioxidants?
5. What is the role of antioxidants in disease prevention?

Answers to Critical Thinking Questions

1. (b); 2. (a); 3. (b); 4. (b); 5. (b)

REFERENCES

1. Khurana, R. K., Kaur, R., Lohan, S., Singh, K. K., & Singh, B. (2016). Mangiferin: a promising anticancer bioactive. *Pharmaceutical patent analyst, 5*(3), 169–181. https://doi.org/10.4155/ppa-2016-0003 (accessed on 12th June 2025).
2. Adji, R. P. (2025). Explores effectivities Asam Galat Sebagian neuroprotective Dallam megabat phenakite Alzheimer: Literature review. *Journal Cakra Wala Academica*. https://www.semanticscholar.org/paper/0804430bca7d10e3fe7a47b80b9d243f970800ce (accessed on 12th June 2025).
3. Akbari, B., Baghaei-Yazdi, N., Bahmaie, M., & Mahdavi Abhari, F. (2022). The role of plant-derived natural antioxidants in reduction of oxidative stress. *Bio Factors, 48*, 611–633. https://doi.org/10.1002/biof.1831 (accessed on 12th June 2025).
4. Akhmedzhanova, A., Ponomarev, S. V., Fedorovykh, Y., Levina, O., & Terganova, N. (2023). The results of tilapia juveniles growing on production compound feeds with the antioxidant astaxanthin addition. *Vatnik of Astrakhan State Technical University. Series: Fishing Industry*. https://www.semanticscholar.org/paper/6ec652bda72e0f1d610e933272fed94e253e4009 (accessed on 12th June 2025).
5. Allison, M. O., Ukor, V. C., Ibrahim, Y. A., & Adeyemo, J. A. (2025). Leveraging natural antioxidants in disease prevention: Investigating the role of medicinal herbs in reducing oxidative stress and chronic disease. *World Journal of Advanced Research and Reviews*. https://www.semanticscholar.org/paper/c5a80c994607aca1f7783033643782cc6387dbaf (accessed on 12th June 2025).
6. Marrocco, I., Altieri, F., & Peluso, I. (2017). Measurement and Clinical Significance of Biomarkers of Oxidative Stress in Humans. *Oxidative medicine and cellular longevity, 2017*, 6501046. https://doi.org/10.1155/2017/6501046(accessed on 12th June 2025).
7. Altunkaya, A. (2014). Potential antioxidant activity of pomegranate peel and seed extracts and synergism with added phenolic antioxidants in a liposome system: A preliminary study. https://core.ac.uk/download/45656515.pdf (accessed on 12th June 2025).
8. Amato, A., Terzo, S., & Mulè, F. (2019). Natural Compounds as Beneficial Antioxidant Agents in Neurodegenerative Disorders: A Focus on Alzheimer's Disease. *Antioxidants (Basel, Switzerland), 8*(12), 608. https://doi.org/10.3390/antiox8120608 (accessed on 12th June 2025).
9. Aryal, B., Kwakye, J., Ariyo, O., Ghareeb, A. F. A., Milfort, M., Fuller, A., Khatiwada, S., et al. (2025). Major oxidative and antioxidant mechanisms during heat stress-induced oxidative stress in chickens. *Antioxidants, 14*. https://www.semanticscholar.org/paper/48f4171b2837a8f7e9cb9117b82db4f33dcf809b (accessed on 12th June 2025).
10. Banerjee, A., Das, D., Paul, R., Roy, S., Bhattacharjee, A., Prasad, S., Banerjee, O., et al. (2020). Altered composition of high-lipid diet may generate reactive oxygen species by disturbing the balance of antioxidant and free radicals. *Journal of Basic and Clinical Physiology and Pharmacology, 31*. https://www.semanticscholar.org/paper/bafe8273c2f689a7c9284380c654fdb80c2aec12 (accessed on 12th June 2025).
11. Cerretani, D., Di Paolo, M., Fineschi, V., Neri, M., Pomara, C., Riezzo, I., & Turillazzi, E. (2015). Cardiac oxidative stress and inflammatory cytokines response after myocardial infarction. https://core.ac.uk/download/54248089.pdf (accessed on 12th June 2025).

12. Chandimali, N., Bak, S., Park, E. H., Lim, H. J., Won, Y. S., Kim, E. K., Park, S. I., et al. (2025). Free radicals and their impact on health and antioxidant defenses: A review. *Cell Death Discovery, 11*. https://www.semanticscholar.org/paper/c285fc80b510073c35181621bac0d5ce5c5e90b3 (accessed on 12th June 2025).

13. Gray, P., Chappell, A., Jenkinson, A. M., Thies, F., & Gray, S. R. (2014). Fish oil supplementation reduces markers of oxidative stress but not muscle soreness after eccentric exercise. *International journal of sport nutrition and exercise metabolism, 24*(2), 206–214. https://doi.org/10.1123/ijsnem.2013-0081 (accessed on 12th June 2025).

14. Che, X., Qi, X., Xu, Y., Wang, Q., & Wu, G. (2021). Using genomic and transcriptome analyses to identify the role of the oxidative stress pathway in renal clear cell carcinoma and its potential therapeutic significance. *Oxidative Medicine and Cellular Longevity, 2021*. https://www.semanticscholar.org/paper/39717220ab4666d01b2a20284aaabcdd07112117 (accessed on 12th June 2025).

15. Choong, Y. S., Deivanai, S., Lachumy, S. J., et al. (2014). Herbal remedies for combating irradiation: A green antiradiation approach. https://core.ac.uk/download/30437851.pdf (accessed on 12th June 2025).

16. Cîrţînă, D., & Popa, R. G. (2024). Study on natural antioxidants: Sources, mechanisms of action and health benefits. *Journal of Research and Innovation for Sustainable Society*. https://www.semanticscholar.org/paper/50ece7f3a5c60c825c8cb5be26910c43c310e6ea (accessed on 12th June 2025).

17. Elpelt A, Lohan SB, Darvin ME, et al. Carotenoids – Effective Radical Scavengers for Healthy and Beautiful Skin. Health Education and Public Health. 2019: 2:4. (accessed on 12th June 2025).

18. David, J. A., Rifkin, W. J., Rabbani, P. S., & Ceradini, D. J. (2017). The Nrf2/Keap1/ARE pathway and oxidative stress as a therapeutic target in type II diabetes mellitus. *Journal of Diabetes Research, 2017*, 1–15. https://doi.org/10.1155/2017/4826724 (accessed on 12th June 2025).

19. Dhalaria, R., Verma, R., Kumar, D., Puri, S., Tapwal, A., Kumar, V., Nepovimová, E., et al. (2020). Bioactive compounds of edible fruits with their anti-aging properties: A comprehensive review to prolong human life. *Antioxidants, 9*, 1123–1123. https://doi.org/10.3390/antiox9111123 (accessed on 12th June 2025).

20. Dias, M. C., Pinto, D. C. G. A., & Silva, A. M. S. (2021). Plant flavonoids: Chemical characteristics and biological activity. *Molecules, 26*, 5377–5377. https://doi.org/10.3390/molecules26175377 (accessed on 12th June 2025).

21. Djabali, S., Barkat, M., Sabba, E., Boussouf, L., Chelaghema, Z., & Haif, N. (2024). Physicochemical analysis and antioxidant benefits of yogurt enriched with betalains from red beet (*Beta vulgaris* L.). *Carpathian Journal of Food Science and Technology*. https://www.semanticscholar.org/paper/e01ea07014ae50bad5142dbf04f08fd442c63aad (accessed on 12th June 2025).

22. Ganeshan, T. K. (2019). Investigating the protective role of the natural hormone melatonin in reducing drug-induced cardiotoxicity in the therapy of chronic diseases. https://core.ac.uk/download/287605215.pdf (accessed on 12th June 2025).

23. Gordon, M. (2011). Significance of dietary antioxidants for health. https://core.ac.uk/download/360108.pdf (accessed on 12th June 2025).

24. Jahan, I., Padhi, A., Sharma, V., Yadav, S., Jyoti, J., & Gupta, V. K. (2024). Quantitative estimation of antioxidant activity in various vegetables by DPPH method. *International Journal of Pharmaceutical Sciences Review and Research*. https://www.semanticscholar.org/paper/0f6fac09af45b0e4a437ea551af78b428e8605ea (accessed on 12th June 2025).
25. Kakako, S., Shuaibu, I., Musa, I. A., Jidda, M. L., Arisegi, S. A., Oyeniyi, J., Tajudeen, I. O., et al. (2025). The impact of cigarette smoking on oxidative stress indices. *Archives of Current Research International*. https://www.semanticscholar.org/paper/bdc538b98d2f05c059c4dd3653fcb2be2cfe2cf4 (accessed on 12th June 2025).
26. Kumari, R. (2023). Role of medicinal plants as antioxidants in the treatment of oxidative stress-related human health disorders. *Journal of Medicinal and Aromatic Plant Sciences*. https://www.semanticscholar.org/paper/1c729e73bff157e1d2390970ab5f79c6b41d166d (accessed on 12th June 2025).
27. Li, J., Cao, F., Yin, H., Huang, Z., Lin, Z., Mao, N., Sun, B., et al. (2020). Ferroptosis: Past, present and future. *Cell Death and Disease, 11*. https://doi.org/10.1038/s41419-020-2298-2 (accessed on 12th June 2025).
28. Lv, Q., Long, J., Gong, Z., Nong, K., Liang, X., Qin, T., Huang, W., et al. (2021). Current state of knowledge on the antioxidant effects and mechanisms of action of polyphenolic compounds. *Natural Product Communications, 16*. https://www.semanticscholar.org/paper/0daec33a6431704453eac5b2c914e8552fb5d4e1 (accessed on 12th June 2025).
29. Nowak, D., Kloskowski, T., Gośliński, M., Buhl, M., Wojtowicz, E., Poplawski, C., Drewa, T., et al. (2025). Antioxidant properties of *Aronia melanocarpa* and *Morinda citrifolia* juices and their impact on bladder cancer cell lines. *Medical Science Monitor: International Medical Journal of Experimental and Clinical Research, 31*. https://www.semanticscholar.org/paper/6902fe3d5c034f40f75c25f6480f2b50ea74bbf6 (accessed on 12th June 2025).
30. Panche, A. N., Diwan, A. D., & Chandra, S. (2016). Flavonoids: An overview. *Journal of Nutritional Science, 5*. https://doi.org/10.1017/jns.2016.41 (accessed on 12th June 2025).
31. Seth, R. (2021). Complementary therapy for periodontal diseases: Antimicrobials and antioxidants. https://core.ac.uk/download/490681814.pdf (accessed on 12th June 2025).
32. Shuja, N. (2025). Iron-catalyzed oxidative stress and atrial conduction delay in β-thalassemia carriers. *Developmental Medico-Life-Sciences*. https://www.semanticscholar.org/paper/3bfa45e5264df09f9310dac3d5d89ddac26edb56 (accessed on 12th June 2025).
33. Sies, H., Berndt, C., & Jones, D. P. (2017). Oxidative stress. *Annual Review of Biochemistry, 86*, 715–748. https://doi.org/10.1146/annurev-biochem-061516-045037 (accessed on 12th June 2025).
34. Tariq, S., Umbreen, H., Noreen, R., Petitbois, C., Aftab, K., Alasmary, F., Almalki, A., et al. (2022). Comparative analysis of antioxidants activity of indigenously produced *Moringa oleifera* seeds extracts. *BioMed Research International, 2022*. https://www.semanticscholar.org/paper/855789a49c05d58043e6656ecb23fdd6febf089e (accessed on 12th June 2025).
35. Tumilaar, S. G., Hardianto, A., Dohi, H., & Kurnia, D. (2024). A comprehensive review of free radicals, oxidative stress, and antioxidants: Overview, clinical applications, global perspectives, future directions, and mechanisms of antioxidant activity of flavonoid compounds. *Journal of Chemistry*. https://www.semanticscholar.org/paper/c6f6a83a8ab562910072c78b9773b0bc913058e5 (accessed on 12th June 2025).

36. Ünsal, V., Çiçek, M., & Sabancılar, İ. (2020). Toxicity of carbon tetrachloride, free radicals and role of antioxidants. *Reviews on Environmental Health, 36*, 279–295. https://doi.org/10.1515/reveh-2020-0048 (accessed on 12th June 2025).

37. Witkop, J. J. (2019). Role of antioxidant supplementation and exercise regimen in handling oxidative stress from natural PM2.5 exposure due to boreal forest fire. https://core.ac.uk/download/222783763.pdf (accessed on 12th June 2025).

38. Yahfoufi, N., Alsadi, N., Jambi, M., & Matar, C. (2018). The immunomodulatory and anti-inflammatory role of polyphenols. *Nutrients, 10*, 1618–1618. https://doi.org/10.3390/nu10111618 (accessed on 12th June 2025).

39. Yong, Y. S. (2007). Determination of synthetic phenolic antioxidants in food items using HPLC and total antioxidants using FIA approaches. https://core.ac.uk/download/32600347.pdf (accessed on 12th June 2025).

40. Zahid, M., Khalid, S., Raana, S., Amin, S., Javaid, H., Arshad, R., Jahangeer, A., et al. (2024). Unveiling the anti-oxidative potential of fruits and vegetables waste in prolonging the shelf stability of vegetable oils. *Future Foods, 10*, 100328–100328. https://doi.org/10.1016/j.fufo.2024.100328 (accessed on 12th June 2025).

41. Zahra, K., Lefter, R., Ali, A., Echaoui, A., Trus, C., Ciobîcă, A., & Timofte, D. (2021). The involvement of the oxidative stress status in cancer pathology: A double view on the role of the antioxidants. *Oxidative Medicine and Cellular Longevity, 2021*. https://www.semanticscholar.org/paper/1ab586fe00ff7d46bc96a0ca18c88050c62225c5 (accessed on 12th June 2025).

XENOBIOTICS AND BIOTRANSFORMATION

5

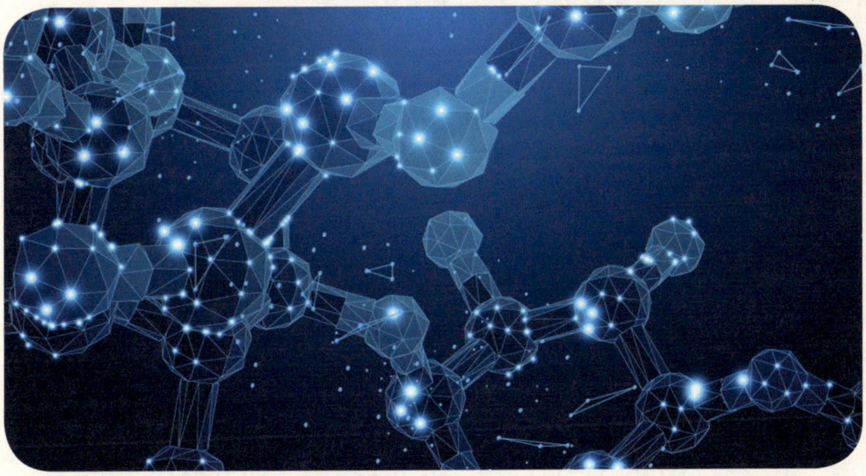

Introduction

The ubiquitous presence of xenobiotics in the environment poses a grave threat to ecosystems as well as to human health. Xenobiotics are foreign chemicals in biological systems and include a wide variety of substances , such as drugs, pesticides, and industrial chemicals. Their widespread use and accumulation later on have caught the interest of scientists to understand their impacts. Biotransformation, the biological process by which living organisms convert xenobiotic substances, plays an important role in overcoming the undesirable consequences of contaminants. Through further learning about how various organisms react to these compounds, scientists can determine means of bioremediation and detoxification and thereby ensure environmental sustainability. Recent studies have proved the remarkable proficiency of certain bacteria in xenobiotic biotransformation. For instance, the environmental bacterial strains *Pseudomonas rhodesiae* KCM-R5 and Bacillus subtilis KCM-RG5 are apt examples of microorganisms that can effectively biodegrade toxic compounds , such as ortho-nitrophenol (o-

LEARNING OBJECTIVES

After studying this chapter, you will be able to:

1. Describe the types and sources of xenobiotics;
2. Know the mechanisms of biotransformation;
3. Know the enzymes involved in biotransformation;
4. Understand the implications of biotransformation.

NP) and 2,4-dichlorophenoxyacetic acid (2,4-D). Upon exposure to xenobiotics, the strains exhibited promising removal efficiency, with a maximum degradation of 86% of o-NP. This capability not only exhibits the potential of bioremediation in contaminated environments but also points to the adaptability of microbial life in overcoming chemical barriers.

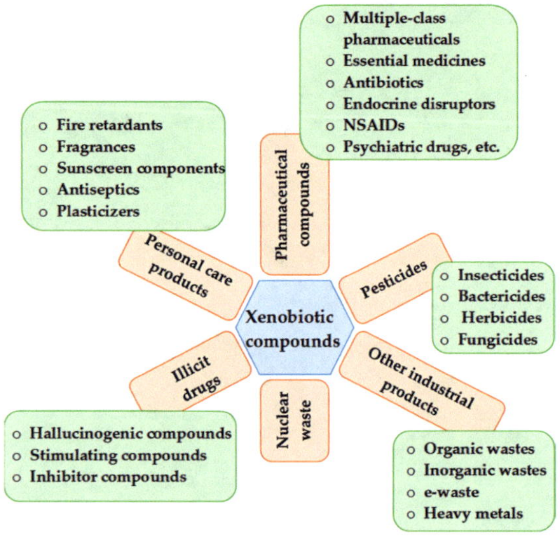

Figure 5.1. Xenobiotic compounds.

Source: https://www.mdpi.com/jox/jox-11-00009/article_deploy/html/images/jox-11-00009-g001.png.

The successful application of such microbes to bioremediation could significantly help efforts toward the recovery of contaminated systems using natural processes to degrade poisonous substances (Golovinsky et al., 2006). The impact of xenobiotics is further enhanced by their ability to cause biochemical responses in living things. Organic pollutants have been known to bioaccumulate in the aquatic environment, leading to harmful impacts on ecosystem integrity and diversity. Induction of the hepatic biotransformation enzyme cytochrome P4501A (CYP1A) has been a widely studied response to organic pollutants, and its use as a fish exposure biomarker. These xenobiotic exposure actions extend beyond acute toxicity to impact ultimate survival and fitness long term through mechanisms of oxidative stress and DNA damage. This biochemistry is essential in addressing the environmental risk posed by xenobiotics, ultimately leading to more intelligent environmental management and policy choices (Livingston et al., 1994) (Figure 5.1).

Definition of Xenobiotics

The xenobiotics is an overarching description of a category of compounds foreign to the living system but encompassing a broad range of chemicals , such as drugs, environmental pollutants, and synthetic chemicals. These compounds possess varying characteristics which can make them potentially toxic or beneficial depending on dosage and duration of exposure. Unlike endogenous substances that are inherently manufactured within living systems, xenobiotics can disrupt homeostasis and trigger a range of biological responses when they enter an organism. Understanding xenobiotic substances is of utmost importance in the field of toxicology, as their interaction with life processes could lead to deleterious or therapeutic outcomes, and thus, it is important to study these substances in more detail. The metabolic elimination of xenobiotics is governed by a process known as biotransformation, which utilizes enzymes to alter the foreign substances to facilitate their excretion from the body. The enzymatic transformation might consist of many reactions that include oxidation, reduction, hydrolysis, and conjugation. The liver holds most of the xenobiotic metabolism, though other tissues , such as skin, do play roles within the pathways. For instance, human skin has the capacity to metabolize xenobiotic chemicals, but little is known about the extent and activity of enzymes responsible for such metabolism. Proteomics has been utilized for the profiling of xenobiotic-metabolizing enzymes in human skin to offer insight into the principal metabolic pathways of xenobiotic compounds (Cupitt et al., 2012). This information is critical for the evaluation of the safety and efficacy of chemicals with which humans come into contact daily. Exposure to xenobiotics in the environment not only impacts human health but also affects ecosystems and wildlife. EDCs are among the compounds that have been reported to enter water bodies, with resultant toxicological impacts on the local biota. Studies on indigenous fish, such as bluegill, have employed biomarkers to assess the effect of EDC exposure, detecting alterations in vitellogenin composition, estrogenic activity in bile, and detoxification process-associated enzyme activity (Truman, 2006). These experiments show the intricate interaction of xenobiotic exposure and biological processes and emphasize the necessity for continued research into how these chemicals exert their effects. By gaining a deeper understanding of xenobiotics and their interactions within biological systems, scientists can make recommendations regarding the reduction of risks from environmental pollution and safeguarding public health (Figure 5.2).

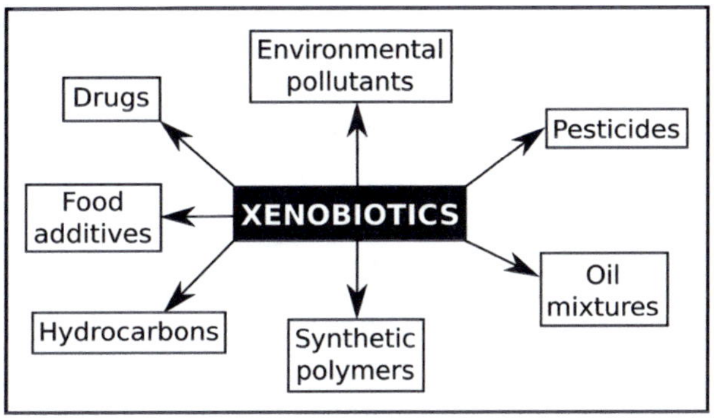

Figure 5.2. Major groups of xenobiotics.

Source: https://biomolecules101.wordpress.com/wp-content/uploads/2018/11/xenobiotics-1.png.

Overview of Biotransformation Processes

Biotransformation reactions are required for the determination of the metabolic conversion of xenobiotics, foreign compounds that are brought into a biological organism, in living things. Biotransformation occurs primarily in the liver, where enzymes change the xenobiotics in a series of reactions, broadly divided into Phase I and Phase II conversions. Phase I reactions involve oxidative, reductive, or hydrolytic transformations that form functional groups or expose latent ones, thereby increasing the compound's reactivity or solubility. And then there are Phase II reactions that involve conjugation with endogenous substrates , such as glucuronic acid or sulfates, to facilitate detoxification and excretion of the compounds. This process of metabolism significantly influences the pharmacological effectiveness and toxicity of xenobiotics and influences both ecological health and human medicine. Besides, biotransformation processes are an important determinant of the bioavailability and bioaccumulation of organic substances, particularly in aquatic organisms. For instance, copper experiments with three-spined sticklebacks reveal that there is oxidative stress in the liver before causing significant metal accumulation, showing complex biotransformation processes. The induction of other antioxidant enzymes , such as catalase and superoxide dismutase (SOD), is a protective mechanism against oxidative damage, indicating the adaptability of the organisms to environmental stress. The interaction between biotransformation and uptake of environmental contaminants demonstrates the harmonious balance between metabolic processes and ecological impact of xenobiotics, again demanding an understanding of biotransformation mechanisms across different species in aid of enlightening conservation and management activities (Sanchez et al., 2005). There is also the field of biotransformation in avian species, where knowledge gaps in organic chemical bioaccumulation and metabolism are considerable. Based on a survey of literature in over 500 studies, heterogeneity of available data for enzymatic activity as well as metabolic pathways is evident. Notable scarcity of robust biotransformation kinetic data limits predictive modeling for avian species, particularly within heterogeneous ecological niches. More emphasis should be on *in vivo* studies and a broader chemical scope for effective risk assessments and environmental assessments. It may thereby bring about strategic advancement in research on biotransformation to offer an avenue towards integrating multiple data sources, enhancing our overall understanding of xenobiotics fate within avian ecosystems (Kuo et al., 2022) (Figure 5.3).

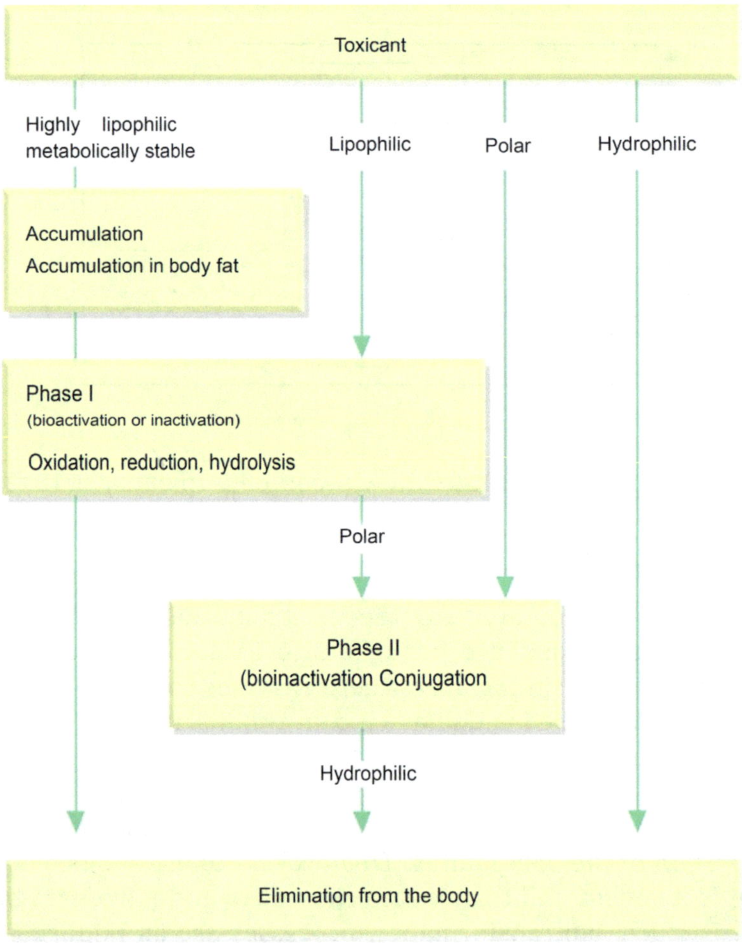

Figure 5.3. The various steps of biotransformation.

Source: https://ars.els-cdn.com/content/image/3-s2.0-B9780128147191000288-f28-09-9780128147191.jpg.

5.1. Types of Xenobiotics

Learning Outcome

1. Learn about natural xenobiotics;
2. Understand the synthetic xenobiotics;
3. Describe the environmental xenobiotics.

Xenobiotics, or chemicals foreign to an organism's biological system, are a broad class of chemical compounds with significant effects on human health and the environment. Some of the principal types of xenobiotics include pharmaceuticals, pesticides, and industrial chemicals. Pharmaceuticals, for example, numerous therapeutic drugs, have a tendency to enter ecosystems through excretion, careless disposal, or agricultural drainage. Pesticides, widely used in agriculture to control pests, have been of concern since they can potentially contaminate soils and water bodies, affecting non-target species. Industrial chemicals like heavy metals and solvents are of great concern since they also have the potential to be stored by living organisms and biomagnify through food chains, ultimately threatening biodiversity and ecosystem resilience, hence the need for effective monitoring and regulation of their application. A very extensive group of xenobiotics is the natural products, for instance, plant constituents that can influence synthetic drugs. Some of the examples include chemicals like St. John's wort and grapefruit juice that were identified as potent drug metabolism modulators due to their influence on biotransformation enzymes. The interactions due to the interaction of these natural products with drugs can lead to altered drug efficacy or increased toxicity, especially in patients on chronic medication for diseases like neurological disorders.

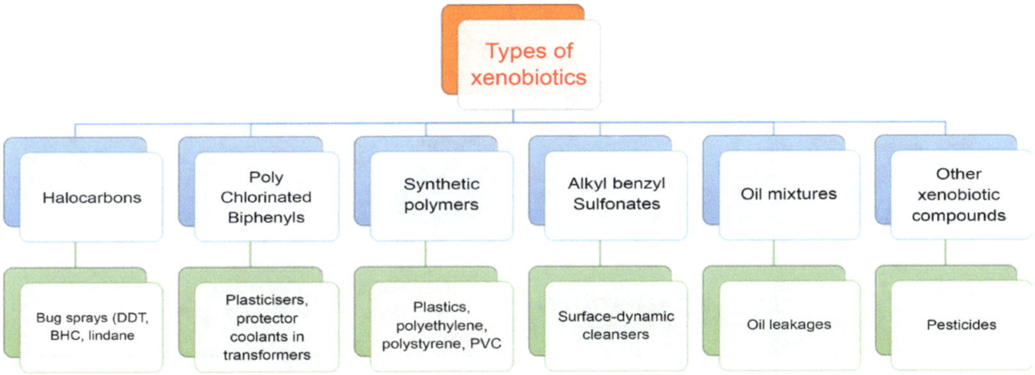

Figure 5.4. Categories of xenobiotics according to key features.

Source: https://www.researchgate.net/publication/382883642/figure/fig3/AS:11431281273402520@1724465393202/Categories-of-xenobiotics-according-to-key-features.png.

Such concern requires cautious use and demands proper patient education regarding likely interactions, thus minimizing the risk of drug-related adverse effects. In understanding the intricacies of such relationships, patients and doctors can decide in an informed manner to conduct safe and effective treatment regimes. The introduction of contaminants of emerging concern (CECs) raises the complexity of classifying xenobiotics since they tend to be man-made compounds that are poorly regulated but have far-reaching ecological effects. Some of the examples of CECs are various personal care items, pharmaceuticals, and nanomaterials, which contaminate water bodies with adverse effects on aquatic life. One of the important effects is the induction of CYP1A, an aquatic organism biotransformation enzyme, associated with chemical carcinogenesis and oxidative stress. The accumulation of such pollutants is a two-pronged threat: inhibiting the physiological functions in impacted organisms and contributing to the loss of aquatic biodiversity. Continued research is needed to elucidate such xenobiotic interactions and apply effective bioremediation to reverse their impact on the environment, highlighting the importance of the integration of ecological well-being into xenobiotic and biotransformation discussion (Figure 5.4).

5.1.1. Natural Xenobiotics

Because natural xenobiotics are prevalent in various ecosystems, it is essential to know about their biotransformation routes for evaluating their ecological significance. Plant and animal metabolism products of naturally occurring compounds tend to seriously derange biological processes when introduced into new environments. For instance, phytochemicals or secondary metabolites, which might be harmless in their indigenous environments, have the tendency to become a nuisance to non-native life forms.

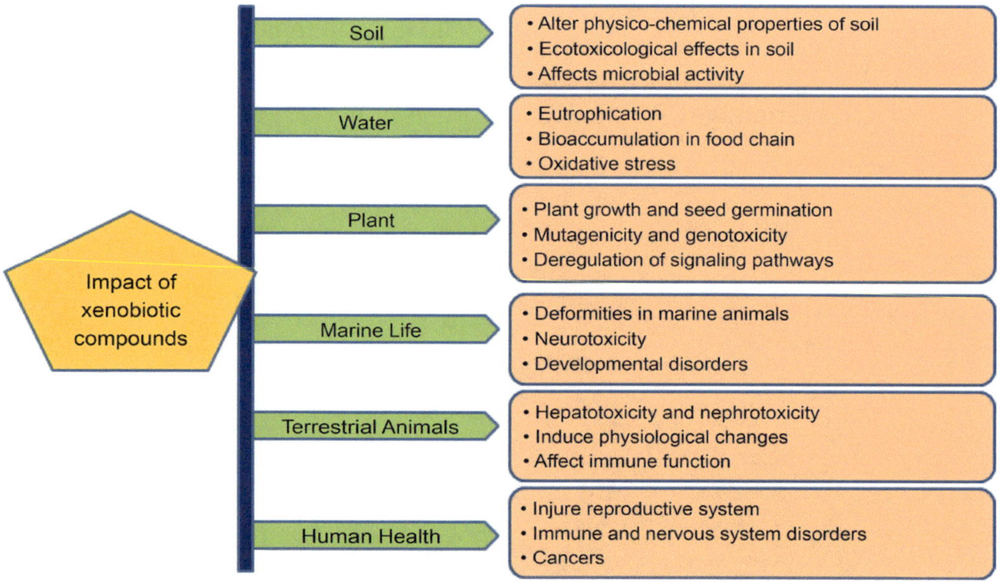

Figure 5.5. Hazardous effects are caused by direct or indirect exposure of xenobiotic compounds on the environment, plants, animals, and human health.

Source: https://www.mdpi.com/metabolites/metabolites-12-00818/article_deploy/html/images/metabolites-12-00818-g001.png.

The mechanisms through which these xenobiotics exert their effects generally involve complex biochemical pathways that result in the binding of such substances to biological macromolecules. An excellent case is the induction of liver cytochrome P450 enzymes, CYP1A, as a biomarker for the exposure of various aquatic animals to numerous organic pollutants, which illustrates the potential for pathological change with exposure to xenobiotics (Livingston et al., 1994). The biological activity of aquatic species in the biotransformation of natural xenobiotics is particularly fascinating, given that some of the species possess the ability to convert such compounds into even more toxic forms. For instance, research on freshwater algae , such as *Chlorella vulgaris* has indicated that natural steroid estrogens are highly biotransformed. Both estradiol and estrone in experiments indicated the potential for being interconvertible, with estrone proving a preferred end-product under certain conditions. Interestingly, the fact that these compounds are persistent in algal culture indicates that the biotransformation process is not only complex but also results in the accumulation of intermediate metabolites, which may have ecological implications by affecting nutrient cycling and predator-prey relationships within aquatic systems (Lai et al., 2002). Additionally, natural xenobiotic biotransformation can impact the fitness and health of organisms within an ecosystem. As highlighted by studies on the induction of CYP1A, the accumulation of organic compounds can lead to oxidative stress and subsequent adverse effects, including reproductive mishaps and increased risk of cancer among aquatic animals. Induction of ROS production as a consequence of xenobiotic exposure is an additional mechanism through which natural xenobiotics can be toxic at the cellular level. Furthermore, the integration of CYP1A induction and ROS-mediated processes in biotransformation science can open the door to more effective biomarkers for monitoring environmental exposure and ecological health, and eventually more insight into the complex relationship between natural xenobiotics and organismal response (Livingston et al., 1994) (Figure 5.5).

5.1.2. Synthetic Xenobiotics

Synthetic xenobiotics are man-made chemicals that do not naturally occur in the environment, and their prevalence has risen exponentially due to industrialization and the development of new technologies. These chemicals can include drugs, pesticides, plasticizers, and many other chemical additives. They are non-biodegradable, and this is a major cause for concern regarding their potential toxicological impact on living organisms. As xenobiotics, they are harmful to the natural process of biotransformation by biological systems, which can be adapted for endogenous substances. Synthetic xenobiotics' biotransformation is a critical determinant of their fate in the environment; whether or not they are excreted and detoxified or are potential toxic metabolites has major environmental and health consequences. The biotransformation processes are crucial to the metabolic handling of synthetic xenobiotics. In the living organism, enzymes facilitate chemical reactions that allow for the biotransformation of these foreign chemicals to less harmful substances. The phase I reactions involve further alteration of the xenobiotics through oxidation, reduction, or hydrolysis that can add or expose functional groups. Phase II reactions can then couple such altered xenobiotics with endogenous substrates to render them more water-soluble and hence easier to excrete. Studies have confirmed that certain synthetic xenobiotics undergo biotransformation reactions, which may yield metabolites of increased toxicity, an indication of the complexity of biointeractions with such compounds. Estradiol and estrone estrogens, for example, after exposure to algal cultures, demonstrate biotransformation activities conducive to transformation into metabolites of indeterminate toxicity (Lai et al., 2002). Moreover, the interaction between synthetic xenobiotics and natural products is of some concern. Several individuals unknowingly consume natural beverages or supplements that can interfere with drugs through biotransformation enzymes. Grapefruit juice, for example, is already renowned for blocking cytochrome P450 enzymes, which are essential in the biotransformation of most man-made drugs. The interactions would lead to different drug potency and efficacy as well as increased risk of side effects, especially among vulnerable populations that are treated for life-threatening illnesses. Knowledge of the interaction is also important as health professionals must educate patients on the effects of combining synthetic xenobiotics with natural compounds to ensure secure and successful treatment procedures (Bacinschi et al., 2020). Awareness of the dynamics of synthetic xenobiotics and their biotransformation helps in policymaking to avoid environmental persistence and enhance public health security.

5.1.3. Environmental Xenobiotics

The increasing prevalence of environmental xenobiotics poses a significant risk to ecosystems and human health due to their synthetic nature and persistence. Such compounds, typically introduced through industrial activities, agricultural use, and urban runoff, are not degraded naturally, leading to their persistence in various environmental matrices. Microorganisms, which typically degrade natural organic compounds, possess diverse capacities when confronted with xenobiotic compounds. Drivers for this decay are microbial community structure, environmental factors, and the xenobiotic's chemical form. The impact of these human-made substances transcends biogeochemical processes, as they can wind up warping trophic relations and affecting biodiversity. Thus, understanding environmental xenobiotics' fate is of utmost significance when developing effective bioremediation processes and reversing their detrimental impacts on living organisms and ecosystem integrity (Kumar, 2023). Of the extensive group of environmental xenobiotics, pharmaceuticals are a new issue, particularly within aquatic ecosystems. For instance, the antidepressant drug citalopram is inadequately removed by conventional wastewater treatment processes, resulting in its ongoing presence in waterways. This raises relevant questions about the ecological risks it imposes on aquatic life, particularly developmental toxicity. Application of methods , such as the fish embryo test (FET) using zebrafish provides a uniform method to screen for the adverse effects of such xenobiotics on developing organisms.

Not only does screening assess the impact of the drug itself, but also the fineness of the extent to which environmental factors , such as pH affect toxicity and biotransformation mechanisms. By describing these interactions, scientists are able to better predict the hazards of such pollutants and design effective management strategies (Heid et al., 2019). Biotransformation by microbial communities of environmental xenobiotics is a complex interaction and plays an important role in regulating the fate of such chemicals in the environment. Microorganisms possess a diverse array of enzymes that are capable of initiating the breakdown of xenobiotics, transforming them into less toxic or more bioavailable forms. This facilitates the final mineralization of such compounds or their incorporation into microbial biomass, thereby limiting ecological impact. However, the effectiveness of microbial degradation is critically dependent on environmental conditions, such as temperature, availability of nutrients, and presence of alternative substrates. Furthermore, some xenobiotics are prone to incomplete breakdown, resulting in potentially harmful metabolites with implications for various organisms in the environment. An understanding of these complex biotransformation processes will become essential to enhancing bioremediation techniques and informing policy regarding environmental xenobiotics (Kumar, 2023) (Figure 5.6).

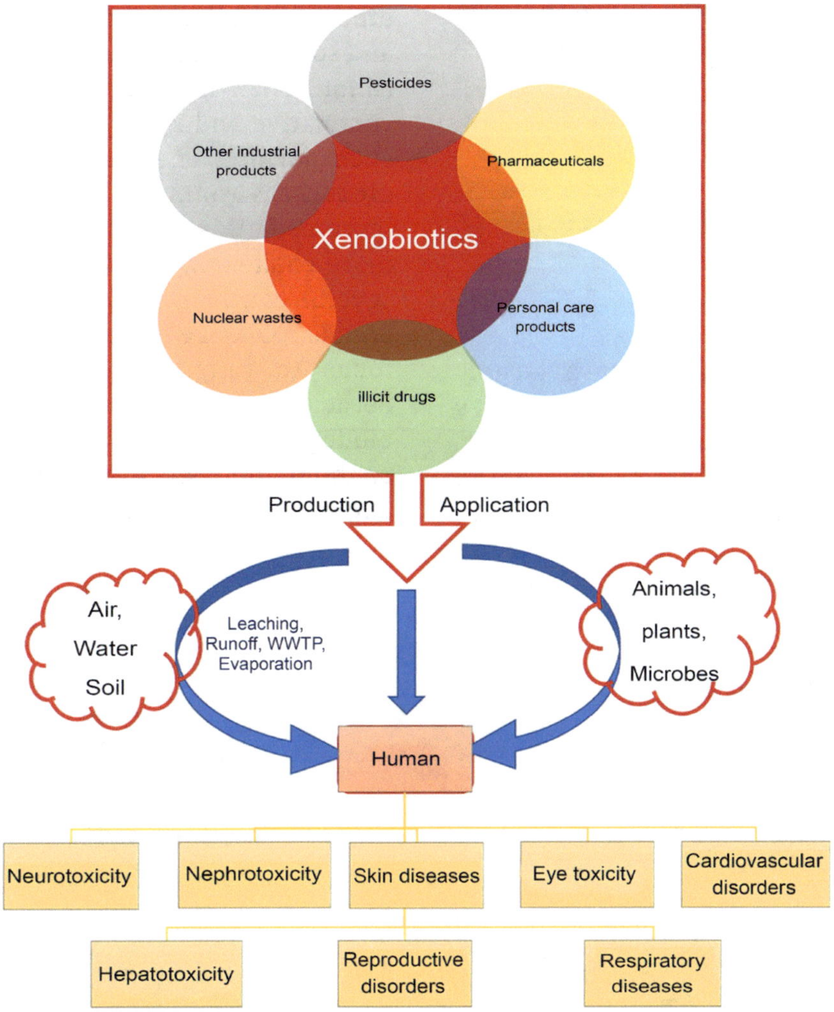

Figure 5.6. Fate of xenobiotics in the environment and their ultimate impacts on humans.

Source: https://www.researchgate.net/publication/382883642/figure/fig4/AS:11431281273344207@1724465393418/Fate-of-xenobiotics-in-the-environment-and-their-ultimate-impacts-on-humans.png.

Test Your Knowledge

1. What are natural xenobiotics?
2. What are environmental xenobiotics?

5.2. Sources of Xenobiotics

Learning Outcome

1. Understand the role of industrial processes in xenobiotics;
2. Know the agricultural practices;
3. Describe the pharmaceutical products.

Their sources are diverse and are largely anthropogenic in nature, which introduces xenobiotics into the environment. Industrialization is a primary source, where factories release diverse chemicals from processing activities into the environment. Volatile organic solvents, heavy metals, and other contaminants find their way into water and soil due to factory effluents and agricultural runoff. Their impacts are further enhanced by cumulative and synergistic interactions among such harmful chemicals, in which they have greater environmental effects. This complicates bioremediation of contaminated places into a more challenging problem since working with several contaminants simultaneously poses a unique challenge. Scientists are giving increasing focus to fungal bioremediation strategies because of fungal metabolic processes, which can biodegrade organic and inorganic xenobiotics in contaminated sites and thus provide a clean and green method for pollution control (Ceci et al., 2018).

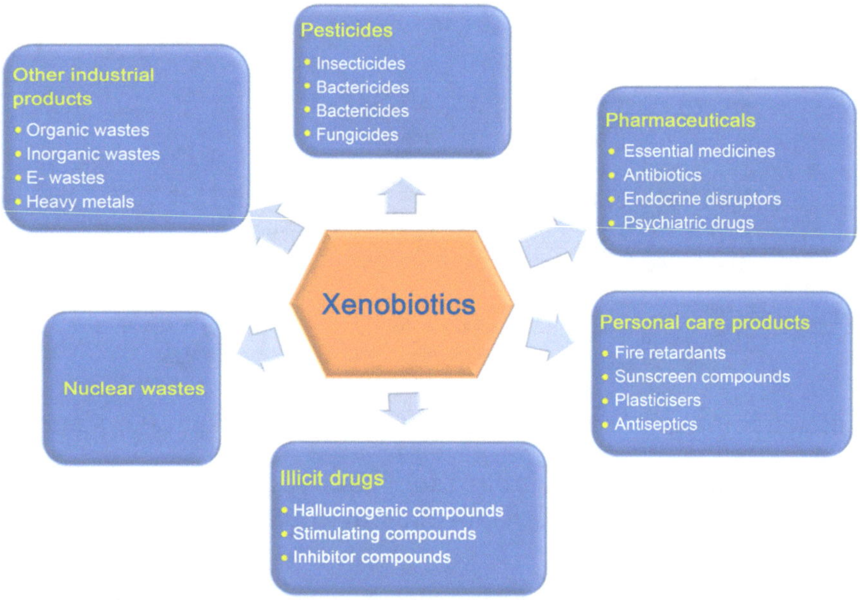

Figure 5.7. Sources of xenobiotics in the environment.

Source: https://www.researchgate.net/publication/382883642/figure/fig2/AS:11431281273328488@1724465392939/Sources-of-xenobiotics-in-the-environment.png.

Pharmaceutical products are a significant source of xenobiotics, particularly for wastewater treatment and agriculture. The presence of antibiotics and other medications in water systems has been a point of concern when it comes to the environment, especially because such medications are known to exhibit persistence and bioaccumulation. Treatment facilities are unlikely to get rid of these medications entirely because they can be converted back into parent medications from conjugated metabolites. This inefficiency will lead to the redeposition of antibiotics into ecosystems, which is concerning given the growing rates of antibiotic-resistant bacteria. Pilot and full-scale wastewater treatment plants have variable removal efficiencies with consideration of factors like solid retention time, as well as influent and effluent loading dynamics. Understanding of removal efficiencies is crucial for the optimization of treatment strategies and the resolution of downstream effects of pharmaceutical pollutants (Andersen et al., 2016). The dissemination of xenobiotics in the environment is also influenced by agricultural practices. The use of fertilizers, herbicides, and pesticides introduces to the environment large numbers of synthetic chemicals used for protection against pests as well as to improve crop yields. Their unforeseen consequences are that they may pollute nearby water bodies and soil ecosystems. Environmental persistence of these chemicals enhances exposure to bioaccumulation in terrestrial and aquatic organisms, which has additional ecological and health implications. This calls for a thorough assessment of farm inputs and their long-term effect on water and soil quality. More sustainable farming practices and bioremediation technologies can be utilized to reduce the use of harmful chemicals, ultimately leading to an environment of good health (Ceci et al., 2018) (Figure 5.7).

5.2.1. Industrial Processes

Industrial processes are a significant source through which xenobiotics gain entry into the environment, where they persist and exert profound ecological effects. Such synthetic substances, typically synthesized during production, pesticide application, or waste management, have the potential to bioaccumulate in living organisms, exerting profound effects on food chains as well as the health of ecosystems. Among these, organic contaminants , such as aromatic hydrocarbons, PCBs, and dioxins are highly toxic due to their potential to cause biochemical effects in aquatic animals. Induction of the liver biotransformation enzyme CYP1A, for instance, is one of the biomarkers utilized as an indicator of exposure to these pollutants. Detection of CYP1A not only shows the presence of poisonous substances but also the potential for chemical carcinogenesis through the build-up of DNA-adducts, pointing towards the importance of witnessing these byproducts of industry in environmental monitoring (Livingston et al., 1994). The facility to biotransform in industrial processes is also demonstrated through some strains of microbes that can break down xenobiotic substances. Experiments have indicated the potential of environmental bacteria , such as *Pseudomonas rhodesiae* and *Bacillus subtilis* to degrade various contaminants , such as phenolic compounds and herbicides. *Pseudomonas rhodesiae* KCM-R5, for instance, removed as much as 86% of ortho-nitrophenol effectively, indicating the potential of bioremediation efforts in polluted environments. Such microbes, in addition to their remarkable tolerance of heavy metals and phenol derivatives, possess enzymatic processes that can allow for the degradation of recalcitrant xenobiotics. The potential of such microbes being used in industry for bioremediation points towards a critical step toward ecologically sustainable environmental management (Golovinsky et al., 2006). Inclusion of biotransformation reactions in production processes is a double benefit: it reduces the toxic effect of xenobiotic chemicals and offers a mechanism of rehabilitation of the environment. The employment of microorganisms as biocatalysts for production can diligently reduce the persistence of industrial wastes. The elucidation of biochemical pathways underlying these conversions may also contribute to the discovery of better processes in chemical manufacture. As emphasized by oxidative stress due to ROS in organisms exposed to pollutants, further studies must be performed to optimize such biotransformation processes. Efforts to include antioxidant measurements as part of traditional monitoring techniques can combine a full assessment of the environmental health, thereby leading to improved regulatory regimes of industrial efflux and enhanced ecological integrity (Livingston et al., 1994) (Figure 5.8).

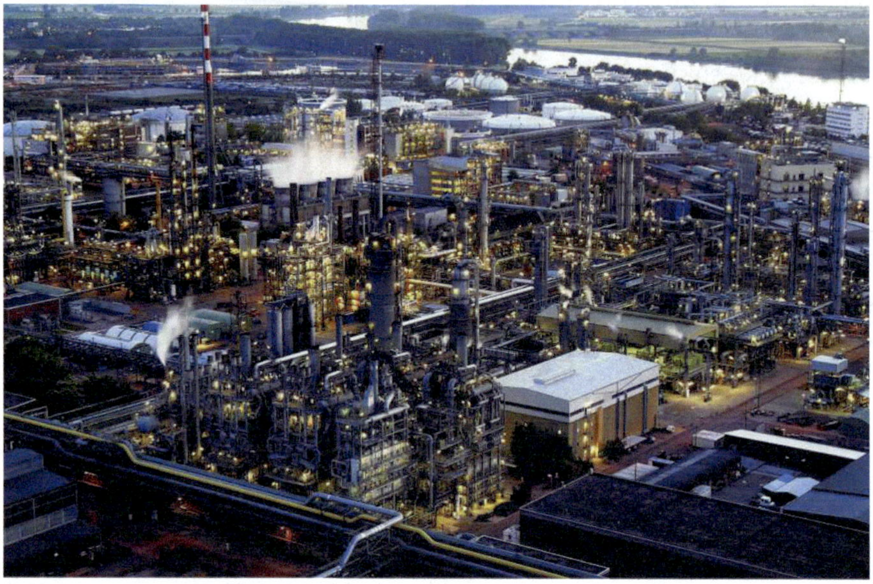

Figure 5.8. Industrial processes.

Source: https://www.essentialchemicalindustry.org/images/stories/040_cracking/01-CrackingFig1Standort.jpg.

5.2.2. Agricultural Practices

Farm practice in agriculture has evolved over time as it adapts to changing social demand, technology, and environmental awareness. Modern practice increasingly uses manufactured herbicides, pesticides, and fertilizers that have been produced to enhance agricultural crops and repel pests. These chemicals can, however, cause accumulation of xenobiotics in agricultural land soils, which is toxic to the environment and human life. Contamination of soil with pharmaceutical and personal care products (PPCPs) has also been observed, particularly through the application of treated wastewater and animal manure. Such contamination can result in the accumulation of such harmful chemicals in crops, offering an immediate entry point for human exposure through the food chain, connecting agricultural farming to increasing public health and environmental sustainability issues (Dudley et al., 2018). The uptake and metabolism mechanism of xenobiotics by crops is central to the comprehension of crop management implications. Research has determined that several plant species may absorb antibiotics, resulting in detectable amounts in edible vegetables eaten by human beings. The process can stimulate risks of antibiotic contamination because transformation products, often present at higher concentrations than the parent compounds, may be unidentified for their toxicological significance. For instance, a study on the absorption of antibiotics by vegetables discovered that certain farm practices, especially where manure is used and water is polluted, resulted in high levels of residues of such chemicals (Tadić, 2020). This intricate interaction between farm practice, crop physiology, and xenobiotic effect demands careful monitoring and regulation for ensuring food safety. Considering these challenges, agricultural practice analysis should be conducted with a focus on new measures for xenobiotic risk control. Integrated methods, such as organic farming, sustainable water resource management, and rotation crops, can prevent the adverse effects of chemical inputs. Besides, public and stakeholder awareness on the implications of xenobiotic persistence in the environment encourages the adoption of practices that are ecological balance-oriented and health safety-oriented. Future research must address the elucidation of the routes of xenobiotic biotransformation in plants and soils so that they can inform best practices for minimizing agricultural contamination. By integrating scientific information and regulatory strategies, agricultural systems can evolve towards safer and more sustainable forms that protect the health of human beings and the environment from the adverse effects of xenobiotics and their metabolites (Dudley et al., 2018; Tadić, 2020) (Figure 5.9).

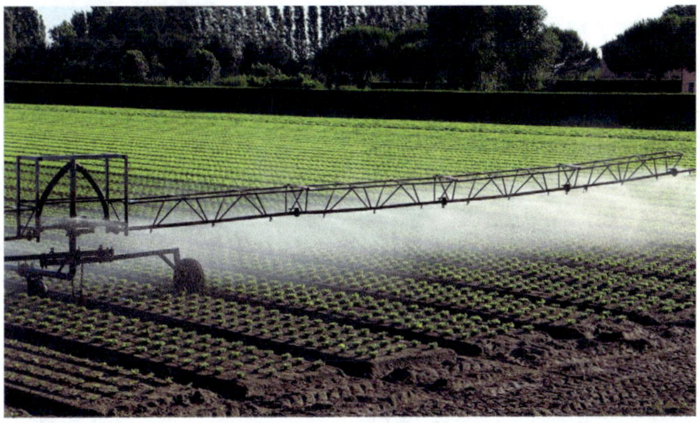

Figure 5.9. Agricultural practices.

Source: https://foodtank.com/wp-content/uploads/2018/06/Crop_Spray.jpg.

5.2.3. Pharmaceutical Products

Pharmaceutical drugs have a close association with the term xenobiotics and their biotransformation in biological systems. Pharmaceutical drugs are known as xenobiotics when they are introduced into an organism, where they undergo a series of metabolic transformations that allow them to be excreted. The organism utilizes biotransformation processes to catalyze lipophilic substances to produce hydrophilic metabolites, thereby enhancing their excretion via urine or bile. It is critical to understand the biotransformation of these drugs because it affects their potency and toxicity. For instance, medicinal active ingredients , such as diclofenac and ibuprofen have documented variable metabolic rates across species, ascertaining the complexities of interspecies variation in drug metabolism as well as implications for both human and environmental health (Hutchinson et al., 2014). The drug products' biotransformation is primarily categorized into two phases. Phase I reactions are characterized by the introduction or exposure of reactive groups of functions on the compound, which is enzyme-catalyzed by proteins , such as cytochrome P450. Phase II reactions, which subsequently ensue, typically consist of conjugation, whereby the metabolites are conjugated to large, hydrophilic molecules in order to further augment their excretion (Hutchinson et al., 2014). An example is the metabolism of common APIs that can yield both active and inactive metabolites, which contribute to therapeutic activity and possible toxicities. In the environment, the metabolism of these chemicals in non-target organisms, like fish in freshwater, demonstrates the extended ecological effect of pharmaceutical release in water ecosystems, influencing not just intended therapeutic uses but also ecosystem and wildlife health (Hutchinson et al., 2014). In addition, the emergence of plant-derived drugs reflects a growing interest in herbal medicines and their unique patterns of metabolism. Familiar herbal drugs , such as St. John's wort and valerian, are being extensively used for neurological disorders without being fully explored in the context of their pharmacokinetics. Preliminary studies indicate that these herbal drugs will exhibit varying extents of absorption and metabolic stability, which could be influenced by how the human gut microbiota modulates them. Such interactions may also impact the pharmacological action of such products by altering the bioavailability of active ingredients. With herbal medicines gaining more popularity, further research becomes necessary to comprehend their biotransformation pathways in detail so that the effects of such products can be enjoyed with no adverse side effects on health or interactions with the body's complex metabolic processes (Figure 5.10).

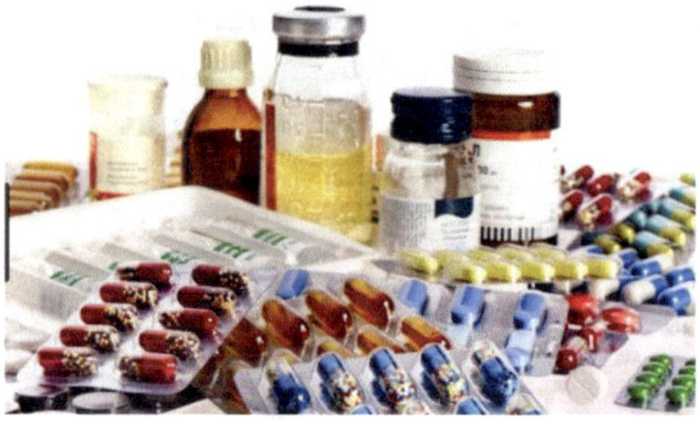

Figure 5.10. Pharmaceutical products.

Source: https://5.imimg.com/data5/QU/XU/MY-22634/pharmaceutical-products.png.

Test Your Knowledge

1. What do you mean by agricultural practices?
2. What is meant by pharmaceutical products?

5.3. Mechanisms of Biotransformation

Learning Outcome

1. Know the phase I reactions in biotransformation;
2. Understand the phase II reactions in biotransformation;
3. Describe the phase III reactions in biotransformation.

The biotransformation processes are critical to account for the metabolism of xenobiotics, such as drugs and pollutants in the environment, in biological systems. The biotransformation reactions tend to take place in two phases: Phase I and Phase II reactions. Phase I reactions are the addition or exposure of the functional groups through enzymatic activity, which are largely carried out by cytochrome P450 enzymes. These reactions may include oxidation, reduction, or hydrolysis, ultimately leading to polar metabolites or more reactive intermediates. This initial process of transformation aids in increasing the solubility of xenobiotics in water and consequently facilitates their excretion by the body. The understanding regarding the role of certain enzymes involved in such Phase I reactions aids in comprehending potential toxicity and metabolism processes—crucial in applications to environmental toxicology and pharmacology. Following Phase I alterations, Phase II biotransformation reactions take place, typically involving conjugation reactions that further enhance the solubility of the resulting metabolites. Such transformations involve the addition of endogenous substrates , such as glucuronic acid, sulfate, or glutathione (GSH), to the polar metabolites formed during Phase I. Conjugation not only serves to detoxify xenobiotics but also to excrete them via bile or urine. The efficiency of these processes varies among species and is determined by numerous factors, including genetic diversity, environmental exposure, and overall health status. Such variability is particularly relevant to wildlife populations, as observed in studies that investigate the response of different species to pollutants. Groundbreaking techniques through biomarker responses, including those in three-spined sticklebacks exposed to heavy metals, have helped illuminate the complex interactions between biotransformation pathways and environmental stressors (Sanchez et al., 2005). In addition to this, xenobiotic biotransformation is also an important area of research among avian species, where large databases and modeling are required to collate information currently available and identify gaps within existing data. A compilation of bioaccumulation and biotransformation data revealed significant fragmentation in our understanding of these phenomena in various avian taxonomic groups. Identification of metabolic pathways and the activity of enzymes remains critical to the development of predictive models for the impact of organic chemicals on birds (Kuo et al., 2022). There is a significant shortage of kinetic data regarding *in vivo* biotransformation since most research relies on *in vitro* methods. This kind of dearth of data may restrict activities in more comprehensive modeling, calling for cross-disciplinary approaches to optimize research efficiency and achieve greater insight into mechanisms of avian biotransformation. Such is required for assessing the ecological hazard of xenobiotics and informing conservation activity (Figure 5.11).

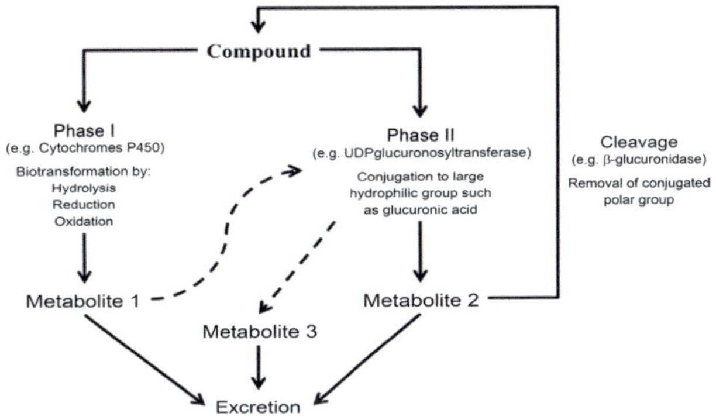

Figure 5.11. Biotransformation of compounds (endogenous and exogenous) into polar metabolites for excretion following Phase I (solid line), Phase II (solid line), or Phase I and II enzyme reactions (dotted line). Conjugated compounds can be regenerated to the parent compound through the cleavage of a large polar group by cleavage enzymes.

Source: https://www.researchgate.net/profile/Luc-Rougee/publication/262572218/figure/fig1/AS:614078309490688@1523419086001/Biotransformation-of-compounds-endogenous-and-exogenous-into-polar-metabolites-for.png.

5.3.1. Phase I Reactions

Phase I reactions are a critical initial phase in xenobiotic biotransformation, in which introduction or exposure of functional groups is accessed through various enzymatic pathways. Predominantly catalyzed by the Enzyme family cytochrome P450, these involve oxidation, reduction, and hydrolysis. It is a step towards improving the hydrophilicity of lipophilic substances and thus their excretion out of the organism. These Phase I-induced alterations also yield metabolites that can have sustained biological activity or are more toxic than the parent molecules, and because of this, the significance of this phase of xenobiotic metabolism cannot be overstated. Such reactions can be highly efficient and result-oriented in one individual versus another due to genetic polymorphism, environmental factors, and lifestyle, the last of which may influence the expression and activity rates of these valuable enzymes. In addition to the cytochrome P450 enzymes, other Phase I enzymes , such as flavin-containing monooxygenases and other oxidoreductases, participate in the metabolic biotransformation of xenobiotics. Though they are fewer in number compared to P450s, they contribute to the rich enzymatic diversity that renders a wide array of xenobiotic substrates available for alteration. The presence of these heterogeneous enzymes brings about metabolic flexibility, in which the organism is able to function in diverse chemical environments and exposures. The final products of the Phase I reactions can further serve as substrates for the following Phase II reactions in order to facilitate conjugation of these metabolites onto more polar groups; a process of primary importance to increase excretion and reduce toxicity. Such dependence reveals the synergistic role of biotransformation phases in detoxification processes of organisms. Phase I reactions may be controlled by numerous extrinsic variables, including diet, drugs, and environmental chemical exposure. For example, certain compounds can induce or inhibit P450 enzyme activity to produce significant changes in the metabolism of concomitantly administered xenobiotics and result in drug interactions. Also, in the process of physiological change, such as pregnancy and lactation, gene expression and enzyme activity for xenobiotic metabolism can be altered, as proven by experiments showing variability in the level of conjugating enzymes and transport systems , such as Mrp2, during these phases of life (Arana et al., 2014). These findings underscore the complexity of Phase I reactions and their coupling with human well-being, in which intersubject and situational variations are able to have substantial impacts on the biotransformation and elimination of xenobiotics and illustrate the role of individualized pharmacology and toxicology. There is a need to comprehend these nuances to be able to institute effective measures for coping with xenobiotic exposure and averting potential harm brought by toxic metabolites that are generated during Phase I reactions (Beaudoin et al., 2004).

5.3.2. Phase II Reactions

Phase II reactions or conjugation reactions constitute an integral component of the mechanisms of biotransformation to facilitate enhanced excretion of xenobiotics. Phase II reactions typically involve the conjugation of endogenous substrates like glucuronic acid, sulfate, or GSH with lipophilic xenobiotic compounds. Phase II reactions make the xenobiotic compounds more polar in nature, enabling them to be excreted from the organism, predominantly through urine or bile. The significance of Phase II metabolism is evidenced by the fact that it detoxifies several toxic substances, thus protecting the body from potential injury. Enzymatic activities are mostly localized in the liver and secondarily in the intestines, where the enzymes UDP-glucuronosyltransferases (UGTs) and glutathione S-transferases (GSTs) operate to catalyze these essential conjugation reactions. The control of Phase II reactions is of critical importance and is governed by physiological states , such as gender and reproductive status. Studies have shown that the expression and activity of Phase II enzymes and transport proteins , such as Mrp2 are significantly reduced during pregnancy, even though these enzymes play a crucial role in the transport of conjugated metabolites. This decrease could be aimed at safeguarding the growing fetus from xenobiotic toxicity by reducing the transfer of xenobiotics. In addition, following birth and during lactation, the levels of these enzymes are elevated, suggesting their adaptive role within a continuously changing physiological system. This dynamic regulation shows that Phase II reactions are not constitutive but adaptive to the life cycle of the organism, which attests to the complexity of xenobiotic metabolism in various circumstances (Arana et al., 2014). Besides, the interaction between aerobic and anaerobic metabolic processes in an organism also reflects the adaptive responses in xenobiotic biotransformation. The use of yeast models for the analysis has shown that changes in anaerobic glycolysis due to xenobiotic ketones can cause various metabolic responses, reflecting the need for multiple modeling approaches for understanding the interactions in detail. These models provide the insight that although simplistic and complex representations of metabolic pathways may result in equivalent mean concentrations and flux predictions, they can differ it concerns oscillatory dynamics that arise following xenobiotic exposure. These results illustrate the complexity inherent in the relationships between metabolic pathways and xenobiotic processing, which consequently shapes how organisms adjust to environmental toxins and manage metabolic needs (Beaudoin et al., 2004) (Figure 5.12).

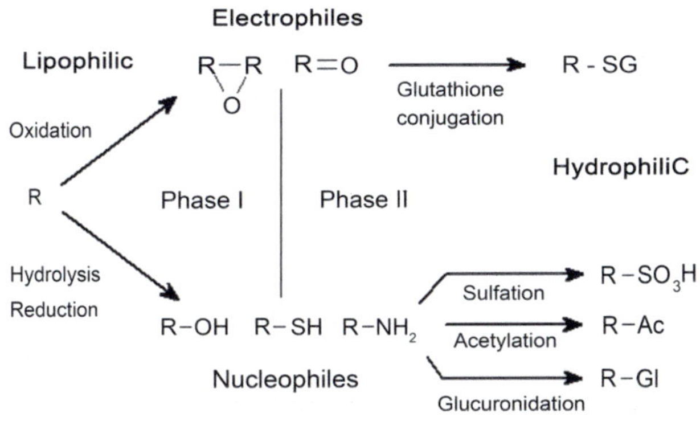

Figure 5.12. Phases I and II of the metabolisms of a lipophilic xenobiotic.

Source: https://upload.wikimedia.org/wikipedia/commons/9/97/Xenobiotic_metabolism.png.

5.3.3. Phase III Reactions

Phase III reactions constitute a crucial phase of biotransformation of xenobiotics, which consists predominantly of conjugation of various metabolites with endogenous substrates to enhance water solubility and facilitate excretion. The phase is also marked by the addition of functional groups , such as glucuronosyl, sulfate, or GSH to the modified xenobiotic or its Phase I or Phase II reaction-formed metabolites. Enzymic pathways, or transferases, play a core role in these reactions, with the conjugation process resulting in metabolites that are typically of lower toxicity and higher hydrophilicity than their parent molecule. This mechanism is as important for detoxification as it is for preventing the build-up of potential toxic substances in biological tissues, thereby maintaining cellular homeostasis (Esteves et al., 2021). In addition, Phase III reactions are not restricted to a single biological system; they occur in a variety of organisms, reflecting their evolutionary significance in xenobiotic metabolism. Specifically, interaction among metabolic pathways is crucial for effective detoxification. For example, the conjugation of several xenobiotics with each other can influence their bioavailability and toxicity. Synergetic effects of the reactions can control the overall metabolic capacity of the organism, determining responses to persistent organic pollutants or heavy metals. Current studies imply that environmental circumstances, such as the occurrence of co-contaminants, can increase or alter Phase III metabolisms with unpredictable ecological effects (Ceci et al., 2018). Knowledge of such interactions is critical for developing strategies that minimize the impact of xenobiotic exposure on human health and the environment. Phase III reaction studies are not only important to pharmacology and toxicology but also to bioremediation. Scientists can utilize microbial systems or fungi with enhanced biotransformation activity by knowing how organisms utilize these metabolic processes. These organisms can be used in bioremediation initiatives, particularly where there is a mixture of complex xenobiotics. The ability of bacteria and fungi to work together in breaking down toxic materials is a good method for degrading pollutants in contaminated environments (Ceci et al., 2018). Further studies on Phase III reactions will enhance the understanding of the process of biotransformation and improve existing biotechnological approaches. By merging knowledge of these metabolic pathways with environmental research, scientists can develop more effective and sustainable means to overcome the risks that xenobiotics pose (Figure 5.13).

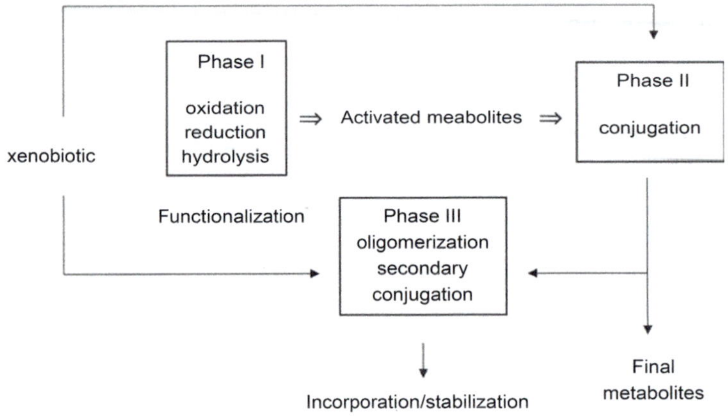

Figure 5.13. The three phases involved in the metabolism of xenobiotics.

Source: https://www.researchgate.net/profile/Christian-Mougin/publication/244586259/figure/fig1/AS:298517231882240@1448183462376/The-three-phases-involved-in-the-metabolism-of-xenobiotics.png.

Test Your Knowledge

1. What are the phase 1 reactions in biotransformation?
2. What are the reactions in phase 2 of biotransformation?

5.4. Enzymes Involved in Biotransformation

Learning Outcome

1. Describe the cytochrome P450 enzymes;
2. Know the transferases;
3. Understand the hydrolases.

Biotransformation is pivotal in the detoxification and removal of xenobiotics from living organisms, primarily by the activity of certain enzymes. Among these, cytochrome P450 enzymes (CYPs) are particularly critical since they can metabolize a broad range of organic chemicals, including drugs and environmental pollutants. The enzymes catalyze oxidation-reduction reactions that transform lipophilic xenobiotics into more hydrophilic species, facilitating their excretion. Particular interest is the CYP1A, which can be induced by exposure to aromatic hydrocarbons and polychlorinated biphenyls (PCBs). Its catalytic function has the capacity to generate reactive intermediates that covalently bind to DNA and cause mutagenic effects as well as potential carcinogenesis. CYP1A is thus not only an essential biotransformation enzyme but also a biomarker for quantifying organic contaminant exposure and toxicity in aquatic life (Livingston et al., 1994). Furthermore, the incorporation of biotransformation enzymes with the production of ROS complicates the xenobiotic effect further. Induction of CYP1A and ROS generation could trigger a series of biological processes culminating in oxidative stress and cell injury, impacting both DNA integrity and the health of the organism as a whole. The mechanisms underline the importance of using biomolecular markers, such as hepatic DNA-adducts and indicators of oxidative stress, for assessing the magnitude of chemical exposure. Such markers will have to be taken into account in an integrated manner, therefore suggesting the likely effectiveness of application of a combination of antioxidant analyses along with pro-oxidant profiling in effectively quantifying biological responses to various pollutants. In addition, ROS-dependent process research can contribute to insight into the broad effects of xenobiotic exposure at a range of levels of biological organization, from cellular physiology to organismal fitness (Livingston et al., 1994). Fungi have been effective agents in biotransformation processes for the remediation of contaminated ecosystems , such as waters and soils, where there is organic and metal poisoning. With enzymatic machinery that is present in fungi, such as lignin peroxidases, manganese peroxidases, and laccases, it is possible to break down recalcitrant xenobiotics. These biodegradation pathways illustrate the capability of fungi to detoxify toxic chemicals and rebalance ecological processes. Fungal-bacterial co-action during these bioremediation processes enhances xenobiotic degradation efficiencies and, therefore, the success of applying biotechnological solutions. As human activities continue to expose the environment to compounds ranging from a broad variety of pollutants, studies on metal and organic contaminant co-occurrence synergistic and antagonistic impacts become essential in formulating sustainable remediation strategies.

5.4.1. Cytochrome P450 Enzymes

The cytochrome P450 enzymes play a crucial role in the biotransformation of xenobiotics, enabling the metabolism of a wide range of foreign substances within the organism. They are predominantly active within the liver, oxidizing the foreign substances, a process that leads to the breakdown and elimination of the substances. The overall versatility of cytochrome P450 (CYP) enzymes is seen in their ability to metabolize a variety of groups of compounds, from drugs to environmental pollutants and dietary components. Importantly, induction of specific CYP enzymes is applied as molecular biomarkers for environmental exposure to toxic xenobiotics, thus providing information on the biochemical responses of aquatic organisms to contaminants. For example, hepatic CYP1A is induced to a considerable extent by organic pollutants , such as aromatic hydrocarbons, in keeping with a well-documented correlation between exposure to environmental toxins and enzyme activity (Livingston et al., 1994). The activity of cytochrome P450 has implications that go beyond detoxification per se, since these enzymes also participate in the pharmacokinetics of drugs and can lead to severe drug interactions. For instance, plant products like grapefruit juice and certain herbal nutritional supplements have been noted to inhibit CYP enzymes, thus modifying drug metabolism and potentially leading to adverse medical outcomes. Research has revealed that the consumption of some natural drinks usually coincides with physician-prescribed medication regimens, which demands more attention from practitioners to such interactions. The principal pathway of such drug-nutrient interactions is frequently associated with inhibition or induction of CYP enzyme activity, which underscores the importance of knowing endogenous and exogenous factors that could influence these biotransformation reactions (Bacinschi et al., 2020). In addition to their role in metabolism, cytochrome P450 enzymes are also implicated in other physiological and disease processes, including carcinogenesis. The catalytic activity of these enzymes converts xenobiotic chemicals into reactive intermediates, which can covalently bind to cellular macromolecules like DNA, leading to mutations and ultimately cancer. In fish, for instance, induction of hepatic CYP1A has been utilized as a commonly employed biomarker to identify the effect of environmental pollution, demonstrating a precise correlation between elevated CYP1A levels and the presence of carcinogenic substances in aquatic ecosystems. This xenobiotic biotransformation not only is the biological xenobiotic response but also points towards a potential application for applying CYP enzyme activity as an indicator of ecological health and organism fitness and thus linking environmental science with public health concerns raised by chemical carcinogenesis research (Livingston et al., 1994) (Figure 5.14).

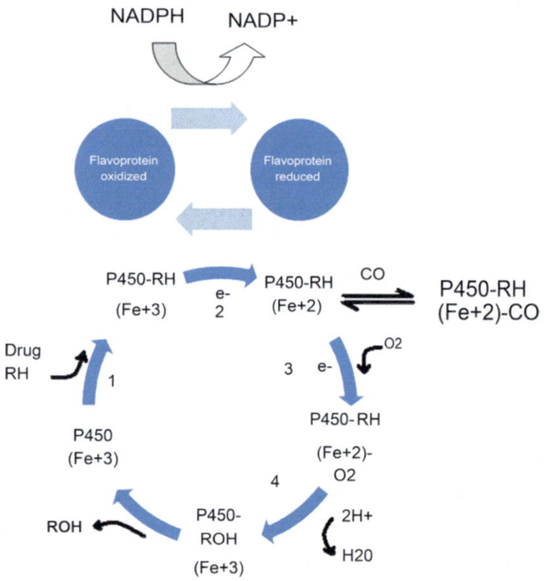

Figure 5.14. Cytochrome P450 cycle, RH is the parent drug, ROH is the oxidized metabolite, e^- is an electron.

Source: https://howmed.net/wp-content/uploads/2012/06/Biotransformation-cycle.png.

5.4.2. Transferases

Transferases play a central role in the biotransformation of xenobiotics, which are foreign substances introduced into the organism, such as environmental pollutants and drugs. The enzymes catalyze the transfer of a functional group of a specific type, such as methyl, acetyl, or glucuronic acid, from highly energetic donor molecules to xenobiotic substrate molecules. Solubility is increased through the process and excretion of potentially toxic compounds, thus preventing toxicity to the organism. Transferase activity is not only essential for xenobiotic detoxification but also for metabolic activation that could lead to the generation of reactive intermediates. Illumination of the intricacy of transferases is key to appreciating their function in drug metabolism and pharmacokinetics, as evidenced by current research revealing a broad spectrum of transferase enzymes present in human tissues, especially in the liver and skin (Cupitt et al., 2012). Different transferase groups have evolved to fit the specific chemical properties of xenobiotics and thus exhibit differing substrate specificity. GSTs, for instance, are implicated in the GSH conjugation of a wide variety of electrophilic substances as protection against toxic metabolites and oxidative damage. Similarly, UGTs catalyze the glucuronic acid transfer from UDP-glucuronic acid onto lipophilic xenobiotics to produce more hydrophilic substances for effective excretion. As these enzymes have distinctive tissue distribution patterns and interindividual variation under the control of genetic factors, their study carries a vital significance for personal medicine. Interestingly, recent research on human skin proteomic profiles has confirmed the presence of numerous xenobiotic-metabolizing enzymes, which denotes the significance of the skin in chemical exposure metabolism and safety testing, an essential step toward enhancing public health measures (Cupitt et al., 2012). Further, understanding transferases in xenobiotic biotransformation is notably important in environmental and biomedical toxicology. As research on them keeps on enhancing, it has now become clear that their activity can be regulated by various agents, e.g., the co-administration of various xenobiotics, nutritional state, and genetic polymorphisms. It may lead to altered metabolic rates, which can affect the pharmacological efficacy and toxicity of drugs. By employing *in vitro* models that simulate human skin and liver enzymatic activity, researchers can better determine the safety and metabolic profiles of novel xenobiotics. These models not only offer a tool for extrapolating human response to chemical exposure but also suggest areas of therapeutic intervention when environmental toxicity is encountered. These findings underscore the vital need for ongoing investigation into transferase enzymology to resolve complex biotransformation processes of xenobiotics and their effects on human health.

5.4.3. Hydrolases

Hydrolases are an essential group of enzymes that catalyze the hydrolysis of numerous biomolecules, and their contribution towards the biotransformation of xenobiotics in biological organisms cannot be overemphasized. By catalyzing the breakdown of organic molecules, hydrolases are central to detoxification and the elimination of potentially toxic compounds that an organism comes into contact with. The most important role these enzymes play is clearly seen in the xenobiotics; alien substances that can disrupt biological processes. Understanding the distinct paths and mechanisms through which hydrolases operate allows for a better understanding of their significance in biological detoxification processes. Furthermore, advances in proteomic tools have allowed for the identification and characterization of several hydrolases and given data on their activities within different environments, including human skin and microbial interaction within ecosystems, which are important for effective xenobiotic management (Cupitt et al., 2012). The role of hydrolases in the process of interacting with xenobiotics underscores the complexity of biotransformation processes. The enzymes not only enable the breakdown of various pollutants but also exhibit specificity as they are directed towards individual chemical groups to hydrolyze. Such specificity is crucial for efficient detoxification of harmful substances because the hydrolytic action of the hydrolases can lead to the formation of less toxic or more excretable metabolites. Extremely notable is the advancement in bioremediation technologies that tap the power of hydrolases for the regulation of xenobiotics in contaminated systems. A case in point, certain fungi species have been found to biosynthesize hydrolases that efficiently convert organic pollutants, thus providing a green, sustainable way of remediation. Such biotransformation reactions are vital, as bioremediation not only restores environmental health but also accumulates ecosystem resistance towards complex cocktails of toxicants (Ceci et al., 2018). Also, hydrolases have a primary role in the study of their environmental and health impact on humans, especially with the increase in the xenobiotic exposure level due to industrialization. Their role in hydrolyzing xenobiotics contributes to the understanding of the metabolic pathway and predictive models for assessing bioaccumulation and toxicity. For example, in human epidermis, a very diverse set of hydrolases has been discovered that potentially dictate the metabolic fate of dermatological xenobiotics, suggesting the skin's potential to be a barrier as well as a metabolic interface. Yet, research on hydrolases provides highly valuable information for risk assessment and safety evaluation of chemicals, particularly for what they do with biological systems. It is key to the development of strategies that negate the damaging effects of xenobiotics and promote public well-being and environmental sustainability (Cupitt et al., 2012) (Figure 5.15).

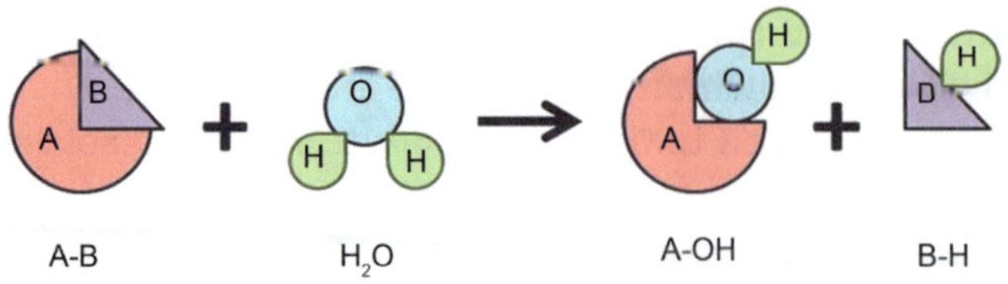

Figure 5.15. Hydrolases are the largest and most diverse class of enzymes, with more than 200 enzymes that catalyze the hydrolysis of several types of compounds.

Source: https://cdnintech.com/media/chapter/80269/1512345123/media/UF1.png.

Test Your Knowledge

1. What are cytochrome P450 enzymes?
2. What is the transferase enzyme?

5.5. Implications of Biotransformation

Learning Outcome

1. Describe the reduction of toxicity associated with xenobiotics;
2. Know the process of drug metabolism;
3. Describe the environmental impact of xenobiotics.

Biotransformation, the chemical alteration of xenobiotics by biochemical means, has significance that extends to the health of humans as well as the safety of the environment. The metabolic activities through different biological mechanisms, such as the gut microbiome, are crucial factors in the determination of the toxicity and bioavailability of xenobiotics. Through the change in the chemical makeup of the compounds, biotransformation can make toxic chemicals less harmful or, alternatively, produce more toxic metabolites. This double nature renders it difficult to assess risks of xenobiotic exposure, particularly in the case of numerous drugs and environmental pollutants that are encountered by humans in daily life. Understanding how biotransformations work is important in designing efficient detoxification mechanisms and pharmacological action, thereby highlighting the need for an integrated approach to both biochemistry and toxicology in solving potential hazards to health due to exposure to xenobiotics. In the field of human health, the role of the gut microbiota in xenobiotic biotransformation is an area of significant research. The multifaceted interactions between gut microorganisms and xenobiotics significantly contribute to drug metabolism, leading to variations in efficacy and safety profiles of drugs. Current data indicate that the gut microbiome can influence pharmacokinetics and, therefore, oral bioavailability and therapeutic effect (Jourov et al., 2016). It causes issues for personalized medicine since differences in the composition of gut microbiota between patients can necessitate customized drug delivery and dosing protocols. Furthermore, the capacity of the gut to metabolize xenobiotics raises issues of impacts triggered by the environment, pointing out that the health of the microbiome needs to be considered in human health and resistance to contaminants' assessments. Biotransformation impacts are not restricted to human health but extend to environmental impacts within interdependent ecosystems. The One Health idea emphasizes interdependence among human, animal, and environmental well-being and how xenobiotic exposure affects a variety of organisms (Haschek et al., 2019). Pesticides and xenobiotics from the environment interact with aquatic organisms, microorganisms, and plants, thereby affecting biodiversity and ecosystem stability. Biotransformation of such xenobiotics could be a significant process in which these pollutants play their role in affecting food security and health effects in all organisms. Therefore, further study of the biotransformation process is imperative while evaluating the environmental risk and planning the control measures, pointing again towards the need for integrated research that accounts for the holistic implications of human activities on the ecosystem and vice versa.

5.5.1. Toxicity Reduction

The reduction of toxicity associated with xenobiotics is one of the main concerns of the area of biotransformation, prompting a perception of the manner in which foreign compounds interfere with biological systems. Biotransformation reactions primarily focus on the activity of converting lipophilic xenobiotic substances into more polar and hydrophilic derivatives that can be easily excreted through the urine or bile. This biotransformation is especially significant in that many of the xenobiotics are very toxic, e.g., they have carcinogenic and/or teratogenic activity. Identification of specific biotransformation pathways, particularly those which lead to detoxification, is a critical factor in formulating interventions that have the ability to regulate the deleterious effects of toxic metabolites. Recent advances in computerized tools for the extraction and assessment of such biotransformation reactions, such as XenoMet, indicate the progress of the compilation and categorization of the various substrates and metabolites involved (Biziukova et al., 2025). They have a key function in lowering the toxic substance load within biological systems and the environment. In terms of environmental and human health, the ability to reduce toxicity through biotransformation is imperative. Xenobiotics, which are prevalent due to industrial activities and agriculture, can become concentrated in ecosystems and result in toxic bioaccumulation. Phase I and Phase II reactions of biotransformation occur synergistically to metabolize such compounds, with Phase I reactions altering the chemical structure of xenobiotics and Phase II reactions conjugating these metabolites with the endogenous substances for excretion. It is, however, crucial to note that in some instances, biotransformation ends up producing even more toxic metabolites, thus diminishing the toxicity reduction objective (Mahanayak, 2024). As such, balanced comprehension of such routes is necessary not only for the evaluation of risk but also for therapeutic action to counteract xenobiotic toxicity effectively. New bioremediation approaches and regulatory mechanisms are also of key relevance to the quest for minimizing toxicity. With the establishment of guidelines, such as the REACH and TSCA acts, resultant risks through xenobiotic exposure can be regulated beforehand. These paradigms are complemented by advances in biotechnological measures, including the application of genetically modified organisms (GMOs) that can decompose some xenobiotic toxins in polluted environments. These approaches, besides minimizing toxicity, also improve the process of environmental rejuvenation. Integration of scientific information obtained from biotransformation studies with regulation and regulation, therefore, optimizes the overall effectiveness of methods to reduce toxicity, safeguarding public health and environmental integrity. Along with a further improvement of the understanding of xenobiotic behavior and biotransformation pathways, an integrated strategy uniting policy and biotransformation science will be required to ensure future success with decreased toxicity (Figure 5.16).

Figure 5.16. Hazard symbol indicating toxic or poisonous substances.

Source: https://images.squarespace-cdn.com/content/v1/612372f65142044df83bb180/1630146808289-9Y2JUTOQR3Y5ZNPWFGGT/Toxicity.jpeg?format=2500w.

5.5.2. Drug Metabolism

Drug metabolism lies at the heart of the pharmacological elimination of xenobiotics, such as drugs administered therapeutically. Metabolism involves biochemical modification of xenobiotics within the body through catalysis by enzymes, permitting the conversion of lipophilic drugs into less lipophilic metabolites. Conversion is significant because it facilitates effective excretion of such xenobiotics through urine or bile. The liver is the primary location of drug metabolism, and specialized enzymes like cytochrome P450 enzymes play a central role in many of the biotransformation reactions. The greater the understanding of the metabolic processes, the better the researchers can anticipate the pharmacokinetics of drugs and the ensuing implications for the treatment of patients, since diverse metabolic processes are accountable for differences in drug efficacy and toxicity. Among the vast array of reactions that drugs experience during processes of metabolism, one important pathway is the creation of carbon-carbon (C-C) bonds, mediated by cytochrome P450 enzymes. Generally seen in organic synthesis, this rare reaction is also of importance when it comes to drug metabolism, inasmuch as it aids in creating new drug metabolites. Recognition of metabolites generated by C-C bond formation can give valuable insights into drug metabolism and ultimately affect their therapeutic profiles. Furthermore, research that detects such mechanisms can not only guide drug design but also assist in mitigating side effects resulting from undesirable metabolites. As pharmacologically active metabolites are capable of possessing novel biological activities when compared to their parent molecules, the in-depth exploration of these C-C forming pathways is imperative to advance the art of drug metabolism (Liu et al., 2025). Metabolites of drugs are much more than the reductionist process of drug excretion; they play a pivotal role in significantly influencing the pharmacological and toxicological characteristics of xenobiotics. The biotransformation of the drug can lead to the formation of metabolites that are more or less active, with a potentiality to exert either therapeutically beneficial or harmful effects. Through thorough investigations of these processes, drug interactions and drug responses in individuals are revealed to be complex because of the differences in metabolic enzymes caused by genetics. As research scientists keep advancing annotated databases and study aids for studying such biotransformation processes, information obtained from there will be instrumental in optimizing drug therapies. In addition, an understanding of the nuances of drug metabolism will be pivotal in creating safer, more effective pharmacological therapies and controlling, on a rational basis, xenobiotics prescribed to individuals (Biziukova et al., 2025).

5.5.3. Environmental Impact

The environmental impact of xenobiotics, particularly those from anthropogenic sources , such as industrialization and agriculture, is a serious challenge to organisms and ecosystems. Xenobiotics come into various environmental matrices, particularly aquatic matrices, and therefore lead to their bioaccumulation in organisms at the local level. The introduction of organic pollutants, including persistent organic pollutants and potentially toxic metals, seriously disturbs the equilibrium of nature. The biotransformation reactions initiated by organisms in response to such pollutants play a critical role in mediating their toxicity. The CYP1A of the liver biotransformation enzyme is an effective biomarker of exposure to organic contaminants since induction has a close correlation with toxic effects in aquatic vertebrates. Also, induction of ROS generation is a sign of the multidimensionality of environmental xenobiotic-induced toxicity, which can potentially lead to harmful health effects, including carcinogenesis in the targeted species (Livingston et al., 1994).

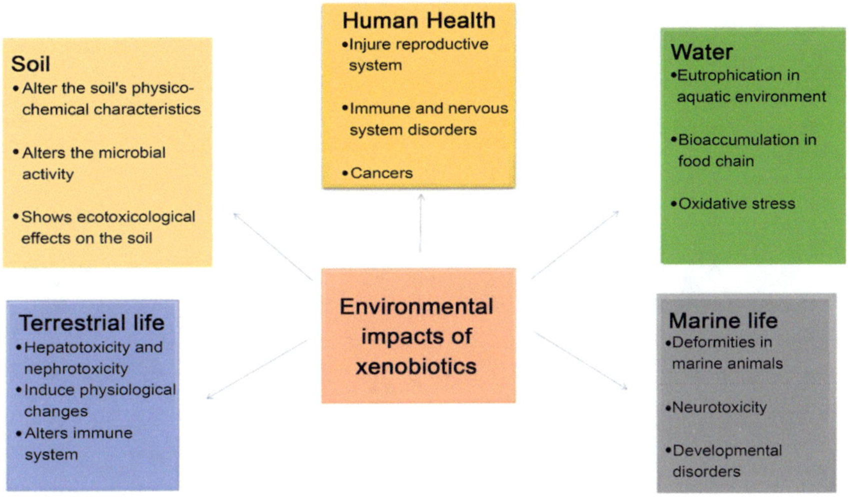

Figure 5.17. Environmental impact of xenobiotics.

Source: https://media.springernature.com/lw685/springer-static/image/chp%3A10.1007%2F978-3-031-35775-6_1/MediaObjects/537248_1_En_1_Fig2_HTML.png.

Also, the coexistence of several toxicants at the same time complicates assessment of their action in the environment because complex chemical interaction can produce synergistic effects that enhance overall toxicity. The simultaneous presence of metals and organic compounds contaminates water and soil, disrupting ecological functions and reducing ecosystem services. For instance, the disruption of biochemical processes in aquatic organisms can hinder their development, reproduction, and survival, eventually threatening biodiversity. In response to the augmenting problem from xenobiotic exposure, innovative bioremediation approaches involving fungi and bacteria have been established. These methods are designed to revitalize contaminated habitats by degrading or transforming toxic compounds to less harmful states. Fungal bioremediation incorporation demonstrates a viable sustainable approach to mitigating the adverse effects of xenobiotic pollution on ecosystems, promoting rehabilitation and resistance in ravaged environments (Ceci et al., 2018). The persistent threat posed by xenobiotics emphasizes the imperative need for comprehensive measures to track and manage their environmental influence. Understanding the biochemical responses of various organisms to xenobiotic exposure could be beneficial to conservation practice and policy designs. Moreover, applying biomarker measurements, e.g., CYP1A activity determination, could help in monitoring the effectiveness of remediation processes. Furthermore, increased research on how fungi and bacteria react with each other during the bioremediation processes to discover maximum means of handling co-contaminated habitats is warranted. By unraveling the complexities of xenobiotic interactions and their biological consequences, scientists and ecologists can better predict longer-term consequences to ecosystems and start procedures for optimizing ecological integrity and sustainability in the face of ongoing anthropogenic pressures (Livingston et al., 1994; Ceci et al., 2018) (Figure 5.17).

Test Your Knowledge

1. What is toxicity reduction?
2. What is the process of drug metabolism?

SUMMARY

In summarizing xenobiotic and biotransformation research, it is evident that these processes are essential in an understanding of foreign compounds' physiological and environmental impacts on biological systems. The highly complex character of xenobiotic-organism interactions emphasizes the worth of systematic investigation with various biological and ecological contexts. Human activities, particularly industrialization and agriculture, have led to widespread pollution of the ecosystem, with compounds potentially harmful and in need of new remediation technologies. In all these cases, the application of bioremediation technologies with fungi and bacteria as a worthy sustainable technology is salient. Through the elaboration of bioremediation processes, we are able to minimize the adverse effects of co-contaminated sites, ultimately leading to improved ecological performance and higher ecosystem services (Ceci et al., 2018). In further enrichment of this discussion of xenobiotics, it is evident that one of the most significant potentials of untargeted metabolomics in toxicology is its ability to comprehensively describe the metabolic responses elicited by xenobiotic exposure. This emerging discipline is enabled through the comprehension of both the fate of the xenobiotic and the biotransformation products. The integration of the measurement of untargeted exposure and measures of physiological response provides an advanced comprehension of how endogenous biochemical processes react to the presence of foreign chemicals. Utilizing a metabolomics platform, researchers are able to discern biotransformation maps, providing an understanding of systemic exposure levels over time and bridging internal doses to metabolic responses. This development paves the way for enhanced risk assessments in environmental health and toxicology (Bowen et al., 2023). Overall, the studies of xenobiotics and biotransformation are of prime importance in an overarching discussion on environmental sustainability and public health. The potential of bioremediation technologies is in line with a growing perception of the need for sustainable means to manage soil and water pollution. Similarly, the application of cutting-edge analytical techniques like untargeted metabolomics enables better insights into xenobiotic metabolism and its implications for human health. With continued research breakthroughs, such transdisciplinary interactions will be key to establishing effective countermeasures against the long-term issues of xenobiotics. Ultimately, more research and transdisciplinarity into these areas will not only enhance ecological resilience but also safeguard human populations against the adverse effects of environmental pollutants.

The interaction between biological systems and xenobiotics is characterized by the complex mechanisms of biotransformation that represent the first line of defense in the conversion of lipophilic compounds into more hydrophilic metabolites. The process of hydrophilic conversion is facilitated by enzymes , such as cytochrome P450, which catalyze oxidative reactions that allow for the elimination of potentially harmful substances. The significance of biotransformation extends beyond detoxification to include the biotransformation of certain xenobiotics into pharmacologically active compounds. This common activity underscores the importance of understanding biotransformation pathways, which are regulated by a large number of factors, including genetic variation and environmental influences, to manage personal drug and environmental toxin responses. Recent studies have also highlighted the acute presentation of liver dysfunction in the context of sepsis, which can significantly alter biotransformation processes. According to studies, hepatobiliary transport and biotransformation dysfunction can be as early as six hours after peritoneal contamination and support the proposition that conventional measures of liver function are not necessarily indicative of the complete degree of dysfunction in the critically ill. Specifically, the disruption of bile acid transport pathways, along with drug metabolism changes, defines a nuanced dynamic between exposure to xenobiotics and hepatic response. These findings support the necessity for the inclusion of new biomarkers, such as plasma bile acids, into clinical practice, since they may provide enhanced predictability about the prognosis and management of liver failure in critically ill patients (Bauer et al., 2012). Understanding the xenobiotic implications and biotransformation mechanisms is necessary to optimize therapeutic intervention and the safety of the patient. An understanding of genetic polymorphisms that affect enzyme activity can inform personalized medicine approaches to maximize drug effect with minimal side effects. Early detection of impaired biotransformation capacity can guide early interventions that may preclude the onset of conditions , such as sepsis. The studies in this field keep progressing not only to advance the theoretical foundation but also to be realized into actual applications in pharmacotherapy and toxic evaluation. As the body of knowledge keeps expanding, it is important to continuously evaluate the clinical usefulness of these discoveries in order to finally improve the management of those disorders that are extremely reliant on xenobiotic interactions and biotransformations (Reinen, 2010).

KEY TERMS FROM THIS CHAPTER

- Biotransformation
- Environmental pollutants
- Hydrolysis
- Organic chemicals
- Pesticides
- Superoxide dismutase
- Synthetic xenobiotics
- Xenobiotics
- Catalase
- Environmental xenobiotics
- Microorganisms
- Oxidation
- Pharmaceuticals
- Synthetic chemicals
- Toxicology

Critical Thinking Questions

1. What are xenobiotics?

a. Naturally occurring biomolecules

b. Foreign substances introduced into the body

c. Endogenous metabolic byproducts

d. Essential vitamins

2. Which organ is the primary site for biotransformation of xenobiotics?

a. Kidney

b. Liver

c. Lungs

d. Stomach

3. Biotransformation of xenobiotics primarily occurs in which two phases?

a. Absorption and distribution

b. Phase I and Phase II reactions

c. Detoxification and excretion

d. Oxidation and hydrolysis

4. Which of the following is a key enzyme in Phase I reactions of biotransformation?

a. Cytochrome P450

b. Glutathione transferase

c. UDP-glucuronosyltransferase

d. Acetyl-CoA synthase

5. The primary function of Phase II reactions in xenobiotic metabolism is:

a. Oxidation of lipids

b. Conjugation to increase water solubility

c. Reduction of reactive intermediates

d. Hydrolysis of proteins

Short Answer Questions

1. Define the xenobiotics.
2. What are the biotransformation processes?
3. List the types of xenobiotics.
4. What are the sources of xenobiotics?
5. What enzymes are involved in biotransformation?

Answers to Critical Thinking Questions

1. (b); 2. (b); 3. (b); 4. (a); 5. (b)

REFERENCES

1. Sanchez, W., Palluel, O., Meunier, L., Coquery, M., Porcher, J. M., & Aït-Aïssa, S. (2005). Copper-induced oxidative stress in three-spined stickleback: relationship with hepatic metal levels. *Environmental toxicology and pharmacology, 19*(1), 177–183. https://doi.org/10.1016/j.etap.2004.07.003(accessed on 12th June 2025).
2. Andersen, H. R., Plósz, B. G., Polesel, F., et al. (2016). Removal of antibiotics in biological wastewater treatment systems—A critical assessment using the activated sludge modeling framework for xenobiotics (ASM-X). https://core.ac.uk/download/83999792.pdf (accessed on 12th June 2025).
3. Arana, M. R., Arias, A., Mottino, A. D., et al. (2014). Hepatic and intestinal biotransformation and transport of xenobiotics during pregnancy and lactation. https://core.ac.uk/download/52482137.pdf (accessed on 12th June 2025).
4. Asif, M., Marques, A. R., Martiniano, H., et al. (2022). A role for gene-environment interactions in autism spectrum disorder is supported by variants in genes regulating the effects of exposure to xenobiotics. https://core.ac.uk/download/553619785.pdf (accessed on 12th June 2025).
5. Bacinschi N, Pogonea I, Podgurschi L, Mihalachi-Anghel M, Ştefănescu E, Socea B, Chianu M. The Role of Biotransformation Processes in Mediating Interactions Between Psychotropic Drugs and Natural Products. *Journal of Mind and Medical Sciences*. 2020; 7(1):9-15. https://doi.org/10.22543/7674.71.P915 (accessed on 12th June 2025).
6. Bauer, M., Carré, J. E., Claus, R. A., et al. (2012). Liver dysfunction and phosphatidylinositol-3-kinase signaling in early sepsis: Experimental studies in rodent models of peritonitis. https://core.ac.uk/download/525035372.pdf (accessed on 12th June 2025).
7. Biziukova, N., Rudik, A., Dmitriev, A. V., Tarasova, O., Filimonov, D., & Poroikov, V. (2025). XenoMet: A corpus of texts to extract data on metabolites of xenobiotics. *ACS Omega, 10*, 2459–2471. https://www.semanticscholar.org/paper/83255d5fdb7f4ef5a157c81e74014971f11cd608 (accessed on 12th June 2025).
8. Bowen, T. J., Hall, A. R., Lloyd, G. R., et al. (2023). Simultaneously discovering the fate and biochemical effects of pharmaceuticals through untargeted metabolomics. https://core.ac.uk/download/577503433.pdf (accessed on 12th June 2025).
9. Brusch, L., Cuniberti, G., & Bertau, M. (2004). Model evaluation for glycolytic oscillations in yeast biotransformation's of xenobiotics. *Biophysical Chemistry, 109*(3), 413–426. https://doi.org/10.1016/j.bpc.2003.12.004 (accessed on 12th June 2025).
10. Ceci, A., Pinzari, F., Russo, F., Persiani, A. M., & Gadd, G. M. (2019). Roles of saprotrophic fungi in biodegradation or transformation of organic and inorganic pollutants in co-contaminated sites. *Applied microbiology and biotechnology, 103*(1), 53–68. https://doi.org/10.1007/s00253-018-9451-1(accessed on 12th June 2025).
11. Cerliani, M. B., & Richard, S. M. (2013). Polymorphism analysis of genes involved in xenobiotic metabolism and circadian rhythm in human breast cancer. https://core.ac.uk/download/159296732.pdf (accessed on 12th June 2025).
12. Chauveau, A. (2023). Intestinal permeability and gut microbiota interactions of phytochemicals from herbal drugs used in the treatment of depressive, anxiety and sleeping disorders. https://core.ac.uk/download/611511666.pdf (accessed on 12th June 2025).

13. Cupitt, J., Edwards, R. J., Fritsche, E., et al. (2012). Elucidation of xenobiotic metabolism pathways in human skin and human skin models by proteomic profiling. https://core.ac.uk/download/29820498.pdf (accessed on 12th June 2025).

14. Kuo, D.T.F., Rattner, B.A., Marteinson, S.C. *et al.* A Critical Review of Bioaccumulation and Biotransformation of Organic Chemicals in Birds. *Reviews Env.Contamination (formerly:Residue Reviews)* **260**, 6 (2022). https://doi.org/10.1007/s44169-021-00007-1 (accessed on 12th June 2025).

15. Dudley, S., Gan, J., Sun, C., al. (2018). Pharmaceutical and personal care products-induced stress symptoms and detoxification mechanisms in cucumber plants. https://core.ac.uk/download/287621692.pdf (accessed on 12th June 2025).

16. Esteves, F., Kranendonk, M., & Rueff, J. (2021). The central role of cytochrome P450 in xenobiotic metabolism—A brief review on a fascinating enzyme family. https://core.ac.uk/download/459213508.pdf (accessed on 12th June 2025).

17. Livingston, D.R.,Förlin, L.,George, S.G.,Sutcliffe, D.W. (2021). Molecular biomarkers and toxic consequences of impact by organic pollution in aquatic organisms.(4), 154-171. http://hdl.handle.net/1834/22821 (accessed on 12th June 2025).

18. Golovinsky, E., Ivanov, I., Satchanska, G., et al. (2006). Xenobiotic biotransformation potential of *Pseudomonas Rhodesia* KCM-R5 and *Bacillus subtilis* KCM-RG5, tolerant to heavy metals and phenol derivatives. https://core.ac.uk/download/12037445.pdf (accessed on 12th June 2025).

19. Haschek, W., Berenbaum, M., Hinton, D., Cora, M., Chernoff, N., Travlos, G., Liu, C. W., et al. (2019). Pathology in ecological research with implications for One Health: Session summary. *Toxicologic Pathology, 47*, 1072–1075. https://www.semanticscholar.org/paper/d9c5bae784230cbd1009804807d3c0a5a34808f6 (accessed on 12th June 2025).

20. Heid, C., Thomaidis, N., Damalas, D., Panagopoulou, E., Aalizadeh, R., Schweizer, M., Köhler, H., et al. (2019). Influence of pH on the toxicity, uptake and biotransformation potential of citalopram in zebrafish (*Danio rerio*) embryos. *Global NEST International Conference on Environmental Science & Technology*. https://www.semanticscholar.org/paper/af9cf7d47831157074c8fbd535c28e3f329d62c5 (accessed on 12th June 2025).

21. Hutchinson, T. H., Madden, J. C., Naidoo, V., et al. (2014). Comparative metabolism as a key driver of wildlife species sensitivity to human and veterinary pharmaceuticals. https://core.ac.uk/download/42478567.pdf (accessed on 12th June 2025).

22. Jourová, L., Anzenbacher, P., & Anzenbacherová, E. (2016). Human gut microbiota plays a role in the metabolism of drugs. *Biomedical Papers of the Medical Faculty of the University Palacky, Olomouc, Czechoslovakia, 160*(3), 317–326. https://www.semanticscholar.org/paper/55f745bdb4a8e00462902973890761 66d33c021f (accessed on 12th June 2025).

23. Khirk, M., Grigorenko, L., Lanskoy, D., et al. (2025). Neutron versus proton scattering on exotic nuclei: The ^{9}He example. https://www.semanticscholar.org/paper/986f5f3df3ac6945149daaf2aaf547cbc0accdaa (accessed on 12th June 2025).

24. Kumar, P. (2023). Degradation of xenobiotics by bacteria and fungi: An overview. *Biopesticides International*. https://www.semanticscholar.org/paper/8f6791f1fc3a4e591cddc810f9a19a438814d80c (accessed on 12th June 2025).

25. Lai, K. M., Lester, J. N., & Scrimshaw, M. D. (2002). Biotransformation and bioconcentration

of steroid estrogens by *Chlorella vulgaris*. https://core.ac.uk/download/333969.pdf (accessed on 12th June 2025).

26. Liu, J., & Zhang, D. (2025). Cytochrome P450-mediated carbon-carbon bond formation in drug metabolism. *Drug Metabolism Reviews, 57*, 51–66. https://www.semanticscholar.org/paper/0ec95868f5f8f021621d6ada081451b7e510ee33 (accessed on 12th June 2025).
27. Mahanayak, B. (2024). Biotransformation reactions of xenobiotics: Mechanisms and implications for environmental and human health. *World Journal of Biology Pharmacy and Health Sciences*. https://www.semanticscholar.org/paper/316ebdd770e940380f80af47be7186c7093d1533 (accessed on 12th June 2025).
28. Reinen, J. (2010). The role of biotransformation in the estrogenicity of xenobiotics. https://core.ac.uk/download/pdf/15463951.pdf (accessed on 12th June 2025).
29. Tadić, Đ. (2020). Uptake and metabolization of antibiotics in crops. https://core.ac.uk/download/365287170.pdf (accessed on 12th June 2025).
30. Truman, P. (2006). Toxicological effects of endocrine disrupting compounds in bluegill. https://core.ac.uk/download/268631559.pdf (accessed on 12th June 2025).
31. Yurchenko, P. O., Shkarupa, V. M., Kakarkin, O. Y., Kovalchuk, A. P., Kovalchuk, B. A., Pechevystiy, O. M., Filchukov, D. O., et al. (2024). Influence of CYP2D6 and its polymorphic forms on the metabolism of tamoxifen in therapy of luminal forms of breast cancer. *Reports of Vinnytsia National Medical University*. https://www.semanticscholar.org/paper/da14915eb63fe7c2d5192284f8ac850d0ae398c2 (accessed on 12th June 2025).

NUTRITION AND METABOLISM

6

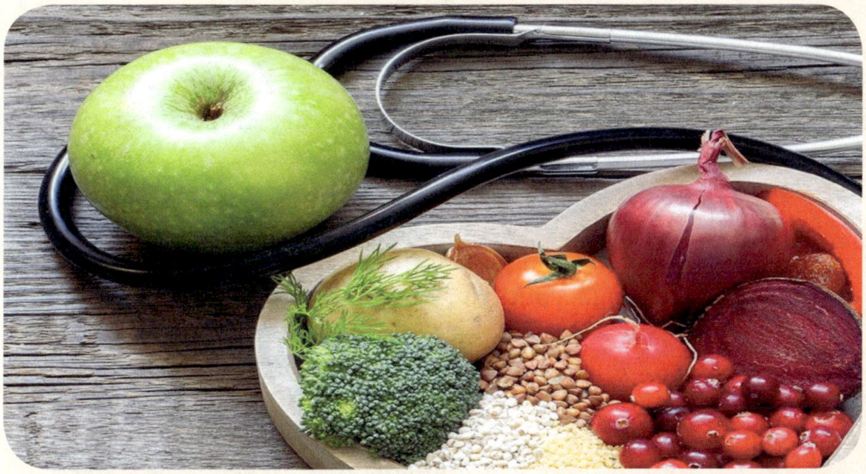

LEARNING OBJECTIVES

After studying this chapter, you will be able to:

1. Understand the role of macronutrients in nutrition and metabolism;
2. Describe the role of micronutrients in maintaining overall health and well-being;
3. Know the role of the digestive system in nutrition and metabolism;
4. Give an overview of metabolism;
5. Understand the concept of energy balance;
6. Describe the nutrition and disease.

Introduction

Understanding human metabolism and the intricacies that come with it is predicated on knowledge of nutrition. Nutrition entails the process of ingesting food and the nutrients that come with it, used to sustain life, optimize health, and grow and develop. Nutrients are categorized as macronutrients, such as carbohydrates, proteins, and fats, used for energy, and micronutrients, comprising vitamins and minerals, used in various physiological processes. When these nutrients are consumed by humans, their bodies produce a complex cascade of biochemical reactions to transform food into energy through metabolic pathways. The bioconversion emphasizes the critical role of proper and balanced nutrition; deficient or unbalanced consumption of nutrients has adverse effects on metabolism and health. Microbes' diverse functionality also requires attention in discussions with a focus towards nutrition, namely the effects on the microbiota-gut-brain axis. These microorganisms, including gut bacteria, have a vital function in maintaining digestive well-being and nutrient uptake. Current evidence highlights the importance of the microbiome in maintaining body weight, insulin sensitivity, and even the creation of short-chain fatty acids (SCFAs), essential for the health of the gut and metabolism. These microbial metabolites can influence systemic inflammation and metabolic reactions directly, demonstrating the intricate interplay between diet, gastrointestinal health, and general metabolic function. By learning about the relationship between nutrition and microbial ecology, one gains a greater insight into the influences of diet on health outcomes through metabolic mechanisms. Secondly, the ever-evolving nature of nutrition science highlights the profound influence of diet on mental health and cognitive function, partly due to the microbiota-gut-brain axis.

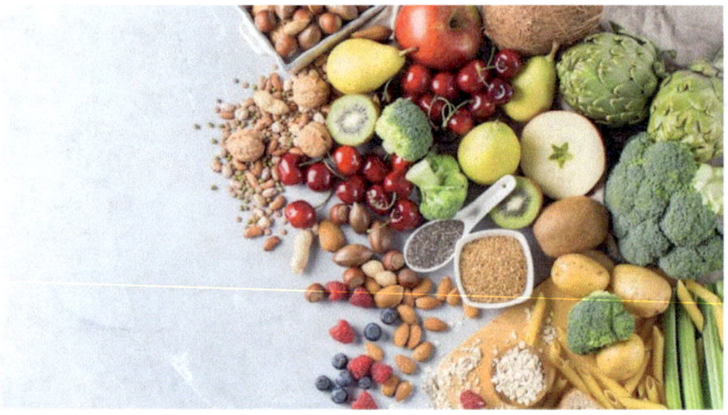

Figure 6.1. Nutrition is crucial to our metabolic health.

Source: https://images.ctfassets.net/mrbo2ykgx5lt/31103/a795427d0596952917 59a0359ffe43b4/nutrition-metabolism-health-diet-cardiovascular-diabetes-obesity-e1567576493654.jpg?&w=912&fm=webp&q=80.

The results show that certain components of the diet can influence brain chemistry and activity, and thereby mood and behavior. For instance, omega-3 fatty acid-dense and standardized antioxidant diets have been correlated with lowered depression and anxiety levels. Conversely, diet rich in processed foods may alter the composition of gut microbiota, which in turn may cause negative impacts on mental health. The liaison between nutrition, metabolism, and mental health is important in pointing out how an integrated approach to a healthy diet is not only vital to one's physical health but also to one's mental resilience, paving the way for future research on microbial-based therapies and therapeutic approaches to enhancing cognitive and emotional well-being (Figure 6.1).

Definition of Nutrition

Nutrition is a complex interaction of varied biochemical activities that are implicated in health promotion and maintenance of overall body functioning. In simple terms, nutrition refers to the intake of food and the ability of the body to digest, process, and utilize nutrients, both macronutrients, including carbohydrates, proteins, and fats, and micronutrients like vitamins and minerals. All nutrient categories have a unifying role to play in cellular functions, energy metabolism, and regulation of physiological homeostasis. To see where the scope of nutrition lies, it is required to know how these nutrients are used in the metabolic processes that sustain life. For instance, the hydrolysis of carbohydrates into glucose provides energy, while proteins provide amino acids for the repair and synthesis of tissue. By means of synthesizing these concepts, an overall understanding of nutrition emphasizes its fundamental significance in metabolism and overall health. The definition of nutrition has also been broadened to include more than merely the physical process of consuming food; it now includes the effect of eating habits upon disease conditions. Recent controversies among scientists emphasize the importance of gut microbiota in nutrition, particularly how diet could modulate the form and function of microbial populations. Such interactions reinforce the importance of a balanced diet in supporting healthy gut bacteria, with improved metabolic health as a consequence. For example, synbiotics are defined by the International Scientific Association for Probiotics and Prebiotics as combinations of live microorganisms and substrates selectively used by host microflora, revealing the intricate relationship between dietary aspects and intestinal wellness (Kelly et al., 2020). These findings confirm the intricacy of nutrition, in which interpreting the interaction between food and the body's metabolism can lead to innovation in dietary guidance and interventions. Also, the concept of nutrition extends further than the realm of individual nutrients to embrace broader diet patterns that support health and prevent disease. Probiotics, since the Food and Agriculture Organization of the United Nations has them as live microorganisms that have a positive effect upon the individual when ingested in adequate amounts, are one such paradigm (Borja et al., 2016). They talk to the gut microbiota and could improve a number of health outcomes through mechanisms like immunomodulation and enhancement of gut barrier functions. This novel emerging field of research emphasizes the intricate interrelationships between nutrition, metabolism, and health that can lead to personalized dietary strategies aimed at optimizing metabolic processes. With the growth in understanding of nutrition, there is an emphasis on the need for inclusive and evidence-informed dietary recommendations based on using scientific understanding of nutrition contribution to health promotion and well-being (Figure 6.2).

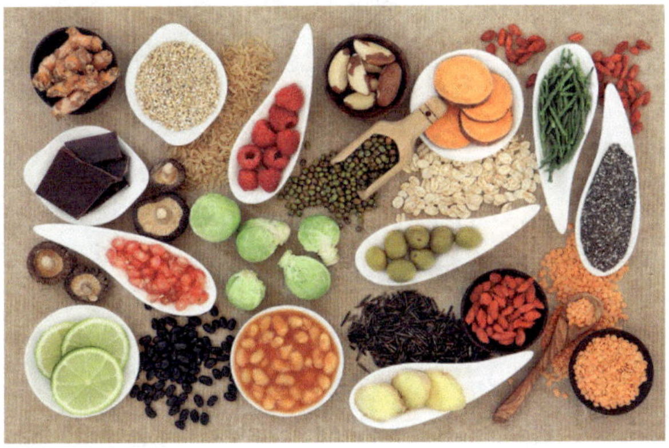

Figure 6.2. Nutrition.

Source: https://domf5oio6qrcr.cloudfront.net/medialibrary/16320/bigstock-health-food-selection-super-foods-fruits-veggies.jpg.

Importance of Nutrition in Health

The contribution of nutrition to the general well-being cannot be overrated since it has a direct impact on the metabolic process of the body. Proper nutrition provides the body with essential nutrients required for tissue growth and repair, enzyme synthesis, and the functioning of the immune system. For instance, the integrity of the intestinal barrier is controlled by a balanced diet with abundant heterogeneous nutrients, particularly those in vegetables and fruits. Deficiency in these factors leads to the impairment of this barrier, which results in vulnerability to a host of ailments due to impaired immunity. In addition, dysbiosis of gut microbiota may arise due to inappropriate food choices, aggravating disease conditions associated with metabolic disorders and compromising the body's defense mechanisms against pathogens (Jopkiewicz et al., 2019). Besides the intestinal barrier, the function of certain nutrients , such as potassium (K) also demonstrates the complex interrelation between nutrition and health. Potassium not only performs the role of muscle function and nerve transmission but is also needed for balance of fluid within cells. Unfortunately, recent patterns of consumption tend to lead to a deficiency of potassium intake, especially via the eating of processed food. These trends are linked with a deleterious rise in sodium consumption simultaneously, which could lead to subsequent health consequences, such as CVD and hypertension. Potassium's role in food yield and plant nutrition emphasizes the importance of considering nutrient composition towards shaping human health. Thus, the availability of adequate potassium-rich foods is significant in preventing nutrient deficiencies from current diets (Barreto et al., 2017). Additionally, the significance of nutrition includes preventing chronic diseases, highlighting its relevance to public health. Nourishment diseases , such as obesity, diabetes, and heart disease are increasing in society, typically due to inappropriate eating habits. By understanding the processes by which nutrition influences metabolism and health, a person can make enlightened choices that decrease their risk for disease. For example, an appropriate diet with whole grains, lean protein, and a combination of fruits and vegetables can maintain blood sugar in check and maximize metabolic function. These dietary modifications not only enhance physical health but also help ensure mental health stability, proving that nutrition is the backbone of effective health measures in today's world (Figure 6.3).

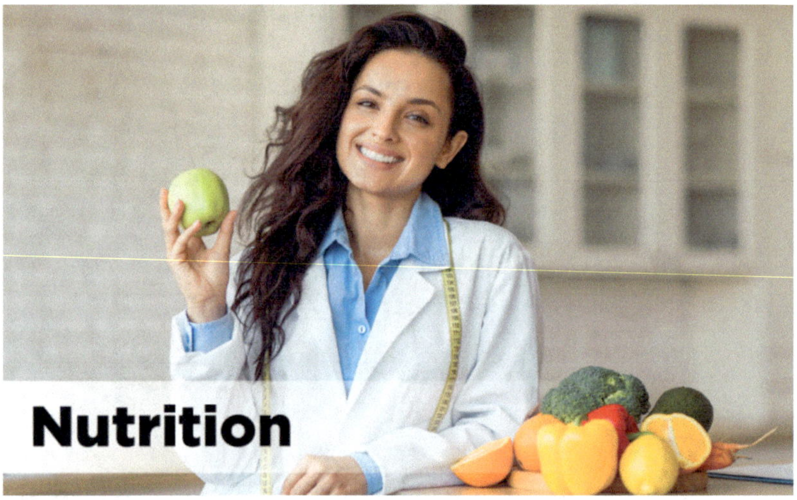

Figure 6.3. The role of nutrition in overall health.

Source: https://saintmarysreno.com/wp-content/uploads/2024/03/Primary-Care-Blog-2-march-2024-01.png.

6.1. Macronutrients

Learning Outcome

1. Describe the types and functions of carbohydrates;
2. Understand the role of proteins in body function;
3. Describe the essential fatty acids and energy in fats.

The role of macronutrients in metabolism and nutrition is at the heart of understanding how the body metabolizes and harnesses energy. Macronutrients, including carbohydrates, proteins, and fats, are the primary sources of energy for all body processes. Carbohydrates are catabolized in a process to provide immediate energy, and they exist in a broad array from simple sugars to complex starches. They are essential to brain function, as glucose is the substrate of choice for energy. The balance between simple and complex carbohydrates is significant in that it affects blood sugar and metabolic health. While proteins, however, are needed to fix tissues and build them up, and as structural components for enzymes and hormones, adequate consumption of protein promotes metabolic processes and can help in better body composition via stimulating the synthesis of muscles, thereby being of significant value in maintaining overall health and warding off disease. Fats are also essential macronutrients that contribute to energy storage and metabolic regulation. Not only do the lipids provide a high-energy source, but they also facilitate the transport of fat-soluble vitamins (A, D, E, and K). Fatty acids, particularly omega-3 and omega-6, are also important for cell membrane integrity and participation in anti-inflammatory processes. Various types of fat influence metabolism in special ways, with unsaturated fats tending to be associated with favorable health outcomes compared to saturated fats. Balancing these macronutrients is essential because excessive intake of any single macronutrient will lead to disruption of the metabolism and diseases , such as obesity and insulin resistance, illustrating the importance of food choice in establishing good health and well-being. In addition to supplying energy and maintaining body functions, macronutrients also impact significantly metabolic health and disease management. Macronutrient make-up of foods influences glycemic and lipid profiles, important chronic condition management parameters, especially in individuals with diabetes or prediabetes. The American Diabetes Association recommends the utilization of medical nutrition therapy for diabetes control, where individualized composition of macronutrients is required to achieve maximum health benefit (Alison et al., 2019). Further, information on macronutrient interactions can guide nutritional counseling in order to enhance metabolic efficiency and rectify health disparities. These results stress the key role that education on macronutrient consumption plays in public health policy and the general strategy for promoting healthier lifestyles and better metabolic health (Figure 6.4).

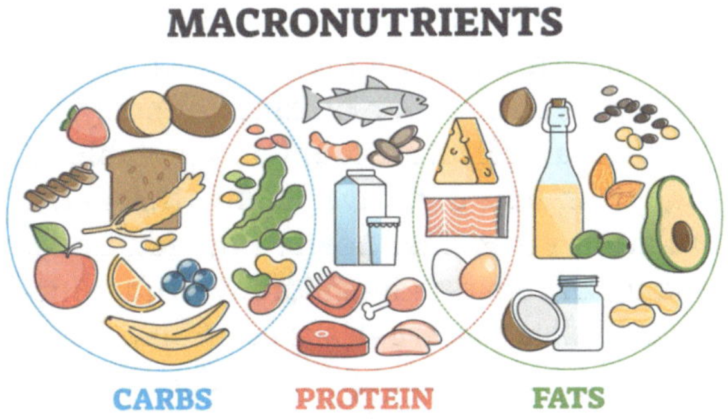

Figure 6.4. Macronutrients.

Source: https://www.cedars-sinai.org/content/dam/cedars-sinai/blog/2022/1/what-are-macronutrients.jpg.

6.1.1. Carbohydrates: Types and Functions

The classification of carbohydrates into simple and complex carbohydrates is significant in their roles in human nutrition. The simple carbohydrates have one or two units of sugar, which they easily assimilate into and yield an instantaneous source of energy. They include glucose and sucrose in fruit, honey, and table sugar. These carbohydrates are generally associated with a quick spike in blood glucose, which leads to a rapid release of insulin. Starch and fiber are complex carbohydrates composed of longer chains of sugar units and are found in whole grains, legumes, and vegetables. These are slower to digest and dump a steady supply of glucose into the system and thus are especially relevant in maintaining energy levels over time. These distinctions are key to grasping the dietary options that favor metabolic health. The functions played by carbohydrates are not merely as a supply of energy, but also very important roles in supporting body function and maintaining overall health. Carbohydrates have a critical role to play in brain function due to the fact that glucose is the major source of energy for the central nervous system (CNS). They also contribute to the regulation of blood sugar and insulin sensitivity, both of which are critical factors in metabolic health and disease prevention. For instance, dietary fiber, a complex carbohydrate found in vegetables and fruits, promotes digestive health through the stimulation of normal bowel function and the avoidance of constipation. Moreover, fiber intake has been linked to lower risks of chronic diseases , such as type 2 diabetes, CVD, and colorectal cancer. The understanding of the action of carbohydrates at various levels—cellular, physiological, and metabolic—is an indicator of the importance of carbohydrates in a balanced diet and a reason why a carbohydrate-based dietary pattern should be recommended. With continuous interaction between carbohydrate and health, research indicates that the interaction between carbohydrate intake and metabolic consequences is sophisticated. Emerging research reveals the significance of the quality of carbohydrate, meaning that carbohydrates consumed are as crucial as how much is consumed. For example, the impact of glycemic index foods, which are also recognized to lead to sharp glucose peaks, has been determined to have adverse health effects, such as insulin resistance and obesity. On the other hand, low-glycemic index foods, including legumes and whole grains, have been associated with sustained energy and improved metabolic state. The correlation between carbohydrate types and long-term health outcomes suggests that there is a demand for dietary interventions highlighting intake of quality rather than calories. Modulation of these elements of carbohydrate consumption may enhance public health campaigns against metabolic disorders and overall well-being, particularly as suggested by the research on food habits of different populations (Çelik et al., 2021; Voroncova et al., 2025) (Figure 6.5).

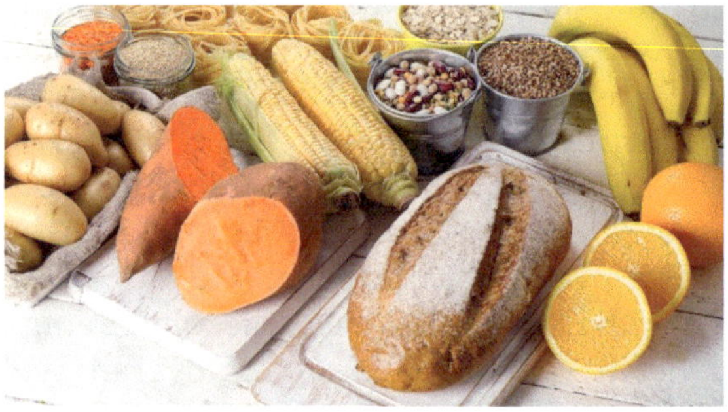

Figure 6.5. Carbohydrates.

Source: https://nutritionsource.hsph.harvard.edu/wp-content/uploads/2024/11/AdobeStock_174798121-1024x580.jpeg.

6.1.2. Proteins: Role in Body Function

Proteins are essential macromolecules that have a vast number of crucial functions in maintaining physiological function and overall wellness. They are basically composed of amino acids, which are the building blocks necessary for varied biological functions. Enzymes, hormones, antibodies, and structural components of cells are all proteins, showing their multifarious functions in the functions of the body. Some examples of such functions are catalysis of biochemical processes by protein enzymes that are essential to metabolism, e.g., production of energy and assimilation of nutrients. The regulatory function of proteins is another important one; they help regulate metabolic processes that maintain homeostasis during fluctuations in diet intake or environmental conditions. Consequently, the role of proteins within the body extends beyond the provision of structural support to encompass dynamic regulatory and catalytic roles necessary for maximal metabolic function. The interaction between proteins and metabolic processes is augmented by dietary intake, highlighting the importance of optimal protein consumption to meet physiological demand. Protein quality, in terms of amino acid profile and digestibility, has a significant bearing on the degree to which the body metabolizes such nutrients. For example, variation in apparent fecal nutrient digestibility, which occurs in various dietary contexts, highlights that not all protein sources are metabolically equivalent. Research indicates that the metabolizable energy (ME) of proteins can differ depending on their dietary context, influencing overall body energy balance (Zou et al., 2007). Moreover, the activity and organization of food proteins can also regulate hormone levels that regulate appetite and metabolism, reflecting the direct link between protein intake and metabolic health. Furthermore, proteins are also seriously involved in the regulation of iron homeostasis, an essential part of metabolic regulation. Hepcidin, a liver-derived protein, regulates dietary iron uptake and cell iron in a direct link of protein activity with nutrient metabolism. In chronic inflammatory conditions, such as obesity, hepcidin may rise and lead to disturbances in iron homeostasis and, consequently, disturbances in the generation of energy within the body (Arefiev et al., 2017). Such dependence highlights the challenges of protein functions beyond structure and enhancing their role as central drivers of metabolic activities. Understanding these interactions shines a light on the broader implications of protein nutrition in preventing and treating disease, again highlighting the merit of proteins as part of an overall balanced diet in terms of nutrition and metabolism (Figure 6.6).

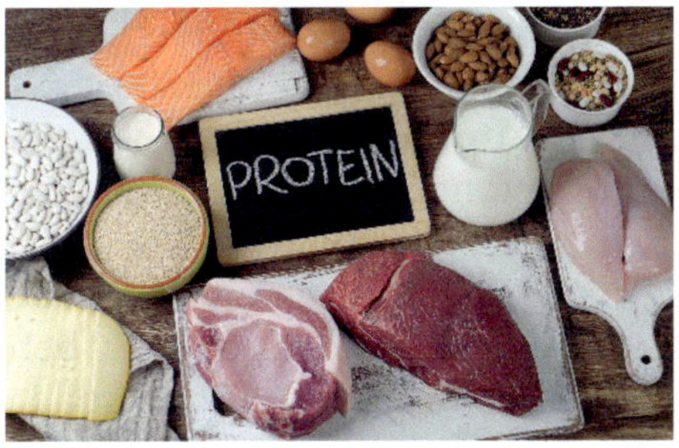

Figure 6.6. Protein.

Source: https://content.dhhs.vic.gov.au/sites/default/files/2022-01/ _0.jpg.

6.1.3. Fats: Essential Fatty Acids and Energy

In metabolism and nutrition, the role of fats, particularly essential fatty acids, plays a pivotal role. Essential fatty acids, i.e., omega-3 and omega-6, are synthesized by the body and must be ingested via diet. These fatty acids are required for numerous physiological processes, like cell membrane structure and hormone synthesis. Apart from that, they have been implicated in inflammatory processes, thus affecting overall health. Biochemistry of such processes presents a complicated interrelation between fats and metabolism, whereby correct intake of essential fatty acids is the cornerstone of cellular homeostasis. Thus, the value of the fatty acids is achieved in the management of metabolic diseases and maintaining proper health through nutrition-oriented approaches based on knowledge, as documented in texts outlining metabolic operations and nutrition requirements (Sarmidi, 2012). Energy production also is an important parameter under the influence of dietary fats, leading to extensive knowledge of their role in human metabolism. Fats are an extremely dense source of energy, with approximately nine calories per gram, compared to carbohydrates and proteins that yield four. This high energy density makes them essential under conditions of high expenditure of energy, for example, where there is excessive body physical activity or prolonged fasting. Dietary lipids have a crucial function in maintaining energy homeostasis such that the body is able to accumulate excess energy but also have an easily accessible source of fuel when needed. Additionally, as individuals progress through various phases of life, especially in children, energy needs can vary, necessitating targeted nutrition interventions according to energy needs and sources of fats utilized (Bauer et al., 2009). Thus, the discussion of dietary fats must involve their unique energetic functions and metabolic impacts. In addition, the interaction of fats and metabolic state cannot be overestimated, particularly with regard to optimum diet compositions. A perturbation of dietary fatty acid balance, in the form of excessive saturated fatty acid composition in relation to that of essential fatty acids, has been linked to the pathogenesis of chronic diseases, including CVD and obesity. Adequate incorporation of sources of essential fatty acids , such as fish, seeds, and nuts can counteract such risks and provide improved health outcomes. Besides, development in the field of nutritional sciences emphasizes the need to understand better the impact of different fats on metabolic pathways. It invokes a shift towards dietary guidelines based on healthy fats for metabolic efficiency. Lastly, an awareness of the intricate relationship between dietary fat and energy metabolism should be the focus of health promotion and disease prevention in heterogeneous populations, in accordance with broader nutritional standards (Bauer et al., 2009; Sarmidi, 2012) (Figure 6.7).

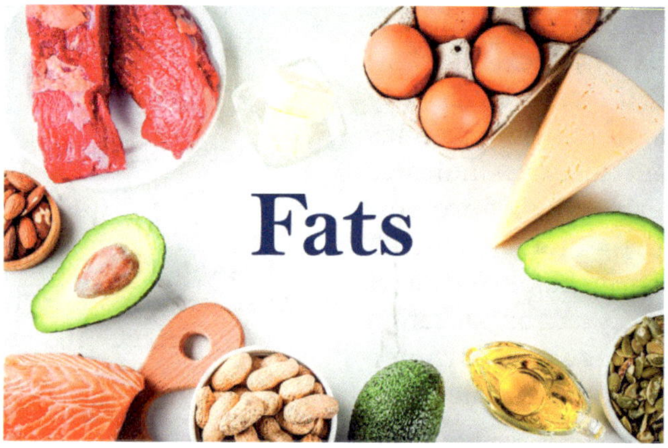

Figure 6.7. Fats.

Source: https://www.doctorkiltz.com/wp-content/uploads/2021/04/Fats-1030x686.jpg.

Test Your Knowledge

1. What are the functions of carbohydrates?
2. What is the role of protein in the human body?

6.2. Micronutrients

Learning Outcome

1. Describe the types of vitamins and their functions;
2. Understand the importance of minerals for metabolic processes;
3. Understand the role of antioxidants in disease prevention.

Micronutrients like minerals and vitamins play a vital role in the maintenance of overall health and wellness and are essential components of many metabolic functions. Micronutrients contrast with macronutrients energy-carrying capacity because they are primarily cofactors for enzymes, making biochemical reactions critical to cell function possible. For instance, several micronutrients play a central role in the synthesis of neurotransmitters and hormones, which regulate body reactions and maintain homeostasis in the body. Additionally, micronutrient shortage can lead to severe health issues, such as impaired immunity or delayed development, to support the significance of adequate dietary nutrition. Alongside, there is also new evidence that establishes the role of gut microbiota as a driving factor in enhancing the bioavailability of such simple nutrients, integrating gastrointestinal well-being with nutrient metabolism and body function as a whole, as detailed in recent literature that identifies the positive effect of certain bacteria in mineral metabolism and bioaccessibility, particularly against the background of evolving dietary practices (Bielik et al., 2021). Selenium, a trace mineral, and vital micronutrient, exemplifies the impact of micronutrients on metabolic health and chronic disease prevention. This essential nutrient is pivotal for various biological processes, including antioxidant defense systems and thyroid hormone metabolism. Studies have indicated that selenium deficiency may have a direct correlation with increased risks of several chronic diseases, including cardiovascular conditions and certain cancers. In response to this condition of public health, numerous biofortification strategies have emerged with the goal of increasing selenium intake in food systems to mitigate deficiency conditions that affect specific groups. Interestingly, selenium supplementation has been supported by robust evidence that reveals its safeguarding against oxidative stress and inflammation, the main drivers of chronic disease development. However, it must be recognized that the relationship between selenium and health outcomes can be complex, demonstrating a U-shaped dose-response relationship where too little or excessive might be hazardous (Hu et al., 2021).

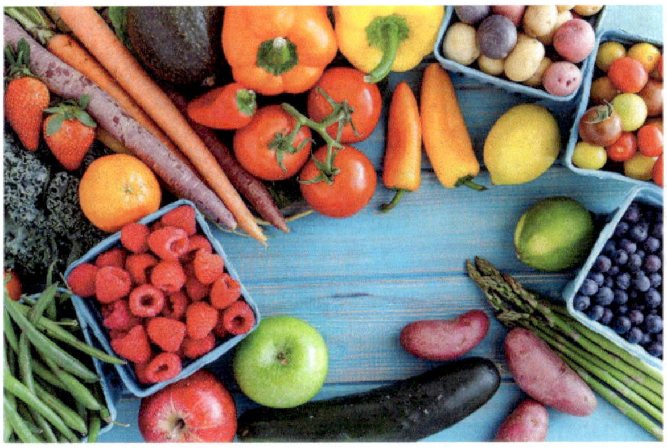

Figure 6.8. Micronutrients.

Source: https://doc.vortala.com/childsites/uploads/3347/files/micronutrients.jpg.

Additionally, the intersection of micronutrients with modern diet habits highlights the importance of considering not only the quantity of micronutrients consumed but also their quality and origin. The contemporary diet is often difficult as processed foods are typically devoid of vital micronutrients, and therefore most individuals have poor nutritional status. This is enhanced by lifestyle factors, which incorporate increased intakes of foods that are calorie-dense but not nutrient-dense and can lead to deficiency despite caloric intake. The growing awareness of the importance of the role of microbiomes in nutrient bioavailability renders the value of a diet rich in varied and whole foods required to guarantee both broad gut flora and sufficient micronutrient absorption. Finally, achieving a balance of micronutrients is crucial, not just for individual health, but also in order to prevent chronic metabolism diseases and build a robust population for decades to come (Bielik et al., 2021) (Figure 6.8).

6.2.1. Vitamins: Types and Their Functions

Vitamins have the critical role of supporting numerous functions and processes of the body, which are divided into two main groups: fat-soluble and water-soluble vitamins. A, D, E, and K are fat-soluble vitamins that are ingested together with dietary fat and stored in fatty tissues and the liver. They play a major role in functions like vision, bone health, antioxidant properties, and blood clotting. For example, vitamin D's unique metabolism occurs in the skin, where it is synthesized as a reaction to sunlight, and is important in the intestinal absorption of calcium, influencing bone density and strength. The complexity of vitamin D metabolism shows the way nutrients and environmental influences might crosstalk, thereby affecting calcium homeostasis in the body and illustrating the complex interaction between vitamins and metabolic processes (Bouillon et al., 2019). Water-soluble vitamins like the B vitamins and vitamin C are necessary for energy metabolism and the generation of metabolic waste. B-vitamins, for instance, are employed as coenzymes within numerous metabolic reactions, which catalyze energy-yielding macronutrient breakdown. Thiamine (B1), for instance, plays a central role in carbohydrate metabolism, while riboflavin (B2) and niacin (B3) are essential for oxidative phosphorylation, an ATP-generating process in mitochondria. This mitochondrial function is also regulated by cofactors and nutrient availability, illustrating pathways that are significant for energy balance within the cell. Deficits of these water-soluble vitamins, thus, can lead to metabolic disorders, affecting both energy availability and overall health, emphasizing their importance in the fields of nutrition and metabolism (Joëlle et al., 2019). In addition to their structural roles in metabolism, vitamins are also signaling molecules involved in gene expression and cell-cell communication. An example is the biosynthesis of metabolites from vitamin metabolism, which can activate or inhibit signaling pathways that control nuclear functions, demonstrating an interactive role between vitamins and cell processes. This connection is also reflected in studies showing that mitochondrial metabolites, under B-vitamin control, have a direct influence on nuclear signaling and, therefore, manage cellular homeostasis and metabolism. Further, an impairment of this interaction has also been linked with various diseases, including metabolic syndrome and diabetes. Consequently, the therapeutic potential of tailoring vitamin intake is gaining attention, as optimizing vitamin levels could provide significant benefits for managing metabolic health and preventing related diseases (Bouillon et al., 2019; Joëlle et al., 2019) (Figure 6.9).

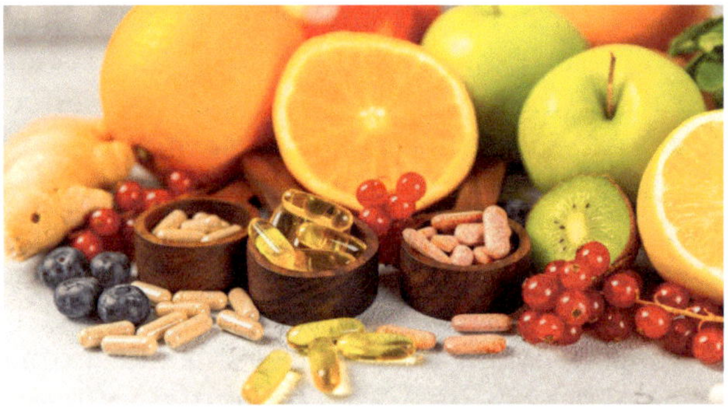

Figure 6.9. Vitamins.

Source: https://www.ewmotiontherapy.com/hubfs/Vitamins.png.

6.2.2. Minerals: Importance for Metabolic Processes

Minerals are the simple components of various metabolic activities, with specific roles in enzyme function, hormone secretion, and physiological regulation. Trace elements, such as zinc, magnesium, and iron, directly participate in catalyzing biochemical reactions and stabilizing cell structures. Iron, for example, plays an essential role in transporting oxygen with hemoglobin, whereas zinc acts as a cofactor for numerous enzymes in nucleic acid metabolism and biosynthesis. The precarious equilibrium of these minerals is vital as deficiencies have been shown to lead to severe metabolic derangements, compromising energy metabolism and general health. While most of the populace may not express frank signs of deficiency, the more subtle effects emerge over time and form the basis of the necessity of a mineral-enriched diet for guaranteeing appropriate mineral levels and normal metabolic processes (Buckton et al., 2014). Their role extends beyond structural involvement; they play active roles in metabolic functions, particularly in energy production and substrate processing. Multivitamin/mineral (MVM) supplementation has been shown to enhance energy metabolism for both mental functioning and physical activity, demonstrating a relationship between mineral availability and metabolic function (Dodd et al., 2020). For instance, it has been shown by studies that certain minerals have the capacity to maximize carbohydrate oxidation, which in turn enhances exercise efficacy and mental performance during hard work. This indicates that sufficient mineral consumption is not only essential for normal body functions but also indispensable in maximizing metabolic adaptation to physical and mental stress. Thus, the addition of a range of essential minerals in one's diet may result in improved metabolic function, establishing their overall significance to health and function. As well, the role of minerals in metabolism also emphasizes the importance of food variety, particularly within the context of modern diets that too often result in micronutrient deficiency. Although many who reside in the developed world are afflicted with overconsumption, they are simultaneously deprived of sufficient minerals to nourish their optimal health. This inconsistency helps to further contribute to the dual risk of both an unhealthy diet along with biochemical needs exceeding available nutrient supplies. This necessitates an intentional dedication to nutrition that entails a lot of whole foods with high mineral content to satisfy their requirements. In so doing, individuals are in a position to establish a well-balanced metabolic status that is favorable to happiness and health, above dependent supplementation whose outcomes do not guarantee the same as varied nutrition (Buckton et al., 2014). The discovery of these nutrients crucial power to influence metabolic processes illuminates their important role in holistic nutrition and metabolism approaches (Figure 6.10).

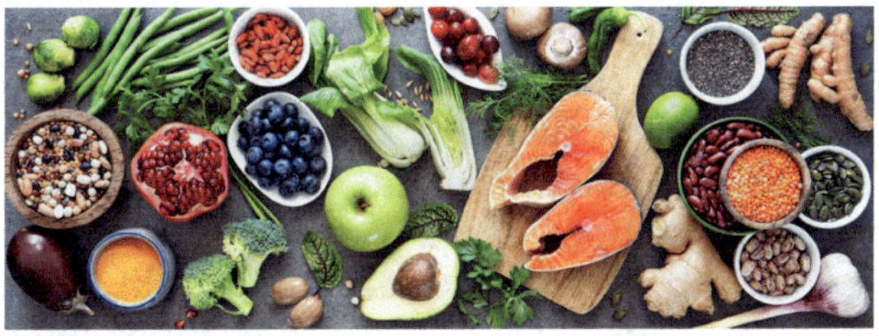

Figure 6.10. Minerals.

Source: https://www.myvitamins.com/images?url=https://blogscdn.thehut.net/app/uploads/sites/3/2023/06/1_1686584276.png&auto=avif&width=1800&fit=crop.

6.2.3. Antioxidants: Role in Disease Prevention

The possible function of antioxidants as anti-disease agents is more and more accepted in nutrition and metabolism. Antioxidants are compounds that inhibit oxidation, a chemical process that generates free radicals, leading to cell damage. This oxidative stress has been linked to a variety of chronic diseases, like cardiovascular disorders, cancer, and neurodegenerative diseases. A diet rich in fruits, vegetables, and whole grains contains a range of antioxidants , such as vitamins C and E, selenium, and phytochemicals, which minimize oxidative damage in the body. While research continues to explore the potential therapeutic uses of these substances, it would seem that understanding antioxidant activity not only protects against disease but also ensures overall health within the metabolic process. Interestingly, studies have emphasized the necessity of antioxidant supplementation in specific groups, more so in individuals with a higher risk for chronic diseases. Overweight and obese individuals, for instance, may have higher oxidative stress, compounded by exercise. In a controlled trial of the effect of pomegranate juice, findings showed reduced post-exercise oxidative markers and reduced blood pressure in participants who consumed this antioxidant-rich drink. This demonstrates that targeted antioxidant interventions can play a key role in maintaining metabolic health and reducing disease risk. Results like this are significant to guide nutritional recommendations and interventions aimed at specific population groups, emphasizing the value of an individualized approach to antioxidant consumption for disease prevention. However, one also needs to consider the counter evidence regarding antioxidant supplements in healthy populations. Studies have established that while dietary sources of antioxidants can provide health-protective benefits, supplements with high intake may not provide the same protective benefits and could, by extension, lead to adverse outcomes. For instance, studies suggest that the use of multivitamin supplements does not necessarily translate into diminished disease incidence and, in some cases, may raise all-cause mortality risks. This paradox points to the need to consume natural food sources of antioxidants in a balanced nutritional regimen. A whole-food approach over supplementation is consistent with the consensus that an eclectic diet, and no single nutrients or chemicals, is the ideal approach to preventing chronic illnesses and maintaining optimal metabolic function (Buckton et al., 2014). In addition, the complexity of nutrient interactions and metabolic pathways underscores that additional research is necessary in order to determine the precise functions of antioxidants for disease prevention within the general framework of metabolism and nutrition (Figure 6.11).

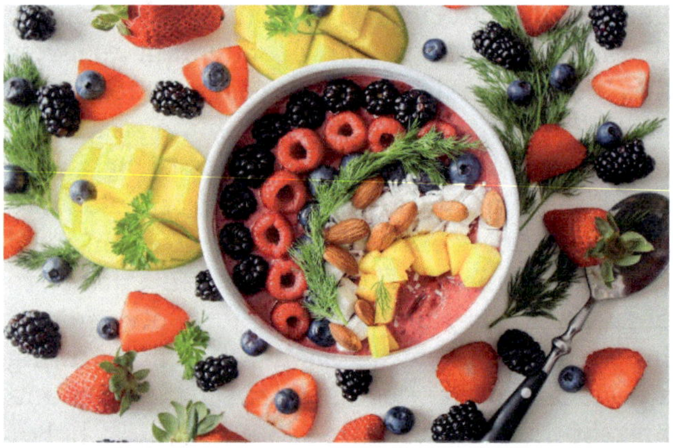

Figure 6.11. The role of antioxidants in disease prevention.

Source: https://cdn.prod.website-files.com/63bf3f41c3bc69578d823f01/67530a38e7f5f0d70bfd601b_pexels-janetrangdoan-1099680.jpg.

Test Your Knowledge

1. What are the categories of vitamins?
2. What is the role of antioxidants in disease prevention?

6.3. The Digestive System

Learning Outcome

1. Give an overview of digestive processes;
2. Describe the process of absorbing nutrients;
3. Describe the impact of gut health on metabolism.

The digestive system plays a role in nutrition and metabolism in the sense that it processes food into nutrients for absorption and utilization by the body. From the mouth, mechanical and enzymatic processes begin digestion, and enzymes in saliva begin to degrade carbohydrates. As food is transported down the esophagus to the stomach, it is subjected to further mechanical churning and chemical breakdown, particularly of proteins, by gastric acids and enzymes. The acid environment within the stomach further conditions food for its ultimate destination in the small intestine, where most of the nutrients are absorbed. Here, the pancreas releases digestive enzymes that further digest macronutrients, and bile from the liver emulsifies fat to enable its digestion. The process is elaborate and points to the digestive system's vital function of converting food into energy and making metabolic processes possible to maintain life. After digestion, the absorptive role of the small intestine plays a vital role in the provision of adequate nutrition. The intestinal lining, covered with microvilli, increases the surface area to achieve maximum nutrient absorption. Carbohydrates are broken down to monosaccharides, proteins to amino acids, and fats are broken down to fatty acids and glycerol, which enter the blood to be distributed to various tissues. The nutrients serve as substrates for metabolic processes to create energy, repair cells, and maintain homeostasis. In a fascinating turn, the function of nutrients goes beyond the provision of energy; they also affect gene expression important to the functioning of the digestive system. For example, varying nutrient levels significantly impact the expression of genes in the intestine and can affect the state of health and resistance to disease. This illustrates the interactive connection between the digestive system and metabolic well-being and suggests that dietary factors can have a significant impact on physiological response. The interaction between nutrition, metabolism, and digestive processes is further complicated under stress conditions, such as heat exposure. Heat stress in certain birds, such as poultry, can negatively affect digestive efficiency and nutrient utilization. Nevertheless, the impact of such stress can be mitigated by adopting specific feeding programs aimed at ensuring that birds still maximize their health and production performance despite adverse conditions.

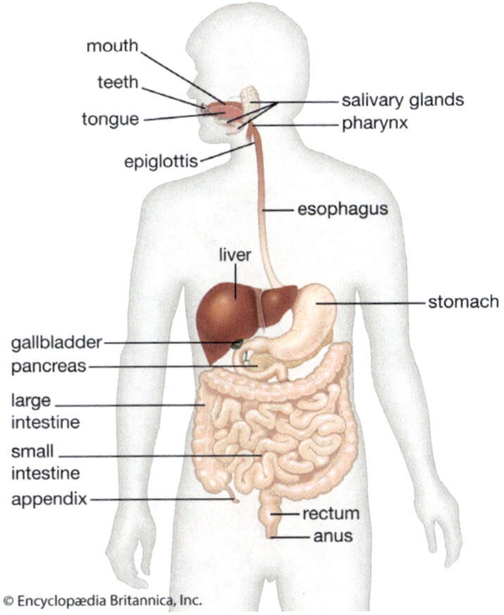

Figure 6.12. Human digestive system.

Source: https://cdn.britannica.com/39/8039-050-B124FC20/human-digestive-system-front.jpg.

For example, delivery of feeds of greater particle size can increase grinding in the gizzard, improving digestion while at the same time minimizing metabolic heat production. In addition, feeding behaviors , such as wet feeding can enhance water consumption, thereby assisting in thermoregulation during heat stress, which is crucial in maintaining performance in the hot tropical climate. Understanding these relationships and methods is important because it highlights the applicability of specialist nutrition to upholding the digestive tract and overall metabolic function, particularly in extreme conditions (Bauer et al., 2011; Kwakkel et al., 2011) (Figure 6.12).

6.3.1. Overview of Digestive Processes

The human digestive system is a sophisticated network designed for the breakdown of food into its basic building blocks, a function necessary for nutrient absorption and metabolism. From the moment food is ingested to the moment it is excreted, every phase of digestion is delicately controlled to promote efficiency and effectiveness. The mouth is the starting point, where mechanical disruption is provided by chewing, with enzymes present in saliva initiating carbohydrate breakdown. As it moves down the esophagus to the stomach, further enzymatic work is performed in an acidic environment to denature and digest proteins. Gastric digestion results in the partially digested food, or chyme, reaching the small intestine, where the majority of nutrient uptake occurs. Here, bile and pancreatic juice secretion assist in the emulsification of fat and neutralization of stomach acid, favoring enhanced breakdown and absorption of nutrients into the bloodstream.

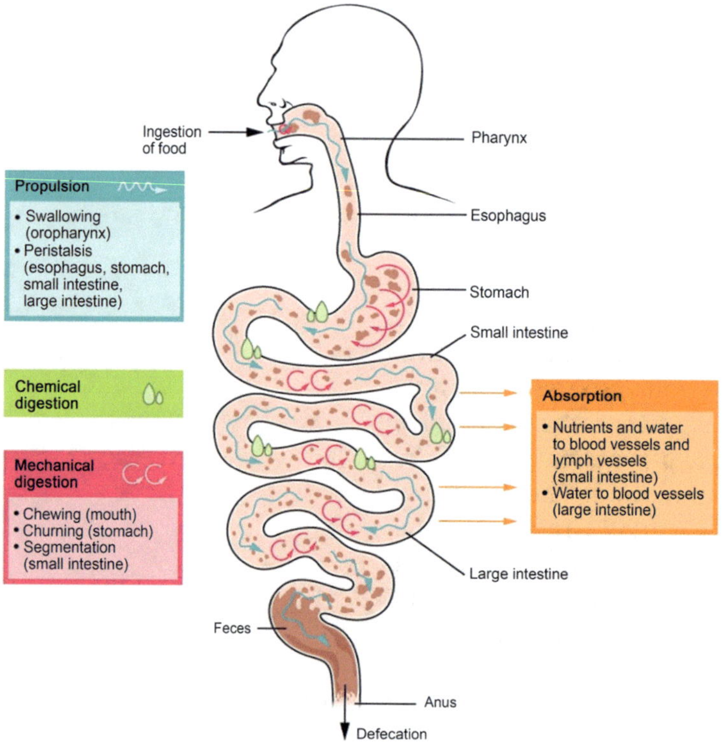

Figure 6.13. The digestive processes are ingestion, propulsion, mechanical digestion, chemical digestion, absorption, and defecation.

Source: https://s3-us-west-2.amazonaws.com/courses-images-archive-read-only/wp-content/uploads/sites/403/2015/04/21031707/2405_Digestive_Process.jpg.

Besides enzymatic digestion, gut microbiota has also been discovered to play a significant role in digestive action in influencing health as well as metabolism. Made up of trillions of microbes of varied composition, the gut microbiome performs vital functions, including the fermentation of indigestible carbohydrates, to lead to the production of SCFAs; essential sources of energy for colon cells. Changes in gut microbiota composition have been linked to various metabolic diseases , such as obesity and type 2 diabetes, suggesting that microbial balance is vital to metabolic health. The interaction of the host physiology and gut microbes shows an exceedingly sophisticated crosstalk that influences energy control and immune function. Using advanced technologies , such as metagenomics, the interactions are being unraveled with significance to comprehend the function of the gut microbiome in developing therapeutic approaches to metabolic diseases (Willem et al., 2022). Finally, digestion terminates in the large intestine, where water and electrolytes are taken up and the remaining of the indigestible material is being prepared to be excreted. The large intestine is not only a reservoir but also an active component of the digestive process, as it has massive amounts of bacteria that further ferment unabsorbed substrates. These products of this fermentation are necessary nutrients and are vital for gut health. In addition, the removal of waste is a central function of overall metabolic activity that has an impact upon many of the body's homeostatic mechanisms. With novel evidence placing the importance of gut health on systemic health and disease in the spotlight, a complete appreciation of digestive processes, including the function of gut microbiota, highlights the intricate relationship between nutrition and metabolism (Campanale et al., 2020) (Figure 6.13).

6.3.2. Absorption of Nutrients

The process of nutrient absorption is pivotal to knowing how the body uses the food components for energy, repair, and growth. Once food is broken down into its nutrient components, these molecules must travel through the intestinal lining to access the blood. This phase of active nutrient uptake is largely conducted in the small intestine, where there are specialized tissues like villi and microvilli that increase the surface area and consequently the uptake of nutrients. Additionally, the interaction of nutrients with gut microbiota plays an important role in it. Research shows that some nutrients can modulate the composition of intestinal microbiota, which in turn influences the efficacy of absorption of other nutrients. This changing interaction brings to prominence the necessity to consider the role of gut microbiomes in nutrition metabolism, and therefore, there is a need for more studies on how nutrition affects both microbiota richness and nutrient assimilation (Ma, 2025). The bioavailability of nutrients, being the portion absorbed and utilized by the body, is another critical characteristic of nutrient absorption. Determinants of bioavailability include nutrient structure, interaction with other nutrients in the food, and individual physiological status. For example, amino acids from proteins may have varying levels of efficiency in absorption depending on origin; studies have shown that sources of tryptophan are of similar bioavailability, meaning consumer experience as well as quality of the source of the nutrient matter (Stéphane et al., 2025). Also, variables , such as gut integrity and overall health affect absorption rates significantly. An impaired gastrointestinal tract, which is typical in most digestive conditions, will significantly reduce nutrient uptake, thus inducing malnutrition despite adequate diet consumption. It is critical to detect and treat these variations to optimize nutritional modalities and obtain better health results. Further, the interaction of nutrients in the gut illustrates human metabolism complexity. The combined uptake of various kinds of nutrients may lead to synergistic actions, which enhance the body's ability to utilize nutrients better. The presence of certain vitamins and minerals may facilitate others absorption; vitamin C can enhance iron absorption, particularly from plant sources. This interdependence indicates the need for a balanced diet with ample quantities of various nutrients to maximize overall nutrient utilization. Conversely, excessive consumption of some forms of nutrients can hinder the absorption of others, leading to deficiencies. As researchers further uncover the secrets of nutrient absorption, including the role of gut microbiome interactions and genetics, the science is poised to deliver breakthroughs that could direct personalized nutrition intervention to achieve optimal metabolism and improve health (Ma, 2025) (Figure 6.14).

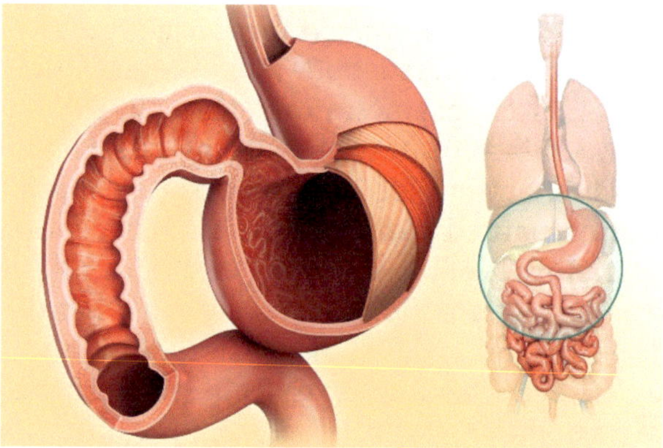

Figure 6.14. Nutrient absorption in the digestive system.

Source: https://www.thoughtco.com/thmb/a-Sv3h9pp_u7hh75E2OFW1LiRic=/1500x0/filters:no_upscale():max_bytes(150000):strip_icc()/stomach_intestines-57ffd6795f9b5805c2ac495f.jpg.

6.3.3. Impact of Gut Health on Metabolism

The intricate relationship between gut well-being and metabolism has been intriguing as a pivotal area of study in the science of nutrition. The gut microbiome, comprised of trillions of microbes, plays a core role in many metabolic processes, influencing energy extraction from food, fat storage, and even insulin sensitivity. An imbalance in gut microbiota, known as dysbiosis, is associated with metabolic diseases like obesity, type 2 diabetes, and metabolic syndrome. Adhering to a high-fiber, prebiotic, and fermented foods diet, the diversity and structure of gut microbiomes can be maximized, potentially contributing to a better metabolic health. These dietary ways are relatively far from the Western diet, characterized by excessive intake of processed and sugary foods, which is capable of exacerbating metabolic dysregulation and inflammation, as indicated in recent reviews (Clemente et al., 2023). An understanding of the impact of such dietary choices on gut microbiota can thus form the foundation for the improvement of metabolic results. As gut microbiota can modulate systemic inflammation, their impact on metabolism should not be overestimated. Prolonged low-grade inflammation, often a result of an unhealthy gut, is implicated in insulin resistance and deranged metabolic function. The consumption of polyphenol-dense foods , such as berries and nuts, has been accused of having a positive effect on gut health and metabolic function. The gut metabolizes these molecules to produce bioactive metabolites that include Urolithin A (UA), which enhances mitochondrial function and activates mitophagy. This is necessary for the maintenance of energy homeostasis and the prevention of age-related metabolic dysfunction. It has been shown that UA administration can reduce inflammatory responses, which are of significant relevance to age-related disease, and further consolidate the guts' role in mediating metabolic well-being (Davide et al., 2021). Thus, gut health may be a promising intervention to reverse metabolic states linked to aging and diet. Lastly, gut health and metabolic health interaction has a potential field for nutritional intervention. Researchers point out that proper eating habits rich in nutrients, along with supplementation with probiotics and prebiotics, can offer significant benefits to gut microbiota, thus supporting maximal metabolic function. This interaction suggests that optimization of gut health can be the most important intervention for maximizing overall metabolic health. Moreover, as more individuals adopt unhealthy eating habits, the need to educate the public about the relationship between microbiota and metabolism is more apparent. A holistic strategy founded on diet, aimed at enabling better gut health, could not only enhance metabolic dysfunction but also enable optimal well-being, and this presents a sound argument for integrated dietary principles in combating metabolic disease (Clemente et al., 2023).

Test Your Knowledge

1. What is the digestive system?
2. What is the process of absorbing nutrients?

6.4. Metabolism Overview

Learning Outcome

1. Understand the definition of metabolism;
2. Describe the anabolism and catabolism;
3. Know the factors influencing metabolic rate.

Metabolism is all the biochemical reactions within an organism that allow food to be turned into energy and the synthesis of compounds needed. This complex system of reactions can be categorized into two broad forms: catabolism, which breaks down molecules to free energy, and anabolism, which utilizes energy to construct cellular entities like proteins and nucleic acids. These metabolic reactions are regulated by several factors, including diet, hormonal levels, and physical activity level (PAL). Metabolism is crucial to comprehend since dysregulation of metabolism can lead to a variety of chronic diseases , such as obesity, diabetes, and CVD, making it crucial to maintain a well-balanced nutrient-rich diet to enable these essential biochemical reactions. As we dive deeper into the metabolic subtleties, we realize that the types of foods we eat have extremely potent roles in determining overall well-being. The impact of food on metabolism is not just about providing energy; it influences systemic inflammation and hormonal homeostasis, which are significant modulators of metabolic health. Dietary components like the quality and quantity of fats play a supportive or non-supportive role in metabolic disturbances. For instance, excessive consumption of saturated fats has been implicated in increased visceral fat accumulation with subsequent metabolic derangements, while high consumption of unsaturated fats , such as in the Mediterranean diet has been associated with improved metabolic profiles and reduced inflammation. In addition, dietary interaction with metabolic pathways is illustrated by the manner in which omega-3 fatty acids may be beneficial for particular metabolic disorders. With novel research dissecting the intricate relationship between diet, inflammation, and metabolic health, there is general urgency to place priority on nutritional education and intervention to achieve optimal public health benefits (Fulton et al., 2021). Besides the linear effects of nutrition on metabolic function, the topic of perinatal programming also illuminates the manner in which nutrition during early life determines the trajectory for a person's metabolic health. Adverse conditions during sensitive developmental periods, such as intrauterine growth restriction due to maternal undernutrition, have been associated with increased risk to chronic disorders later in life, including asthma and other respiratory conditions. This further underscores the importance of optimal maternal nutrition not merely for fetal development but for constructing an efficient metabolic framework. Current evidence is beginning to reveal the exact mechanisms responsible for such long-term effects, such as the role of inflammation and nutrient sensing in lung growth and metabolic health. Clarification of such connections is important to inform the development of preventive and therapeutic strategies to restore metabolic derangement from infancy into adulthood (Kuiper-Makris et al., 2021) (Figure 6.15).

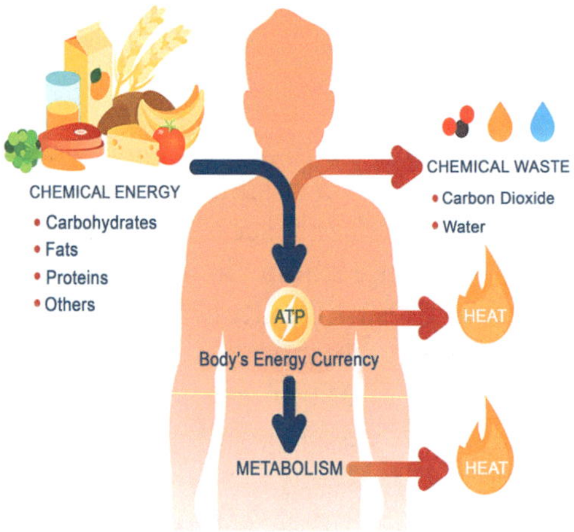

Figure 6.15. Metabolism.

Source: https://assets.lybrate.com/imgs/tic/enadp/image-of-the-metabolism.jpg.

6.4.1. Definition of Metabolism

It is necessary to know the definition of metabolism to be aware of how it participates in nutrition and health. Metabolism refers to all biochemical events within the organism that are responsible for sustaining life, such as the processes that convert food into energy and processes that are involved in biomolecule synthesis and decomposition. These processes are typically divided into two major categories: catabolism, which breaks down molecules to produce energy, and anabolism, which uses that energy to build cellular structures. This intricate set of reactions not only plays a vital part in the production of energy but also keeps homeostasis intact, controlling vital processes like temperature, nutrient availability, and waste removal. Furthermore, metabolic processes are influenced by a number of factors, including age, sex, physical fitness, and external environmental factors, which emphasizes the individuality and complexity of metabolic functions. The significance of metabolism cannot be stressed enough, particularly when nutrition is taken into consideration. Peak metabolic efficiency is inextricably interdependent with the access and intake of nutrients since the body depends on a number of vitamins, minerals, and macronutrients to create enzymatic processes and energy creation. Lack or disruption of these essential nutrients can lead to metabolic impairment, impacting anything from weight management to mental functioning. In addition, metabolic science also improves the knowledge of broad health issues, including obesity and metabolic syndrome, which are becoming common in contemporary society. Dysregulated metabolic processes can lead to these diseases, where excessive caloric intake accompanied by sedentary life leads to adipose tissue deposition and associated health issues, emphasizing the close relationship between nutrition and metabolic well-being. In exploring the modern notion of metabolism, a crucial task is to recognize new phenomena, such as sarcopenic obesity, which characterizes the co-occurrence of low muscle mass and overweight body fat. Sarcopenic obesity highlights the need for a comprehensive exploration of challenges in metabolic health. As noted by experts, sarcopenic obesity is characterized by changes in metabolism because of lifestyle, comorbidities, and aging, necessitating specifically tailored nutrition and exercise strategies for prevention and management. Recent activities, including those of the European Society for Clinical Nutrition and Metabolism (ESPEN), advocate for clear diagnostic criteria and better insight into weighted factors of metabolism on the patient outcome. These complexities need to be addressed to improve effective intervention that maximizes metabolic function and quality of life, thus filling the important interstice between nutrition and metabolism in health care (Lorenzo et al., 2022).

6.4.2. Anabolism vs. Catabolism

The subtle balance of anabolism and catabolism is a central component of nutrition and metabolism and plays a major role in defining an organism's total health and energy balance. Anabolism is the metabolic process that constructs molecules from smaller units, which aids in the accumulation of tissues and their repair. It involves constructing proteins out of amino acids and constructing carbohydrates and lipids out of simpler substances. On the other hand, catabolism involves the breakdown of complex molecules to simpler ones, a process that reveals energy necessary in supporting physiological activities as well as responding to temporary energy requirements. The continuous interaction of these two metabolic activities indicates the body's adjustment to varied nutritional conditions, as it highlights the need for a perfect balance to enable appropriate growth, repair, and energy supply in organisms. Understanding the processes that control anabolism and catabolism holds important relevance to nutrition, particularly in activity level and food intake. Various dietary content has the ability to change the balance of these two processes. A diet consisting of a high quantity of proteins and calories, for instance, will enhance anabolic reactions, promoting the building of muscle and general growth. Conversely, caloric deficit or insufficient nutrition encourages more catabolic processes, which may develop muscle loss and energy insufficiency and lead to low metabolism. These pathways are also influenced by age, gender, and genetic constitution, such that individual variability warrants customized nutrition for optimal metabolic health and prevention of disorders caused by an imbalance in metabolism. In animal farming and agriculture, the principles of anabolism and catabolism are significant considerations for improving efficiency and profitability. For example, growth functions mathematically quantify the body weight of animals , such as poultry, as a mathematical relationship between age and food intake, allowing producers to predict growth and nutrient requirements effectively. The relationship helps in the effective management of feed resources while avoiding wastage and enhancing animal well-being. Alongside this, mathematical modeling of such metabolic processes enables farmers to modulate feeding strategies based on stages of growth, optimizing anabolic processes and managing catabolic requirements in conditions of illness or stress. Advances in nutritional science further develop these models to permit more accurate forecasts and interventions in securing the health of livestock, simultaneously with securing economic dimensions of production systems (Dumas et al., 2008; Kuhi et al., 2010) (Figure 6.16).

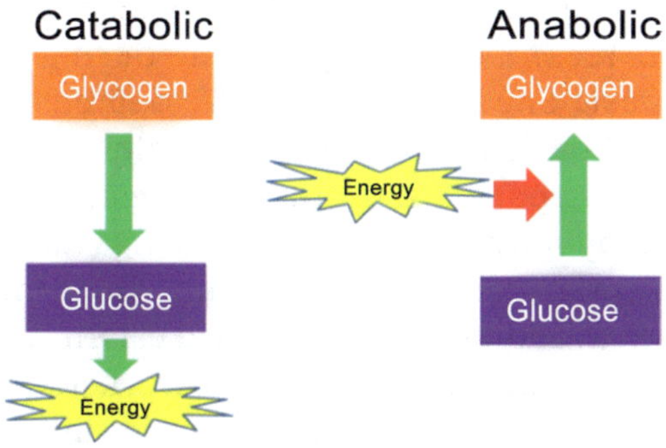

Figure 6.16. The breakdown of glycogen to glucose is catabolic. The glucose can then be used to produce energy. The synthesis of glycogen from glucose is anabolic and requires energy.

Source: https://med.libretexts.org/@api/deki/files/1537/Figure_6.12.png?revision=1&size=bestfit&width=479&height=319.

6.4.3. Factors Influencing Metabolic Rate

Metabolic rate, or how fast the body expends energy, is influenced by a wide range of variables that could be intrinsic or extrinsic to an individual. Most likely the most significant ones are age, gender, body composition, and heredity. As one ages, the basal metabolic rate (BMR) falls primarily due to a reduction in lean body mass. On the other hand, men typically have a higher BMR than women because of differences in muscle and fat distribution. Second, individuals who have higher muscle mass also have a higher metabolic rate, as muscle tissue is more metabolically active than fat. The integration of all these factors points to the complexity of energy expenditure and how there must be approach-specific nutrition and fitness programs that are addressed based on an individual's unique metabolic profile. The influence of PAL on metabolic rate should not be overstated. PAL, or the proportion of total energy expenditure (TEE) to BMR, is an integral measure to take into account in recognizing the impact of physical activity on energy requirements. Physical activity daily contributes not just to BMR but also to TEE, which means the energy spent during work and rest. Shetty et al. (2005) demonstrates that although BMR is proportionally the same in various populations, the difference brought about by physical activities brings about a differential requirement picture in terms of energy. In addition, pattern-based classifications of physical activity help health workers in the formulation of focused intervention in weight management and metabolic health. Since individuals adopt different lifestyles, monitoring PAL may help identify diet changes that are needed to realize optimal energy balance. New findings have further highlighted the role of gut microbiota in affecting metabolic health and opening a new channel to the controversy surrounding determinants of metabolic rate. Current literature suggests that the composition and function of gut microbiota may affect energy harvesting from ingested food and regulatory hormonal response. Edwards et al. (2016) emphasizes the potential of gut microbiota to contribute to obesity and metabolic diseases through mechanisms , such as production of SCFAs and the modulation of inflammation. The interaction between diet and gut microbiota composition needs a closer focus, particularly on how they interlink with metabolic rate. Such knowledge might be brought forth as new nutritional strategies that not only cause weight reduction but also provoke a healthier metabolic phenotype by modulating the complex interactions between diet, microbiome, and metabolism (Figure 6.17).

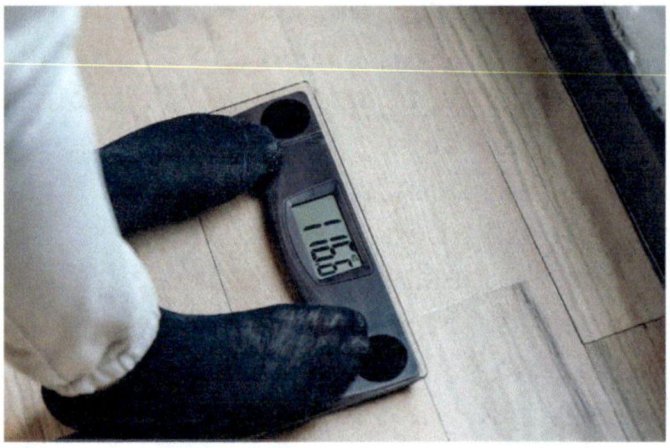

Figure 6.17. Individual measuring body weight using a digital scale.

Source: https://longevity.technology/lifestyle/wp-content/uploads/2023/12/closeup-on-person-wearing-socks-stepping-on-weighing-scale.jpg.

Test Your Knowledge

1. What is a simple definition of metabolism?
2. What are the factors affecting the metabolic rate?

6.5. Energy Balance

Learning Outcome

1. Understand the concept of caloric intake and expenditure;
2. Describe the role of physical activity;
3. Describe the impact of metabolism on weight management.

Energy balance is the central idea to identify the role of nutrition on metabolism and general health. Energy balance is the balance between energy derived from food and beverages and energy expenditure due to metabolic actions and exercise. Energy balance is achieved when calories taken are balanced by calories spent, which is crucial for body weight and metabolic health. Disruption of this balance can lead to obesity or malnutrition and thus affect various components of physiological function. Remarkably, dietary composition and lifestyle are critical determiners of energy balance. Understanding the role of individual nutrients in affecting energy balance contributes to the development of strategic dietary recommendations for optimizing metabolic processes. The role of SCFAs in energy equilibrium is particularly fascinating in that they are produced by the fermentation of dietary fibers by intestinal bacteria. SCFAs like acetate, propionate, and butyrate contribute to energy homeostasis through the regulation of glucose and lipid metabolism and thus act as a key bridge between diet and energy regulation. Research indicates that dietary fibers that promote SCFA-producers are capable of inhibiting the growth of pathogenic gut bacteria, favoring an improved gut environment (Li et al., 2024). Gut microbiota modulation is significant not just because it influences energy food extraction but also because it impacts metabolic health and the etiology of energy imbalance-related diseases , such as type 2 diabetes and CVD. In addition to SCFAs, bile acids also become essential regulators of energy metabolism, considering the polyvalent role they play in digestion and nutrient absorption. Secreted from the liver, bile acids facilitate emulsification of dietary fats such that they become more accessible in the body (Jia et al., 2024). Beyond the influence of the gut microbiota and bile acids on each other, modulation of bile acid metabolism is significant because it has the potential to shape the composition and formation of bile acid intestinal ecosystem, linking gut health to energy metabolism. Finally, understanding how bile acids can be modified through nutrition illuminates the optimization of livestock energy intake and how that could have broader implications for human health. The intersection of these metabolic pathways is evidence of the intricate interaction between nutrition and energy balance, highlighting the significance of increased research in this topic to develop effective nutritional interventions (Figure 6.18).

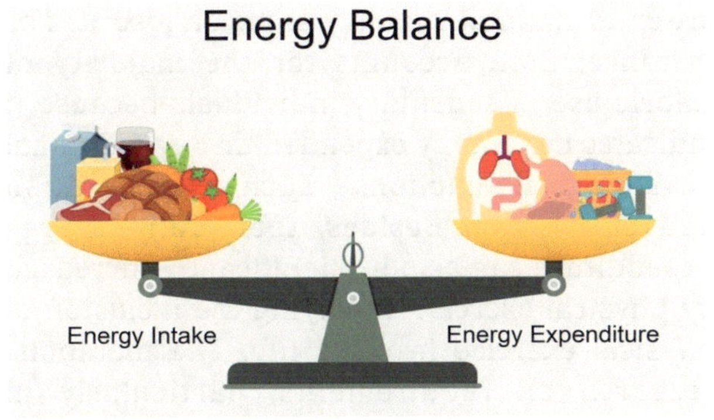

Figure 6.18. Energy balance.

Source: https://www.fitpaa.com/wp-content/uploads/2023/07/Untitled-design-2023-07-03T205457.373.jpg.

6.5.1. Concept of Caloric Intake and Expenditure

The caloric intake and expenditure are the basis of nutrition and metabolism learning because they establish the energy balance crucial in maintaining body functions and health. Caloric intake refers to the calories received from food and beverages, while caloric expenditure is the caloric loss from metabolic processes, body movement, and thermogenesis. Equilibrium between both elements is necessary; where intake is larger than expenditure, the body stores the excess energy as fat and gains weight, as well as experiences connected health effects. A caloric deficit, where expenditure is larger than intake, usually results in weight loss. Thus, the balance of caloric intake and expenditure becomes pivotal in effective diet planning and management, particularly when dealing with specific groups like astronauts, for whom nutritional adequacy is paramount in space travel according to studies by LSRO. Furthermore, the differences among individuals' caloric needs arise from a variety of factors including age, sex, body composition, and activity level. Metabolic rate, influenced by these variables, is significant in the determination of how many calories a person will need in order to maintain their weight or lose it. For instance, BMR accounts for the majority of caloric use in sedentary individuals because it indicates the energy expended through minimal physiological functions , such as respiration and circulation. Besides, total daily energy expenditure can also be significantly increased by physical exercise, justifying the inclusion of physical exercise in one's life. The metabolic research on requirements, particularly in controlled situations like in space, emphasizes the intricate relationship between caloric supply and adaptation of the body and has applications in nutrition therapy in extreme environments (Altman et al., 1986). Moreover, dietary composition directly affects calorie utilization and metabolism. Different macronutrients , such as fat, protein, and carbohydrates contain different caloric values and impact on satiety and energy expenditure. For instance, protein will have a higher thermic effect compared to carbohydrates and fats and more energy will be required for breakdown and metabolism and consequently impact total caloric balance. This concept is particularly appropriate where persons have specific nutritional needs, such as those who are about to embark on long-duration space travel, and in which nutrition must be precisely designed to sustain energy levels and prevent metabolic disruption. Furthermore, understanding adaptive metabolic processes to fluctuating caloric intake and nutrient composition is essential for the formulation of effective dietary recommendations, as evidenced by studies that determine the physiological adaptation to spaceflight (Chen et al., 2017). Overall, an insightful understanding of caloric intake and energy expenditure, and macro- and micronutrient variables, is essential to optimize health and performance in a wide range of environments (Figure 6.19).

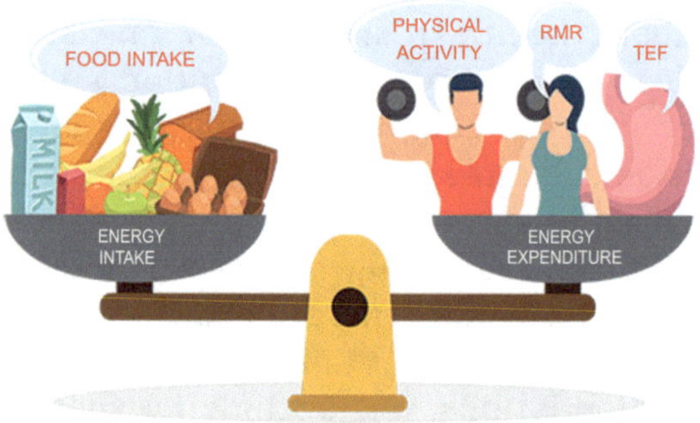

Figure 6.19. Active health energy balance.

Source: https://www.activesgcircle.gov.sg/hubfs/Active%20Health%20Website/Energy%20Balance/AH-Nutrition-Resource-Energy-Balance.png.

6.5.2. Role of Physical Activity

Physical exercise is extremely vital in enhancing various aspects of nutrition and metabolism, particularly the utilization of nutrients by the body. Exercise activates metabolic pathways that lead to higher energy expenditure and utilization of nutrients. Surprisingly, studies have shown that active subjects use more carbohydrate oxidation during exercise, leading to a more efficient utilization of dietary carbohydrates. This is particularly evident in men, who exhibit increased energy expenditure and elevated carbohydrate metabolism following MVM supplementation, thereby highlighting the inter-relationship between exercise, nutrition, and overall metabolic health. Hence, the incorporation of physical activity into daily living not only adds to the achievement of fitness goals but also optimizes the metabolic response of the body to the consumption of nutrients, creating a synergistic relationship between physical activity and dietary habits that improves general well-being (Dodd et al., 2020). Apart from acute metabolic benefits, the effect of physical activity extends to long-term health outcomes. Consistent physical exercise has been associated with improved muscle strength and loss of mass, important in metabolic functions, particularly with increasing age or in the context of medical conditions , such as cancer. Evidence further indicates that muscle loss among cancer patients can produce negative effects on physical function and quality of life, making sustained exercise an essential component to maintain muscle integrity and metabolic health. Amino acid metabolism is enhanced in cancer patients undergoing chemotherapy, which suggests that active participation in exercise may prevent muscle loss through a mechanism of heightened protein synthesis and reduced muscle breakdown. Including exercise in the conversation regarding nutrition and metabolism is, therefore, essential since it not only optimizes metabolic function but also inspires resistance against ailments that drain the body of its bodily strength (Deutz et al., 2018). In addition, the psychological and behavioral factors of physical exercise contribute significantly to nutrition outcomes. Regular exercise as a habit means improved eating and a motivation towards choosing healthier food, thus positively affecting nutrition in general. The conjunction of exercise and eating habits translates into less mental fatigue, further encouraging improved performance in physical activities. For instance, studies have indicated that multivitamin supplementation has the potential to augment energy expenditure under high-intensity cognitive tasks, particularly in physically active humans. Such findings imply that exercise is not only efficient in enhancing metabolic efficiency but also creates a context that is conducive to embracing healthy lifestyle behaviors. Lastly, the intricate relationship between nutrition and physical activity emphasizes the necessity of an integrated health concept where exercise is not simply a means to an end but rather an essential component of metabolic and nutritional well-being (Dodd et al., 2020) (Figure 6.20).

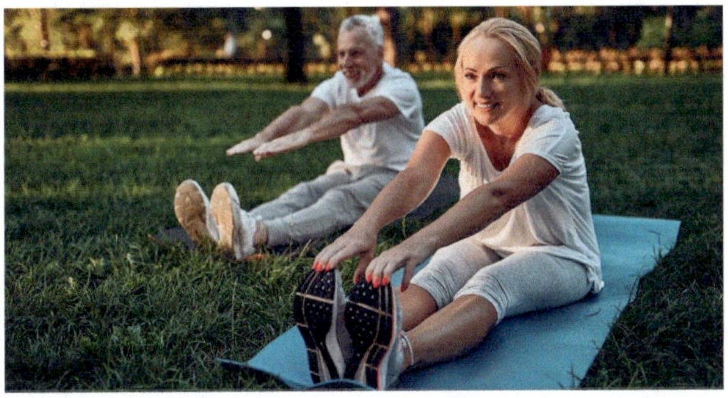

Figure 6.20. Older adults performing stretching exercises outdoors.

Source: https://assets.firstbeat.com/firstbeat/uploads/2019/09/header-blog-ukfitnessday.jpg.

6.5.3. Impact of Metabolism on Weight Management

Metabolism is a critical part of weight regulation, as it governs the manner in which the body uses food for energy and accumulates fat. Metabolism rate, or the speed at which these processes are executed, varies widely among individuals depending upon their genetic, hormonal, and lifestyle characteristics. For instance, people whose BMR is higher tend to burn more calories while at rest, which makes it relatively easier to control weight in comparison to people with lower BMR. Further, muscle tissue significantly influences metabolism; lean muscular tissue consumes more calories than fat tissue even when at rest.

Thus, physical exercise and strength training can contribute to increased muscle mass, with the added benefit of enhanced metabolic rate, together with improved body composition. The link between weight regulation and metabolism speaks volumes for the necessity for individually tailored methods in nutritional and exercise regimens for optimizing individual outcomes. Diet composition is another extremely crucial element that impacts metabolism and weight regulation. The macronutrient make-up of an individual's diet, the ratio of carbohydrates, proteins, and fats, directly influences metabolic function. For instance, diets high in protein are known to increase metabolic rate by inducing thermogenesis, the creation of heat in the body as a secondary effect of consuming food, as well as the preservation of muscle mass during weight loss. Also, certain dietary therapies , such as high high-protein diet, have been linked with increased satiety and reduced total energy consumption, allowing for effortless weight loss or maintenance in individuals. This is particularly relevant to disease control , such as diabetes, where individualized nutrition practices can lead to optimal glycemic control in addition to effective weight management, elucidating the nexus between diet choice and metabolic health (Olorunfemi et al., 2025). Also, the metabolic health issues extend beyond weight regulation to the prevention of chronic diseases. NAFLD is directly associated with metabolic dysregulation and obesity. There is evidence that proper dietary control, particularly with adequate protein provision, can exert a strong influence on metabolic processes and reduce the development of NAFLD. Increased protein intake not only aids in reducing fat deposits in the liver but also assists in overall metabolic functions, which are essential for weight control. Plant proteins, in particular, have additional metabolic advantages over animal proteins, illustrating the importance of the diversity of proteins in one's diet. Hence, metabolic health management through deliberate nutritional choices is of utmost significance not only for the regulation of weight but also for enhancing the establishment of long-term wellness and reducing the incidence of chronic disease in the population (Shariq et al., 2025) (Figure 6.21).

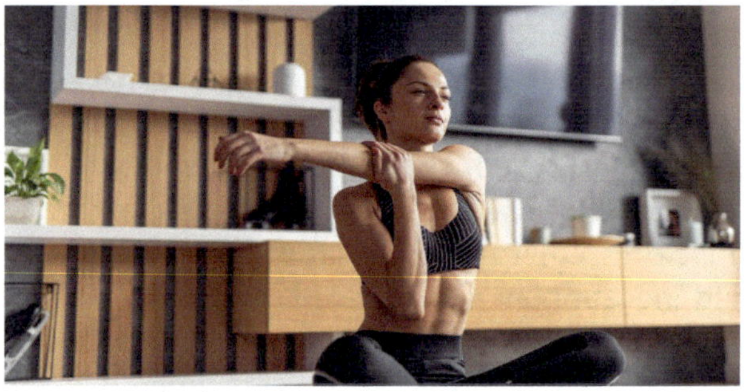

Figure 6.21. Understanding the vital role of metabolism in weight management.

Source: https://setu.in/cdn/shop/articles/24-May-blog-images_970x.jpg?v=1716791081.

Test Your Knowledge

1. What is the role of physical activity?
2. How does metabolism affect weight management?

6.6. Nutrition and Disease

Learning Outcome

1. Describe the relationship between nutrition and chronic diseases;
2. Understand the role of nutrition in immune function;
3. Know the nutritional interventions for disease prevention.

Interactions between disease and nutrition have increasingly shown themselves in modern public health discourse. Given the alarming rise in obesity at a global level, the World Health Organization declared obesity as a global epidemic on the basis of overwhelming statistics pointing to over 1.5 billion adults being classified as overweight and approximately 500 million as clinically obese, defined by body mass indexes over 25 kg/m^2 and 30 kg/m^2, respectively (Kyrou et al., 2010). This trend is not limited to adults but also applies to children and teenagers, and the problem is of increasing concern to future health trends in youth. It is thus important to explicate the mechanisms linking poor diet with obesity pathologies , such as type 2 diabetes and CVD in order to develop interventions to reverse these trends and foster improved health outcomes. The interaction between food intake and disease development including type 2 diabetes is mediated to a large degree by the metabolic consequences of dietary consumption. Resistance to insulin has become one of the major predictors of the onset of type 2 diabetes, as well as combined chronic energy overconsumption and physical inactivity. This is a lifestyle trend that leads to risk factors including abdominal adiposity and metabolic syndrome. Weight loss has been shown to reduce insulin resistance effectively; however, the long-term maintenance of weight loss poses a significant barrier to public health intervention. It has been determined by scientific findings that modifications in the macronutrient content of diets may provide additional metabolic benefits through the treatment of insulin resistance independent of weight loss, which may contain promising data on the treatment of obesity and diabetes prevention (Weickert, 2012). For tackling the negative impacts on health owing to unhealthy eating patterns, an overall solution towards nutrition education is the way forward. The shift should include not only emphasizing the importance of consuming healthy foods rich in whole foods but also the need for long-term behavioral changes that result in more physical activities and awareness in eating. Preventative interventions need to surpass personal dietary choices, addressing broader socio-economic determinants of nutrition inequalities, especially among vulnerable groups. By equipping individuals with the knowledge and assistance to make correct food decisions, public health initiatives are well-placed to address the double epidemics of obesity and type 2 diabetes, hence yielding a healthier population as well as reduced accompanying healthcare expenditures. Managing diet-related disease through education and policy has the potential to create an environment supportive of healthier food and improved metabolic health, laying a groundwork for long-term change (Figure 6.22).

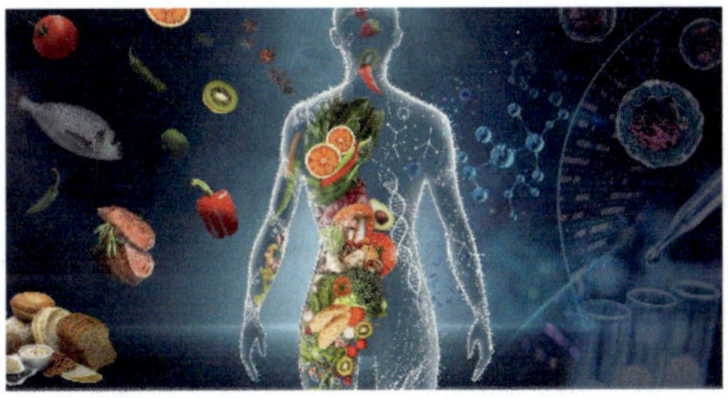

Figure 6.22. Nutrition and disease.

Source: https://magazine.einsteinmed.edu/wp-content/uploads/sites/4/2024/10/SF24-Food-Header-Full-FPO-2.jpg.

6.6.1. Relationship Between Nutrition and Chronic Diseases

The intricacy of the interaction between dietary

patterns and chronic diseases underscores the relevance of eating habits in controlling good health and the prevention of metabolic diseases. Modern diet lifestyles involving high-calorie intake and minimal nutrient content have contributed to a rise in obesity that has been described as a world epidemic. Obesity is causally related to various chronic diseases, most of which include CVD, type 2 diabetes, and certain cancers. Moreover, obesity is not only a standalone condition, but it also exacerbates other medical threats , such as hypertension and dyslipidemia, to become a multifaceted dynamic that is challenging to address by public health measures. Interventions focused on nutrition education and promotion of healthy diets are required to offset these dangers. Through employing whole diet guidelines that focus on nutrient-rich foods , such as fruits, vegetables, and whole grain cereals, a significant amount of prevention may be achieved against limiting the prevalence of obesity and other chronic diseases (Stasi et al., 2022). In addition to maintaining adequate control of caloric intake, some nutrients play vital roles in disease prevention. For instance, carotenoids, which occur in abundance in pigmented fruits and vegetables, are associated with lower risks of many chronic conditions, including CVD and obesity. While positive correlations with dietary consumption have been noted, intervention trials using isolated carotenoid supplements have produced mixed findings, an indication that supplementation with these compounds alone does not replicate the health advantage gained through foods. Their complexity of metabolic interactions and processes in the diet shows that the intricate interactions of the different nutrients can be crucial to achieve maximum health effects. Thus, the understanding of such mechanisms is significant in the development of evidence-based dietary recommendations that can successfully counteract chronic disease (Bohn et al., 2021). Further, chronic diseases often have multiplex etiologies, like lifestyle and genetic susceptibility. To optimally address such complexity, nutritional strategies must be personalized and consider variability in health status and genetics. For example, the Mediterranean diet, with its emphasis on healthy fat, lean protein, and plentiful vegetables and fruit, has been effective in managing conditions related to obesity and CVD. It is worth mentioning, however, that responses to diets , such as these may vary with pre-existing medical conditions and individual metabolic responses. Therefore, the integration of nutrition interventions in integrated health care models has the ability to provide personalized interventions for vulnerable populations. Based on an interdisciplinary model with nutrition, genetics, and lifestyle change, it is possible to promote preventive behaviors with significant impacts on the prevention of and development of chronic diseases (Stasi et al., 2022) (Figure 6.23).

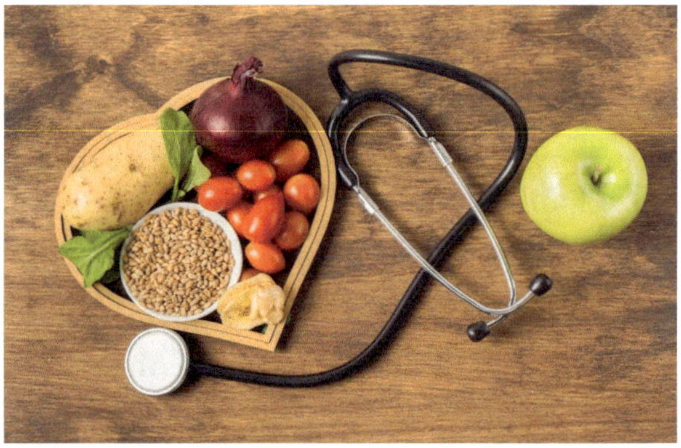

Figure 6.23. Conceptual image highlighting the role of nutrition in heart health and chronic disease prevention.

Source: https://www.euroschoolindia.com/blogs/wp-content/uploads/2024/04/nutrition-chronic-diseases.webp.

6.6.2. Role of Nutrition in Immune Function

The intricate interplay between nutrition and immune response is underscored by the powerful role that food nutrients play in the body's defense against infection. Optimal nutrition is required for maintaining the integrity of the immune system. Deficient consumption of certain key nutrients, such as vitamins A, C, D, and E, and minerals zinc and selenium, can compromise immune function and lead to increased susceptibility to infections. Moreover, the role of macronutrients, carbohydrates, proteins, and fats, in immune function regulation cannot be overestimated. Proteins, for instance, bring precursors to antibodies and immune response enzymes, while balanced carbohydrates power immune cell function. Thus, proper attention to food structure is of highest importance in the maintenance of optimal immune health, especially among risk populations like the aged, whose immune functions naturally decline with increasing age. When the body grows older, the relationship between diet and immune function is more complex. Aging comes together with changes in metabolism, along with diminished immune responsiveness, or immune senescence. Diet is significant in influencing this state through lifestyle that alters not only nutrient consumption but also gut microbiome composition. New research indicates that high-fiber eating, protein, and specific fatty acids, such as omega-3s, can have a positive influence on immune function, particularly in the elderly. Such diets promote the growth of gut-friendly bacteria that enhance immune function and overall well-being. It is essential to appreciate the dynamic interaction between nutrient intake, gut microbiome, and immune function in establishing dietary guidelines for aging populations. It aims to reverse the effects of aging on immunity through applying nutrition as a strategic intervention in health care, enhancing the quality of life of individuals as they age (Babakhani et al., 2025). Nutrition is more than the mere delivery of macronutrients and micronutrients; it is also the broader context of determinants of lifestyle that might influence immune efficacy. For example, environmental exposure to toxic agents , such as secondhand smoke has been shown to disrupt immune signaling mechanisms and can counteract the benefits of a normal diet. In individuals who are already experiencing compromised health, such as patients with cystic fibrosis, further deterioration of immune function by extrinsic factors is especially problematic. Moreover, emerging evidence highlights the pathological effects of e-cigarette smoking, which disturb immune function, adding to the complexity in nutritional approaches to promote healthy outcomes within exposed populations. As more studies continue to unravel these complex relationships, a greater focus on a comprehensive approach that integrates both nutrition and the environment is critical to establishing immune resilience within diverse populations (Wisniewski et al., 2025) (Figure 6.24).

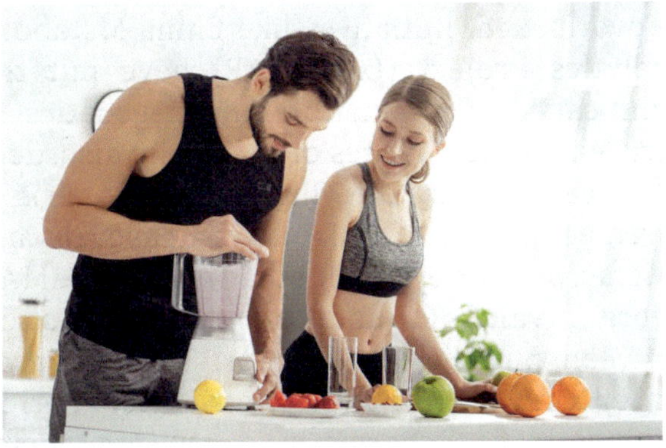

Figure 6.24. The role of nutrition in boosting immunity.

Source: https://www.fasttrackurgentcare.com/wp-content/uploads/2024/02/The-Role-Of-Nutrition-In-Boosting-Immunity-A-Deep-Dive.jpg.

6.6.3. Nutritional Interventions for Disease Prevention

The synergy of metabolism and nutrition has received increasing scrutiny for its therapeutic potential for disease prevention of chronic diseases. The most recent approach is time-restricted feeding (TRF), which exploits the physiological events underlying the body's circadian rhythms. By restricting caloric intake to a regular interval of less than 12 hours, TRF disrupts the usual dieting regimens that underlie metabolic derangement. Research has demonstrated that such a regimen is effective in controlling a variety of metabolic processes, hence reducing the possibility of obesity, diabetes, and CVD. Specific mechanisms have been affirmed by preclinical research, which laid down possible mechanisms behind the metabolic health effects of TRF. With growing comprehension of circadian biology, TRF represents a viable intervention through nutrition, a new chapter in understanding how eating patterns could regulate overall health and suppress disease (Emily et al., 2021). In concert with data on TRF, the strong influence of genetic factors in metabolic disorders cannot be overlooked. Initiatives like China Metabolic Analytics Project (ChinaMAP) have put the significance of population-human genetics in unravelling the nuances of metabolic disorders into focal point. By studying the genetic basis of parameters , such as blood glucose levels and BMI across different populations, ChinaMAP offers invaluable data on the interaction between nutrition and genes. This research underscores that nutrition intervention tailored to each person's genetic tendencies can lead to enhanced prevention of disease. This comprehensive approach of combining nutritional and genetic factors is aided by today's consensus that individual genetic variations can influence reaction to diet and long-term health (Cao et al., 2020). This combination of nutritional intervention and genetics calls for an integrated approach to disease prevention. As society is confronted with increasing incidence of metabolic disorders, embracing personalized nutritional approaches, like TRF, may represent the key to prevention. Not only do such approaches target intervening in existing health patterns, but they also enable individuals by offering practical eating advice grounded in both genetic information as well as in metabolic science. Besides, with the scientific community progressing in understanding the intricate connections between our metabolism and genes, ongoing study will be necessary to make these treatments more accurate. Ultimately, a complete practice that melds together nutritional science with genetics is most important to formulate individualized dietary regimens that avoid not just disease but also promote lifelong health (Cao et al., 2020; Emily et al., 2021) (Figure 6.25).

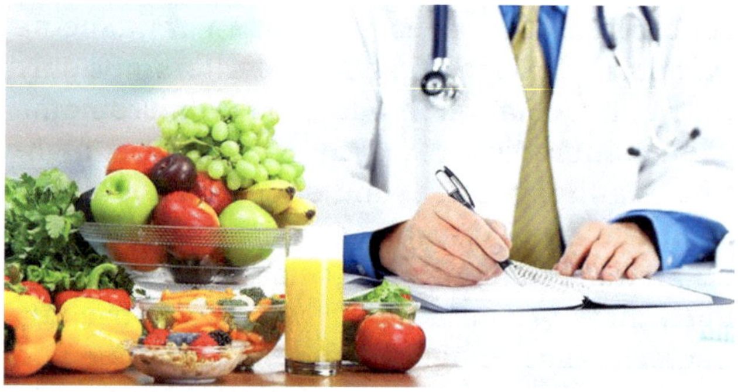

Figure 6.25. The role of diet and nutrition in disease prevention and management.

Source: https://caresupp.in/cdn/shop/articles/tregtytr.jpg?v=1702977100.

Test Your Knowledge

1. What is the relationship between nutrition and chronic diseases?
2. What is the role of nutrition in immune function?

SUMMARY

In drawing conclusions regarding the relationship between metabolism and nutrition, it is evident that dietary selection plays a crucial role in affecting metabolic processes and health. As human diet structure would directly affect the gut microbiota, dietary nutrients , such as dietary polysaccharides and oligosaccharides have been found to strongly modulate microbial structure and metabolic activities. For instance, evidence indicates that the intake of wheat bran arabinoxylan oligosaccharides (AXOS) can lead to an increase in populations of health-promoting bacteria, such as Bifidobacterium species, which themselves are associated with improved metabolic health and potentially lower risk of disease. The confluence of nutrition and metabolism both emphasizes the importance of planning meals and provides an opportunity to tailor nutritional interventions to maximize returns for health. Furthermore, the consequences of diet extend far beyond individual health to affect broader public health concerns, particularly in light of global imperatives like food security. With the population of the world predicted to rise to 9 billion by 2050, sustainable strategies for food production must become an urgent priority. That imperative renders it essential to develop dietary strategies that are both nutritionally appropriate and environmentally sustainable. Policies that favor the cultivation of nutrient-dense crops, in addition to access/utilization balance, are integral. These measures will create the needed pathway for every community to achieve optimal nutrition and therefore metabolic health. These interdependent problems require resolution by a multidisciplinary approach in nutritional science that synergizes epidemiologic data with innovative means of farming. Lastly, a comprehensive understanding of metabolism and nutrition must be a reflection of the dynamism of dietetics and its impact on wellness. Current research indicates the importance of continually exploring the impact of certain nutrients on metabolic processes and general health in various populations. Personalized nutrition can become an integral method in optimizing metabolic health as evidenced by the action of prebiotic supplementation on gut microbiota composition. However, this field needs more research to understand the long-term impact of food interventions. It is most crucial that research scientists, medical professionals, and policymakers work together to bridge the gap between new nutritional science and daily practice in public health. By forming such partnerships, society can transition to a healthier future where informed food decisions play their part in the proper manner towards individual and public metabolic health (Matthew et al., 2017; Chung et al., 2020).

The intricate relationship between nutrition and metabolism is underlined by the powerful effect of nutritional patterns on metabolic performance. One of the most significant issues within this field is malnutrition, particularly among the most vulnerable groups, such as cancer patients. Malnutrition has severe implications, including prolongation of hospital stay, increased treatment-related toxicity, and diminished quality of life, ultimately affecting the prognosis of the patient. Studies have shown that the majority of cancer patients are nutritionally under-nourished, and routine nutritional screening with established instruments , such as the Nutritional Risk Screening 2002 and the Mini Nutritional Assessment, is essential. Screening should occur at the time of diagnosis and then regularly during the course of treatment to provide timely intervention for those who are at nutritional risk. A tailored nutritional management, in the form of counseling, is critical in maximizing the outcome for this group (Beretta et al., 2016). Metabolic reactions to nutrition interventions are significant in understanding the health status. For instance, sleep is a significant parameter that affects insulin sensitivity as well as metabolic function. Experimental evidence has established that deprivation in sleep leads to decreased insulin sensitivity, a parameter that is not desirable for metabolic health. Surprisingly, exercise has been shown to reverse some of these adverse effects. A single session of sprint interval exercise is shown by studies to significantly increase insulin sensitivity after nocturnal sleep deprivation. Comparison of late-phase insulin response during exercise versus a control condition gives valuable insight into metabolic resilience under challenge. This finding points to the possibility of incorporating ordered physical activity into daily life, particularly in susceptible individuals at risk of metabolic disorder (Ellis et al., 2020). Overall, the interplay between food and metabolism is central to enhancing well-being, particularly in susceptible groups. Personalized nutritional care for cancer patients and interventions to enhance metabolic health through regular physical activity are promising opportunities for the optimization of therapeutic outcomes. The need for comprehensive approaches , such as nutritional evaluation, customized dietary counseling, and constant exercise patterns heightens as medical professionals seek to treat the dual concerns of malnutrition and metabolic disturbance. By taking these variables into account comprehensively, treatment professionals are able to make significant contributions to both short-term recuperation and final prognosis in patients confronting challenging health challenges. Thus, ongoing research is essential to further enhance these strategies and their effective implementation in clinical settings for the overall well-being of the patients (Beretta et al., 2016; Ellis et al., 2020).

KEY TERMS FROM THIS CHAPTER

- Biochemical reactions
- Carbohydrates
- Enzymes
- Fats
- Hepcidin
- Macronutrients
- Metabolizable energy
- Metabolism
- Micronutrients
- Minerals
- Nutrition
- Prebiotics
- Probiotics
- Proteins
- Vitamins

CRITICAL THINKING QUESTIONS

1. **Which macronutrient provides the highest amount of energy per gram?**
   a. Carbohydrates
   b. Proteins
   c. Fats
   d. Vitamins
2. **The basal metabolic rate (BMR) primarily measures:**
   a. Energy expended during exercise
   b. Energy required for digestion
   c. Energy needed for basic physiological functions at rest
   d. Energy consumed from dietary sources
3. **Which of the following vitamins is water-soluble?**
   a. Vitamin A
   b. Vitamin D
   c. Vitamin C
   d. Vitamin E
4. **Which mineral is essential for the synthesis of hemoglobin?**
   a. Calcium
   b. Magnesium
   c. Iron
   d. Zinc
5. **The primary storage form of carbohydrates in the human body is:**
   a. Glucose
   b. Glycogen
   c. Starch
   d. Cellulose

Short Answer Questions

1. Why is nutrition important to health?
2. What are macronutrients?
3. What are micronutrients?
4. What is the role of the digestive system in nutrition?
5. What is metabolism?

Answers to Critical Thinking Questions

1. (c); 2. (c); 3. (c); 4. (c); 5. (b)

REFERENCES

1. Al-Dujaili, E., Good, G., & Tsang, C. (2016). Consumption of pomegranate juice attenuates exercise-induced oxidative stress, blood pressure and urinary cortisol/cortisone ratio in human adults. https://core.ac.uk/download/305121376.pdf (accessed on 12th June 2025).
2. Altman, P. L., & Fisher, K. D. (1986). *Research Opportunities in Nutrition and Metabolism in Space*. https://core.ac.uk/download/pdf/10458014.pdf (accessed on 12th June 2025).
3. Arefiev, Y., Chao, R., Chaudry, H., et al. (2017). Heme oxygenase induction suppresses hepatic hepcidin and rescues ferroprotein and ferritin expression in obese mice. https://core.ac.uk/download/129592561.pdf (accessed on 12th June 2025).
4. Babakhani, K., Kucinskas, A. L., Ye, X., Giles, E. D., & Sun, Y. (2025). Aging immunity: Unraveling the complex nexus of diet, gut microbiome, and immune function. *Immunometabolism (Cobham, Surrey), 7*, e00061–e00061. https://www.semanticscholar.org/paper/5500305979172731f2e3c8b527b97dc8b49097d2 (accessed on 12th June 2025).
5. Barreto, R. F., Cruz, F. J. R., Felisberto, G., et al. (2017). Potassium nutrition in fruits and vegetables and food safety through hydroponic system. https://core.ac.uk/download/322434200.pdf (accessed on 12th June 2025).
6. Bauer, E., Metzler-Zebeli, B. U., Mosenthin, R., et al. (2011). Intestinal gene expression in pigs: Effects of reduced feed intake during weaning and potential impact of dietary components. https://core.ac.uk/download/pdf/29230036.pdf (accessed on 12th June 2025).
7. Bauer, K., Böhles, H., Fusch, C., et al. (2009). Neonatologie/Pädiatrie–Leitlinie Parenterale Ernährung, Kapitel 13. https://core.ac.uk/download/14527634.pdf (accessed on 12th June 2025).
8. Beretta, G. D., Caccialanza, R., Cereda, E., et al. (2016). Nutritional support in cancer patients: A position paper from the Italian Society of Medical Oncology (AIOM) and the Italian Society of Artificial Nutrition and Metabolism (SINPE). https://core.ac.uk/download/74324933.pdf (accessed on 12th June 2025).
9. Bielik, V., & Kolísek, M. (2021). Bio accessibility and bioavailability of minerals in relation to a healthy gut microbiome. *International Journal of Molecular Sciences, 22*, 6803–6803. https://doi.org/10.3390/ijms22136803 (accessed on 12th June 2025).
10. Bohn, T., Bonet, M. L., Borel, P., Keijer, J., Landrier, J. F., Milisav, I., Ribot, J., et al. (2021). Mechanistic aspects of carotenoid health benefits–Where are we now? *Nutrition Research Reviews, 34*, 276–302. https://doi.org/10.1017/s0954422421000147 (accessed on 12th June 2025).
11. Bonner, M. R., & Alavanja, M. C. R. (2017). Pesticides, human health, and food security. *Food and Energy Security, 6*, 89–93. https://doi.org/10.1002/fes3.112 (accessed on 12th June 2025).
12. Bouillon, R., & Bikle, D. D. (2019). Vitamin D metabolism revised: Fall of dogmas. *Journal of Bone and Mineral Research, 34*, 1985–1992. https://doi.org/10.1002/jbmr.3884 (accessed on 12th June 2025).
13. Buckton, C., & Combet, E. (2014). Micronutrient deficiencies, vitamin pills and nutritional supplements. https://core.ac.uk/download/42357992.pdf (accessed on 12th June 2025).
14. Campanale, C., Massarelli, C., Savino, I., Locaputo, V., & Uricchio, V. F. (2020). A detailed

review study on potential effects of microplastics and additives of concern on human health. *International Journal of Environmental Research and Public Health, 17*, 1212–1212. https://doi.org/10.3390/ijerph17041212 (accessed on 12th June 2025).

15. Cao, Y., Li, L., Xu, M., Feng, Z., Sun, X., Lu, J., Xu, Y., et al. (2020). The ChinaMAP analytics of deep whole genome sequences in 10,588 individuals. *Cell Research, 30*, 717–731. https://doi.org/10.1038/s41422-020-0322-9 (accessed on 12th June 2025).

16. Çelik, Z., Akduman, G., Özen, H., Daşdemir, Ş., & Güneş, F. (2021). Determining the possible effect of diabetes on the nutritional status of hemodialysis patients. *Journal of International Health Sciences and Management*. https://www.semanticscholar.org/paper/58994554515b3cc479885975375c605732712097 (accessed on 12th June 2025).

17. Chen, L., Delville, C., Derous, D., et al. (2017). The effects of graded levels of calorie restriction: VIII. Impact of short-term calorie and protein restriction on basal metabolic rate in the C57BL/6 mouse. https://core.ac.uk/download/80685984.pdf (accessed on 12th June 2025).

18. Chung, W. S. F., Walker, A. W., Bosscher, D., Garcia-Campayo, V., Wagner, J., Parkhill, J., Duncan, S. H., et al. (2020). Relative abundance of the *Prevotella* genus within the human gut microbiota of elderly volunteers determines the inter-individual responses to dietary supplementation with wheat bran arabinoxylan-oligosaccharides. *BMC Microbiology, 20*. https://doi.org/10.1186/s12866-020-01968-4 (accessed on 12th June 2025).

19. Clemente-Suárez, V. J., Beltrán-Velasco, A. I., Redondo-Flórez, L., Martín-Rodríguez, A., & Tornero-Aguilera, J. F. (2023). Global impacts of Western diet and its effects on metabolism and health: A narrative review. *Nutrients, 15*, 2749–2749. https://doi.org/10.3390/nu15122749 (accessed on 12th June 2025).

20. Cryan, J. F., O'Riordan, K. J., Cowan, C. S. M., Sandhu, K. V., Bastiaanssen, T. F. S., Boehme, M., Codagnone, M. G., et al. (2019). The microbiota-gut-brain axis. *Physiological Reviews, 99*, 1877–2013. https://doi.org/10.1152/physrev.00018.2018 (accessed on 12th June 2025).

21. D'Amico, D., Andreux, P. A., Valdés, P., Singh, A., Rinsch, C., & Auwerx, J. (2021). Impact of the natural compound urolithin A on health, disease, and aging. *Trends in Molecular Medicine, 27*, 687–699. https://doi.org/10.1016/j.molmed.2021.04.009 (accessed on 12th June 2025).

22. Darmani Kuhi, H., Dijkstra, J., Dumas, A., et al. (2010). A review of mathematical functions for the analysis of growth in poultry. https://core.ac.uk/download/pdf/29241478.pdf (accessed on 12th June 2025).

23. de Vos, W. M., Tilg, H., Van Hul, M., & Cani, P. D. (2022). Gut microbiome and health: Mechanistic insights. *Gut, 71*, 1020–1032. https://doi.org/10.1136/gutjnl-2021-326789 (accessed on 12th June 2025).

24. Deutz, N. E. P., Engelen, M. P., Rodriguez, R. E., et al. (2018). Increased amino acid turnover and myofibrillar protein breakdown in advanced cancer are associated with muscle weakness and impaired physical function. https://core.ac.uk/download/196606826.pdf (accessed on 12th June 2025).

25. Dodd, F., Haskell-Ramsay, C., Jackson, P., et al. (2020). Acute and chronic effects of multivitamin/mineral supplementation on objective and subjective energy measures. https://core.ac.uk/download/305121296.pdf (accessed on 12th June 2025).

26. Donini, L. M., Busetto, L., Bischoff, S. C., Cederholm, T., Ballesteros-Pomar, M. D., Batsis, J. A.,

Bauer, J. M., et al. (2022). Definition and diagnostic criteria for sarcopenic obesity: ESPEN and EASO consensus statement. *Clinical Nutrition, 41*, 990–1000. https://doi.org/10.1016/j.clnu.2021.11.014 (accessed on 12th June 2025).

27. Dumas, A., Dijkstra, J., & France, J. (2008). Mathematical modelling in animal nutrition: A centenary review. https://core.ac.uk/download/pdf/29258963.pdf (accessed on 12th June 2025).

28. Edwards, C. A., Gerasimidis, K., Khan, M. J., et al. (2016). Role of gut microbiota in the aetiology of obesity: Proposed mechanisms and review of the literature. https://core.ac.uk/download/74229906.pdf (accessed on 12th June 2025).

29. Ellis, J., Harkes, T., Kyza, I., et al. (2020). Impaired insulin profiles following a single night of sleep restriction: The impact of acute sprint interval exercise. https://core.ac.uk/download/286359281.pdf (accessed on 12th June 2025).

30. Estevão, S. C. O., da Silva, G. H. N., Oliveira, L. R. R., dos Santos, L. O., Raimundo, E., Vieira, R. B., Rodrigues, T. A., et al. (2025). Bioavailability of tryptophan biomass for laying hens. *Animals: An Open Access Journal from MDPI, 15.* https://www.semanticscholar.org/paper/878e6056c428f6a50ef2c8a8fb83e3387a1dd7f4 (accessed on 12th June 2025).

31. Evert, A. B., Dennison, M., Gardner, C. D., Garvey, W. T., Lau, K. H. K., MacLeod, J., Mitri, J., et al. (2019). Nutrition therapy for adults with diabetes or prediabetes: A consensus report. *Diabetes Care, 42*, 731–754. https://doi.org/10.2337/dci19-0014 (accessed on 12th June 2025).

32. Fulton, S., Décarie-Spain, L., Fioramonti, X., Guiard, B. P., & Nakajima, S. (2021). The menace of obesity to depression and anxiety prevalence. *Trends in Endocrinology and Metabolism, 33*, 18–35. https://doi.org/10.1016/j.tem.2021.10.005 (accessed on 12th June 2025).

33. Hu, W., Zhao, C., Hu, H., & Yin, S. (2021). Food sources of selenium and its relationship with chronic diseases. *Nutrients, 13*, 1739–1739. https://doi.org/10.3390/nu13051739 (accessed on 12th June 2025).

34. Janssen, J. J. E., Grefte, S., Keijer, J., & de Boer, V. C. J. (2019). Mito-nuclear communication by mitochondrial metabolites and its regulation by B-vitamins. *Frontiers in Physiology, 10.* https://doi.org/10.3389/fphys.2019.00078 (accessed on 12th June 2025).

35. Jia, H., & Dong, N. (2024). Effects of bile acid metabolism on intestinal health of livestock and poultry. *Journal of Animal Physiology and Animal Nutrition.* https://www.semanticscholar.org/paper/d1f92a37c4c4d9479eca252d28d3871978ec6723 (accessed on 12th June 2025).

36. Jopkiewicz, S. P. (2019). The barrier and the intestinal microflora–The factors determining the state of human health. https://core.ac.uk/download/587243125.pdf (accessed on 12th June 2025).

37. Kuiper-Makris, C., Selle, J., Nüsken, E., Dötsch, J., & Alejandre Alcázar, M. A. (2021). Perinatal nutritional and metabolic pathways: Early origins of chronic lung diseases. *Frontiers in Medicine, 8.* https://doi.org/10.3389/fmed.2021.667315 (accessed on 12th June 2025).

38. Kwakkel, R. P., Syafwan, W., & Verstegen, M. W. A. (2011). Heat stress and feeding strategies in meat-type chickens. https://core.ac.uk/download/pdf/29231768.pdf (accessed on 12th June 2025).

39. Kyrou, I., & Weickert, M. O. (2010). Clinical problems caused by obesity. https://core.ac.uk/download/46324.pdf (accessed on 12th June 2025).

40. Li, J., Zhao, J., Tian, C., Dong, L., Kang, Z., Wang, J., Zhao, S., et al. (2024). Mechanisms of regulation of glycolipid metabolism by natural compounds in plants: Effects on short-chain fatty acids. *Nutrition & Metabolism, 21*. https://www.semanticscholar.org/paper/a93757d78d965823703f5484e4e1ef95519ad111 (accessed on 12th June 2025).

41. Ma, Y. (2025). The relationship between gut microbes and nutrient absorption and its application status. *Theoretical and Natural Science*. https://www.semanticscholar.org/paper/ed88d10acf5e1112493612747496 4f3873f8bf35 (accessed on 12th June 2025).

42. Manoogian, E. N. C., Chow, L. S., Taub, P. R., Laferrère, B., & Panda, S. (2021). Time-restricted eating for the prevention and management of metabolic diseases. *Endocrine Reviews, 43*, 405–436. https://doi.org/10.1210/endrev/bnab027 (accessed on 12th June 2025).

43. Olorunfemi, O., Oni, O. F., & Owoyomi, D. O. (2025). Transforming diabetes care through self-care: The role of customized nutrition plans and carbohydrate tracking in achieving weight regulation and improved clinical outcomes. *Bangladesh Journal of Endocrinology and Metabolism*. https://www.semanticscholar.org/paper/4573d46cb1399c1294b383dd07b209b5e9d8f704 (accessed on 12th June 2025).

44. Parreño, M. A., Alaux, C., Brunet, J. L., Buydens, L., Filipiak, M., Henry, M., Keller, A., et al. (2021). Critical links between biodiversity and health in wild bee conservation. *Trends in Ecology & Evolution, 37*, 309–321. https://doi.org/10.1016/j.tree.2021.11.013 (accessed on 12th June 2025).

45. Sánchez, B., Delgado, S., Blanco-Míguez, A., Lourenço, A., Gueimonde, M., & Margollés, A. (2016). Probiotics, gut microbiota, and their influence on host health and disease. *Molecular Nutrition & Food Research, 61*. https://doi.org/10.1002/mnfr.201600240 (accessed on 12th June 2025).

46. Sarmidi, M. R. (2012). *Food is Our Medicine.* https://core.ac.uk/download/11801185.pdf (accessed on 12th June 2025).

47. Shariq, A., Khan, S., & Usmani, S. U. R. (2025). The role of dietary protein in mitigating the risk of nonalcoholic fatty liver disease. *Nutrition Reviews*. https://www.semanticscholar.org/paper/8f9676f77fdcf00be8ea9de515a48c17b0be8bf2 (accessed on 12th June 2025).

48. Stasi, A., Cosola, C., Caggiano, G., Cimmarusti, M. T., Palieri, R., Acquaviva, P. M., Rana, G., et al. (2022). Obesity-related chronic kidney disease: Principal mechanisms and new approaches in nutritional management. *Frontiers in Nutrition, 9*. https://doi.org/10.3389/fnut.2022.925619 (accessed on 12th June 2025).

49. Swanson, K. S., Gibson, G. R., Hutkins, R., Reimer, R. A., Reid, G., Verbeke, K., Scott, K. P., et al. (2020). The International Scientific Association for Probiotics and Prebiotics (ISAPP) consensus statement on the definition and scope of symbiotic. *Nature Reviews Gastroenterology & Hepatology, 17*, 687–701. https://doi.org/10.1038/s41575-020-0344-2 (accessed on 12th June 2025).

50. Voroncova, T., Konyk, T., Trokhymenko, M., & Mudryk, Y. (2025). Breast milk: Its components and special effects on newborns and infants. *Journal of Education, Health and Sport*. https://www.semanticscholar.org/paper/44cea209d22ce3a4236be9ed2515311458969019 (accessed on 12th June 2025).

51. Weickert, M. O. (2012). Nutritional modulation of insulin resistance. https://core.ac.uk/download/18328007.pdf (accessed on 12th June 2025).

52. Wisniewski, B., Shrestha, M., Bojja, D., Shrestha, C., Lee, C. S., Ozuna, H., Rayner, R., et al. (2025). Secondhand vape exposure regulation of CFTR and immune function in cystic fibrosis. *American Journal of Physiology. Lung Cellular and Molecular Physiology*. https://www.semanticscholar.org/paper/d796ce1303cc49d90f0e1f6ddfbf67bbbc3a5017 (accessed on 12th June 2025).

53. Zheng, J., Wittouck, S., Salvetti, E., Franz, C. M. A. P., Harris, H. M. B., Mattarelli, P., O'Toole, P. W., et al. (2020). A taxonomic note on the genus *Lactobacillus*: Description of 23 novel genera, emended description of the genus *Lactobacillus* Beijerinck 1901, and union of *Lactobacillus* and *Leuconostocaceae*. *International Journal of Systematic and Evolutionary Microbiology, 70*, 2782–2858. https://doi.org/10.1099/ijsem.0.004107 (accessed on 12th June 2025).

54. Zou, M. L. (2007). *Variation in the Apparent Fecal Digestibility of Macronutrients and Urinary Energy Excretion for Three Diets Varying in Fat and Fiber Content—Assessment of the Atwater Factors and Related Energy Conversion Factors: A Thesis Presented in Partial Fulfillment of The Requirements for The Degree of Master of Science in Nutritional Science at Massey University, Palmerston North, New Zealand.* https://core.ac.uk/download/162617248.pdf (accessed on 12th June 2025).

METABOLISM OF SPECIALIZED TISSUES

7

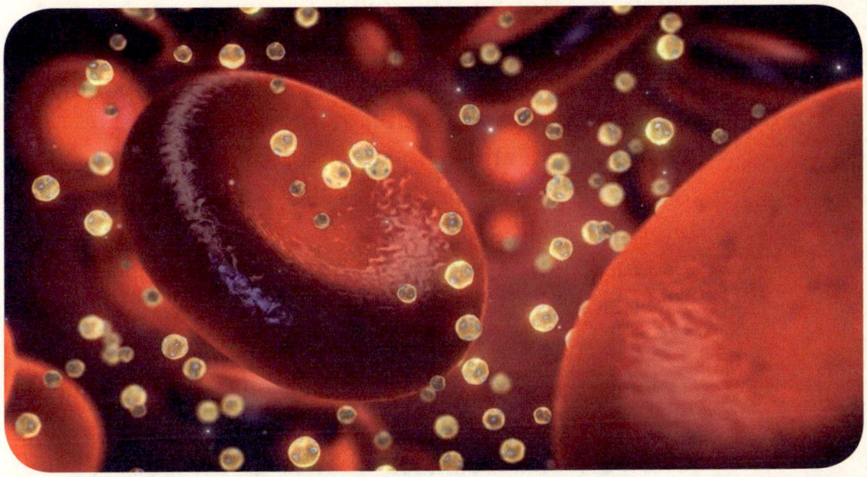

LEARNING OBJECTIVES

After studying this chapter, you will be able to:

1. Describe the muscle and adipose tissue metabolism;
2. Understand the liver and brain metabolism;
3. Understand the metabolism in endocrine tissues.

Introduction

The study of metabolic process in specialized tissues is part of the knowledge of how organisms adapt to internal and external stimuli and regulate homeostasis. Metabolism, in general as the summation of biochemical reactions occurring in a living organism, differs significantly between various types of tissues. This is due to the individual functions and environmental conditions of each tissue, which dictate various metabolic pathways. For example, in plant cells, leaf, stem, and fruit tissues possess unique metabolic adaptations that allow them to perform activities , such as photosynthesis, nutrient storage, and defense against disease. By examining these metabolic profiles, researchers can learn about how tissues communicate and orchestrate their behavior in response to developmental cues and environmental stresses, providing a context for the investigation of metabolic activities in specialized tissues. Understanding the reason why specialized tissues have unique metabolic pathways often involves exploring their molecular and genetic foundation. A few recent studies demonstrated how transcriptomic analyses, such as those involving RNA sequencing, capture profound changes in gene expression that are associated with various metabolic activities. Transcriptomic modulation in fruit tissues can potentially cause upregulation of genes associated with sugar metabolism and starch biosynthesis, which serves as an indication of complex interplay between disease symptomatology and metabolism. For instance, infection response in the plant can reveal alterations in source-sink relations that reorganize metabolic patterns to indicate how external stressors can compromise tissue function and plant health.

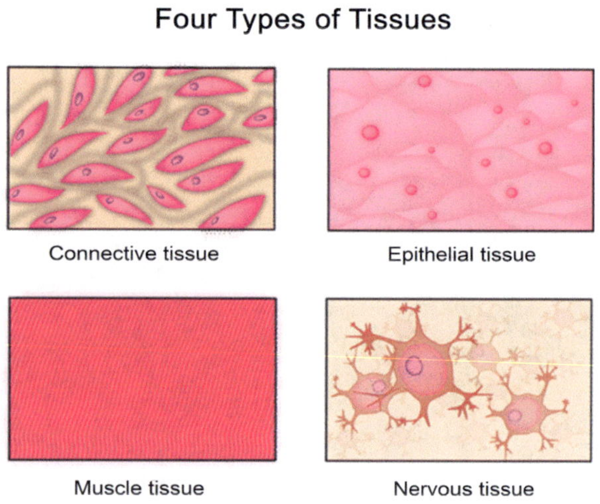

Figure 7.1. Four types of tissues.

Source: https://dr282zn36sxxg.cloudfront.net/datastreams/f-d%3A2d8ce980735ced00cf17c661eea81cbc3ab7e5054a8b27972a21ffd8%2BIMAGE_THUMB_POSTCARD_TINY%2BIMAGE_THUMB_POSTCARD_TINY.1.

These findings are crucial to establishing the molecular mechanisms underlying metabolic regulation and promising pathways to intervention in disease outbreaks, further elucidating complex interactions within specialized tissue. Besides plants, in model organisms , such as Caenorhabditis elegans, metabolic adaptation within specialized tissues is shown, providing a simpler system for the investigation of metabolism during developmental periods. The nematode's metabolic response to environmental attacks proves the conservation throughout evolution of fundamental metabolic processes, in agreement with higher eukaryotic systems. Notably, metabolic function alterations during the Dauer stage, characterized by a definite hypometabolic condition, point to the relevance of metabolic flexibility in surviving stressful environments. Such metabolic plasticity to environmental stressors enhances long-term survival and can be useful in shedding light on aging and longevity. Through the combination of data from plant and animal systems, studies of specialized tissue metabolism not only advance our knowledge of the biological processes involved but also enable applied research in both agriculture and medicine (Figure 7.1).

Importance of Specialized Tissues in the Body

The role of specialized tissues in the body of human beings cannot be overstated, as they carry out distinct roles that are crucial in maintaining the body's health and homeostasis. Specialized tissues , such as epithelial, connective, muscular, and nervous tissues, all have distinct functions in the body's integrated system. For instance, epithelial tissues form protective covering and facilitate absorption and secretion functions, while connective tissues provide strength and enable the transport of wastes and nutrients. Furthermore, muscular tissues bring about movement, and nervous tissues coordinate responses to internal and external stimuli. This intricate system of specialized tissues allows the body to successfully perform complex functions necessary for survival, underlining the importance of each tissue type in performing metabolic processes essential to life. Understanding the metabolic function of specialized tissues offers vital information regarding their role in health and disease. For example, skeletal muscle tissue, which accounts for a large proportion of body weight, is essential to locomotion and metabolic regulation. Far from being an inert contractile organ, as traditionally supposed, new proteomic analyses have highlighted, skeletal muscle is an active tissue involved in complex biochemical processes governing energy utilization and substrate use. These investigations uncovered over 10,000 proteins, shedding light on the intricate signaling pathway web that governs glucose and lipid metabolism. Such detailed metabolic mapping demotes the scepter of importance from the heart, suggesting how the normal function of skeletal muscle is not merely required for mobility but for overall metabolic balance and prevention of diseases like obesity and type 2 diabetes (Deshmukh et al., 2015). In addition, specialized tissue health is intricately linked with their respective systems, as evidenced by Ayurvedic Dhātu that aligns with our understanding of the different tissue types. According to Ayurvedic physiology, these special tissues, or Dhātus, are important for the attainment of balance between two or more body systems, such as the cardiovascular and immune systems, each contributing to dynamic homeostasis interaction. Tridosha theory is meant to emphasize how Vāta, Pitta, and Kapha balance explains the intricate control mechanisms of the body, including neural, endocrine, and immune activity (Patwardhan, 2008). A deeper understanding of how the metabolism of such specialized tissues governs larger physiological outcomes will enhance our ability to intervene in instances of disease and improve therapeutic approaches, thereby proving the generalized significance of specialized tissues to human health (Figure 7.2).

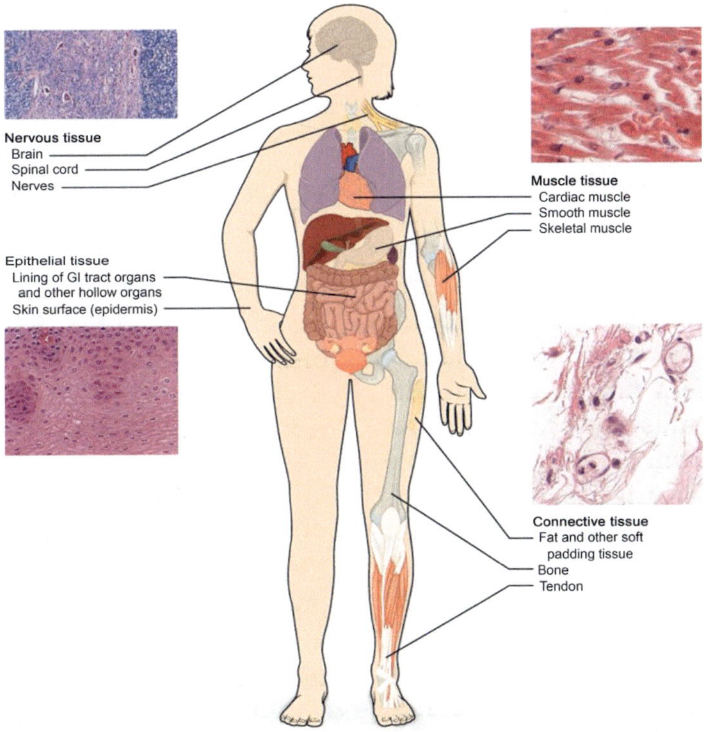

Figure 7.2. The four primary tissue types: Examples of nervous tissue, epithelial tissue, muscle tissue, and connective tissue found throughout the human body.

Source: https://open.oregonstate.education/app/uploads/sites/157/2019/07/401_Types_of_Tissue-768x815.jpg.

7.1. Muscle Tissue Metabolism

Learning Outcome

1. Describe the aerobic vs. anaerobic metabolism in muscles;
2. Understand the role of glycogen in muscle energy;
3. Describe the impact of exercise on muscle metabolism.

Muscle tissue metabolism is a dynamic and complex process that is primarily charged with the role of maintaining overall body homeostasis. About 40% of body weight consists of skeletal muscle, which not only facilitates movement but is also predominantly involved in the regulation of systemic metabolism. The tissue is highly heterogeneous, containing proteins involved in various metabolic processes, including glucose uptake and lipid metabolism. Emerging proteomic technologies have established a total of 10,218 skeletal muscle proteins, which show the presence of specific transcription factors regulating muscle differentiation and function. By measuring absolute protein abundances, researchers have been in a position to gain valuable insights regarding how these proteins associate with each other in metabolic pathways, specifically the intricate regulation of AMP-activated protein kinase and insulin signaling pathways in muscle tissue and how this is beneficial towards understanding how these pathways function under varying physiological conditions (Deshmukh et al., 2015). Furthermore, constructing functional models of muscle metabolism is enhanced by large-scale measurements of its transcriptome and proteome. Such an integrative strategy leverages massive datasets, allowing scientists to construct highly detailed models that account for the multitiered functions of skeletal muscle. By classifying proteins into specific functional families, e.g., those required for excitation, mechanical transmission, metabolic bioenergetics, and signaling, researchers can appreciate how muscle tissues respond to both regular physiological needs and disease states. Each functional family contains subfamilies that work in synergy, which emphasizes the interdependence feature of muscle metabolism. This analytical method not only contributes to the explanation of healthy muscle function but also serves as an instrument for the analysis of the etiopathogenesis of muscle diseases and metabolic disease, providing avenues for intervention (Subramaniam et al., 2012).

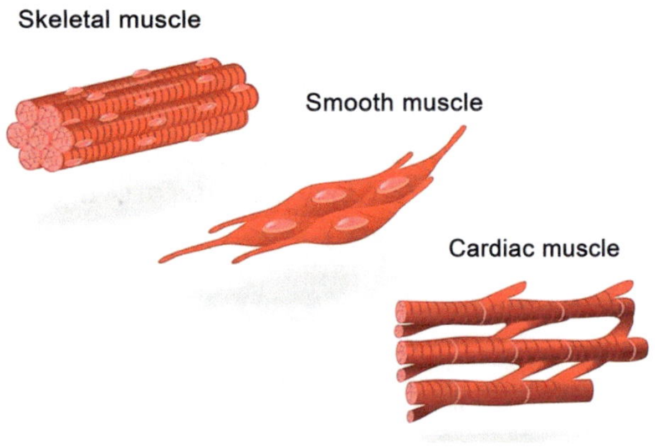

Figure 7.3. Types of muscle tissue.

Source: https://www.sciencelearn.org.nz/_next/image?url=https%3A%2F%2Fwww.datocms-assets.com%2F117510%2F1722387917-types-of-muscle-tissue20161111-16640-1c2x74o.jpg&w=3840&q=75&dpl=dpl_4n9pVfrF4H6vbtWLHqt8okXU1ahu.

In brief, the intricate muscle tissue metabolism is due to a heterogeneous population of proteins and biochemical pathways that respond to energetic demands on skeletal muscle. As new studies continue to uncover the details of muscle tissue proteomics and transcriptomics, the functional models developed enhance our ability to describe muscle behavior under various physiological conditions. The complex inter-mapping of the metabolic, signal, and mechanical networks is essential and can lead to improved strategies for therapeutic intervention in diseases of the muscle. Deciphering the metabolic intricacies of the muscle tissue is a vital endeavor within the broad framework of specialized tissue metabolism, and it will open doors to further studies that can utilize these complexities to the benefit of muscle health and longevity (Figure 7.3).

7.1.1. Aerobic vs. Anaerobic Metabolism in Muscles

In muscle physiology, one must first understand the independent pathways of aerobic and anaerobic metabolism to grasp the generation of energy in different types of physical activity. Aerobic metabolism that occurs in an oxygen-rich environment relies upon the process of oxidative phosphorylation in mitochondria in generating adenosine triphosphate (ATP)—the cell's primary energy currency.

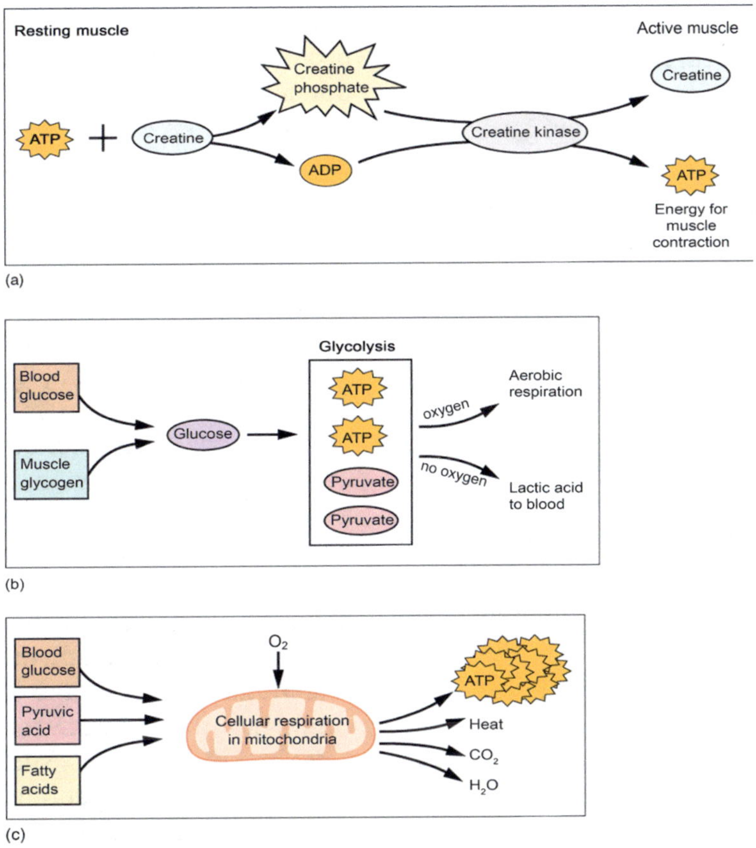

Figure 7.4. Cellular respiration during muscle metabolism.

Source: https://me-pedia.org/w/images/a/ab/Cellular-respiration.jpg.

This pathway utilizes glucose and fatty acids efficiently and generates a high ATP yield for long, moderate-intensity exercise, such as running or cycling a distance. Anaerobic metabolism, or oxygen-free metabolism, is mechanistically based heavily on glycolysis, which metabolizes glucose to pyruvate, leading to the production of lactic acid when oxygen is in short supply. It is a fast process that supplies immediate bursts of energy but with decreased yield of ATP compared to aerobic metabolism and thus also emphasizing the functional importance of each system under different physiological conditions. The proper adjustment between aerobic and anaerobic metabolism has a tremendous influence on the degree of athletic performance and muscle efficiency. Under long-endurance, high-intensity work, such as running sprints, anaerobic systems become predominant to enable nearly simultaneous supply of ATP. As time does come to pass and oxygenation is refilled, however, muscle becomes aerobic in metabolism, relying on mitochondrial oxidative mechanisms for continued energy production and recovery. Recent research has demonstrated the interplay between these mechanisms. For instance, lactate, previously solely regarded as a byproduct of anaerobic metabolism, has a key energy substrate during recovery and is also involved in signaling pathways that promote the regeneration and adaptation of muscles. The dual function of lactate indicates its significance in the overall metabolic composition of muscle tissue and exhibits how seemingly disparate energy systems can work synergistically according to various physical stresses (Glancy et al., 2020). The implications of aerobic and anaerobic metabolism extend beyond mere energy production; they play critical roles to have in the health of muscles and in physiological adaptation in general. Understanding the mechanisms of these metabolic processes can be translated to training regimens and rehabilitation methods in athletes. Increased knowledge of lactates role, as pinpointed by current research, has far-reaching implications for optimizing performance and health in various athletic populations. Also, the difference between such metabolic pathways can lead to disease conditions , such as muscle fatigue or increased oxidative stress, compromising overall muscular function. Hence, investigation into how different tissue types generate energy by aerobic and anaerobic metabolism provides insight into athletic performance as well as into therapeutic interventions in metabolic disease and age-dependent decline of muscle (Critchley et al., 2020) (Figure 7.4).

7.1.2. Role of Glycogen in Muscle Energy

The role of glycogen within muscle energy metabolism is most crucial, particularly during exercise. Glycogen, a stored polysaccharide located primarily in the liver and skeletal muscle, is an energy reservoir for storage. During intense exercise periods, such as strength training or prolonged endurance sports, glycogen is broken down into glucose units by glycogenolysis. This glucose is then utilized in glycolysis, a metabolic reaction that produces ATP, the currency of energy for the cell. Mobilization of glycogen stores at a high rate is essential to keep muscle contractions and performance intact. Therefore, understanding glycogen metabolism is crucial for athletes and those who receive high-intensity training because depletion of these stores leads to fatigue and decreased performance. The function of glycogen extends beyond mere provision of energy; it is also a regulatory component in many metabolic processes in muscle tissues. Skeletal muscle contributes approximately 40% of the body mass of an individual and is the controlling factor in locomotion and metabolic homeostasis. The metabolic landscape of the muscle involves complex interplay between glucose uptake and signaling mechanisms, such as those facilitated by AMP-activated protein kinase and insulin signaling, which are extremely responsive to glycogen content. A proteomics analysis led to the disclosure of complex regulation of these pathways, highlighting dynamic relationships in charge of governing muscle metabolism under opposite nutritional conditions (Deshmukh et al., 2015). This demonstrates the extent to which the muscle's ability to store and release glycogen is not just the determining characteristic for energy availability but for the health of the metabolism generally. In professional sports, a managed glycogen strategy is essential to performance.

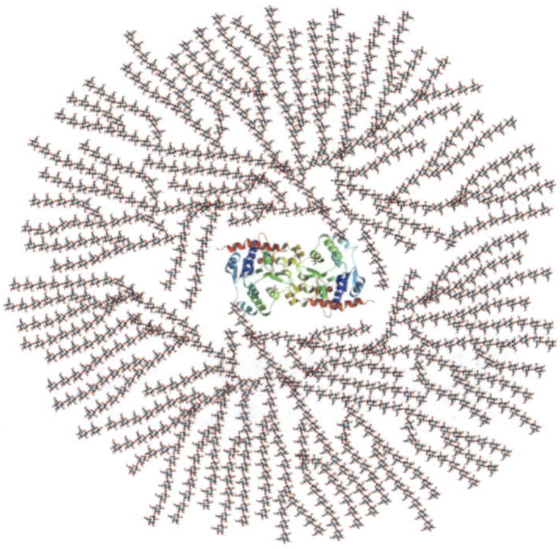

Figure 7.5. Schematic two-dimensional cross-sectional view of glycogen: A core protein of glycogenin is surrounded by branches of glucose units. The entire globular granule may contain around 30,000 glucose units.

Source: https://upload.wikimedia.org/wikipedia/commons/4/47/Glycogen_structure.svg.

Recommended nutritional guidelines encourage personalized dietary plans tailored to coordinate around the athlete's precise training and competition schedules. Appropriate intake of carbohydrates (CHO) is necessary, varying in amounts around exercise to either enhance energy supply or induce adaptations through low-CHO training (Nattiv et al., 2020). Also, storage of glycogen must be maintained in the scenario of endurance events where expenditure is high. Nutritional strategies also require care concerning the timing of carbohydrates to assist sportsmen in storing their glycogen adequately before competition. Thus, a clear understanding of glycogen's role in the energy of muscle not only impacts training schedules but also informs nutrition intake crucial to sporting success (Figure 7.5).

7.1.3. Impact of Exercise on Muscle Metabolism

Exercise plays a crucial role in muscle metabolism, and it significantly influences the biochemically mediated process of energy production and consumption in skeletal muscle. During exercise, the muscles draw primarily on glucose and lipids as energy sources, which highlights their dual metabolic role. When energy demands are high, for example, during intense exercise, there is increased use of glycogen stores and fatty acids and an impressive increase in mitochondrial biogenesis. This accommodation is crucial since augmented mitochondrial capacity translates to enhanced ATP production capability, resulting in enhanced endurance and performance. The ability of skeletal muscle to adapt or remodel itself in response to exercise is thus an important part of overall muscle health and metabolic adaptation (Duszka et al., 2020). These adaptations not only improve athletic performance but also reverse the effects of muscular atrophy that are potentially associated with aging, inactivity, or certain disease states. Furthermore, exercise modulation of muscle metabolism extends beyond energy substrate use to include sophisticated hormonal regulation and signal cascades. Resistance training uniquely induces activation of signaling cascades that promote protein synthesis and muscle hypertrophy. Some of the key actors in the process include insulin and growth factors, which regulate the activation of the mTOR pathway, a central pathway for the regulation of muscle protein anabolism. Further, the activity of peroxisome proliferator-activated receptors (PPARs), which respond to fatty acids and affect genes involved in metabolism and inflammation, enters the scene during and after exercise. Specifically, PPARβ/δ is involved in energy metabolism, mitochondrial biogenesis, and fiber type switching, in alignment with the metabolic stress imposed on the muscle during exercise (Duszka et al., 2020). Understanding such pathways, therefore, sheds light on how to optimize exercise adaptation to muscle function as well as general metabolic health. Finally, the addition of nutritional interventions to exercise can also optimize muscle metabolism and function. The athletes are encouraged to follow personalized nutrition programs that support intense training regimens and recovery needs. Adequate fueling during exercise plays a key role; changing carbohydrate availability can bring about different metabolic adaptations according to training goals, either for strength or endurance. Adequate consumption of good-quality protein distributed throughout the day becomes relevant in an effort to optimize recovery and muscle adaptation. Consequently, nutrition supplements may support such efforts, that is, in the prevention of deficiencies in nutrients that would hinder sport performance. Thus, the synergistic interaction between exercise and food points to the complexity of muscle metabolism as a platform for adaptive responses that maximize metabolic efficiency and muscular resilience over time.

Test Your Knowledge

1. What is the difference between aerobic and anaerobic metabolism?
2. What is the impact of exercise on muscle metabolism?

7.2. Adipose Tissue Metabolism

Learning Outcome

1. Know the function of adipose tissue in energy storage;
2. Describe the lipolysis and fatty acid oxidation;
3. Understand the hormonal regulation of adipose metabolism.

Adipose tissue metabolism is important for the homeostasis of energy in the body. Comprising WAT and BAT, adipose tissue not only acts as an inactive lipid storage depot but is actively involved in various metabolic processes. WAT is primarily an energy reservoir and is needed for the storage and mobilization of lipids in the event of an excess or shortage of calories. In contrast, BAT possesses a thermogenic role, producing heat from deposited fat and thus regulating body temperature. Advances in imaging techniques, such as the STRIDE approach, have provided insights into the metabolic functions of adipose tissues, revealing the intricate dynamics of glucose-based macromolecule production. Through such findings, researchers are gaining insights into the function of adipose tissues in systemic metabolism beyond mere fat storage (Liu et al., 2019). Additionally, the novel field of beige adipocyte science once again unveiled the complexity of adipose tissue metabolism. Beige adipocytes, containing both WAT-like and BAT-like features, possess the unique ability of being thermogenically activated by certain stimuli, such as cold exposure or specific hormonal stimulation. Recent research has explored recent findings that have identified a variety of endogenous factors permitting white adipocytes to become browning cells, initiating a thermogenic program in them. This transformation enables beige adipocytes to enhance energy consumption, and hence, it has therapeutic potential for lowering obesity and related metabolic disorders. Through the discovery of regulation of beige adipocyte biology, researchers are exploring how to stimulate beige adipogenesis and white-to-beige adipocyte transdifferentiation, which holds promising prospects for the treatment of metabolic health (Koliwad et al., 2018). Clarifying the metabolic processes and regulatory mechanisms in adipose tissue is essential for controlling metabolic dysfunctions of type 2 diabetes and obesity. The bidirectional interactions among adipocytes of different types and their secreted factors heavily influence systemic insulin sensitivity, glucose metabolism, and overall energy homeostasis. As research continues to advance, techniques for investigating the metabolic heterogeneity of adipose tissues are becoming increasingly sophisticated. Techniques , such as the STRIDE imaging not only reveal utilization of glucose-derived products but also identify the adaptive mechanisms employed by adipose tissue according to environmental and physiological perturbations (Liu et al., 2019). An integrated view of adipose tissue metabolism thus holds promise for new therapeutic targets to promote metabolic health and mitigate the metabolic disease burden (Figure 7.6).

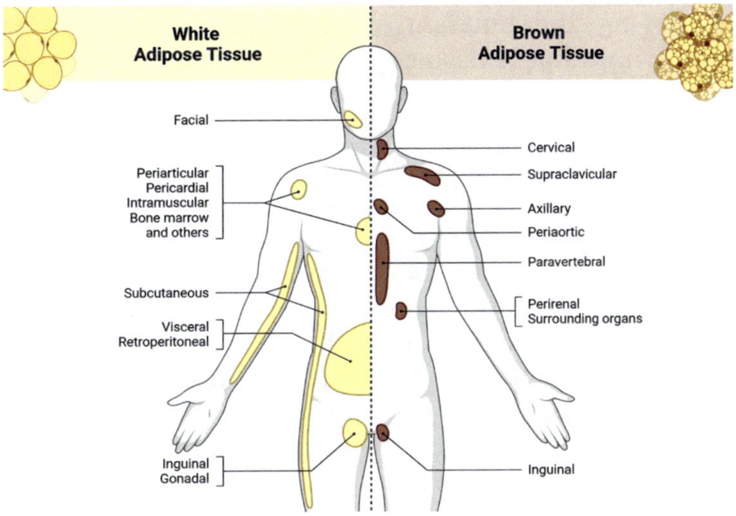

Figure 7.6. Adipose tissue.

Source: https://endoconsult.b-cdn.net/wp-content/uploads/adipose-tissue.png.

7.2.1. Function of Adipose Tissue in Energy Storage

Adipose tissue has a crucial function in energy storage as the central depot for triglycerides, the body's highest form of energy density. Composed largely of adipocytes, this distinctive tissue not only stores excess energy from the diet but also regulates the output of fatty acids when energy is low. When blood glucose is low or caloric inputs are insufficient, adipose tissue mobilizes fatty acids into the circulation where other tissues utilize them as energy. Thus, adipose tissue plays a critical role in maintaining energy homeostasis by alternating between storage and release modes of function, a process that is crucial in ensuring the body functions uninterrupted even when fasting or undergoing increased physical activity. Aside from basic energy storage, adipose tissue also acts as an endocrine organ, which secretes many bioactive molecules, known as adipokines, that play important roles in metabolic regulation. The adipokines like leptin and adiponectin, aside from regulating appetite and energy expenditure, influence insulin sensitivity and inflammation. In obesity, the surplus adipose tissue may lead to dysregulation of the signals and cause systemic insulin resistance and metabolic syndrome. The pro-inflammatory state of adipose tissue is also significant; pathologic adipocytes can produce pro-inflammatory cytokines that enhance insulin resistance and other metabolic disease. Thus, knowledge of the balance between energy storage and endocrine function of adipose tissue is key to understanding the impact of obesity on overall metabolism and health outcomes, as documented in studies of the subtleties of this tissue (Gutierrez et al., 2017). Further, the interaction between maternal obesity and adipose tissue emphasizes the tissue's role in energy metabolism in critical physiological states , such as pregnancy. Maternal obesity could predispose an individual to the development of conditions , such as gestational diabetes mellitus (GDM), owing to imbalanced energy storing and nutrient transport mechanisms involving adipose tissue. The alterations in adipose tissue functioning during pregnancy have effects on both maternal and fetal health, emphasizing the need for energy balance from the maternal perspective. Certain factors , such as inflammation in obesity-related adipose tissues, may even contribute to further complications, affecting the hormonal environment necessary for pregnancy and metabolism regulation (Jayabalan et al., 2017). This intricate interaction between energy storage, hormonal regulation, and metabolic adjustment emphasizes the role of adipose tissue as more than an inactive reservoir of energy and hence a point of interest in the study of specialized tissues and their metabolic importance.

7.2.2. Lipolysis and Fatty Acid Oxidation

Lipolysis and fatty acid oxidation are crucial pathways in the context of metabolic regulation, particularly in specialized tissues , such as adipose tissue and skeletal muscle. Lipolysis refers to the hydrolysis of triglycerides into glycerol and free fatty acids by enzymes known as lipases. Hormone-sensitive lipase (HSL) is a key enzyme in this catabolic process, whereby hormonal stimuli (e.g., catecholamines) initiate the discharge of stored fats. These free fatty acids are then transported to tissues for the generation of energy, which underscores the significance of lipolysis not just in energy homeostasis but also in the maintenance of metabolic flexibility. Understanding the mechanism of how the processes are regulated provides insight into such conditions as obesity and metabolic syndrome, where lipolytic activity may be abnormal, which underscores the need for further studies on their mechanistic frameworks. The regulation of lipolysis has been linked to a group of proteins, particularly the PAT family, which includes perilipin and ADRP. These proteins are key to regulating the accessibility of lipases to lipid droplets, and as such, they influence the rate of lipolysis. PAT proteins are positioned at the lipid droplet surface and act as regulators that respond to metabolic cues signaling the need for increased liberation of fatty acids. Genetic variations that affect these proteins, particularly perilipin, have also been associated with metabolic phenotypes , such as type 2 diabetes and obesity, highlighting their importance in energy balance and fat metabolism. The rules and interactions of these proteins show the complexity of lipid metabolism in differentiated tissues, whose disruption can lead to severe metabolic disruptions, making them a therapeutic target for metabolic disease (Bickel et al., 2009). The second process utilized by the released free fatty acids is fatty acid oxidation, where they are formed mainly in the mitochondria for ATP. This process is well regulated and involves activation of fatty acids to acyl-CoA and subsequent transport to the mitochondrial matrix for β-oxidation. It has been proven through research that elements of energy expenditure, such as thermogenesis, play a decisive role alongside lipolysis in determining metabolic effects. For instance, TRIP-Br2 has been identified as a co-transcriptional regulator that activates lipolytic activity and enhances oxidative metabolism, implying an evident synergetic interaction of the two processes. The potential for increased energy expenditure through increased fatty acid oxidation offers a therapeutic challenge in treating obesity and insulin resistance and highlights the importance of elucidating these metabolic processes within specialized tissues (Blüher et al., 2014) (Figure 7.7).

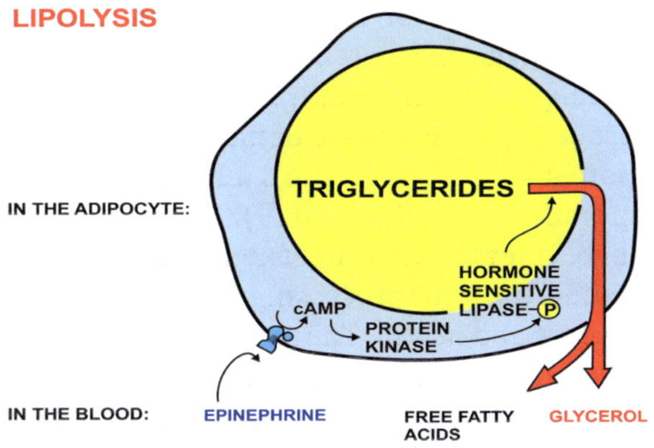

Figure 7.7. Illustration of the activation of lipolysis in an adipocyte.

Source: https://upload.wikimedia.org/wikipedia/commons/5/5f/Metabolism1.jpg.

7.2.3. Hormonal Regulation of Adipose Metabolism

The hormonal regulation of adipose metabolism is a critical component in the understanding of the mechanisms by which energy homeostasis is controlled in specialized tissues. Various hormones, including insulin, glucagon, and adipokines, all play crucial roles in controlling the activity of adipose tissue. Insulin, for instance, promotes the storage of lipids by stimulating glucose uptake and lipogenesis and concurrently suppressing lipolysis. Conversely, glucagon's action is to enhance lipolysis under fasting states to enable fatty acids to be mobilized in the circulation so that they may be utilized for energy. This fine balance is important to enable normal metabolic functions and is impaired in states of metabolic illnesses , such as obesity and type 2 diabetes mellitus (T2DM). A nuanced understanding of these hormonal interactions not only sheds light on energy homeostasis but also highlights potential therapeutic targets for intervention in adipose tissue dysregulation disorders. The CNS is another important factor involved in hormonal regulation of adipose metabolism. The CNS detects and integrates signals from plasma hormones as well as nutrient status and helps to coordinate substrate utilization and energy expenditure. It has been demonstrated in recent studies that the CNS further regulates postprandial glucose levels by communicating with adipose tissue. Such coordination enables the CNS to regulate glucose output from the liver and peripheral tissue glucose uptake according to the body's energy needs. The system is most efficient under the condition of external stress , such as a high-fat diet, which disrupts normal homeostatic function. Current research shows that the treatment of CNS dysfunction may provide a greater impact on managing the relationship between obesity and T2DM, potentially to provide effective therapy for diseases with a systemic nature (Arble et al., 2013). Furthermore, the activity of adenosine monophosphate-activated protein kinase (AMPK) establishes the complexity of hormone regulation in adipose tissue. AMPK is a master metabolic regulator, modulating many cellular processes to maintain energy homeostasis. AMPK coordinates the adipocyte's metabolic responses under hormonal stimuli, activating fatty acid oxidation and inhibiting lipogenesis when energy stores are replete. Aberration in AMPK function is associated with numerous metabolic disorders, including diabetes and metabolic syndrome, underlining its pathophysiological significance in these conditions. While the role of AMPK in metabolism is well understood, interactions with hormones in the CNS and fat tissue remain an open field. The understanding of the nuances of AMPKs regulation could unveil new windows of opportunity for overcoming metabolic disease's costs (Fioramonti et al., 2016).

Test Your Knowledge

1. What is lipolysis and fatty acid oxidation?
2. What is the hormonal regulation of adipose metabolism?

7.3. Liver Metabolism

Learning Outcome

1. Understand the role of the liver in glucose homeostasis;
2. Know the detoxification processes in the liver;
3. Describe the synthesis of proteins and lipids in the liver.

The liver is a central player in the metabolism of specialized tissues, playing the role of biochemical hub for many processes crucial in maintaining homeostasis. The unique structure of the liver allows for the incorporation of disparate metabolic pathways, reflective of its pivotal role in nutrient perception, energy storage, and detoxification. For instance, the liver catalyzes the deposition of surplus glucose into glycogen during periods of high carbohydrate intake, referred to as glycogenesis. Conversely, during increased energy demand, the liver hydrolyzes the glycogen reserves via glycogenolysis and thereby regulates blood glucose levels. The liver also synthesizes essential proteins like albumin and coagulation factors that are necessary in order to maintain osmotic equilibrium and hemostasis. This multifaceted function points to the liver's active role in coordinating metabolic responses to various physiological states. What can be learned about the metabolism of the liver is used to show the complexity of its cellular processes, particularly in terms of anabolism and catabolism. Newer technologies, such as spectral tracing of deuterium (STRIDE), have contributed significantly to the understanding of how glucose-derived metabolites are metabolized via various metabolic pathways. For example, this technique enables researchers to observe the synthesis of lipids, proteins, and DNA macromolecules, revealing the biochemical pathways that take place in cells of the liver. The ability of the liver to modify its metabolic pathways depending on food intake and energy requirements is of utmost importance in regulating overall metabolism. Research applying high-level microscopy has revealed that such dynamic metabolic activities are often regionally localized within the liver, revealing a heterogeneous landscape of metabolic activities responsible for the organ's functionality and adaptability (Liu et al., 2019). Drawing further on liver metabolism, its extension is beyond individual nutrient processing to systemic effects on disease and health. The significance of hepatic function in glucose homeostasis directly impacts metabolic diseases , such as Type 2 diabetes and non-alcoholic fatty liver disease (NAFLD). Liver metabolism necessitates integrating physiological concepts from various schools, including Ayurveda's notions that emphasize harmony among body systems as being vital. The metabolism of the liver is inextricably integrated with the body's general homeostasis, controlled by mechanisms that oversee multiple functions of the body, reflecting principles inherent in contemporary and conventional physiological paradigms (Patwardhan, 2008). With an understanding of the interaction of liver metabolism with the body's health, we are better able to comprehend the holistic nature by which metabolic dysregulation can initiate disease, highlighting the need for further research in this critical field (Figure 7.8).

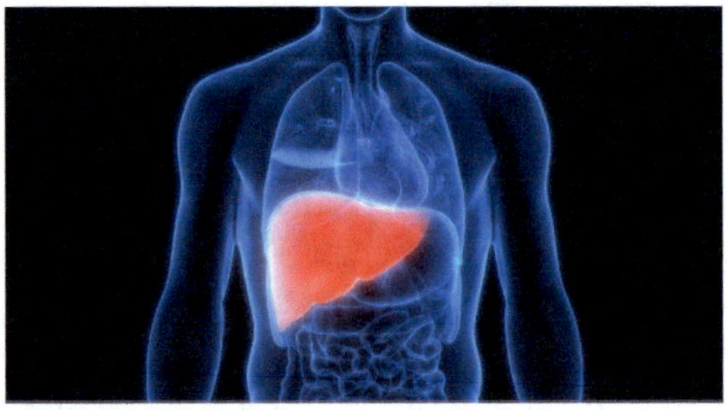

Figure 7.8. Digital illustration highlighting the human liver within the torso.

Source: https://www.medstarhealth.org/-/media/project/mho/medstar/blogs/blogmedstar2021/thomas-liver-disease-desktop.jpg.

7.3.1. Role of the Liver in Glucose Homeostasis

The liver maintains glucose homeostasis, which is critical to overall metabolic health. The organ is an integrative hub for the creation and storage of glucose through processes , such as gluconeogenesis and glycogenolysis. Following ingestion of a meal, the liver offsets elevated blood glucose levels by storing glucose in excess as glycogen for subsequent use to maintain energy as instantly available when fasting. However, during longer periods of fasting, the liver can instantly transform glycogen into glucose and release it into the circulation and thereby maintaining a stable amount of glucose. This dual role is indicative of the importance of the liver in controlling metabolic response and illustrates its pivotal role in regulating energy stores, especially in energy-consuming states. In addition to that, the liver's control of blood glucose is tightly linked with hormonal regulation, specifically insulin and glucagon. Insulin promotes the extraction of glucose from blood by liver cells and the production of glycogen, while glucagon stimulates gluconeogenesis and glycogenolysis to provide a balanced response to glucose availability. This ensures the avoidance of both hyperglycemia and hypoglycemia, which can have fatal health effects. According to recent research, the CNS is also involved in modulating hepatic glucose production according to postprandial nutrient levels (Arble et al., 2013). This intricate liver-CNS relationship is a well-evolved regulatory process necessary for the maintenance of glucose homeostasis. Also, disruptions in the liver's glucose-regulating capacity can contribute to severe metabolic derangements, including insulin resistance and type 2 diabetes mellitus (T2DM). The liver's ability to respond to extrinsic stresses like high-fat diets and environmental stress is of growing interest in light of metabolic dysregulation (Villalobos et al., 2016). Understanding how these external factors modulate hepatic function is critical to designing more effective therapeutic strategies. Furthermore, emerging results on the role of the CNS in glucose homeostasis raise the postulate that CNS intervention would offer new avenues to improve glucose metabolism and curative therapy for related diseases more effectively. The liver, with its multitasking functionality and interaction with other systems, remains pivotal in research on the struggle against metabolic disorders.

7.3.2. Detoxification Processes in the Liver

The liver is one of the body's fundamental detoxification organs and is in charge of metabolizing every substance that is ingested by the body. With specific cellular processes, this complex organ converts poisonous materials into less toxic substances that can be efficiently excreted. Hepatocytes, the major functional cell types of the liver, are equipped with sophisticated enzymatic pathways, such as the cytochrome P450 enzyme system, to facilitate biotransformation of xenobiotics. These pathways not only detoxify the toxins but also metabolize lipophilic substrates to hydrophilic products, which are rendered more water-soluble to be excreted by the kidneys. Through these active processes of detoxification, the liver protects the body from potential damage caused by environmental toxins, drugs, and metabolites, thereby creating homeostasis. Beyond its metabolic functions, the liver's processes of detoxification also possess genetic determinants that control differential drug and environmental toxin responses. Pharmacogenetics, with its focus on how genetic variation affects drug metabolism, has highlighted the contribution of liver enzymes to the regulation of therapeutic response and toxicity. For example, certain polymorphisms in genes for cytochrome P450 affect the metabolism rates of some drugs and thus vary between patients in efficacy and toxicity. This integration of detoxification and genetics demonstrates the liver's function not only in drug metabolism but also in modulating the therapeutic approach to the patient. These advances promulgate the potential of pharmacogenetic-guided therapy, optimizing the benefit-to-risk ratio of drug dosing as well as enhancing personalized medicine practice as physicians try more effective treatment protocols (Fenech et al., 2014). Its distinctive anatomical structure also helps enable its detoxification function, in which blood from the digestive system is carried through the hepatic portal vein to hepatocytes, which are supplied with materials to be processed. This positioning of liver cells in the circulatory system aids the quick metabolism of nutrients and toxins, demonstrating the organ's dual nature. Moreover, the liver's ability to regenerate and adapt to various physiological conditions ensures its continuous capacity to manage detoxification demands. However, chronic exposure to excessive toxins or a high-fat diet can impair these detoxification processes, potentially leading to liver diseases. Thus, understanding liver metabolism in the context of detoxification is important as it emphasizes the significance of liver function to the integrity of overall metabolic stability and acts to reinforce the significance of individual interventions to persons at risk (Bratty et al., 2012) (Figure 7.9).

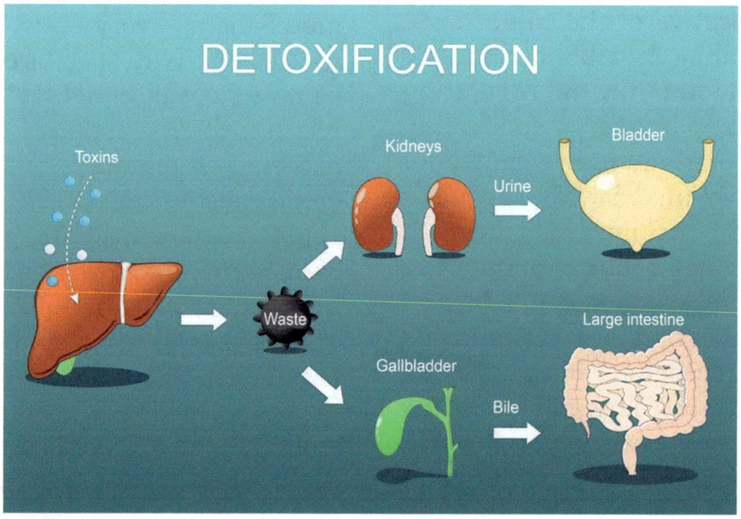

Figure 7.9. The liver detoxification process.

Source: https://www.detoxplusuk.com/wp-content/uploads/2024/10/detoxification-process-body-organs-diagram-1.jpg.

7.3.3. Synthesis of Proteins and Lipids in the Liver

The liver is a central organ in protein and lipid synthesis, coordinating numerous metabolic events that have a profound impact on overall-body homeostasis. The hepatocytes are the main workhorse cells of the liver, producing a variety of proteins including clotting factors, enzymes, and serum albumin, crucial for osmotic balance and transport. Protein synthesis is intimately related to the supply of amino acids, which depends on nutritional intake and the overall metabolic status. When there is an excess of dietary protein, the liver increases its translational activity so that protein synthesis coupled with energy metabolism and immune response is augmented. The liver also efficiently controls the export of synthesized proteins into the bloodstream so that peripheral tissues can have access to elements that ensure their best function. Thus, the understanding of the liver's capacity for protein synthesis is critical to appreciating its role in the overall scheme of metabolic processes of specialized tissues. Besides its protein synthetic role, the liver also plays a critical role in lipid metabolism, regulating the synthesis and degradation of various species of lipids. Mechanisms through which lipids are synthesized involve *de novo* lipogenesis, where excess glucose and carbohydrates are converted to fatty acids. These fatty acids can subsequently be esterified to form triglycerides, serving as an energy storage pool in fat or released into the bloodstream as very-low-density lipoproteins (VLDL). Lipid synthesis and degradation should be balanced to prevent lipotoxicity resulting from the accumulation of toxic lipid intermediates within tissues like the liver and muscle. When metabolic stress occurs, such as with obesity or insulin resistance, the liver's role in controlling lipid metabolism is tested with subsequent ectopic fat accumulation that is damaging to liver function and systemic metabolism (Ertunc et al., 2016). This complex interaction of lipid metabolism pathways with overall health illustrates the significance of the liver in maintaining metabolic homeostasis. In addition, the liver's signaling to other specialized tissues is mediated by lipids and proteins synthesized in the liver, emphasizing the livers integration role in systemic metabolism. To illustrate, pro-inflammatory cytokines synthesized by the liver modulate immune responses in adipose tissue, linking lipid metabolism to inflammation. Moreover, the liver's adaptation to altered dietary fat and carbohydrate intake directly impacts synthesis of apolipoprotein and transport protein, the latter for which the former is needed to facilitate lipid delivery and metabolism in peripheral tissues. The liver may become dysfunctional during periods of prolonged nutrient excess, by way of change in protein function and lipid buildup to fuel a vicious cycle of metabolic dysregulation. These mechanisms highlight the importance of the liver as both a center of metabolism and a master controller of homeostasis, with far more to explore in order to determine the underlying mechanisms behind diseases like fatty liver disease and metabolic syndrome (Deanna et al., 2017).

Test Your Knowledge

1. What is the role of the liver in glucose homeostasis?
2. What is protein synthesis in the liver?

7.4. Brain Metabolism

Learning Outcome

1. Describe glucose as the primary energy source for the brain;
2. Know the metabolic adaptations during fasting;
3. Understand the impact of neurotransmitters on brain metabolism.

Metabolic processes within the brain are key to understanding its complex functions and overall well-being. The substrate for brain metabolism is glucose, which is its preferred energy substrate. The reason is due to the high energy demands of neurons, that is, to maintain ion gradients essential for action potential and neurotransmission. However, advances in imaging techniques, such as STRIDE, have allowed researchers to probe deeper into the intricate brain metabolic patterns instead of merely glucose uptake. STRIDE is able to visualize different macromolecules derived from glucose, i.e., DNA, proteins, lipids, and glycogen, and therefore reveal an entire picture of how the brain is utilizing glucose to perform various anabolic processes. The ability to follow these metabolic pathways is crucial in uncovering the brains plasticity and effects of altered metabolism on neurodegenerative disease (Liu et al., 2019). In specialized tissues, the brain illustrates the manner in which metabolic heterogeneity influences physiological processes. Diverse regions in the brain contain various metabolic patterns due to functional specialization. For instance, brain areas that are involved in sensory processing may have higher metabolic activity under the influence of a stimulus, whereas cognitive areas may have differential patterns under cognitive tasks. Even the STRIDE imaging method provides depth to such findings through temporal resolution in metabolic observation, showing how different groups of glucose are involved in dynamic brain functions. This heterogeneity of brain metabolism across space and time accentuates the complexity of its energy demands and how such processes may change in disease states. Fluctuations need to be understood as they are direct likely therapeutic interventions for conditions , such as Alzheimer's disease or traumatic head injury where metabolic processes are disrupted (Liu et al., 2019). Furthermore, consequences of brain metabolism extend to broader debates over neurological health and disease progression. Metabolic disorder, characterized by deranged glucose utilization, is linked to mental impairment and various neurodegenerative illnesses. Advances in sophisticated techniques like STRIDE emphasize the potential of novel methodologies to measure and image metabolic phenomena *in vivo* and, in the process, illuminate the relationship between metabolism and brain health. Exploring enzyme function with respect to glucose metabolism, along with new imaging technology, may result in targeted treatment approaches to the correction of metabolic balance in those with the condition. As research continues to progress, brain metabolism will not only expand our knowledge of its physiological processes but also guide prevention and therapy options for neurological diseases (Figure 7.10).

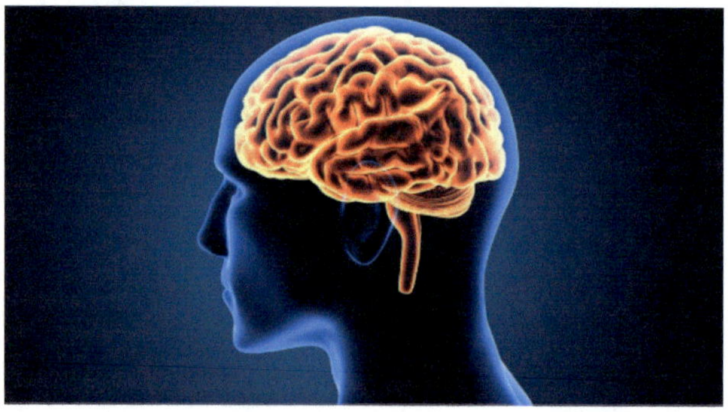

Figure 7.10. Side view illustration of the human brain within a transparent head profile.

Source: https://neurospinesurgical.com/wp-content/uploads/2018/01/5-facts-that-you-didnt-know-about-the-human-brain-neurospine-surgical-consultants.jpg.

7.4.1. Glucose as the Primary Energy Source for the Brain

The human brain, weighing roughly 2% of body weight, consumes approximately 20% of the body's energy reserves, nearly entirely derived from glucose. This tremendous requirement marks glucose's status as the primary energy substrate for neuronal functioning and metabolism. Neurons require a continuous supply of glucose to facilitate their extensive networks and function optimally. In normal physiological conditions, the brain relies on glucose metabolism by glycolysis and oxidative phosphorylation to produce ATP for synaptic transmission as well as overall neuronal health. The fine regulation of glucose uptake is particularly essential as any change in glucose availability can have a profound impact on brain function, translating into symptoms of hypoglycemia or other metabolic disorders. Furthermore, the CNS plays a role in glucose homeostasis via complex networks combining metabolic inputs and neuronal activity. As has been elucidated by recent literature, the CNS dictates the production of glucose by the liver and stimulates glucose entry into peripheral tissues, exemplifying the interconnection of brain metabolism and systemic glucose control. The dynamic interactions between the CNS and glucose metabolism are of relevance, particularly in response to external stimuli, including the nutritional content of the diet and circadian rhythm. These interactions are being explored today as potential therapeutic strategies for diseases , such as type 2 diabetes mellitus (T2DM), where CNS pathology contributes to dysregulation of blood glucose levels, complicating the management of the disease (Arble et al., 2013). There is also evidence that specialized cells in the hypothalamus, such as tanycytes, play a central role in glucose sensing and response. The presence of GK in these cells enables them to sense the plasma glucose and subsequently to modulate the hypothalamic circuit for the regulation of appetite and energy expenditure. Evidence shows that manipulation of GK in these cells alters the expression of hunger and satiety neuropeptides and feeding behavior and metabolic control (Barahona et al., 2017). Thus, glucose not only serves as a critical source of energy but also as a signaling molecule able to modulate a vast array of physiological responses, validating the importance of glucose metabolism in specialized brain tissues (Figure 7.11).

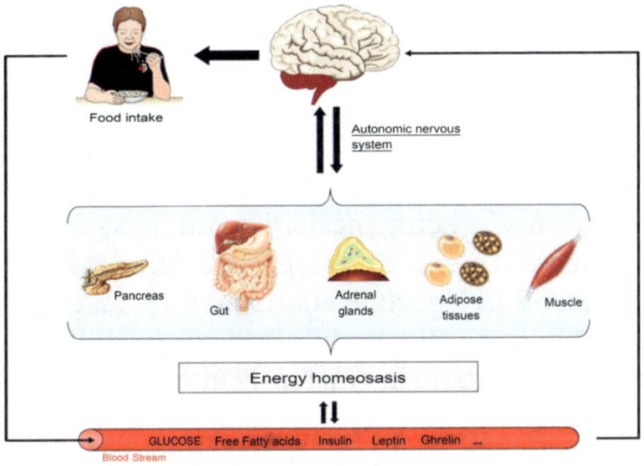

Figure 7.11. Role of the brain in the control of energy homeostasis.

Source: https://cdnintech.com/media/chapter/68362/1512345123/media/F1.png.

7.4.2. Metabolic Adaptations During Fasting

Fasting triggers a series of metabolic changes that ensure the conservation of energy and homeostasis in specialized cells. When fasting, the body shifts from a glucose-dependent to a fatty acid- and ketone body-dependent state for energy. This metabolic adaptation not only ensures the maintenance of blood glucose but also spares muscle protein from catabolism. The liver is central to this process, since it hydrolyses stored glycogen and produces glucose through gluconeogenesis, besides triggering the production of ketone bodies from fatty acids. These processes are crucial in supporting energy supplies in extended fasted conditions without food consumption, allowing organisms to endure fasting situations without causing untoward effects on muscle and organ functions. Further research into fasting metabolic adaptations reveals fundamental changes in the hormonal milieu that enhance these metabolic shifts. Insulin decreases during fasting, promoting lipolysis and increasing the discharge of free fatty acids from adipose tissue stores. Concomitantly, glucagon and cortisol increases enhance gluconeogenesis and lipolysis, respectively, creating a milieu conducive to the utilization of stored fat as fuel. The activity of hormones , such as growth hormone (GH) and norepinephrine is also engaged since they have other effects to further enhance fatty acid oxidation and ketogenesis. The fineness of such hormonal interactions reflects the adaptive processes of specialized tissues to fasting, a testament to the body's amazing ability to manage metabolism efficiently under conditions of nutrient deficiency. Specialized tissues like the brain and muscle have unique adaptations during fasting.

The brain, which is otherwise glucose-dependent, adapts to utilizing ketone bodies due to their neuroprotective nature and as a good source of energy. Increased expression of monocarboxylate transporters in neuron cells makes this adaptation possible so that the brain can produce its requirements even when there is no glucose. Similarly, muscle tissues prefer fatty acid oxidation during fasting, which is coupled with downregulation of glucose uptake mechanisms. This metabolic flexibility decreases protein breakdown, enabling muscle structure to be preserved. This combination of metabolic adaptations during fasting and specific requirements of specialized tissues demonstrates the body's intricate regulating systems, emphasizing the necessity of the adaptations to overall maintenance of body function during periods of nutrient limitation.

7.4.3. Impact of Neurotransmitters on Brain Metabolism

The intricate relationship between neurotransmitters and brain metabolism is one of the prime targets for the identification of what controls metabolic events in specialized tissues. Neurotransmitters, such as glutamate and gamma-aminobutyric acid (GABA), have a significant influence on synaptic activity and energy demands in the brain. For instance, increased activity of neurons is associated with increased release of glutamate that leads to increased glucose usage in order to meet the high energy demands of neurons. These changes in metabolism are not passive but are intimately connected with the signals communicated by neurotransmitters to enhance glucose from the periphery and control glycogen synthesis in astrocytes, the primary brain glial cells. This adaptation of metabolism underscores the central role of neurotransmitters in the control of energy supply and demand in harmony with cognitive demands, which recognizes a very sophisticated regulatory system vital to maintaining homeostasis in brain processes. Furthermore, research highlights the regulatory role of CNS in modulating postprandial glucose metabolism via neurotransmitter-mediated pathways. CNS is reported to synthesize multimodal inputs from peripheral tissues, including circulating hormones and metabolizable nutrients, to control glucose release from the liver and peripheral tissue uptake, based on current research. Balance of neurotransmitter signaling is key, and dysregulation has been implicated in metabolic pathologies , such as type 2 diabetes mellitus (T2DM). In particular, neurotransmitters may influence the perception of energy states by the brain, thus controlling metabolic pathways that govern glucose availability. Insight into interactions between glial and neuronal cells further highlights such neurotransmitter-controlled functions and suggests that therapeutic intervention in the CNS may significantly affect metabolic disease, determining the need for well-characterized strategies to the treatment of T2DM with the brain regulatory role taken into consideration (Arble et al., 2013). The relationship between metabolism and neurotransmitters in the brain is also complicated by the activity of neuronal plasticity, as non-neuronal and neuronal cells adapt to shifting functional demands and environmental stimuli. The ability of astrocytes to communicate with neurons by releasing neurotransmitters is particularly important because glial cells react not only to neuronally derived information but also influence metabolic events by controlling extracellular milieus. For instance, astrocytic neurotransmitter uptake can modulate lactate release, aligning synaptic activity with brain energy metabolism. The novel identification of extracellular vesicles (EVs) highlights additional levels of communication by which neuronal and glial cells exchange regulatory molecules governing adaptive metabolic responses. Therefore, it is imperative to understand these intricate interactions in order to uncover metabolic regulation in expert tissues, gaining insight into potential therapeutic opportunities for a variety of disorders (Liegro et al., 2019) (Figure 7.12).

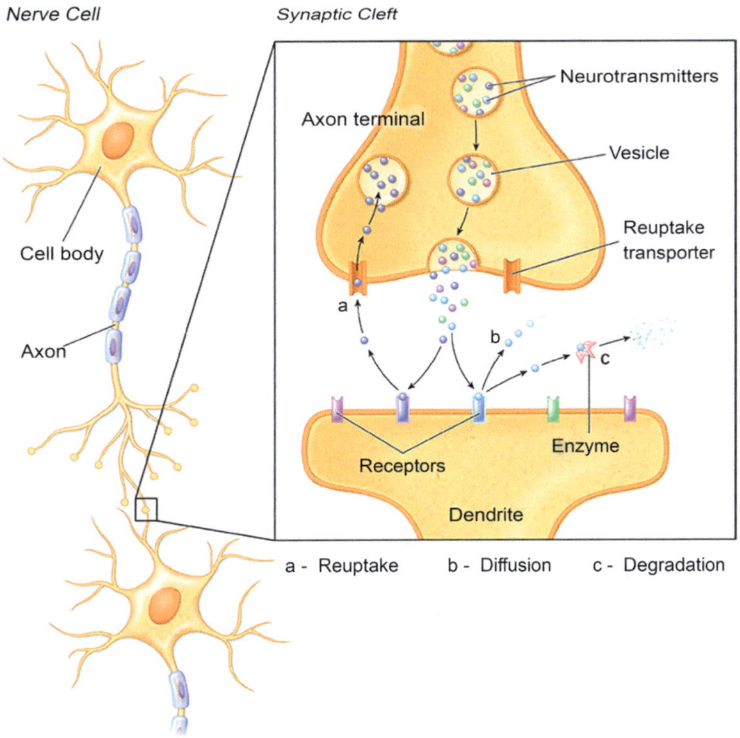

Figure 7.12. Neurotransmitters carry chemical signals ("messages") from one neuron (nerve cell) to the next target cell.

Source: https://my.clevelandclinic.org/-/scassets/images/org/health/articles/22513-neurotransmitters.

Test Your Knowledge

1. What is the primary source of energy of the brain?
2. What is the impact of neurotransmitters on brain metabolism?

7.5. Metabolism in Endocrine Tissues

Learning Outcome

1. Understand the hormonal regulation of metabolic processes;
2. Describe the role of the pancreas in glucose metabolism;
3. Know the thyroid hormones and their effect on metabolism.

Understanding endocrine tissue metabolism is critical in knowing the function that such specialized organs serve in homeostasis and in metabolic regulation. Endocrine tissue metabolism, as in organs , such as the pancreas and adrenal glands, involves intricate biochemical processes to facilitate the secretion and production of hormones. Such hormones, in turn, control various physiological functions in the body, influencing metabolic processes of glucose, lipids, and proteins. For example, the pancreatic islets secrete insulin, which decreases blood glucose levels and makes energy available for use. Such intricate regulation is crucial as disturbances in hormone secretion lead to metabolic disorders , such as diabetes and obesity, making such metabolically active tissues extremely important. In addition, the physical and functional asymmetries exhibited in such glands point towards an adaptive mechanism whereby their metabolic profiles are suited to their specialized physiological environments, as indicated in studies on the topic (Bratty et al., 2012). The interrelationship between endocrine metabolism and environmental factors, such as exposure to endocrine-disrupting chemicals (EDCs), also needs close scrutiny. Recent research has indicated that compounds like polybrominated diphenyl ethers (PBDEs) exert an enormous influence on hormone secretion and metabolism by endocrine organs. For instance, studies indicate that PBDE exposure can compromise immune function by inhibiting the release of pro-inflammatory cytokines by alveolar macrophages, an immune system element (Hennigar et al., 2010). These immune deficits may indirectly affect metabolic health, suggesting an integrated relationship between environmental toxins and the metabolic function of endocrine tissue. The biochemical mechanisms targeted by endocrine disruptors reinforce the need to think about metabolic responses not in isolation but as within an ecological and physiological context.

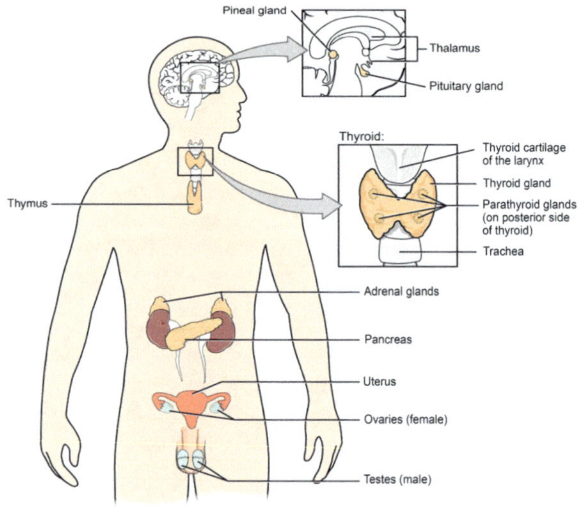

Figure 7.13. The endocrine system.

Source: https://www.physio-pedia.com/images/1/15/1801_The_Endocrine_System.jpg.

To clarify, the metabolism of specialized endocrine tissues is not only limited to hormone secretion but also encompasses regulation of systemic metabolic processes and communication with other tissues. For instance, the thyroid gland controls the metabolism by the release of thyroid hormones that adjust basal metabolic rate (BMR) and energy expenditure. The thyroid hormones control metabolic activities in many tissues , such as muscle and liver, affecting how these tissues can metabolize glucose and fatty acids. In addition, the feedback mechanisms controlling these hormones emphasize the importance of maintaining metabolic equilibrium throughout the endocrine system. An imbalance within this intricate regulating system could lead to considerable impacts , such as altered metabolism and increased susceptibility towards diseases , such as hypothyroidism and hyperthyroidism. This complexity further underscores the necessity of an integrative approach when considering the metabolism of endocrine tissues within the context of overall metabolic well-being (Figure 7.13).

7.5.1. Hormonal Regulation of Metabolic Processes

Hormonal regulation of metabolic processes is a primary function during the metabolism of specialized tissue, where hormones , such as auxins, gibberellins, and cytokinins play a central role in coordinating growth and development. These phytohormones act as mediators of varied physiological processes by influencing metabolic pathways that are essential for tissue differentiation and growth. For instance, during organogenesis, cell division and elongation are induced by auxins, leading to the formation of specialized tissues , such as roots and shoots.

Particularly, the interaction between the hormone-metabolic network drives the partitioning of the resources, thus tissue-specific functions , such as respiration and photosynthesis. Because plant tissues are dynamic in their responses to environmental cues, the regulated hormonal interactions allow a responsive metabolic process that maximizes survival and productivity. The fine balance of the concentrations of hormones and their individual impacts on metabolic processes highlights the complexity of plant growth and adaptation systems. Furthermore, regulation of assimilate distribution in high-quality tissues , such as seeds and fruits highlights the significance of hormonal signals in metabolic processes. Hormones like auxins and gibberellins are important in fruit setting and seed development because they regulate cellular respiration and nutrient distribution. Sucrose transporters have now been identified by recent research as pivotal in regulating assimilate partitioning during such stages as directly associated with yield potential. Hormonal interactions, for example, can prevent stress-induced seed and fruit abortion by enhanced sugar transport and storage. This raises the question of an advanced interaction between hormonal signaling and the regulation of metabolic pathways, where there is a necessity to inquire about how these activities are orchestrated to maximize reproductive success. Notably, the perception of these associations in specialized tissues proves helpful in maximizing crop yields and tolerance to environmental stresses.

Furthermore, coordination of metabolic networks via hormone regulation goes beyond primary growth to include secondary growth and wood development in specialized tissues. In the studies of xylogenesis, it has been shown that organellar carbon metabolism transcriptional modules are regulated by hormonal cues tightly during developing tissue, indicative of a high level of control in developing tissues. It is particularly crucial in direct response to environmental stimuli on the growth rates, requiring dynamic remodeling of the metabolic activities.

The intersection of the metabolic pathways of plastids and mitochondria in wood formation is an excellent example of coordinated response to internal and external stimuli to ensure effective carbon distribution for primary and secondary growth processes. By describing these hormone actions on metabolic regulation, researchers can gain an understanding of the mechanisms that drive tissue specialization development and functioning, which will eventually lead to more applications in agricultural and plant biology (Bouzayen et al., 2012; Gutierrez et al., 2019).

7.5.2. Role of the Pancreas in Glucose Metabolism

The pancreas plays a pivotal role in glucose metabolism regulation and is a preponderant organ to maintain homeostasis by both its endocrine and exocrine secretions. The pancreatic islets, or islets of the pancreas, are composed of multiple cell types, and alpha and beta cells are particularly crucial in glucose control. Beta cells secrete insulin, a hormone that enables peripheral tissues , such as muscle and adipose tissue to absorb glucose, activate glycolysis and lipogenesis. Alternatively, alpha cells secrete glucagon, which triggers glycogenolysis and gluconeogenesis in the liver when blood glucose is low. This tightly controlled hormonal balance ensures that glucose levels remain steady, crucial for the body's overall metabolic health and state of energy, particularly in specialized tissues with high glucose dependency for proper function. Besides this, the recent advances in imaging technology have also emphasized the pancreas multifunctional role in glucose metabolism. With methods , such as stimulated Raman-scattering imaging, researchers can now see the dynamic utilization of glucose within tissues as diverse as the pancreas itself.

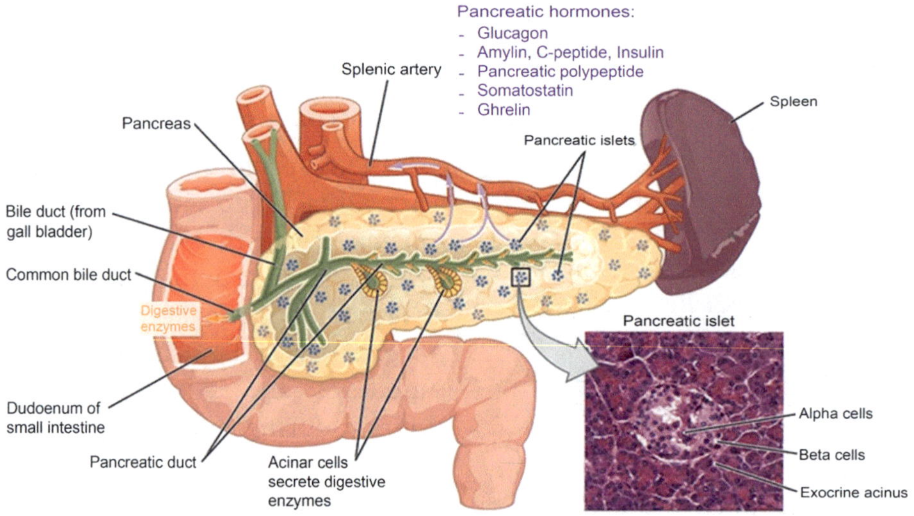

Figure 7.14. Anatomical organization of the pancreas.

Source: https://media.springernature.com/full/springer-static/image/art%3A10.1038%2Femm.2016.6/MediaObjects/12276_2016_Article_BFemm20166_Fig1_HTML.jpg?as=webp.

This type of technological capability enables measurement of recently synthesized macromolecules from glucose, such as proteins and lipids, and how these activities are controlled differentially across specialized tissues. These findings point towards the dynamic interactions between glucose utilization and insulin signaling pathways, showing that the pancreas is not merely reacting to blood glucose fluctuations but instead actively contributes to regulating more widespread metabolic responses within the body (Liu et al., 2019). The introduction of such technologies sheds light on diabetic complications and other pancreatic-related metabolic diseases. Also, the effects of pancreatic function are not confined to glucose regulation, as evidenced by the participation of numerous diverse metabolic processes. An important characteristic of this relationship is tracing element participation, such as zinc, which has been shown to play a role in glucose metabolism and pancreatic secretions. Zinc supplementation has been promising in modifying oxidative stress and its accompanying renal morbidity in diabetic patients, showing the manner in which disturbance of glucose metabolism cascades into more diffuse health issues, including CKD. These findings highlight the pancreas key role not just in glucose metabolism but also in overall welfare of specialized tissues affected by metabolic derangement. It is this awareness of these intricacies that can enable a more comprehensive management of diabetes and its associated complications (Figure 7.14).

7.5.3. Thyroid Hormones and Their Effect on Metabolism

The effect of thyroid hormones on metabolism is a major one, with the hormones playing a crucial role in regulating energy expenditure and metabolic rate in most tissues. Thyroid hormones, triiodothyronine (T3) and thyroxine (T4), control the metabolic processes that enable the cells to use nutrients to generate energy. Through the regulation of gene expression, the hormones elevate the BMR, affecting the metabolism of carbohydrates, lipids, and proteins. The interactive play between thyroid hormones and the metabolic machinery is an insidious web of endocrine regulation required to maintain homeostasis in specialized tissues. Disturbances in this hormonal balance can lead to metabolic disturbances, underscoring the crucial role of thyroid hormones not just in energy metabolism but in overall physiological well-being as well. These are metabolic adverse effects that are apt to occur when thyroidal dysfunction, for example, hypothyroidism, sets in. This is in the event of a deficiency in thyroid hormones.

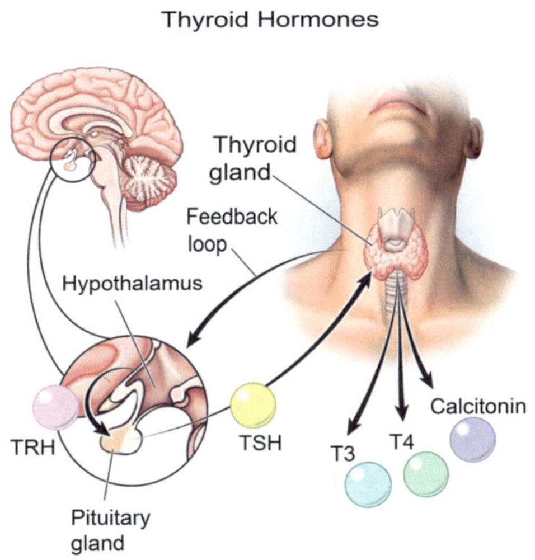

Figure 7.15. Your body controls your thyroid hormone (T3 and T4) levels through a complex feedback loop. Your hypothalamus releases thyrotropin-releasing hormone (TRH), which triggers your pituitary gland to release thyroid-stimulating hormone (TSH), which stimulates your thyroid to release T3 and T4.

Source: https://my.clevelandclinic.org/-/scassets/images/org/health/articles/22391-thyroid-hormone.

The clinical presentation of this hormonal inadequacy is an accelerated decline in metabolic rate with a consequent weight gain, fatigue, and alteration in lipid metabolism. Recent studies have also enlightened us about the significance of iodothyronine deiodinases, those enzymes that effect the conversion of T4 to the more active T3, crucial to maintaining adequate levels of thyroid hormone in target tissues. Of special interest, studies have demonstrated that failure to develop normal serum levels of T3 in hypothyroid patients on levothyroxine therapy can be attributed to genetic polymorphism of the *DIO2* gene, which again obscures the physiological effect of thyroid hormone therapy. These observations are a reminder of the intricate regulatory networks behind metabolic processes and the necessity of unraveling them for clinical management to be potent (Gereben et al., 2015). Moreover, the setting of thyroid hormones in the grand scheme of metabolism helps to remind us of their role in specialized tissues, where they exert specific actions based on cell requirements. For instance, thyroid hormones in the fat tissue control lipolysis to release stored fat for energy when there is increased demand. In muscle tissue, thyroid hormones cause the oxidation of fatty acids to help in enhanced physical performance and endurance. Their interaction with energy metabolism in these specialized tissues not only highlights their importance for exercise physiology but also illuminates possibilities for interventions in metabolic disease , such as obesity and insulin resistance. As scientists unravel the complexity of thyroid function, the therapeutic promise of thyroid hormones in determining metabolic outcome is an exciting frontier for future research (Patwardhan, 2008) (Figure 7.15).

Test Your Knowledge

1. What is the role of the pancreas in glucose metabolism?
2. What are thyroid hormones and their effect on metabolism?

SUMMARY

In describing the study of specialized tissue metabolism, one must consider the intricate biochemical processes by which these tissues are able to perform their specific physiological activities. The recent discoveries regarding the metabolomics of Drosophila melanogaster provide a compelling example of how different tissue types have unique metabolite profiles that are suited to their function. This work not only speaks to the interdependence of tissue specialization and metabolism but also to the potential for using model systems to elucidate human metabolic disease. The identification of 242 polar metabolites and 251 lipids in various tissues reveals the specificity and complexity of the metabolic processes, proving that each tissue has evolved to meet the specific demands of its environment and biological function, as the elevated level of acylcarnitines in alimentary canal testifies, characteristic of its central position in the metabolism of fats (Kamleh et al., 2013). Secondly, the data obtained from metabolomic studies are not merely a listing of metabolites; they form the foundation for insights into the interaction of different tissues within the collective metabolism network of an organism. The holistic perspective presents a clearer picture of the tissue-specific processes, which can be applied to guide research in aging, metabolic disease, and modeling human diseases. The ability to associate metabolite profiles with tissue functions also deepens our knowledge of pathology and suggests therapeutic targets. For instance, the high abundance of GSH in the cuticle suggests oxidative defense function, demonstrating how tissue-specific metabolism is able to affect overall health and disease susceptibility (Kamleh et al., 2013). Reflecting on the advancements in this research area, it is clear that continued exploration in the area of specialized tissue metabolism can help to elucidate complex biological interaction mechanisms in organisms. Future studies should be directed toward expanding the model organism types and linking results with transcriptomic data to form a multidimensional view of metabolism. In addition, the applications of this research extend into clinical practice, where an understanding of tissue metabolism can inform the treatment of inborn errors of metabolism and other metabolic abnormalities. As the support provided by NHS Grampian testifies to the desirability of continuing this research, the academic world must utilize these results to further the creation of new methodologies and treatments that can contribute to improved human health.

The metabolism of specialized tissues is an extremely advanced and basic area of investigation that reveals how various cellular milieus determine metabolic pathways. One of the most important pieces of information is the role of lactate metabolism in high-grade prostate cancer. A study using hyperpolarized 13C magnetic resonance spectroscopy illustrated that increased lactate production, fueled by upregulated lactate dehydrogenase (LDH) activity and overexpression of monocarboxylate transporter 4 (MCT4), is able to segregate high-risk and low-risk prostate cancer. The significant metabolic differences between high-grade cancer tissue and benign tissue underscore the potential of non-invasive imaging modalities to provide critical diagnostics for locoregional disease and thereby expand our knowledge in the progression of disease and therapeutic targets (Ahamed et al., 2020). Beyond cancer metabolism, the intricate regulation of plant metabolic processes underscore the contribution of specialized tissue metabolism in different biological contexts. The study of Eucalyptus xylogenesis has revealed the nuclear-encoded genes that regulate subcellular localization of carbon metabolism in plastids and mitochondria. With the use of targeted systems genetics coexpression network, researchers unveiled interconnected transcription modules that regulate organellar activity. Not only does this demonstrate the complexity of metabolic interactions, but also underscores the concurrent mechanisms that could possibly regulate primary growth and secondary development in wood formation. These findings suggest that a thorough understanding of metabolic processes has the potential to lead to fundamental agricultural and biotechnological advances (Gutierrez et al., 2019). The integration of findings from both plant biology and cancer biology puts the bigger picture in focus for understanding metabolic specializations within different tissues. These unique metabolic pathways are not only limited to their respective systems but also echo a universal message of regulation and adaptation to cellular and environmental signals. The capacity to unravel these sophisticated interactions adds to our expanding knowledge of tissue-specific metabolism and identifies potential pathways for innovation in targeted therapies and sustainable agriculture practices. By integrating knowledge from various biological systems, researchers have been able to gain insights into the metabolic topography that governs disease and health, paving the way for the next generation of investigations into metabolic intervention strategies and biotechnological innovation.

KEY TERMS FROM THIS CHAPTER

Adipose tissue	Brain metabolism
Brown adipose tissue	Caenorhabditis elegans
Fatty acid oxidation	Gluconeogenesis
Glycogenolysis	Lipolysis
Metabolic dysregulation	Muscle tissue metabolism
Nervous tissues	RNA sequencing
Skeletal muscle	Specialized tissues
White adipose tissue	

Critical Thinking Questions

1. **Which tissue is primarily responsible for the storage of triglycerides?**
   a. Muscle tissue
   b. Adipose tissue
   c. Liver
   d. Brain
2. **Which specialized tissue can carry out gluconeogenesis?**
   a. Adipose tissue
   b. Muscle
   c. Liver
   d. Brain
3. **Cardiac muscle primarily derives energy from:**
   a. Glucose
   b. Ketone bodies
   c. Fatty acids
   d. Amino acids
4. **Which enzyme is highly active in brown adipose tissue to produce heat?**
   a. ATP synthase
   b. Hormone-sensitive lipase
   c. Uncoupling protein 1 (UCP1)
   d. Hexokinase
5. **What is the role of white adipose tissue in metabolism?**
   a. Heat generation
   b. Storage and release of energy as triglycerides
   c. Protein synthesis
   d. Gluconeogenesis

Short Answer Questions

1. What is the importance of specialized tissues in the body?
2. Describe the role of glycogen in muscle energy.
3. What is the function of adipose tissue in energy storage?
4. What is the detoxification process?
5. What is the brain metabolism?

Answers to Critical Thinking Questions

1. (b); 2. (c); 3. (c); 4. (c); 5. (b)

REFERENCES

1. Ahamed, F., Bok, R. A., DeLos Santos, J., Keshari, K. R., et al. (2020). Elevated tumor lactate and efflux in high-grade prostate cancer demonstrated by hyperpolarized 13C magnetic resonance spectroscopy of prostate tissue slice cultures. https://core.ac.uk/download/323073589.pdf (accessed on 12th June 2025).
2. Albrecht, U., Bowman, K. D., Dandekar, A. M., Davis, M. J., et al. (2013). Gene regulatory networks elucidating Huanglongbing disease mechanisms. https://core.ac.uk/download/323070988.pdf (accessed on 12th June 2025).
3. Al-Gubory, K., Arianmanesh, M., & Fowler, P. A. (2016). The sheep conceptus modulates proteome profiles in caruncular endometrium during early pregnancy. https://core.ac.uk/download/131024953.pdf (accessed on 12th June 2025).
4. Arble, D. M., & Sandoval, D. A. (2013). CNS control of glucose metabolism: Response to environmental challenges. https://core.ac.uk/download/213087639.pdf (accessed on 12th June 2025).
5. Barahona, M. J., Elizondo Vega, R., García Robles, M. de los Á., Martinez, M. J., et al. (2017). Adenovirus-mediated suppression of hypothalamic glucokinase affects feeding behavior. https://core.ac.uk/download/159286728.pdf (accessed on 12th June 2025).
6. Becu Villalobos, D., Coirini, H., Cornejo, M. P., Elias, C. F., et al. (2016). Neuroendocrine regulation of metabolism. https://core.ac.uk/download/159290530.pdf (accessed on 12th June 2025).
7. Gereben, B., McAninch, E. A., Ribeiro, M. O., & Bianco, A. C. (2015). Scope and limitations of iodothyronine deiodinases in hypothyroidism. Nature reviews. Endocrinology, 11(11), 642–652. https://doi.org/10.1038/nrendo.2015.155 (accessed on 12th June 2025).
8. Bich, L., Moreau, J. F., & Pradeu, T. (2019). Understanding multicellularity: The functional organization of the intercellular space. https://core.ac.uk/download/228134961.pdf (accessed on 12th June 2025).
9. Bickel, P. E., Tansey, J. T., & Welte, M. A. (2009). PAT proteins, an ancient family of lipid droplet proteins that regulate cellular lipid stores. https://core.ac.uk/download/46715477.pdf (accessed on 12th June 2025).
10. Blüher, M., Boucher, J., Cheong, J. K., Doria, A., et al. (2014). Ablation of TRIP-Br2, a novel regulator of fat lipolysis, thermogenesis and oxidative metabolism, prevents diet-induced obesity and insulin resistance. https://core.ac.uk/download/28946336.pdf (accessed on 12th June 2025).
11. Bouzayen, M., Fernie, A. R., Osorio, S., Patrick, J. W., et al. (2012). Molecular regulation of seed and fruit set. https://core.ac.uk/download/12043888.pdf (accessed on 12th June 2025).
12. Braeckman, B., Houthoofd, K., & Vanfleteren, J. (2009). Intermediary metabolism. https://core.ac.uk/download/84042477.pdf (accessed on 12th June 2025).
13. Bratty, M. A., Chintapalli, V., Davies, S. A., Dow, J. A. T., et al. (2012). Functional correlates of positional and gender-specific renal asymmetry in *Drosophila*. https://core.ac.uk/download/6175807.pdf (accessed on 12th June 2025).
14. Calota, D., Calota, F., Mesina, C., Mogoanta, L., et al. (2019). Oncogenesis—Kaleidoscopic and

multi-level reality. https://core.ac.uk/download/216811042.pdf (accessed on 12th June 2025).

15. Deshmukh, A. S., Murgia, M., Nagaraj, N., Treebak, J. T., Cox, J., & Mann, M. (2015). Deep proteomics of mouse skeletal muscle enables quantitation of protein isoforms, metabolic pathways, and transcription factors. *Molecular & cellular proteomics : MCP, 14*(4), 841–853. https://doi.org/10.1074/mcp.M114.044222 (accessed on 12th June 2025).
16. Critchley, H., Babayev, E., Bulun, S. E., Clark, S., Garcia-Grau, I., Gregersen, P. K., Kilcoyne, A., et al. (2020). Menstruation: Science and society. *American Journal of Obstetrics and Gynecology, 223*, 624–664. https://doi.org/10.1016/j.ajog.2020.06.004 (accessed on 12th June 2025).
17. De Rosa, V., Marelli-Berg, F., Mauro, C., Solito, E., et al. (2015). Metabolic syndrome and the immunological affair with the blood-brain barrier. https://core.ac.uk/download/30697111.pdf (accessed on 12th June 2025).
18. Di Liegro, C. M., Di Liegro, I., & Schiera, G. (2019). Cell-to-cell communication in learning and memory: From neuro- and glio-transmission to information exchange mediated by extracellular vesicles. https://core.ac.uk/download/286528528.pdf (accessed on 12th June 2025).
19. Duszka, K., Manickam, R., & Wahli, W. (2020). PPARs and microbiota in skeletal muscle health and wasting. https://core.ac.uk/download/427409477.pdf (accessed on 12th June 2025).
20. Ebenhoeh, O., Matthaeus, F., & Salazar, C. (2008). Biosynthetic potentials of metabolites and their hierarchical organization. https://core.ac.uk/download/25497442.pdf (accessed on 12th June 2025).
21. Ertunc, M. E., & Hotamışlıgil, G. S. (2016). Lipid signaling and lipotoxicity in metaflammation: Indications for metabolic disease pathogenesis and treatment. *Journal of Lipid Research, 57*, 2099–2114. https://doi.org/10.1194/jlr.r066514 (accessed on 12th June 2025).
22. Fenech, A. G., & Grech, G. (2014). Pharmacogenetics: The science of predictive clinical pharmacology. https://core.ac.uk/download/46602555.pdf (accessed on 12th June 2025).
23. Fernando, J., & Zhou, S. (2015). The role of zinc in renal pathological changes in diabetic status. https://core.ac.uk/download/130975189.pdf (accessed on 12th June 2025).
24. Fierro Gutierrez, A. C. E., Marchal, K., Mizrachi, E., Myburg, A. A., et al. (2019). Organellar carbon metabolism is coordinated with distinct developmental phases of secondary xylem. https://core.ac.uk/download/195331582.pdf (accessed on 12th June 2025).
25. Fioramonti, M., Fracassi, A., Marangoni, M., Rosso, M., et al. (2016). AMPK in the central nervous system: Physiological roles and pathological implications. https://core.ac.uk/download/188827766.pdf (accessed on 12th June 2025).
26. Glancy, B., Kane, D. A., Kavazis, A. N., Goodwin, M. L., Willis, W. T., & Gladden, L. B. (2020). Mitochondrial lactate metabolism: History and implications for exercise and disease. *The Journal of Physiology, 599*, 863–888. https://doi.org/10.1113/jp278930 (accessed on 12th June 2025).
27. Hennigar, S. R. (2010). Exposure to polybrominated diphenyl ethers (PBDEs) suppresses the release of pro-inflammatory products by alveolar macrophages *in vitro*. https://core.ac.uk/download/215515896.pdf (accessed on 12th June 2025).
28. Jayabalan, N., Nair, S., Sobrevia Luarte, L., Zuñiga, F. A., et al. (2017). Cross talk between

adipose tissue and placenta in obese and gestational diabetes mellitus pregnancies via exosomes. https://core.ac.uk/download/132469732.pdf (accessed on 12th June 2025).

29. Kamleh, A., Malmendal, A., Jackson, A. A., Jeulin, C., Watson, D. G., et al. (2013). Mapping an atlas of tissue-specific *Drosophila melanogaster* metabolomes by high resolution mass spectrometry. https://core.ac.uk/download/16462998.pdf (accessed on 12th June 2025).

30. Koliwad, S. K., McQueen, A. E., & Wang, J. C. (2018). Fighting obesity by targeting factors regulating beige adipocytes. https://core.ac.uk/download/323311252.pdf (accessed on 12th June 2025).

31. Liu, Y., Miao, Y., Min, W., Qian, X., et al. (2019). Spectral tracing of deuterium for imaging glucose metabolism. https://core.ac.uk/download/323065665.pdf (accessed on 12th June 2025).

32. Longstaffe, F. J., Metcalfe, J. Z., Schwartz-Narbonne, R., Zazula, G. D., et al. (2015). Solving the woolly mammoth conundrum: Amino acid 15N-enrichment suggests a distinct forage or habitat. https://core.ac.uk/download/286714021.pdf (accessed on 12th June 2025).

33. Nattiv, A., Philp, A., Loucks, A. B., Jeukendrup, A. E., et al. (2020). Nutrition strategies for triathlon. https://core.ac.uk/download/249364290.pdf (accessed on 12th June 2025).

34. Patwardhan, K. (2008). Concepts of human physiology in Ayurveda. https://core.ac.uk/download/pdf/87482.pdf (accessed on 12th June 2025).

35. Plubell, D. L., Wilmarth, P. A., Zhao, Y., Fenton, A. M., Minnier, J., Reddy, A. P., Klimek, J., et al. (2017). Extended multiplexing of tandem mass tags (TMT) labeling reveals age and high fat diet specific proteome changes in mouse epididymal adipose tissue. *Molecular & Cellular Proteomics, 16*, 873–890. https://doi.org/10.1074/mcp.m116.065524 (accessed on 12th June 2025).

36. Prado, C. M., Landi, F., Chew, S. T. H., Atherton, P. J., Molinger, J., Ruck, T., & González, M. C. (2022). Advances in muscle health and nutrition: A toolkit for healthcare professionals. *Clinical Nutrition, 41*, 2244–2263. https://doi.org/10.1016/j.clnu.2022.07.041 (accessed on 12th June 2025).

37. Saito, R. de F., Andrade, L. N. de S., Bustos, S. O., & Chammas, R. (2022). Phosphatidylcholine-derived lipid mediators: The crosstalk between cancer cells and immune cells. *Frontiers in Immunology, 13*. https://doi.org/10.3389/fimmu.2022.768606 (accessed on 12th June 2025).

38. Schermerhorn, T. (2013). Normal glucose metabolism in carnivores overlaps with diabetes pathology in non-carnivores. https://core.ac.uk/download/33353526.pdf (accessed on 12th June 2025).

39. Subramaniam, S., Wang, Y., & Winters, J. (2012). Functional classification of skeletal muscle networks. I. Normal physiology. https://core.ac.uk/download/213080019.pdf (accessed on 12th June 2025).

IMMUNOCHEMISTRY

8

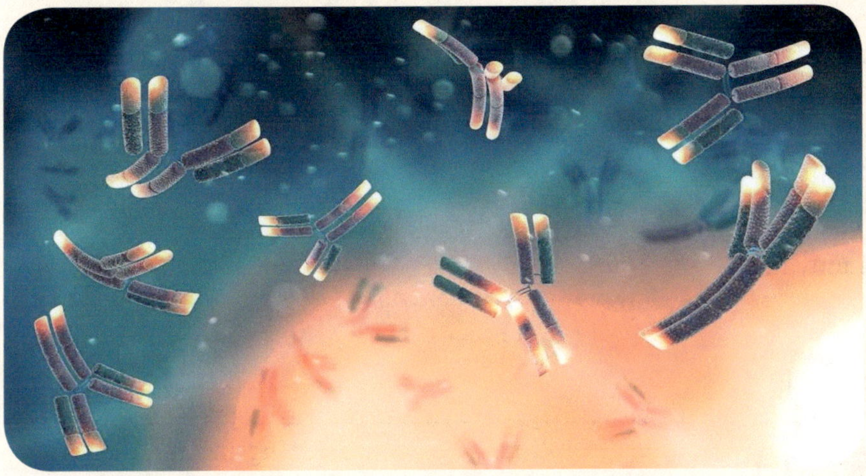

LEARNING OBJECTIVES

After studying this chapter, you will be able to:

1. Understand the fundamental concepts of immunochemistry;
2. Know the techniques of immunochemistry;
3. Describe the clinical diagnostics applications;
4. Know the application of immunochemistry in research;
5. Understand the advances in immunochemical techniques.

Introduction

Immunochemistry is an active interdisciplinary field between immunology and biochemistry that concerns the investigation of immune phenomena and the molecules responsible for such processes. Immunochemistry is important as it reveals the intricate interactions between antibodies and antigens, which shed light on biological systems. Applying methodologies , such as ELISA and Western blotting, scientists can detect and quantify certain proteins or molecules from various samples. This methodological foundation enables an individual to investigate further in terms of cellular processes involved in immunity, hence enhancing the comprehension of health and disease. With the appreciation of the pivotal role that immunochemistry is playing in diagnosis and therapy, students and practitioners need to comprehend such analytical techniques. Such knowledge serves as a foundation for extending immunologic research and devising new treatments for numerous diseases. Advances in immunochemistry have been advanced by new technologies that enhance the specificity and sensitivity of detection methods.

Among the significant advances is the marriage of genetic engineering and X-ray crystallography, whereby scientists can obtain precise structures of ligand-receptor complexes, which assists in the understanding of their affinities and mechanisms. Furthermore, advances in computing power and simulation techniques have enabled it to be possible to investigate macromolecular interactions at unprecedented resolution. The multi-dimensional character of the study expands the research scope by providing new avenues towards understanding kinetic and mechanical aspects of cell membrane receptors leading to novel hypotheses as well as experimental approaches (Alder et al., 2008). Consequently, immunochemistry develops progressively, broadening theoretical knowledge and practical methods across broad fields , such as clinical diagnostics, vaccine development, and therapeutic antibody design.

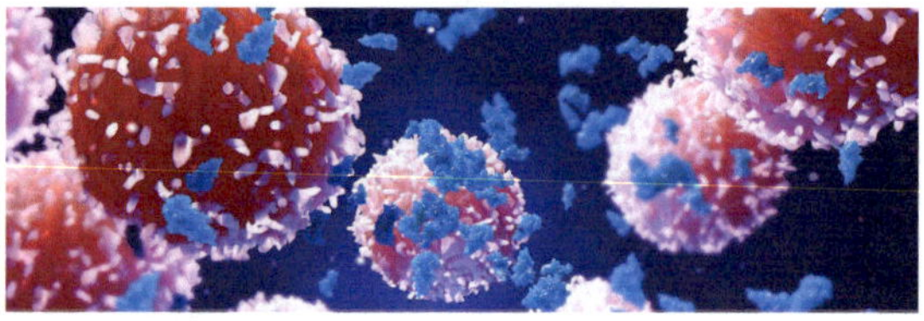

Figure 8.1. Immunochemistry.

Source: https://www.elgalabwater.com/sites/default/files/2020-05/GettyImages-972355096%20%281%29_0.jpg.

In schools, the incorporation of laboratory experiments has proven to be highly beneficial in reinforcing students' understanding of immunochemistry principles. One such example is the application of Western blotting in undergraduate laboratory courses with the goal of teaching students' protein detection and localization in model organisms , such as *Drosophila melanogaster* (Gogia et al., 2017). This laboratory exercise not only exposes students to biochemical techniques but also demonstrates the use of immunochemistry in biological problem-solving. By actively involving students in protein isolation steps, gel electrophoresis, and immunodetection, educators can impart a deep sense of respect for how immunochemistry is used in research. These exercises eventually enable the students to make a lasting contribution to the discipline, enabling them to work on creative solutions to serious biological issues in the future (Figure 8.1).

8.1. Fundamental Concepts of Immunochemistry

Learning Outcome

1. Describe the antibodies and their structure;
2. Understand the antigens and their role in immune response;
3. Know the principles of antigen-antibody interactions.

Essentially, immunochemistry is an interdisciplinary science bridging immunology and biochemistry, with the focal point being the interaction between antigens and antibodies. The intricate interaction is fundamental to understanding how the immune system recognizes and neutralizes pathogens. Antibodies or immunoglobulins are glycoproteins secreted by B cells as the body's defense mechanism against infectious agents. The antibodies' specificity to specific antigens emphasizes their pivotal position in natural immunity as well as in immunological memory. In addition, the specificity forms the basis for the design of different diagnostic and therapeutic agents in contemporary medicine. Techniques , such as ELISA and Western blotting are based on these interactions between antigens and antibodies, demonstrating how concepts in immunochemistry can be translated to practical applications in disease therapy and diagnosis and eventually learn more about immunological responses to an enormous scope of diseases. Complementing the central role of antibodies is the complexity of the complement system. This cascade of plasma proteins complements the activity of antibodies in removing microbes and eliciting inflammation and, therefore, serves a very crucial role in innate immunity. Complement pathway is triggered by three main pathways: classical pathway, alternative pathway, and lectin pathway. These three pathways diverge but eventually converge to one point—membrane attack complex (MAC) that degrades cell integrity of pathogens. Clarification of these pathways is essential to the development of therapeutics that will be capable of modulating immune responses. For instance, enhancement of complement activity is therapeutic in some cancers, where the immune response is amplified and targeted against killing tumor cells. Thus, interaction of antibodies with the complement system emphasizes the complex and dynamic character of immunological events observed during health and disease.

Moreover, immunochemistry advancements have significantly impacted the advancement of vaccines and immunotherapy. Using immunochemical techniques, scientists can now create more potent vaccine platforms that evoke strong immune responses. For example, the addition of adjuvants can enhance antigens that can trigger immunogenicity, hence leading to vaccines that generate long-term immunity. This is particularly relevant in emerging infectious disease situations, where the quick production of vaccines can be lifesaving. In addition, the application of immunotherapy in the form of monoclonal antibody therapy has transformed cancer therapy to ensure that targeted treatment is attained with little harm inflicted on normal tissues and yet sufficient efficacy against tumors. This treatment depends on the concepts of immunochemistry, demonstrating the applicability of elementary principles into novel medical treatments. In essence, the fundamental concepts of immunochemistry not only enhance our understanding of the immune process but also provide the foundation for groundbreaking healthcare innovations (Association, 1960; Moorhead, 2022) (Figure 8.2).

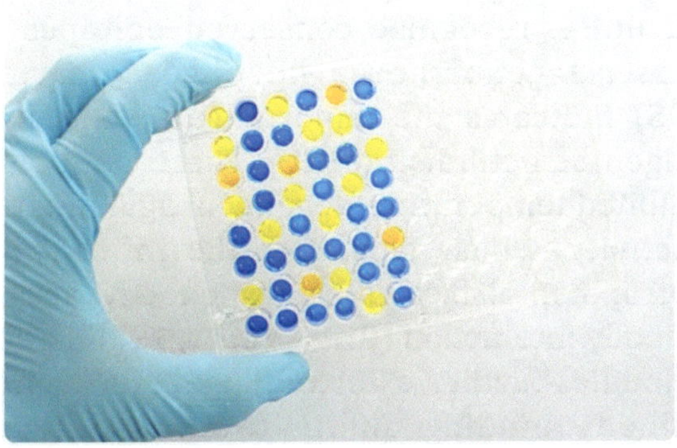

Figure 8.2. Enzyme-linked immunosorbent assay (ELISA) is an immunology testing method in 96 96-well microplate.

Source: https://www.azolifesciences.com/image-handler/ts/20180824125932/ri/673/picture/2018/8/shutterstock_324073772.jpg.

8.1.1. Antibodies and Their Structure

Antibodies or immunoglobulins are glycoproteins derived from B cells that specialize in the immune response. The proteins are highly specific and bind to particular antigens, foreign particles that trigger an immune reaction. There are four polypeptide chains with two heavy and two light chains constituting the antibodies, which are coupled to each other through disulfide linkages to form a Y-shaped molecule. The variation in the amino acid sequences of the variable regions of these chains is the cause of the vast antibody variability. Every antibody can recognize particular epitopes on an antigen, so that antibodies are capable of targeting pathogens specifically. Not only does this structural organization enable antigen recognition, but it also determines the general function of the immune response, an ideal illustration of the functional dependency of antibody structure and immunological function. Antibody antigen binding is regulated by interactions that are very specific and can be modulated by structural manipulation of the antibody and the antigen. As such, an article demonstrating how particular mAbs, say 3F11 and 06B4, recognize conserved epitopes on Neisseria gonorrhoeae lipooligosaccharides (LOS) indicates the importance of antibody-antigen structural integrity. These antibodies exhibited temperature-dependent agglutination reactivity, which highlights the influence of environmental factors on the effectiveness of antibody interaction (Griffiss et al., 1988). These antibodies further exhibited highly differential antibody binding ability towards different glycosphingolipid molecules present on human erythrocytes, which highlights that subtle variations in antigen structure can considerably influence immune recognition. The ability of antibodies to adapt to differential structural features of antigens is crucial for an effective humoral immunity. Furthermore, antibodies undergo post-translational modification (PTM) processes , such as glycosylation that have the ability to influence their specificity and function even further. The presence of sialic acid residues, for instance, plays an important role in creating specific antigenic structures to facilitate enhanced pathogen recognition. Investigation into how gonococci treated with cytidine monophospho-N-acetyl-neuraminic acid (CMP-NANA) displayed alteration of the lipooligosaccharide structure illustrates the dynamic relationship between microbial adaptation and antibody specificity (Apicella et al., 1990). Such adaptability is of prime significance for pathogens that evolve mechanisms for avoidance of immune detection, providing further impetus to the importance of an understanding of antibody structure and function in immunochemistry. Finally, the intricate interaction between antibody structure and the oscillating nature of antigenic motifs plays a crucial role in the immune landscape, making the humoral immune system effective (Figure 8.3).

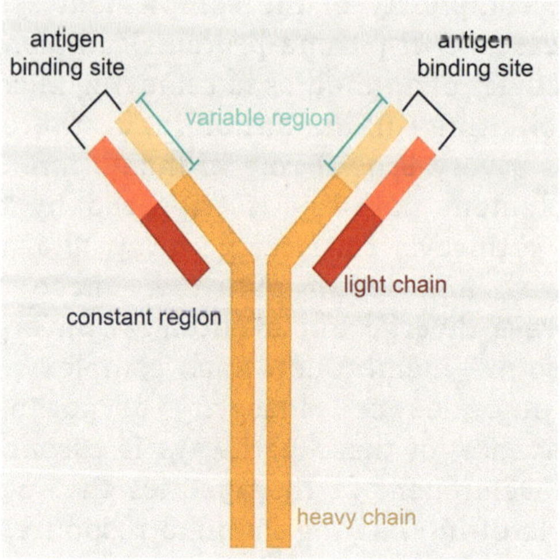

Figure 8.3. Diagram of an antibody structure showing its key components, including antigen binding sites, variable and constant regions, light chains, and heavy chains.

Source: https://www.news-medical.net/image-handler/ts/20250203015838/ri/950/src/images/Article_Images/ImageForArticle_16427_17386091169636892.jpg.

8.1.2. Antigens and Their Role in Immune Response

Antigens are critical components of the immune system, designed to recognize foreign substances that trigger an immune response. These polysaccharide molecules or proteins can be derived from a variety of sources, including infectious agents , such as bacteria and viruses, or non-infectious agents , such as pollen and transplanted tissues. Immune cells, particularly B lymphocytes and T lymphocytes, respond to antigens when they invade the body. This recognition sets off a cascade of immune responses to neutralize or kill the invading foreign agent. Immune response specificity depends mainly on the unique structures of antigens, enabling the design of antibodies that are specifically crafted to recognize these unique motifs. These interactions form the basis of immunochemistry, demystifying the mysteries of how the immune system detects danger and mounts defenses against it. The role of antigens is not just identification; they stimulate a complicated play of the immune system. Phrases like idiotype, which refer to the antigen-binding site on an antibody unique to it, reflect the specificity of the reaction. Display of the idiotype of a given antigenic monoclonal antibody, 14-4-4S, for instance, has been linked with the effectiveness of immune responses against specific antigens, such as the Ia antigen (Bluestone et al., 1981). This link implies that genetic determinants, in addition to influencing the presence of antibodies, also influence the quality and magnitude of the immune response. The nuances of the idiotype-specific responses demonstrate how antigens can shape the immune landscape in such a manner that it is enhanced or specific immune protection based on genetic background and prior exposure. In addition to causing an immune response, antigens are also reported to cross-react with respective structures in the host, a characteristic that largely favors autoimmune responses. For example, in antibody tests using *Neisseria gonorrhoeae* LOS, the antibodies have caused these to agglutinate human erythrocytes, indicative of structural homologies (Griffiss et al., 1988). This cross-reactivity is also perilous in that the failure of the immune system to distinguish self from non-self can lead to injury to tissues. This points to the importance of antigenic structure and the differential capacity of the immune system to recognize. This study thus not only discusses how immune protection is built but also highlights salient issues regarding the potential for autoimmune reactions resulting from these complex interactions (Figure 8.4).

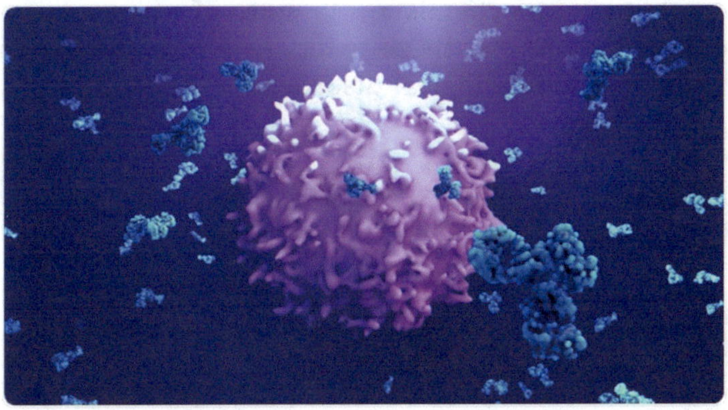

Figure 8.4. 3D rendering of a cancer cell interacting with antibodies.

Source: https://www.news-medical.net/image-handler/ts/20201005071709/ri/673/picture/2020/10/shutterstock_1476281402.jpg.

8.1.3. The Principles of Antigen-Antibody Interactions

One of the fundamental rules of immunochemistry within the field of biochemistry is the intricate relationship between antigens and antibodies. Antigens, i.e., foreign molecules typically proteins or polysaccharides, induce the immune system to generate a particular antibody. These B cell-secreted antibodies are very specific in that they specifically bind tightly to their cognate antigens by virtue of highly specific noncovalent interactions like hydrogen bonds, van der Waals, and ionic bonds. It is the specificity of these interactions that enables pathogen recognition and immune response, enabling the body to target and inactivate a wide range of infectious organisms without damaging its own tissues. An understanding of such interactions not only sheds light on basic immune mechanisms but also aids in optimizing diagnostic reagents and treatment methods in immunology. Environmental conditions and conformational alteration of the interacting molecules also affect antigen-antibody interactions. As an example, in the higher glucose levels that are common with diabetes, the binding ability of some C-type lectins to specific oligosaccharides has been shown to be significantly altered, potentially to increase the susceptibility of people to infection (Ahmed et al., 2011). This competitive inhibition is a sign of the need to have a correct study of how physiological alterations could influence the fundamental premises of such interactions. In addition, high-tech experiments employing atomic force microscopy have provided information on the kinetics and physical properties of the binding reactions, emphasizing the importance of physical environments in mediating the effectiveness of immune responses. Such interdisciplinarity continues to elevate our understanding of antigen-antibody interactions in health and disease. Moreover, the new methodologies of research have enhanced the accuracy with which such interactions can be viewed and controlled. Advances in X-ray crystallography and genetic design have allowed researchers to delineate the true structures and affinities of numerous ligand-receptor systems and so enormously improve our knowledge of macromolecular interaction (Alder et al., 2008). These breakthroughs not only describe how small variations in molecular structure influence binding specificity but also create the potential for creating targeted immunotherapies that can maximize or modulate immune response. Overall understanding across several fields of research reinforces the complexity and significance of antigen-antibody interactions, reasserting their preeminent place within immunochemistry. As more of this evolving research continues to be developed, increased understanding of these tenets will undoubtedly continue to advance our capacity to address a variety of immunological disorders (Figure 8.5).

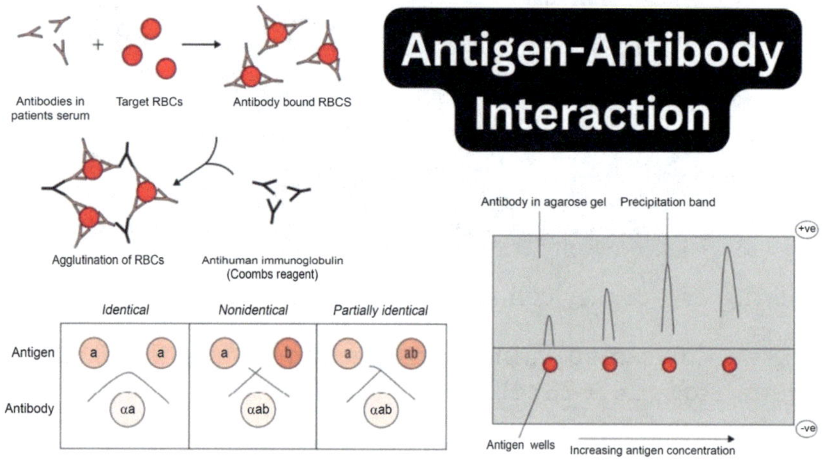

Figure 8.5. Antigen-antibody interaction.

Source: https://biologynotesonline.com/wp-content/uploads/2022/10/Antigen-Antibody-Interaction-1024x576.jpg.

Test Your Knowledge

1. What antibody has 4 polypeptide chains?
2. What are the antigens?

8.2. Techniques in Immunochemistry

Learning Outcome

1. Understand the enzyme-linked immunosorbent assay (ELISA);
2. Know the Western blotting and its applications;
3. Describe the immunofluorescence microscopy.

Immunochemistry is the investigation of a variety of methods through which immune responses can be investigated at the molecular level. One of the fundamental methods is ELISA, which allows one to detect and quantify the antigens or antibodies in body fluids. The method involves the use of enzyme-labeled antibodies to generate a measurable response through substrate conversion, thereby allowing one to assess immune markers for research and diagnostic purposes in the clinic. Optimization of conditions , such as temperature and pH, allows the researchers to enhance the sensitivity and specificity of the assay. Novel forms of ELISA, such as competitive and sandwich formats, also satisfy a range of analytical needs. The flexibility of the ELISAs has made it an immunochemical laboratory standard for applications ranging from disease diagnosis to biomarker identification. The second most common technique in immunochemistry is Western blotting, which has widespread use in the detection and characterization of proteins. This method is the union of gel electrophoresis and antigen-specific antibody binding in that researchers separate proteins based on size and then identify them using antibodies against specific epitopes. This method involves blotting separated proteins onto a membrane and incubation with primary and secondary antibodies for the amplification of the signal. Western blotting is particularly useful for studying protein expression and PTMs and is therefore invaluable in unraveling cellular processes and disease pathology. Visualization of proteins in complex mixtures provides insight into the state of various diseases and the efficacy of therapeutic interventions, and our understanding of immunity accordingly. Immunohistochemistry (IHC) is also a critical technique within the discipline, which allows for the localization of antigens in tissue sections. Through the application of labeled antibodies that bind particular targets in situ, IHC provides precious data about protein distribution and expression in tissue structure. IHC finds significant utility in oncology, wherein it facilitates the diagnosis and prognosis of tumors by identifying particular malignancy-linked markers. The essence of IHC is to get maximum staining with minimal background signal; thus, the selection of the best antigen retrieval steps and detection systems is critical. Moreover, utilization of IHC in combination with other approaches, such as fluorescence microscopy, can enhance spatial resolution and multiplexing capacity and enable extensive analysis of protein interactions and tissue microenvironments, which are critical in advancing immunological research and therapeutic strategies (Figure 8.6).

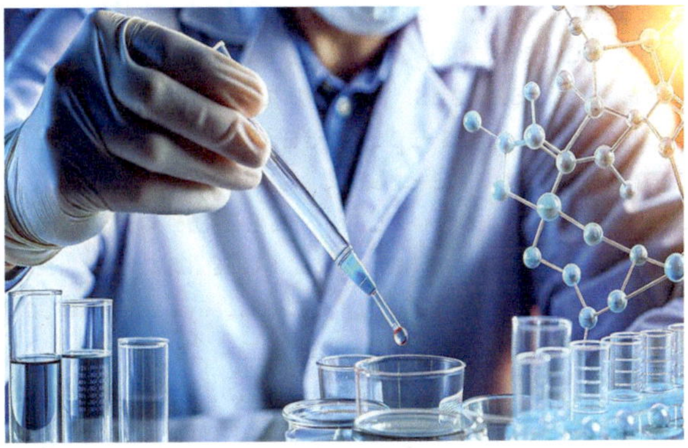

Figure 8.6. Scientist conducting laboratory research in immunochemistry.

Source: https://medicalbuyer.co.in/wp-content/uploads/2025/04/Immunochemistry-%E2%80%93-Pioneering-diagnostics-and-therapy-frontiers.jpg.

8.2.1. Enzyme-Linked Immunosorbent Assay (ELISA)

The ELISA is an immunochemistry method of central importance with unparalleled flexibility in the measurement and detection of antibodies and antigens. ELISA depends on the immobilization of an antibody or antigen on a solid support, such as a microplate, followed by the addition of a homogeneous antibody conjugated to an enzyme. After adding the substrate, enzymatic activity generates a detectable signal, usually a color reaction, which allows researchers to quantify the presence of the target molecule. The method is most valuable due to its high specificity, which allows accurate results in serological analysis and research applications in various fields , such as medicine, veterinary medicine, and food security. ELISA tests have evolved using various formats, including direct, indirect, sandwich, and competitive ELISA. Each of them possesses distinct strengths depending on the target of interest. Sandwich ELISA employs two antibodies that react to different epitopes of a shared antigen in order to increase sensitivity and specificity. Competitive ELISA is more adapted for small antigens that are not easily captured. Monoclonal production has enhanced the sensitivity and reproducibility of ELISA tremendously, particularly in research involving broad-spectrum pathogens. For example, in bovine enteric coronavirus research, the co-application of mAbs in ELISA format gave better detection than with standard methods, emphasizing ELISA's versatility in various diagnostic scenarios (Czerny et al., 1989). In avian virology, the application of ELISA has provided new standards beyond standard serological methods, including the hemagglutination inhibition (HI) test. For instance, ELISA has been found to be more efficient as an early marker of antibodies to avian influenza virus (AIV) subtypes H5 and H7. Studies indicated that these specific ELISAs were identified to possess higher sensitivity and specificity than HI tests, allowing for better screening of poultry flocks. The reproducibility of the assay also reflects its viability with high correlation factors testifying to consistent operation under different experimental conditions (Comin et al., 2013). As the need for speedy and efficient diagnostic procedures remains, ELISA remains ahead of immunochemical applications with ongoing innovation in disease monitoring and control procedures (Figure 8.7).

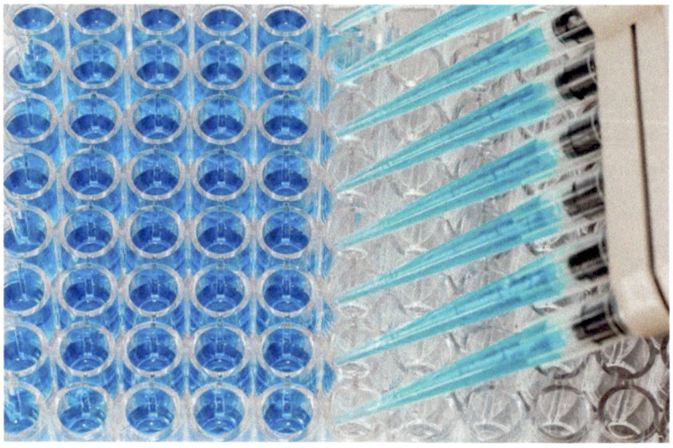

Figure 8.7. An enzyme-linked immunosorbent assay (ELISA) being performed in a laboratory.

Source: https://cdn.britannica.com/53/193053-050-8DEBAA0B/assay-laboratory.jpg.

8.2.2. Western Blotting and Its Applications

Western blotting is an important technique in immunochemistry primarily applied for detecting and measuring specific proteins in intricate mixtures. It involves the separation of proteins based on their molecular weight by sodium dodecyl sulfate-polyacrylamide gel electrophoresis (SDS-PAGE). Then, proteins are transferred to a membrane where they can be detected using antibodies against the protein of interest. Its dual capability to measure and characterize clearly points to the broad number of applications for Western blotting in various biological research settings. Its adaptability is observed as it is used in research areas like cancer research, research in infectious diseases, and therapeutic intervention measurement, allowing researchers to characterize protein expression patterns and PTMs under experimental conditions. In educational settings, Western blotting is not just a research tool but an effective teaching resource in biology classes. As a specific example, an undergraduate laboratory session founded upon Drosophila melanogaster permits students to isolate and pinpoint proteins within the fruit fly compound eye. This hands-on session gives students a chance to work with the reality of protein biochemistry, from protein isolation to the final detection on membranes. The course centers on the fundamental principles of protein chemistry and how they can be applied to practical research, thereby developing an informed appreciation of immunochemical techniques. Through this experiential learning, students gain essential skills and an appreciation of methodologies behind current biological advances, hence linking theory and practice. Applications of Western blotting also extend towards the study of new biomaterials and how they interact with the immune system. Recent studies in the interaction of carbon nanotubes with human serum complement reveal the high potential of the method. With the help of Western blot and SDS-PAGE, researchers can examine the activation pathways of complement proteins when they interact with novel materials like carbon nanotubes. The outcomes indicate that these nanotubes can activate complement via classical and alternative pathways, and this is also an area for continued research in immunological reactions. This research demonstrates that Western blotting, apart from assisting in the explanation of fundamental biological processes, provides insight into novel applications, such as drug delivery systems and vaccine construction, thereby highlighting its pivotal role in the advancement of immunochemistry (Salvador-Morales et al., 2006; Gogia et al., 2017) (Figure 8.8).

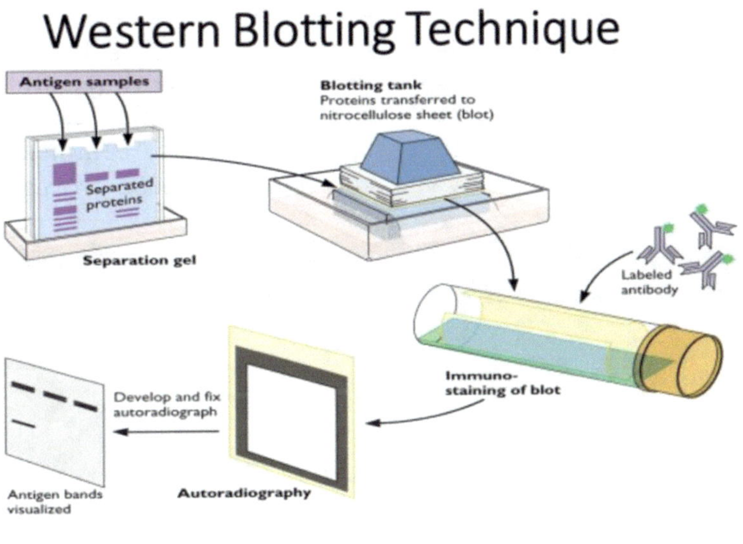

Figure 8.8. Western blotting technique.

Source: https://www.mybiosource.com/learn/wp-content/uploads/2018/06/western-blotting-feature-678x381.jpg.

8.2.3. Immunofluorescence Microscopy

Immunofluorescence microscopy is an essential technique in immunochemistry that allows one to visualize specific antigens in biological tissues using fluorescently labeled antibodies. It is a technique stemming from the pathbreaking work that appeared during the 1940s, allowing researchers to localize proteins with high sensitivity and specificity. The use of fluorescein-conjugated antibodies marked a significant milestone that led to the optimization of many immunohistochemical techniques to enhance the reliability of antigen detection (Linnoila & Petrusz, 1984). Choosing appropriate methods of fixation is vital since it preserves cellular morphology as well as antigen immunoreactivity, allowing antibodies to penetrate tissue sections. Consequently, this technique has gained interest while studying complex biological samples and has provided insights that are useful for gaining insight into disease mechanisms and tissue anatomy. Application of immunofluorescence microscopy is particularly beneficial in lung tissue analysis, which is predisposed by nature due to its extensive surface area and many cell types. By employing this technique, researchers have been successful in analyzing critical components like collagen, enzymes, and tumor markers in the respiratory airway (Linnoila & Petrusz, 1984). These results emphasize the worth of the method in disclosing details about lung health effects from the environment and identifying the earliest symptoms of respiratory sickness. Immunofluorescence microscopy also helps to complement other immunochemical methods to expand the information for clinicians and scientists to apply. It is thus key to productive areas of biomedical research that require an intuitive understanding of cell response to disease and environmental stimuli. New developments, particularly the introduction of spectral imaging methods, have also enhanced the utility of immunofluorescence microscopy. With superior optics and labeling reagents, researchers can now detect an array of parameters in parallel at unprecedented molecular and cellular resolution. This multi-modal strategy provides high-resolution diagnostic and prognostic information that supports improved analyses in pre-clinical and clinical investigations. The spectrum of multispectral technologies accessible, while providing unique strengths and limitations, expands the range of applications for immunofluorescence microscopy to many areas of study. As the demand for precise, high-throughput imaging technologies has grown, the improvement of immunofluorescence approaches remains essential to further our understanding of complex biological systems and related disease processes.

Test Your Knowledge

1. What is ELISA?
2. What is immunofluorescence microscopy?

8.3. Applications in Clinical Diagnostics

Learning Outcome

1. Understand the role of immunochemistry in disease detection and monitoring;
2. Describe the use of immunochemistry in the diagnosis of autoimmune diseases;
3. Know the applications in infectious disease testing.

In clinical diagnosis, immunochemistry is critical in that it facilitates the measurement and determination of particular biomarkers by antigen-antibody reactions. The very sensitive method is central in diagnosing several illnesses, such as infections including HIV, where the determination of anti-HIV antibodies is indispensable. With advanced techniques, e.g., piezoelectric quartz sensors, scientists have shown it is possible to detect antibodies with the aid of synthetic peptides immobilized on sensor surfaces. For instance, using this technique, it is possible to record frequency changes that reflect the antibody-target binding, thus enabling fast diagnostic processes. The stability and sensitivity in such methods are evidence of the revolutionary impact that immunochemistry has on clinical diagnostics, offering clinicians reliable means of preclinical disease detection and control that are essential in increasing patient outcomes and public health programs (Chi-Shun et al., 1992). Moreover, advancements in the multiplex immunoassay have maximally enhanced the detection of a variety of analytes from a single biological sample, which has bridged the gap for efficiency in clinical labs. The techniques employed previously, like ELISA, are focused basically on the detection of one analyte; however, advancements in multiplex technology paved the way for including varied biomarkers. This adjustment is necessary not only to reduce cost and sample size but also to improve diagnosis speed, hence allowing clinicians to make informed decisions in a timely manner. With more laboratories using multiplex immunoassays, the possibility of improved diagnosis of complex diseases like cancer and autoimmune diseases becomes apparent, revealing the potential of immunochemistry to fight complex health conditions (Ahsan & Ahmad, 2020). Although the advantages provided by multiplex technologies are enticing, the implementation of these high-level immunoassays is not free from complications.

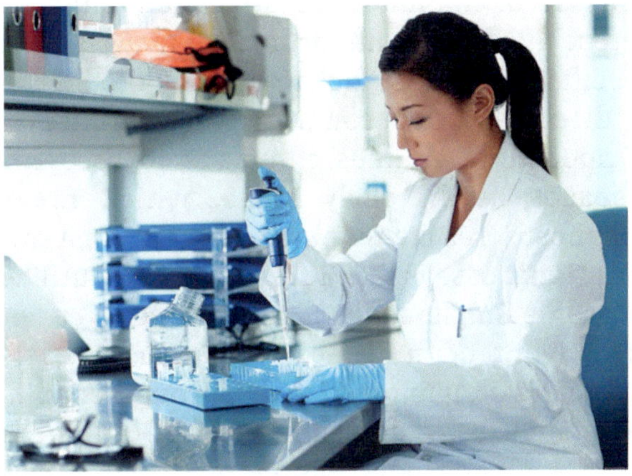

Figure 8.9. Researcher using a micropipette in a clinical laboratory setting.

Source: https://sciex.com/adobe/dynamicmedia/deliver/dm-aid--d054a129-5983-4e55-b335-45b3f17173cf/clinical-compendium-2000x1500.jpg?quality=75&width=1920.

Issues regarding the potential for cross-reactivity, reduced specificity, and the complexity of assay validation can go a long way towards discouraging widespread application of multiplex assays within the clinical setting. The cost of analysis bioanalyzers that enable multiplex detection can similarly go a long way towards limiting access among some medical centers. But constant research to enhance these systems hopes to overcome these barriers by enhancing assay performance to the maximum and offering reliability for broader applications. The future is set to require harmonization among clinicians, scientists, and technologists who are trying to come up with solutions for these challenges that will eventually enhance the application of immunochemistry in clinical diagnosis and assist in promoting individualized medicine (Ahsan & Ahmad, 2020) (Figure 8.9).

8.3.1. Role in Disease Detection and Monitoring

The use of immunochemistry to monitor and detect diseases is important, as it utilizes the specificity of antibodies to identify biomarkers of disease-related conditions. The utilization of specificity enables clinicians to recognize diseases at an early stage, which means enhanced treatment outcomes. For instance, traditional assays like ELISA have been utilized to profile single analytes for decades, yet with the advent of multiplex immunoassays, this has made a significant step. Through enabling the concurrent determination of numerous analytes in a single sample, multiplexing not only minimizes the need for large-scale sampling but also optimizes resource utilization within clinical settings. As outlined, these techniques not only optimize diagnostic performance but also streamline monitoring of disease advancement, with the potential to remodel the diagnostic paradigm for various health ailments (Ahsan & Ahmad, 2020). Further opportunity for disease monitoring is also provided by the use of specific and selective sensors in immunochemistry. These sensors have been designed to detect the presence of specific molecules with great fidelity so that the results obtained are both consistent and relevant. The use of synthetic arrays brings further complexity to this because increased selectivity in the detection of biomarkers of disease is possible. With a combination of the best of selective as well as specific sensing approaches, researchers are now creating new sensing platforms that take advantage of the strengths of each method. Such a hybrid facilitates not only better reliability of assay results but also enables the manufacture of complex monitoring systems that can track disease trends over time (Peveler et al., 2016). While the promise of multiplex immunoassays and sensor technologies is enormous, however, it cannot be overlooked that problems with their usage in clinical practice are significant. Purchase and operation costs of sophisticated analytical apparatus, as well as multi-probe costs, which are often discouraging, are of great hindrance to the wide applicability of these methodologies. Furthermore, the complexity of handling multiplex assay results is a concern among clinicians, particularly in the maintenance of test specificity and sensitivity. Despite these difficulties, ongoing technological advancements are more likely than not to ease these difficulties, paving the way towards broader utilization of immunochemical methods for disease monitoring and detection. The continuous improvement of these techniques reflects the necessity for ongoing research and investment in this vital branch of medical science (Ahsan & Ahmad, 2020).

8.3.2. Use in Autoimmune Disease Diagnosis

The use of immunochemistry in the detection of autoimmune diseases is a foundation achievement in clinical practice, through which autoantibodies that play a pivotal role in disease cause are detectable and quantifiable. Autoantibodies are biomarkers that can indicate the presence and severity of autoimmune disease. For example, in type II autoimmune polyendocrine syndrome (APS II), some antibodies , such as those directed against glutamic acid decarboxylase (GAD) isoforms, have been shown to be implicated in the development of concomitant type 1 diabetes mellitus (IDDM) in sufferers. It has been demonstrated that GAD65 and GAD67 antibodies appear much more commonly in APS II patients with IDDM compared to healthy controls, suggesting that these autoantibodies can be important for distinguishing disease subtypes and informing treatment (Baekkeskov et al., 1994). Thus, identification of these autoantibodies improves accuracy and allows specific patient management. Aside from their use as biomarkers, immunochemical assays, and even more so multiplex immunoassays, have transformed the diagnosis of autoimmune disorders by allowing the detection of many autoantibodies in a single sample at one time. Not only is this more effective, but it also reduces the need for frequent venipuncture, which is not pleasant for patients. The new multiplexing technology offers a significant advantage in the simultaneous detection of several biomarkers of autoimmune diseases at a lower cost and consumption of samples. Notwithstanding, there are challenges, such as high levels of expensive advanced analytical instruments and the inability to detect low-abundance analytes (Ahsan & Ahmad, 2020). Despite these challenges, multiplex immunoassays are unlocking doors to global autoimmune disease profiling, which can lead to earlier diagnosis and improved patient outcomes. The value of immunochemistry in the diagnosis of autoimmune diseases is not limited to individual biomarkers but also includes a larger appreciation of immune dysregulation. Measurements of autoantibody profiles can delineate the pathophysiology of autoimmune diseases and guide clinical management. For instance, the detection and specificity of GAD antibodies can distinguish between different types of diabetes and other autoimmune syndromes. Furthermore, additional research on the development of new biomarkers will continue to expand the array of diagnostic equipment that will be available to practitioners. With the advancement in immunochemistry, it will enhance the precision with which autoimmune diseases will be diagnosed, facilitating early interventions and individualized treatment regimens for individuals suffering from such diseases (Baekkeskov et al., 1994; Ahsan & Ahmad, 2020). The marriage of emerging technologies and ongoing research will only advance the diagnostic instruments in this highly relevant area of clinical immunology (Figure 8.10).

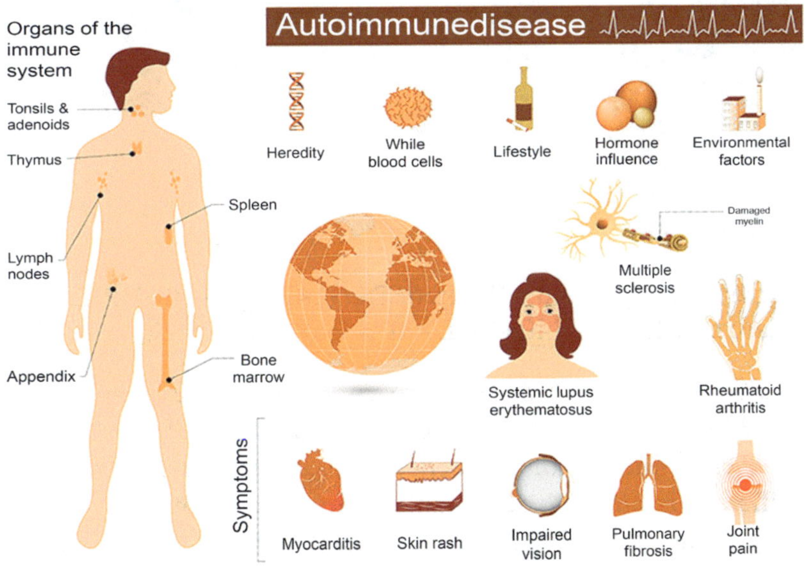

Figure 8.10. Autoimmune disease.

Source: https://www.niehs.nih.gov/sites/default/files/health/assets/images/autoimmune_disease.jpg.

8.3.3. Applications in Infectious Disease Testing

The capacity to diagnose infectious diseases with accuracy and efficiency is paramount in current healthcare, and immunochemistry plays an important role in such uses. One of the major developments in this field has been the development of multiplex immunoassays, wherein it is possible to examine more than a single biomarker in the same sample. This enhances efficiency significantly, reducing time and cost incurred in diagnosis. For instance, while traditional ELISAs have been widely used to determine the presence of a single analyte, multiplex assays with the capability of detecting several infectious pathogens in parallel are now trending in laboratories. Technological advances in clinical immunochemistry not only increase diagnostic capability but also facilitate the certification of new biomarkers to support correct and timely diagnosis of disease, ultimately improving patient outcomes in infectious disease management (Ahsan & Ahmad, 2020). Of particular interest in infectious disease testing is the application of specific-purpose immunoassays directed against individual pathogens. For example, the detection of AIV subtypes H5 and H7 demonstrates immunochemistry use for public health. The laborious HI test has been traditionally used for serological identification of these subtypes; however, advances are such that ELISAs offer a promising alternative.

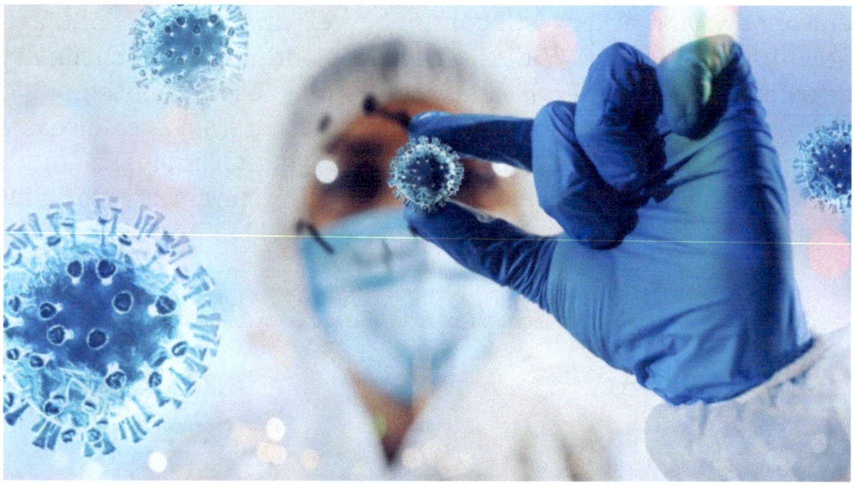

Figure 8.11. Infectious diseases testing.

Source: https://www.invitek.com/-/media/Invitek/Tier-1-Images---COMPRESSED/Genomics--MDx/Infectious-Diseases/Carousel-Images_Infectious-diseases/AdobeStock_419105002.jpeg.

Research has confirmed that such ELISAs are very sensitive and specific in the detection of H5 and H7 antibodies, which usually detect serological reactions before the HI test. Such enhanced diagnosis confirms the capability of immunochemical techniques in screening massive samples of avian sera in an efficient manner, hence enabling the identification of impending threats from infectious pathogens (Comin et al., 2013). In summary, the application of immunochemistry in infectious disease tests is progressing rapidly, bearing witness to the worth of new diagnostic techniques within contemporary medicine. Multiplex assays as a trend represent a more overarching shift toward integrating efficiency with accuracy in disease screening, with the specific case studies , such as screening for AIV testing, proving the relevance of tailored immunoassays. With further research improving these technologies, the potential for improved diagnostic capacity in dealing with infectious diseases becomes more feasible. These advancements not only allow for rapid identification of pathogens but also make enhanced surveillance and response options available for public health. By embracing such innovations, the healthcare professionals will be able to more effectively prevent the menace posed by infectious diseases to become better prepared and stronger in the presence of ongoing challenges (Ahsan & Ahmad, 2020; Comin et al., 2013) (Figure 8.11).

Test Your Knowledge

1. What is the role of immunochemistry in disease detection and monitoring?
2. What is the use of immunochemistry in the diagnosis of autoimmune diseases?

8.4. Immunochemistry in Research

Learning Outcome

1. Understand the role of immunochemistry in biomarker discovery;
2. Know the applications of immunochemistry in cancer research;
3. Describe the use of immunochemistry in vaccine development.

The application of immunochemistry in scientific research permeates into a wide range of disciplines, impacting cell biology, immunology, and diagnostics. With the use of antibodies as critical tools, researchers have been able to specifically detect and measure biomolecules, particularly proteins and antigens, at very specific locations in complex biological samples. An example of such a landmark is the development of new immunochemical reagents, which are antibodies coupled to small latex particles. These reagents serve as visual markers for the identification of antigens on cell surfaces through methods , such as scanning electron microscopy. Definition of a specific cellular structure provides deeper insight into mechanisms of cell signaling and interaction and, therefore, a clearer understanding of immune reactions and cellular abnormalities. Thus, the advances have provided opportunities of great impact to health diagnostics and therapeutic intervention in pathology and immunological diseases (Dreyer et al., 1975). Immunochemical techniques have also been applied to exhibit structural homologies in different biological samples, which proves their versatility and applications for comparative study. For instance, research employing mAbs has identified immunochemically corresponding Neisseria gonorrhoeae lipooligosaccharide structures on human erythrocytes. The investigation not only identifies the presence of conserved epitopes that may serve as diagnostic markers but also proves the functional relevance of immune recognition. Systematic agglutination evidenced in erythrocytes shows that antibodies mimic the role of human cold agglutinins, which identifies their application in the study of immune mechanisms at the cellular and molecular levels. In addition, differential reactivity of antibodies with specific glycosphingolipids demonstrates the complexity of immune interactions and the potential for the use of these discoveries in the design of targeted therapies for the treatment of autoimmune and infectious diseases (Griffiss et al., 1988). Also, the application of immunochemistry together with other biochemical methodologies has significantly revolutionized research methods, improving disease mechanisms and therapeutics in research. Researchers are now able to couple immunochemical assays with high-throughput screening (HTS) technologies in order to facilitate rapid discovery and qualification of novel biomarkers. Such a combination enhances quantitative cell surface receptor and antigen studies, and our understanding of pathophysiological processes is advanced. As demonstrated by the employment of latex beads tagged with fluorescent molecules for the detection of a variety of antigens, these developments have the potential to improve diagnostic reagents and therapeutic targets. Finally, continued development of immunochemistry will extend its usefulness on the continuum of research problems, from basic science to the clinical setting, and extend our capacity to solve new health problems (Dreyer et al., 1975) (Figure 8.12).

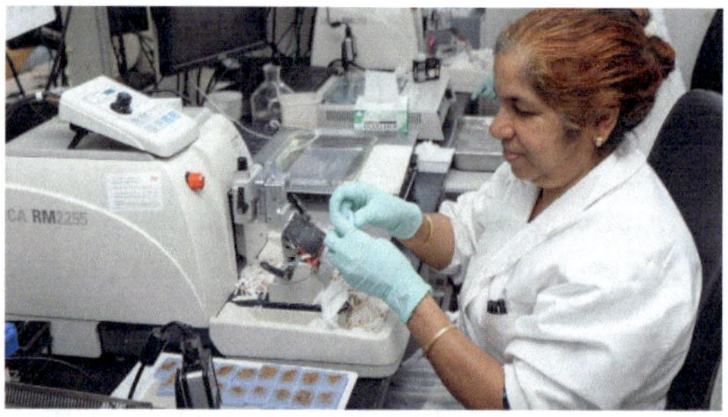

Figure 8.12. Immunohistochemistry laboratory.

Source: https://www.pathology.columbia.edu/sites/default/files/styles/cola_media_1280_16_9/public/media/images/2020-02/3881_pathology-170421-0031.jpg?itok=QPWyqzq2.

8.4.1. Role in Biomarker Discovery

The role of immunochemistry in the discovery of biomarkers is important, particularly for multiplexed assays. The traditional immunoassay platforms, such as ELISA, are primarily set to detect a single analyte at a time. Technology has advanced, and it has brought about the capacity to analyze various biomarkers from a single sample all at once using multiplex immunoassays. This not only increases throughput but also conserves resources by minimizing the number of samples and reagents used. The sophistication of disease mechanisms necessitates the identification of multiple biomarker candidates to provide more accurate diagnostic information. As is evident, progress towards multiplexing in immunochemistry is challenging but significantly enhances the sensitivity and specificity of biomarkers and thus Personalized Medicine and clinical performance in most conditions of health (Ahsan & Ahmad, 2020). Application of biomarkers to clinical decision-making requires the effectiveness and trustworthiness of solid immunochemical techniques. In the area of CVD in type 2 diabetes, targeted biomarker panels like apolipoprotein CIII (apoCIII) and N-terminal prohormone B-type natriuretic peptide (NT-proBNP) have been demonstrated to enhance risk stratification. It has been established through studies that measurement of these biomarkers predicts new-onset CVD accurately and therefore informs clinical strategies and therapy. For instance, when combined, NT-proBNP and apoCIII significantly improve models from conventional risk factors. This is a testament to the central role played by immunochemistry in biomarker discovery, in assisting clinical professionals to identify patients who are at a heightened risk of severe cardiovascular events (Aroner et al., 2018). The more such methods evolve, the better they will assist in streamlining diagnostic and treatment plans across various diseases. Furthermore, biomarker discovery in immunochemistry is characterized by a constant see-saw between technology development and clinical usefulness. With multiplex assays becoming more prevalent, the laboratory is challenged with the twin task of ensuring accuracy within the complexity of multiple interactions among biomarkers. Despite technical hurdles inherent in multiplexing, such as interference between incumbent antibodies and the necessity of sophisticated detection systems, the benefits far outshine these challenges. High-throughput technologies have enabled new biomarkers to be validated and incorporated into clinical applications. So, the constant advancements in multiplex immunoassays usher in more comprehensive diagnostic models, transforming disease prevention and treatment approaches among clinicians (Ahsan & Ahmad, 2020). With the continually evolving immunochemistry, its role in biomarker discovery is bound to increase, shaping the future of precision medicine.

8.4.2. Applications in Cancer Research

The area of cancer research has witnessed tremendous advances with the application of immunochemistry, particularly in identifying and manipulating tumor antigens. Immunochemistry techniques enable scientists to see specific proteins in tissues such that they can identify malignancies based on their distinct antigenic signatures. Using numerous markers and antibodies, researchers are capable of distinguishing between cancerous and normal tissues and eventually towards proper diagnosis and treatment planning. In addition, the techniques can evaluate cancer therapy effectiveness by quantitating antigen alterations. Therefore, immunochemistry not only enhances our understanding of tumor biology but also enhances therapy by providing a clear definition of tumor kinetics within the course of treatment cycles, which reflects its central role in contemporary oncology. Incorporation of advanced sensing technologies into immunochemistry has also further promoted cancer study. By employing selective and specific receptors, novel sensor platforms have been developed that may identify cancer biomarkers with high selectivity and sensitivity. This two-pronged approach—using both synthetic arrays and specific sensors—is effective in notable case studies and has proven useful for discovering tumor markers in different matrices of biological fluids. This is important since early cancer detection by serum biomarkers has the ability to greatly enhance the outcomes of patients. As showcased in the results of existing research, studies of integrated sensor approaches enable efficient diagnostics processes, which have the potential to transform the area of precision medicine. Existing research in the domain shows a revolution in the approach of cancer diagnosis and therapy, necessitating more research into more effective sensor designs (Peveler et al., 2016). Furthermore, cancer research has been revolutionized by the application of sophisticated materials, such as gold nanoparticles.

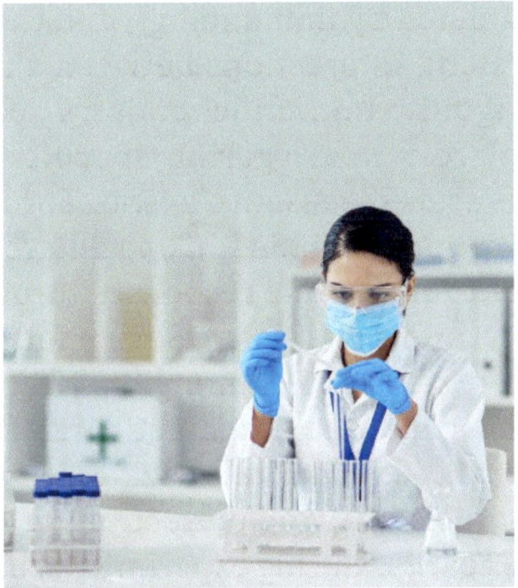

Figure 8.13. Cancer research.

Source: https://cancer.stonybrookmedicine.edu/sites/default/files/CancerResearch-Mobile-1080x1240.jpg.

Gold nanoparticles possess unique properties that can be tailored to be applied in targeted therapy and imaging modalities. Cytotoxicity of gold nanoparticles, particularly in their various forms and encapsulations, suggests their therapeutic potential. Research has shown that certain formulations, e.g., cetyltrimethylammonium-bromideencapsulated gold nanorods, are more cytotoxic and therefore effective in selectively inducing cancer cell apoptosis without causing damage to normal cells. This illustrates the importance of particle surface chemistry and functionality over simple parameters like size or charge. Continuing research into such nanoscale materials in conjunction with immunochemical techniques opens up new frontiers to targeted drug delivery systems, the way ahead being paved for new forms of cancer treatment to ensure maximum efficacy and minimum side effects (Chen et al., 2012) (Figure 8.13).

8.4.3. Use in Vaccine Development

The area of vaccine production is increasingly being regulated by immunology, and this makes us understand interactions between antibodies and antigens. Immunochemistry plays an important role in triggering specific immune responses against causative agents. For instance, the application of ELISAs has facilitated easier assessments of immune responses through high specificity and sensitivity. Such methods are helpful in quickly determining the effectiveness of vaccine candidates against viral diseases, as evidenced in avian influenza research. New methods facilitate the detection of specific antibodies earlier during experimental infections than conventional methods, and this speeds up the evaluation process and also improves public health interventions. By making it easier to detect immune responses, immunochemistry dramatically enhances the process of creating successful vaccines to meet the rapid demands of newly encountered infectious diseases like avian flu and COVID-19. Also, the evolution of social media as a public health vehicle has given way to monitoring vaccine sentiment and discussion within different populations. As has been highlighted in recent research into public responses to COVID-19 vaccine messages, platforms like Twitter and Reddit are rich repositories for real-time sentiment tracking. Through the observation of millions of social media comments and posts, public health campaigns and vaccine policy can be informed. Through analysis of the data, the sociology of vaccine uptake, hesitation, and mythmaking is uncovered and provides health authorities with priceless feedback loops.

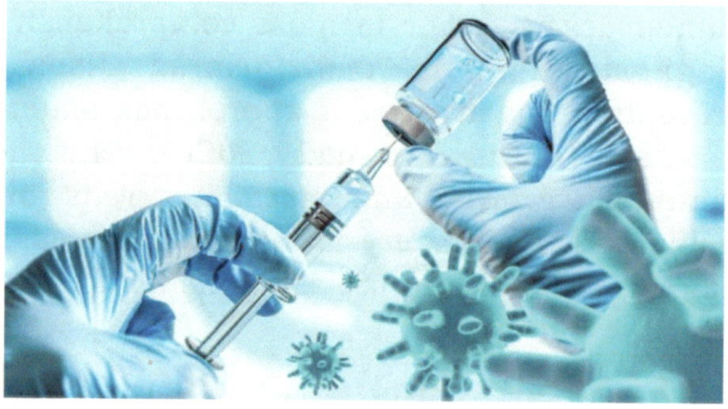

Figure 8.14. COVID-19 vaccine development.

Source: https://static.biospace.com/dims4/default/b6e7f67/2147483647/strip/true/crop/622x350+1+0/resize/1440x810!/quality/90/?url=https%3A%2F%2Fk1-prod-biospace.s3.us-east-2.amazonaws.com%2Fbrightspot%2Flegacy%2FBioSpace-Assets%2FFF893178-9FFA-4B80-943E-1D8EB6E3A783.jpg.

By correlating immunochemistry with such sociological consciousness, vaccine developers can couch their message in a way that responds to immediate questions, generating more public confidence and participation in vaccination programs, especially in the era of skepticism and disinformation. Beyond this, immunochemistry is utilized in vaccine design and manufacture. Monoclonal antibody technologies have enabled researchers to create extremely targeted antibodies that may be added to vaccines to improve immune response. The bird flu vaccine illustration illustrates the potential for employing antibody technology in creating more potent immunizations. By using mAbs to develop highly specific ELISA tests, researchers can quantify vaccine efficacy more precisely, allowing for the rapid adjustment of vaccine strategy when faced with emerging or expanding infectious agents. This two-pronged vaccine development approach, applying both immunochemical techniques and leveraging social media analysis, is a robust platform for pushing forward public health in the realm of emerging complex global health threats, with vaccine development staying abreast of the nature of contemporary pathogen challenges (Figure 8.14).

Test Your Knowledge

1. What is the role of immunochemistry in biomarker discovery?
2. What is the use of immunochemistry in vaccine development?

8.5. Advances in Immunochemical Techniques

Learning Outcome

1. Explain the development of monoclonal antibodies;
2. Know the innovations in imaging techniques;
3. Describe the high-throughput screening methods.

Improved immunochemical techniques have revolutionized therapeutic monitoring and diagnostics. These involve the development of biosensors that make use of selective and specific receptors to provide accurate detection of analyte targets. These biosensors present two complementary strategies: specific sensors that provide high selectivity and synthetic arrays that provide wider capability of recognition. The ongoing discussion regarding the benefits and drawbacks of such novel methods spells out their fruitful applications in clinical monitoring and environmental monitoring, emphasizing their importance in enhancing diagnostic accuracy. The potential to merge the two strategies in a one-platform sensor can deliver unprecedented enhancement in immunochemical applications and solve long-standing problems in sensor functionality and design, which is critical for future biomedical diagnostics and therapeutic research (Peveler et al., 2016). While the intricacies of molecular interactions were deciphered through groundbreaking techniques , such as genetic engineering and X-ray crystallography. These methods give a molecular-level understanding of ligand-receptor relationships and thus play a critical role in the optimization of immunochemical techniques. By resolving the structural and affinities of various macromolecular interactions, researchers can build more efficient antibodies or antigens suitable for specific immunochemistry purposes. Moreover, the advancement of computational approaches now makes it possible to simulate realistic macromolecular interactions, which allows research on binding kinetics and immunological reaction. This multi-dimensionality significantly enhances the individual understanding of the ligand and receptor dynamics, paving the way for new immunochemical applications in disease therapy and diagnostics (Alder et al., 2008). This research is also seen in the advancement of experimental protocols that facilitate direct observation of single molecule interactions. Techniques , such as atomic force microscopy, optical tweezers, and hydrodynamic flow have provided unparalleled insights into the dynamic nature of ligand-receptor bonds at the single-molecule level. Such experimental information is crucial for the design of more sensitive new immunochemical assays and also permit biological processes to be tracked in real-time. With continued investigation of well-characterized cell systems, the mechanical and kinetic properties of cell membrane receptors of interest, reaffirming the importance of such motion in immunochemistry. Overall, the intersection of these new techniques demonstrates the vibrant, interdisciplinary nature of immunochemistry and its broad range of implications for future biomedical research and clinical application (Figure 8.15).

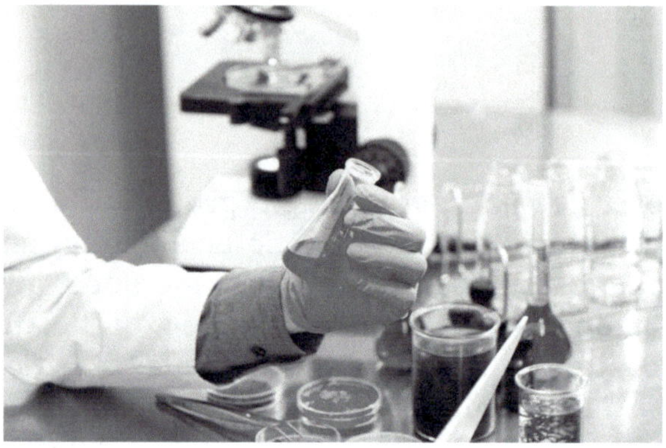

Figure 8.15. Researcher handling a flask in a laboratory setting with various glassware and a microscope.

Source: https://area9lyceum.com/laboratorymedicine/wp-content/uploads/2020/05/pexels-chokniti-khongchum-2280571.jpg.

8.5.1. Development of Monoclonal Antibodies

The discovery of mAbs is a breakthrough in immunochemistry that enables targeted therapy and diagnostics. Revolution began with the technology of hybridomas in the 1970s, where cells from the spleen of immunized mice are fused with myeloma cells to produce hybrid cells that are able to proliferate indefinitely but produce a specific antibody. This method allows for the generation of mAbs with high specificity to particular antigens, which increases their efficacy in therapeutic applications. For instance, the successful production of anti-RAGE antibodies illustrates how mAbs could be employed to inhibit processes related to chronic inflammatory disorders. The high specificity and reproducibility of mAbs bring additional value in research and clinical uses, thus transforming the face of immunotherapeutics and diagnostic reagents in modern medicine (Jyoti et al., 2013). Greater research on mAbs has become increasingly essential in expanding their use, such as multiplex immunoassays that facilitate the detection of multiple analytes from one sample in parallel. This advancement plays a critical role in maximizing efficiency in clinical diagnosis, particularly in the detection of numerous biomarkers associated with diseases. As laboratories and healthcare institutions continue to adopt multiplexing strategies, it is evident that the benefits of mAbs for facilitating these assays become apparent. Multiplex immunoassays can potentially reduce costs, minimize test duration, and optimize utilization of samples, thus making it possible for comprehensive disease profiling. This technological innovation is part of an overarching trend towards high-throughput analytical capacity in clinical sciences that improves the accuracy and specificity of medical diagnostics (Ahsan & Ahmad, 2020). Notwithstanding this, there remain limitations on assay development and validation that need ongoing research and development. mAbs are not only utilized for diagnostics but also for preventative and therapeutic interventions in several diseases , such as cancer and autoimmune diseases. mAbs can be capable of exerting their effects through multiple mechanisms, including through receptor blocking, induction of apoptosis in target cells, or by guiding cytotoxic species directly into the target tissues. Use of anti-RAGE antibodies is significant as a demonstration of their therapeutic efficacy for inflammation-related conditions, wherein their efficacy has been shown to block tumor growth and modulate immune responses in preclinical models. The increasing recognized role of mAbs emphasizes their completeness and the importance of continued research in their design. As scientists are deciphering more pathways and mechanisms of action, mAbs will continue to reshape medical treatment and diagnostics, thereby emphasizing their central role in the future of immunochemistry (Jyoti et al., 2013) (Figure 8.16).

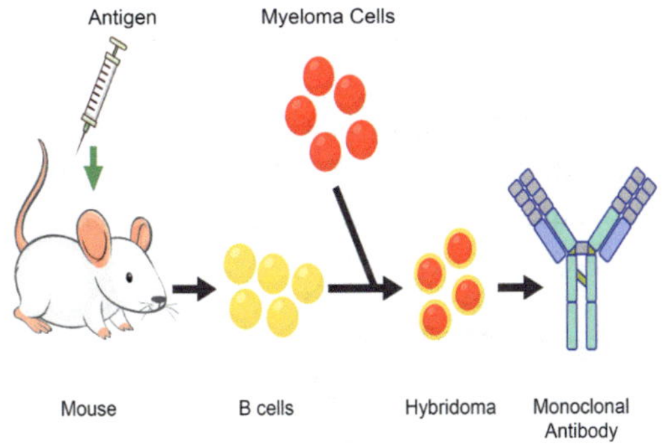

Figure 8.16. Monoclonal antibody.

Source: https://media.geeksforgeeks.org/wp-content/uploads/20221219104058/Monoclonal-Antibody.png.

8.5.2. Innovations in Imaging Techniques

Imaging techniques have progressed significantly during the past few years, particularly in immunochemistry, where they are essential for exploring cellular and molecular dynamics. Technologies , such as intravital imaging allow researchers to track biological processes in living organisms, which is crucial to better comprehending immunological interactions. One of the strongest applications of intravital imaging is in observing in real time calcium signaling, which is paramount in studying cell communication and behavior in tumor microenvironments. Intravital imaging, in combination with more advanced methodologies, has recently proven to reveal mechanisms in which therapies can induce cellular responses, i.e., increased intracellular concentrations of calcium, which causes cell death. Such approaches provide useful information to enhance our knowledge of immune responses and therapeutic efficacy in most diseases, including cancer (Bonora et al., 2014). Moreover, the integration of imaging techniques with lab-based research is revolutionizing the way students and researchers engage with complex biological concepts. For instance, the creation of undergraduate laboratories focused on protein localization provides important hands-on experience, including Western blotting. This technique not only facilitates the detection of proteins in particular tissues but also fosters a sophisticated knowledge of protein chemistry and its use in immunological research. By including laboratory practice along with theoretical instruction, students acquire fundamental proficiency in applying imaging techniques that form the foundation for future research work. This educational advancement is placing special emphasis on filling the gap between clinical practice and classroom instruction, readying future generations of scientists to respond to complex immunological questions (Gogia et al., 2017). Lastly, the scope of imaging advances extends beyond traditional laboratory boundaries and has implications for the clinic. New imaging technologies enable accurate diagnosis and customized medicine, tending toward directed therapy based on patient-specific profiles. By applying advanced imaging methods, clinicians are able to view immune dynamics in real time and better assess the effectiveness of therapeutic interventions. This movement toward the inclusion of cutting-edge imaging technology in research as well as in health care underscores the synergistic relationship between immunochemistry and technical advances. Ultimately, these innovations not only streamline research approaches but also provide gateways to improved patient care through more effective tailoring of treatments to a patient's personalized immunological environment.

8.5.3. High-Throughput Screening Methods

High-throughput screening (HTS) technologies have revolutionized the field of immunochemistry by giving the ability to analyze numerous analytes in one sample at the same time. Traditional immunoassays, such as ELISA, are usually optimized for single-target analysis and therefore restricted by throughput and efficacy. Multiplex immunoassays, however, allow scientists to analyze multiple biomarkers at once, enabling thorough profiling of biological samples. This capability not only conserves reagents and samples but also greatly reduces the expense and time involved in analysis. Furthermore, advances in technology, including high-resolution imaging and sophisticated detection systems, facilitate the increased complexity and sensitivity required to accomplish effective multiplexing. Thus, HTS methods are at the forefront of research to provide more information on disease mechanism, therapeutic response, and biomarker validation as outlined in today's challenges and opportunities of immunoassays (Ahsan & Ahmad, 2020).

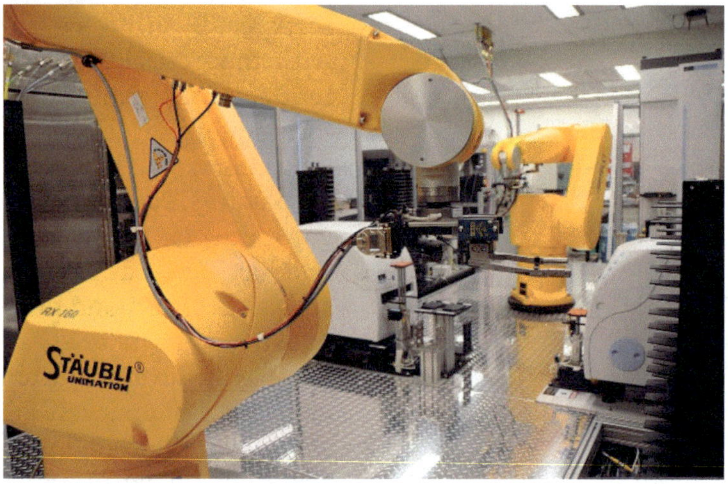

Figure 8.17. High-throughput screening robots.

Source: https://upload.wikimedia.org/wikipedia/commons/2/27/Chemical_Genomics_Robot.jpg.

Even though the use of high-throughput methods is invaluable, their utilization is not without issues. One such area of concern lies in the cross-reactivity between assays in a multiplex setting that could lead to false results. These interferences must be carefully designed and verified for multiplex immunoassays, as evidenced by studies demonstrating how feed extracts can degrade assay sensitivity (Haasnoot et al.). Moreover, the initial expenditure of creating and implementing HTS technology could be prohibitive, especially for small laboratories or research institutes. Despite all this, demand for fast, low-cost screening alternatives still fuels research into immunochemical technologies. Researchers are beginning to examine more closely how to make assay conditions more optimal and discover good calibration strategies to decrease some of the complexities of multiplex assays. The future of multiplexing in HTS of immunochemistry is promising with the incorporation of artificial intelligence (AI) and machine learning algorithms to enhance interpretation and analysis of the data. With the application of such next-generation computational algorithms, scientists can better manage the large volumes of data generated in multiplex assays, discovering significant patterns and correlations that result in discovery. Further, as the technology advances, there will be greater demand for harmonized methods and validation protocols upon which results are replicable and trustworthy on different platforms and laboratories. Collaborative approaches to best practice and benchmark sharing will become critical in addressing the inherent limitations present in HTS methods, ultimately allowing for their widespread adoption within research and clinical settings. This coming event will continue our understanding of complex biological systems and improve the diagnostic utility of immunochemical assays, reinforcing the central role played by HTS methodologies in modern biomedicine (Figure 8.17).

Test Your Knowledge

1. When was hybridoma technology invented?
2. What are the methods for high-throughput screening?

SUMMARY

In recapitulating the immunochemistry discussion, it is clear that immunochemistry is at the center of helping develop a better understanding of intricate biological systems. Immunochemical methods have changed diagnostic strategies in most medical specialties, especially in the evaluation of disease status and interpretation of biological processes. By applying biomarkers , such as the cerebrospinal fluid (CSF)/serum ratio of albumin (QAlb), researchers have made important data regarding blood–CSF barrier permeability for neurologic diagnosis. Data gathered in studies on sex-differences in QAlb thresholds highlights the role of precision medicine, in which the diagnostic criteria are optimized to account for patients' biological variability, thereby enhancing clinical performance (Alessi et al., 2020). Besides neurological diseases, immunochemistry has also extended its implications far beyond and has profoundly impacted oncology research. The role of cancer-associated fibroblasts (CAFs) in tumor development clearly exemplifies this extensive application of immunochemistry in oncology. Identification of specific protein markers in tumor tissue through high-level techniques like real-time PCR and IHC provides the platform to develop prognostic markers of gastric cancer patients. The correlation between tumor characteristics and the prevalence of CAF indicates not only the importance of immunochemistry in tumor biology but also new possibilities for targeted therapy and tailored patient management (Noel et al., 2010). Overall, the overview obtained from previous studies emphasizes the revolutionary potential of immunochemistry both as a diagnostic and therapeutic measure. The continued search for biomarkers and cell-to-cell interactions has the potential to further reveal the intricacies of different diseases, better allowing us to diagnose, treat, and forecast patient outcomes in an effective manner. With advancements in the field, it is crucial to continue developing methodologies as well as increasing our knowledge on immunochemical markers to enable the advances of personalized medicine. Lastly, the union of immunochemistry with emerging technologies will be decisive in shaping the course of future medical science, in such a way that medical practice will be informed by the most accurate and relevant biological data.

Immunchemistry is an important analytical tool in the diagnosis and management of most medical diseases, particularly through the testing of CSF samples. One of the main concepts of this science is visual inspection for xanthochromia, a sign of intracranial bleeding. Older techniques have relied on this observation by eye, which remains the method of choice in most labs worldwide. However, newer studies show that this technique may not be as reliable as was once thought. The findings suggest that the spectrophotometric techniques offer a more accurate determination of bilirubin concentration in CSF, especially when low levels of bilirubin or hemolyzed blood make visual examination problematic. Thus, shifting to spectrophotometry is warranted, considering the demands for newer methods offering improved diagnostic precision and patient care (Keir et al., 2005). Beyond the establishment of CSF analysis, the use of immunochemistry is further applied in the examination of neurological disease through the measurement of neuronal differentiation processes. A central focus in neuroscience is the process by which stem and progenitor cells differentiate into various types of neurons within the vertebrate CNS. Molecular regulation, including those encompassing pathways like Notch, Shh, and Wnt, has been shown to play a fundamental role in differentiation. Of these pathways, the Notch signaling pathway has been of particular interest due to its pivotal position in neuronal identity specification. By studying proteins , such as delta like 1-homologue (DLK1), the mechanisms by which the signaling molecules control the development of neural progenitor cells (NPCs) to neurons have been established. This establishes immunochemistrys clear role in developmental biology and also in understanding neurological pathologies (Surmacz et al., 2010). Furthermore, integration of data from both clinical and basic research significantly enhances insight into disease processes, ultimately progressing to better therapy. The study of DLK1 in neuronal differentiation shows how certain signaling molecules can regulate progenitor cell behavior and eventually direct neuronal development. Importantly, studies have noted that DLK1 expression is linked with increased neuronal differentiation, while its effects on progenitor cell growth stay low. Thus, this provides a preview of targeted therapies that can possibly use molecular pathways to enhance neuronal well-being. Such collective knowledge supports the importance of immunochemistry not only as a diagnostic technique but also as a key element in the establishment of therapeutic techniques and information on intricate neurological diseases, paving the way for novel treatment modalities (Surmacz et al., 2010).

KEY TERMS FROM THIS CHAPTER

- Antibodies
- Atomic force microscopy
- Drosophila melanogaster
- Immunochemistry
- Immunohistochemistry
- Infectious diseases
- Plasma proteins
- X-ray crystallography
- Antigens
- Avian influenza virus
- Genetic engineering
- Immunoglobulins
- Immunology
- Lipooligosaccharides
- Western blotting

Critical Thinking Questions

1. What is the primary function of antibodies in the immune response?

a. To digest pathogens

b. To neutralize antigens

c. To synthesize proteins

d. To secrete hormones

2. The immunoglobulin most abundant in the blood is:

a. IgA

b. IgE

c. IgG

d. IgM

3. Which immunoglobulin is involved in allergic reactions?

a. IgG

b. IgA

c. IgE

d. IgM

4. The complement system is activated during which type of immune response?

a. Humoral immune response

b. Cellular immune response

c. Innate immune response

d. All of the above

5. The antigen-binding region of an antibody is known as:

a. Constant region

b. Variable region

c. Fc region

d. Hinge region

Short Answer Questions

1. What is immunochemistry?
2. What is the principle of antigen-antibody interaction?
3. Describe the techniques of immunochemistry.
4. What are clinical diagnostic applications?
5. What is immunohistochemistry used for in research?

Answers to Critical Thinking Questions

1. (b); 2. (c); 3. (c); 4. (d); 5. (b)

References

1. Ahsan H, Ahmad R. Multiplex Technology for Biomarker Immunoassays [Internet]. Innate Immunity in Health and Disease. IntechOpen; 2021. Available from: http://dx.doi.org/10.5772/intechopen.91730 (accessed on 12th June 2025).
2. Ahmed, B. K. T., Botto, M., Bouyain, S., Caparros, E., Carlow, D., Ceriello, A., et al. (2011). High glucose disrupts oligosaccharide recognition function via competitive inhibition: A potential mechanism for immune dysregulation in diabetes mellitus. https://core.ac.uk/download/44215.pdf (accessed on 12th June 2025).
3. Alder, B. J., Alon, R., Amit, A. G., André, P., Antosiewicz, J., Ashkin, A., Atherton, A., et al. (2008). Ligand-receptor interactions. http://arxiv.org/abs/0809.1926 (accessed on 12th June 2025).
4. Alessi, F., Baldi, E., Bellini, T., Caniatti, M., et al. (2020). Increased age and male sex are independently associated with higher frequency of blood–cerebrospinal fluid barrier dysfunction using the albumin quotient. https://core.ac.uk/download/287848476.pdf (accessed on 12th June 2025).
5. Apicella, M. A., Cole, J. A., Griffiss, J. M., Lesse, A. J., et al. (1990). *In vitro* and *in vivo* modification of *Neisseria gonorrhoeae* lipooligosaccharide epitope structure by sialylation. https://core.ac.uk/download/323073300.pdf (accessed on 12th June 2025).
6. Aroner, B., Farran, B., Battistoni, G., Charlton-Menys, G., Colhoun, H., Crosby, J., et al. (2018). Apolipoprotein CIII and N-terminal prohormone b-type natriuretic peptide as independent predictors for cardiovascular disease in type 2 diabetes. https://core.ac.uk/download/195287899.pdf (accessed on 12th June 2025).
7. Baekkeskov, S., Banga, J. P., Boehm, B. O., Betterle, C. F., Bjork, E., Bottazzo, G. F., et al. (1994). Association between antibodies to the Mr 67,000 isoform of glutamate decarboxylase (GAD) and Type 1 (insulin-dependent) diabetes mellitus with coexisting autoimmune polyendocrine syndrome Type II. https://core.ac.uk/download/12166925.pdf (accessed on 12th June 2025).
8. Beechem, J., Levenson, R., & McNamara, G. (2012). Spectral imaging in preclinical research and clinical pathology. https://core.ac.uk/download/323068082.pdf (accessed on 12th June 2025).
9. Bluard-Deconinck, J. M., Evans, R. W., Massont, P. L., Osinski, C., et al. (1978). Iron-binding fragments from the N-terminal and C-terminal regions of human lactoferrin. https://core.ac.uk/download/336805.pdf (accessed on 12th June 2025).
10. Bluestone, J. A., Epstein, S. L., Ozato, K., Sachs, D. H., et al. (1981). Idiotypes of anti-Ia antibodies. I. Expression of the 14-4-4S idiotype in humoral immune responses. https://core.ac.uk/download/323075189.pdf (accessed on 12th June 2025).
11. Bonora, M., Giorgi, C., Mammano, F., Missiroli, S., et al. (2014). Intravital imaging reveals p53-dependent cancer cell death induced by phototherapy via calcium signaling. https://core.ac.uk/download/53517674.pdf (accessed on 12th June 2025).
12. Chen, Y., Li, W., Xu, D., Yu, M., et al. (2012). Effect of size, shape, and surface modification on cytotoxicity of gold nanoparticles to human Hep-2 and canine MDCK cells. https://core.ac.uk/download/9559163.pdf (accessed on 12th June 2025).

13. Chi-shun, C., Kößlinger, C., Davis, F., Aberl, H., Wolf, H., Kanazawa, N., Modrow, S., et al. (1992). A quartz crystal biosensor for measurement in liquids. https://core.ac.uk/download/11549704.pdf (accessed on 12th June 2025).

14. Comin, A., Moreno, A., Shafer, A. L., Lebarbenchon, C., Upadhyay, C., Dlugolenski, D., et al. (2013). An enzyme-linked immunosorbent assay for detection of avian influenza virus subtypes H5 and H7 antibodies. https://core.ac.uk/download/18495521.pdf (accessed on 12th June 2025).

15. Czerny, C. P., & Eichhorn, W. (1989). Characterization of monoclonal and polyclonal antibodies to bovine enteric coronavirus: Establishment of an efficient ELISA for antigen detection in feces. https://core.ac.uk/download/12164367.pdf (accessed on 12th June 2025).

16. Dreyer, W. J., Molday, R. S., Rembaum, A., Yen, T., et al. (1975). New immunolatex spheres: Visual markers of antigens on lymphocytes for scanning electron microscopy. https://core.ac.uk/download/9124353.pdf (accessed on 12th June 2025).

17. Salvador-Morales, C., Flahaut, E., Sim, E., Sloan, J., Green, M. L., & Sim, R. B. (2006). Complement activation and protein adsorption by carbon nanotubes. *Molecular immunology*, *43*(3), 193–201. https://doi.org/10.1016/j.molimm.2005.02.006 (accessed on 12th June 2025).

18. Gogia, Neha; Sarkar, Ankita; and Singh, Amit, "An Undergraduate Cell Biology Lab: Western Blotting to Detect Proteins fromDrosophila Eye" (2017).Biology Faculty Publications. 236. https://ecommons.udayton.edu/bio_fac_pub/236brought to you by COREView metadata, citation and similar papers at core.ac.ukprovided by University of Dayton

19. (accessed on 12th June 2025).

20. Griffiss, J., Macher, B., & Mandrell, R. (1988). Lipooligosaccharides (LOS) of *Neisseria gonorrhoeae* and *Neisseria meningitidis* have components that are immunochemically similar to precursors of human blood group antigens. Carbohydrate sequence specificity of the mouse monoclonal antibodies that recognize cross-reacting antigens on LOS and human erythrocytes. https://core.ac.uk/download/323079362.pdf (accessed on 12th June 2025).

21. Gros, D. B., Hood, L. E., Kent, S. B. H., Nicholson, K., et al. (1985). The Mr 28,000 gap junction proteins from rat heart and liver are different but related. https://core.ac.uk/download/4878506.pdf (accessed on 12th June 2025).

22. Haasnoot, W., Peters, J., Ploum, M. E., Rijk, M., et al. (2025). Development of a multiplex flow cytometric microsphere immunoassay for mycotoxins and evaluation of its application in feed. https://core.ac.uk/download/pdf/29236614.pdf (accessed on 12th June 2025).

23. Jyoti, F. (2013). Development of new antibody-based theragnostic agents targeting the receptor for advanced glycation end-product (RAGE). https://core.ac.uk/download/211298927.pdf (accessed on 12th June 2025).

24. Keir, G., Petzold, A., & Sharpe, T. L. (2005). Why human color vision cannot reliably detect cerebrospinal fluid xanthochromia. https://core.ac.uk/download/1687748.pdf (accessed on 12th June 2025).

25. Linnoila, I., & Petrusz, P. (1984). Immunohistochemical techniques and their applications in the histopathology of the respiratory system. *Environmental health perspectives*, *56*, 131–148. https://doi.org/10.1289/ehp.8456131 (accessed on 12th June 2025).

26. Melton, C. A. (2022). *Mining Public Opinion on COVID-19 Vaccines Using Unstructured Social Media Data*. https://core.ac.uk/download/552579819.pdf (accessed on 12th June 2025).

27. Minnesota State University Moorhead. (2022). *Undergraduate Bulletin, 2022–2023*. https://core.ac.uk/download/580007976.pdf (accessed on 12th June 2025).

28. Noel, A., Orimo, A., Olumi, A. F., Santos, A. M., Anderson, C., Townsend, C. M., Vindrieux, D., et al. (2010). Cancer-associated fibroblasts are positively correlated with metastatic potential of human gastric cancers. https://core.ac.uk/download/pdf/8423401.pdf (accessed on 12th June 2025).

29. Peveler, W. J., Rotello, V. M., & Yazdani, M. (2016). Selectivity and specificity: Pros and cons in sensing. *ACS Sens.* 2016, 1, 11, 1282–1285 https://core.ac.uk/download/132211233.pdf (accessed on 12th June 2025).

30. Special Libraries Association. (1960). *Special Libraries, October 1963*. https://core.ac.uk/download/70425351.pdf (accessed on 12th June 2025).

31. Surmacz, B. (2010). Role for DLK1 in neuronal differentiation of mouse and human embryonic stem cells.

ENDOCRINOLOGY

9

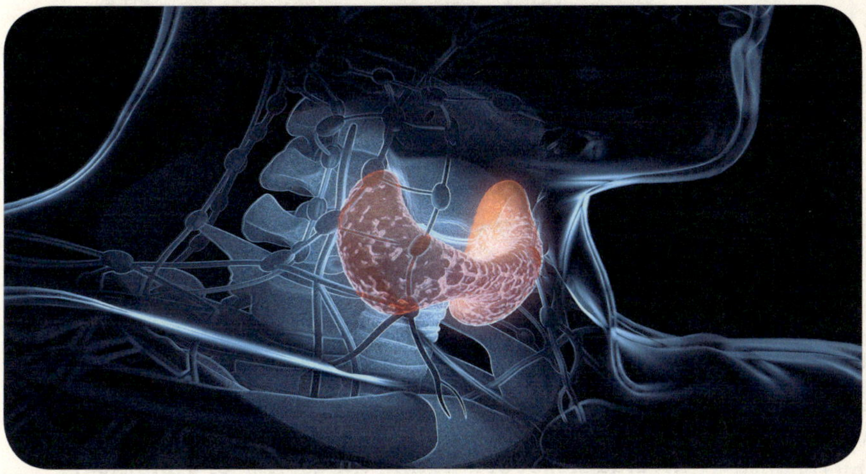

Introduction

Endocrinology is the study of the intricate specifics of hormones, how they function, and their vital role in keeping body functions in a wide range of physiological systems. Endocrinology shows how glands , such as the pituitary, thyroid, adrenal, and pancreas work together to provide homeostasis by secreting hormones directly into the circulatory system. Hormones are chemical messengers that influence processes from metabolism and growth to mood regulation and reproductive health. Where the hormonal communication intersects with the body's response, it demonstrates the complexity of the human body, and the necessity for precise regulatory processes in order to gain maximum functioning. With increased understanding on the complexity of endocrine interactions, it is found that such knowledge is of major importance in the understanding of normal physiology as well as disease process pathophysiology. Endocrinology is characterized by hormonal imbalance effects being quite far-reaching, especially given that such effects are

LEARNING OBJECTIVES

After studying this chapter, you will be able to:

1. Know the endocrine system;
2. Understand the hormonal regulation;
3. Describe the common endocrine disorders;
4. Describe the diagnostic techniques in endocrinology;
5. Know the treatment approaches in endocrinology;
6. Learn about advances in endocrinology.

being experienced on the level of reproductive function and fertility. For instance, in dairy cattle, selection for yield of milk has been termed one of the causes of decreased fertility, which is highly involved with the regulation of estrous behavior. Estradiol is a key hormone regulating such endocrine and behavioral phenomena, but interaction with other hormones , such as progesterone and insulin-like growth factor-1, complicates its function. Existing literature highlights the fact that gene expression changes involved in these hormonal interactions have the potential to ultimately impact estrous behavior and fertility outcomes. Although research is still being sought, the use of mathematical models in conjunction with physiology and genomic data may advance our understanding of biological networks that regulate the control of estrus, and further research to be conducted within this field (Beerda et al., 2010).

A second critical area of endocrinology is the study of those hormones affecting calcium homeostasis and bone, i.e., PTH, calcitonin, and vitamin D. The field has been advanced by recent improvements in radio assay methods, allowing us to understand how such hormones operate under different states of physiology, both normal and unusual , such as weightlessness in space flight.

Alterations in the pattern of hormonal secretion may now be regarded as causing severe metabolic derangements, which can lead to such conditions as osteoporosis. The focus laid on how such hormones cope with exceptional circumstances, like the lack of gravitational forces, speaks volumes about their vital roles in ensuring the integrity of bones and overall health. Moreover, an understanding of these factors is central to remedying endocrine failure-induced disorders, and hence the utility of endocrinological research for both space and clinical medicine (Potts, 2025) (Figure 9.1).

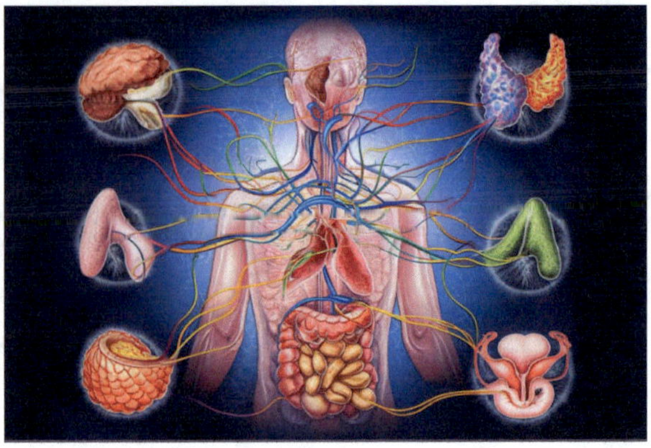

Figure 9.1. Endocrinology.

Source: https://vijaysuperspecialityhospital.in/wp-content/uploads/2024/08/a-captivating-and-educational-illustration-of-the-WRC8-LHTRKOHzEbV76x5Ug-a0JXnm_NT7ygxOblUMTjUA-1024x576.jpeg.

Importance of Hormones in Human Physiology

The role of hormones in human physiology is invaluable, coordinating thousands of biological events to lead to homeostasis and health. The biochemical messengers that are manufactured by the different endocrine glands influence various functions, which include growth, metabolism, immune functions, as well as reproductive functions. Of particular note are thyroid hormones , such as triiodothyronine (T3) and thyroxine (T4), which play significant roles in governing development and metabolic processes throughout the body. The recent research has shown their incredible influence on the process of reproduction, meaning the interdependence of sexual health and metabolic functioning. The interconnection outlines the superiority of thyroid function in keeping reproduction at its best and reproduction outcomes, since derangement of thyroid hormone levels can lead to adverse effects on male and female reproductive systems, evidence which is corroborated in recent literature (Carosa et al., 2018). The adrenal hormones (cortisol) also depict the complex controlling nature of the hormones in the endocrine system. The stress hormone or cortisol does not only mediates the response of the body to a stressful situation but also plays an imperative role in maintaining blood pressure, immune response, as well as carbohydrate metabolism. Research in red deer stags has demonstrated seasonality and circadian rhythms of cortisol release, demonstrating that feedback regulation of hormones is able to adapt to environmental stimuli and physiological requirements (Crockford et al., 1999). Such inherent flexibility bears witness to the versatility of management of the hormones and to the degree that this is in the interests of the needs of body homeostasis. The fact that adrenal responsiveness varies in different seasons implies the complexity of the hormone interaction and the potential influence on health and behavioral patterns at different life periods. Besides the mentioned metabolic and stress response roles, hormones play a significant role in growth and development at different periods in life, starting with puberty through to adulthood. Growth hormone (GH), for instance, not only induces linear growth in children but also muscle and bone mass in adults, showing its sustained impact on body growth. Hormone interactions during adolescence are of particular importance, meaning that they prepare the body to be able to reproduce by initiating secondary sex characteristics and the development of reproductive organs. Moreover, the deregulation of these hormonal interventions results in the occurrence of growth disorders or late puberty, which underlines the necessity of a clear understanding in the area of endocrinology. All these attributes describe why the actions of different hormones are naturally linked to key life processes, which prove their significance in human physiology (Figure 9.2).

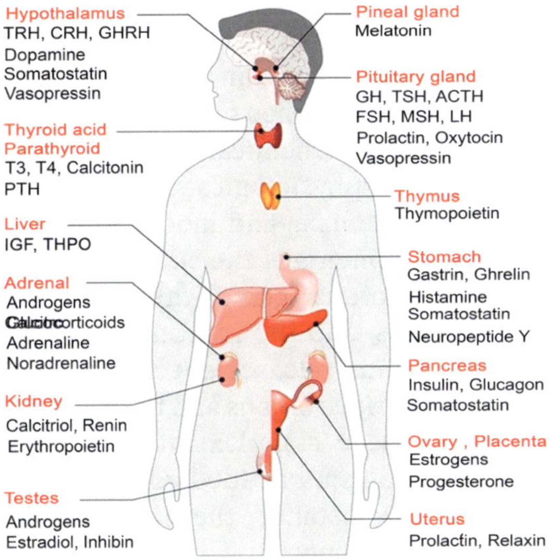

Figure 9.2. Human hormonal system.

Source: https://www.news-medical.net/image-handler/ts/20180620110232/ri/673/picture/2018/6/shutterstock_430118209.jpg.

9.1. The Endocrine System

Learning Outcome

1. Describe the major glands of the endocrine system;
2. Know the hormones produced by various glands;
3. Understand the interaction between the endocrine and nervous systems.

The endocrine system plays a vital role in maintaining homeostasis in the body through the secretion of hormones from various glands. The hormones are chemical messengers that affect numerous physiological functions, such as growth, metabolism, and mood. Some of the most vital components of the endocrine system include the pituitary gland, thyroid, adrenal glands, pancreas, and the reproductive glands. Each of the glands releases specific hormones that influence various organs and tissues, making it possible to have complex interactions and feedback mechanisms needed to enable body functioning. For instance, the pituitary gland, referred to as the master gland, regulates the functioning of numerous other glands and plays an important role in the regulation of hormone levels, thereby emphasizing the interrelationship between the glands in the endocrine system. This intricate network of hormones highlights the fine balance required for normal function within the body and illustrates the way imbalances in the levels of hormones can generate disease. Recent research has begun exploring the relationship between the endocrine system and gut microbiota, particularly through the gut-brain axis. This novel field of study centers on the impact of the microorganisms within the gut on various neurochemical and endocrine functions, which in turn influence health. SCFAs, the metabolites of gut bacteria of dietary fiber, are presumed to play a major role in enhancing neuro-immunoendocrine regulation. These findings suggest that the integrity of the gut microbiota can substantially influence hormonal equilibrium and metabolic health. Furthermore, this axis possesses therapeutic applications for the treatment of diseases induced by endocrine disturbances, such as obesity and mood disorders. By leveraging the knowledge of microbiota-gut-brain interaction, researchers hope to develop new strategies that could enhance endocrine system function and overall well-being, promising a future in endocrinology (Silva et al., 2020). The gut-brain-endocrine interaction has immediate implications that extend beyond physiological functions, influencing various psychological and neurological diseases. The studies on animal models have established that the gut microbiota can modulate neurogenesis and myelination through mechanisms that include modulation of the immune response, as well as the secretion of some of the microbial metabolites. This is an insight into how dysfunctions of the endocrine system can exacerbate conditions like anxiety, depression, as well as neurodegenerative conditions like Alzheimer's and Parkinson's (John et al., 2019). Moreover, other stimuli , such as stress, diet, and antibiotics have been shown to affect the composition of gut microbiota, making the interaction between the two systems even more intricate. Hence, there is a need for further translational research in studying microbial-based therapies aimed at restoring endocrine system homeostasis with a focus on how integrated treatment approaches may revolutionize endocrinology treatment paradigms (Figure 9.3).

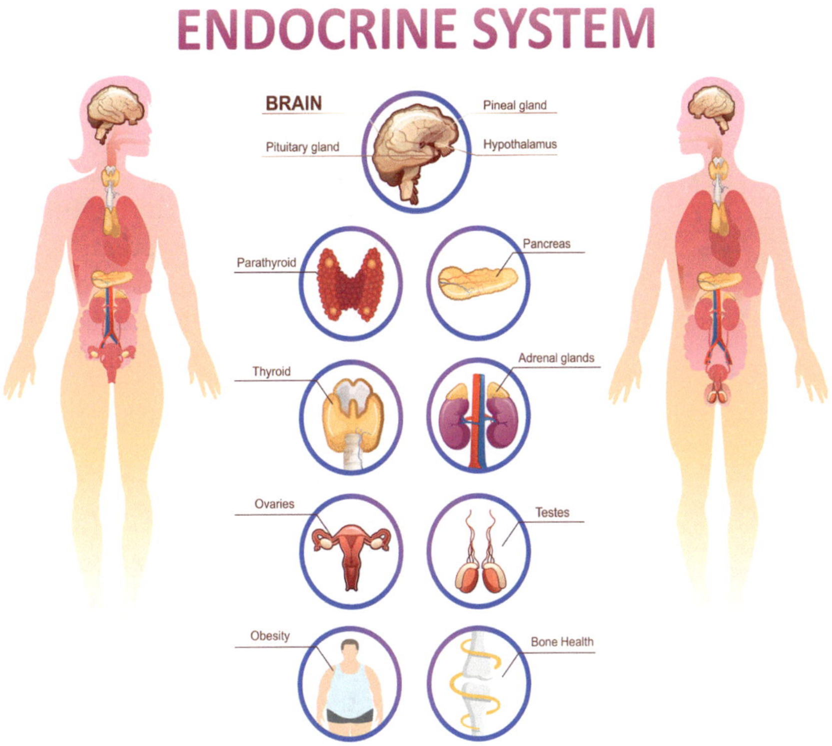

Figure 9.3. Endocrine system.

Source: https://www.wh.com.sg/ClinicalCareServices/MedicalDepartmentsServices/PublishingImages/WH-Website_Endocrinology.png.

9.1.1. Major Glands of the Endocrine System

The endocrine system consists of a complex network of glands that are all interrelated to perform vital roles in the maintenance of physiological homeostasis through hormone production. These interrelated glands include the pituitary gland, or the master gland, which regulates numerous functions of the body by affecting other endocrine glands. It releases hormones , such as GH, required for growth and metabolism, and adrenocorticotropic hormone (ACTH), which stimulates the release of cortisol from the adrenal glands. This hierarchical structure emphasizes the interconnectedness of the endocrine organs and reveals how disturbances in one gland will trigger universal hormonal imbalances affecting overall health and well-being. The significance of the pituitary glands regulatory role reaffirms the complexity of endocrine interaction so vital to normal and disease states within the human body. The second significant endocrine structure is the thyroid gland, with its deep impact upon metabolic processes through the production of thyroid hormones, thyroxine (T4) and triiodothyronine (T3). These hormones also play a significant role in the regulation of metabolism and influencing energy expenditure and growth and development of most tissues. Alteration of thyroid hormone levels can lead to hypothyroidism or hyperthyroidism, both of which have varied clinical presentations affecting many organ systems.

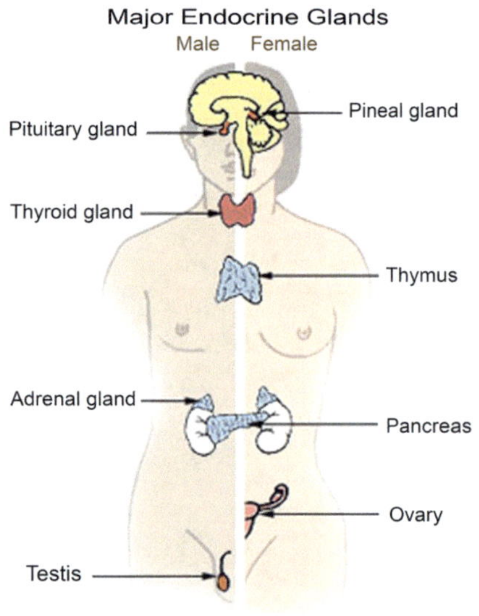

Figure 9.4. Major endocrine glands.

Source: https://training.seer.cancer.gov/images/anatomy/endocrine/endocrine_system.jpg.

The sensitivity of thyroids to the hypothalamic-pituitary axis demonstrates the complexity of the endocrine system since it relies on signals from the anterior pituitary to regulate its hormone production. Understanding these interactions accounts for the development of endocrine disease and emphasizes the importance of early detection and treatment of thyroid failure. The adrenal glands, situated above the kidneys, also play a key part in the endocrine system, releasing a variety of hormones that allow the body to handle stress and maintain metabolic balance. The two parts of the glands are distinct: the cortex and the medulla, which secrete different hormones for synthesis, like cortisol and adrenaline. Cortisol is a glucocorticoid and plays a very significant role in keeping blood glucose constant, immunity, and inflammation. Adrenaline, synthesized based on stress, generates fight or flight by increasing cardiac rate and the availability of energy. The interaction between these hormones is reflective of an elegant adaptive process that is crucial for survival in times of stress. As explained in more recent research, hormonal interactions at the cellular level underscore the endocrine systems' central function not just in the regulation of the body but also in broader psychological and emotional responses to environmental stimulations (Steinhart et al., 2001) (Figure 9.4).

9.1.2. Hormones Produced by Each Gland

The endocrine system regulates a very complex ballet of hormones produced by numerous different glands that regulate critical physiological processes. One of the chief glands is the pituitary gland, referred to also as the master gland, since it releases hormones , such as GH, prolactin, and ACTH. Growth, lactation, and the stress response are regulated by these hormones, respectively. GH induces tissue growth and metabolism and prolactin allows for milk secretion in females. Additionally, ACTH regulates the release of cortisol from the adrenal glands, showing intricate feedback mechanisms that take place in the endocrine system. Additionally, contemporary studies show that transforming growth factor-alpha (TGF-α) in the anterior pituitary enhances the effects of estrogen to induce cell division, harmonizing hormonal action to adjust general health and homeostasis (Kloehn et al., 2016). The adrenal glands have central functions as metabolism, immune response, and stress adaptation regulators through their hormone secretion. The glucocorticoids, like cortisol, secreted by the adrenal cortex, regulate glucose metabolism in stress responses. Aldosterone, however, regulates sodium and potassium balance, thereby affecting blood pressure regulation. Research has demonstrated that sex differences exist in the secretion of adrenal hormones, particularly glucocorticoids, which vary according to the physiology of the individual as well as the environment. Notably, testosterone has been observed to boost circadian amplitudes of hormone production in male adrenal glands, unveiling the refined enjoyment of sexual dimorphism in adrenal function and its resultant effect on stress reactivity in both men and women (Kakeya et al., 2003). The observation says a lot about the role of the adrenal glands in relation to maintaining metabolic stability and emotional well-being. The thyroid gland plays an essential role in regulating metabolic processes by the release of thyroid hormones, primarily thyroxine (T4) and triiodothyronine (T3). Thyroid hormones are essential for the metabolism of energy, growth, and development. The levels of thyroid hormone are precisely controlled by thyroid-stimulating hormone (TSH) of the anterior pituitary, showing the interaction of different endocrine glands. Dysregulation in the production of thyroid hormones may result in diseases , such as hyperthyroidism and hypothyroidism, impacting overall health. Additionally, the thyroid also secretes calcitonin, which aids in the regulation of blood calcium by suppressing osteoclast activity. This dual function highlights the profound impact on both metabolic and skeletal well-being, demonstrating the intricacy of hormonal interactions in the endocrine system (Kakeya et al., 2003; Kloehn et al., 2016).

9.1.3. Interaction Between the Endocrine and Nervous Systems

The endocrine-nervous coordination is a central part of human physiology, enabling the body to control its internal world and adaptively respond to the external environment. Coordination is based primarily on chemical communication, such as the role of hormones as messengers that are conveyed via the circulatory system to affect target tissues, and the nervous system, using quick electrical impulses for the coordination of rapid responses. The hypothalamus is instrumental in this integration in linking the two systems together; it releases hormones that signal the pituitary gland to release hormones that have direct effects on other endocrine glands. This exchange illustrates the cooperation required for both immediate responses and long-term adjustments, illustrating how integrated the activities of the two regulatory systems are in ensuring overall physical well-being. Further exploration of this interaction reveals significant biochemical pathways that underlie various physiological functions. The metabolic and stress regulation, as well as the influence on neuronal function and cognition by hormones , such as cortisol, released from the adrenal glands, are just a few examples. Neurotransmitters and hormones interact on various levels, as in the case of the activity of chromogranin A (CGA), a protein stored in large quantities in endocrine and neuronal secretory vesicles. Recent studies have established that CGA mRNA is present in CNS neurons and adrenal tissues and that it could be a factor in signal transduction in the motor system. This double presence indicates the importance of some proteins in making communication between the endocrine and nervous systems possible (Bergmann et al., 1992). The impact of this communication is vast, from mood regulation to reproductive functions. Endocrine disorders can have serious neurological consequences, as hypothyroidism or adrenal insufficiency, which cause dysfunction of cognition and emotional status. All the systems are connected in complex feedback circuits, and the nervous system can adjust endocrine activities suitably to maintain homeostasis. This adaptability is also crucial when responding to stressors in which the body needs to quickly assess and react. Understanding these nuances of bidirectional interaction illuminates the complexity of disease as well as health and highlights the worth of holism as an approach to the study of endocrinology and neuroscience (Gross et al., 2001) (Figure 9.5).

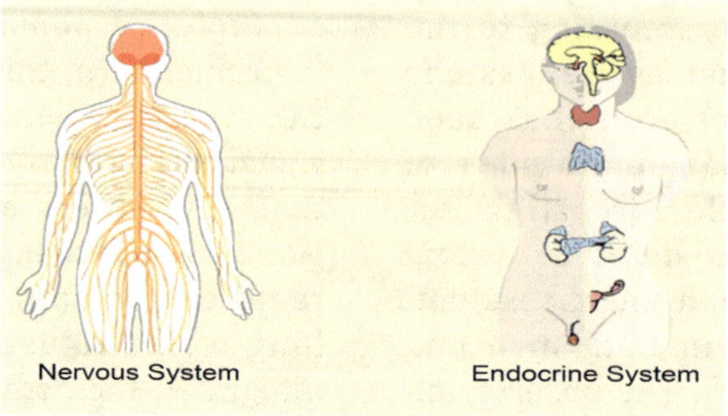

Figure 9.5. Nervous system and endocrine system.

Source: https://knyamed.com/cdn/shop/files/Desktop_-_2024-05-15T171056.228.jpg?v=1715773622&width=1600.

Test Your Knowledge

1. What are the major glands of the endocrine system?
2. What is the interaction between the endocrine and nervous systems?

9.2. Hormonal Regulation

Learning Outcome

1. Know the mechanisms of hormone action;
2. Describe the feedback loops in hormone regulation;
3. Understand the role of receptors in hormone signaling.

Endocrine hormonal regulation is at the heart of the body's homeostasis, encompassing various functions and systems. The endocrine hormones are released into the blood by glands like pituitary, thyroid, adrenal glands among others to control target tissues so as to control metabolism, growth, and reproductive process. For instance, the interaction between luteinizing hormone (LH) and follicle-stimulating hormone (FSH) plays a significant role in the reproductive health of men. The testes have sensitivity to these hormones through Leydig and Sertoli cells thus controlling the release of testosterone and spermatogenesis. A violation of the balance of this hormone can cause fertility or developmental disorders, which determines the importance of hormonal signaling in physiology. The complexity of hormonal control testifies to the complexity of the endocrine system and its central role in human health. Neural processes and hormonal interactions also demonstrate the many-sidedness of hormonal regulation. The example of thermoregulation development in birds shows the coordination of the hormonal messaging and the neural pathways in birds. The thermoregulatory adaptation in the embryonic and post-hatching period is coordinated by the HPT and HPA axes. An example would be the precocial birds that have an early activation of the HPT-axis, enabling them to respond faster to environmental changes compared to the altricial species that activate this axis after hatching. The thyroid hormones, which were previously considered to directly influence thermoregulation, have been demonstrated to interact with other hormonal messages in a more complicated way in a bid to achieve successful body temperature regulation. This interchange underlines the significance of hormonal control in cross-species and evolutionary changes in endocrine capability. Hormonal dysregulation can have quite dramatic effects, and so it serves as an example of how hormone balance is required to permit normal physiology.

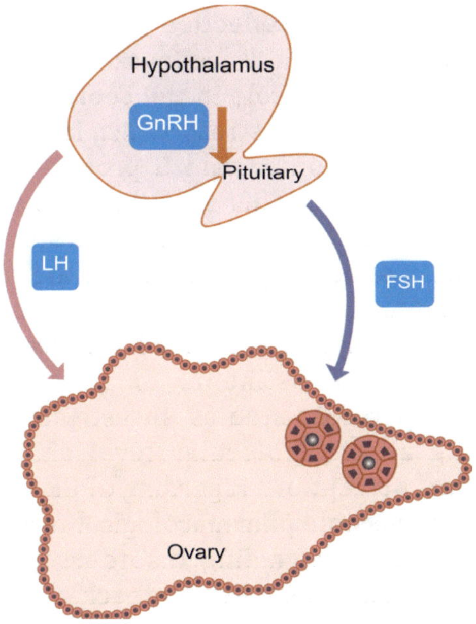

Figure 9.6. Hormonal regulation.

Source: https://cms-media.bartleby.com/wp-content/uploads/sites/2/2021/06/05150456/Hormonal-Regulation-1-770x1024.jpg.

Within the male reproductive axis, FSH and LH act in functional synergy to control key events, including testosterone synthesis and spermatogenesis. Hormonal activities are not limited to the reproductive processes; they also herald the converging routes of growth and development, metabolism, and stress response. In exploring the disorders like hypogonadism or adrenal insufficiency, the fact is clear that hormone regulation leads to serious health problems. As an illustration, the sexual dysfunction, muscle mass, and general health can be negatively impacted by the violation of the balance of the testosterone level. Accordingly, the study of the mechanism of hormone regulation is not only of theoretical but also of great clinical significance and therapeutic value because endocrine diseases need to be managed properly to restore a healthy state and ensure wellness (Figure 9.6).

9.2.1. Mechanisms of Hormone Action

Hormones exert action through intricate mechanisms involving binding to their specific receptors, thereby initiating biochemical cascades ultimately leading to physiological effects. The action mechanism of hormones can be classified into two general categories: classic endocrine signaling and paracrine signaling. In classic endocrine signaling, the hormone is secreted into the bloodstream and transported to distant targets, controlling activities , such as metabolism, growth, and reproduction. For example, estradiol plays a significant role as a key regulator of the estrous cycle in dairy cows, influencing both endocrine and behavioral events, as documented in the literature on control of estrous behavior, where gene expression changes responsive to hormonal status are apparent (Beerda et al., 2010). Understanding these pathways illuminates the complex interaction involved, showing the role of each hormone in homeostasis and the regulation of the body's mechanisms. In addition, the interaction of the hormones with their receptors can lead to more than one outcome depending on the cellular context as well as the presence of co-regulators. For instance, the glucocorticoid receptor can regulate gene transcription via an interaction with transcription factors that react to a range of stimuli. This could account for how some hormones, like cortisol, play multifaceted roles in stress response, affecting not only metabolism but also immunity and the brain. Pharmacological approaches could also be employed to study hormonal interactions, as is the case with the research on reboxetine and mirtazapine, where the latter antagonist activity affects cortisol release and other pituitary hormones. These investigations shed light on the mechanisms of negative feedback and regulatory processes controlling the action of hormones, specifically highlighting the intricate modulation of hormone action in the endocrine system (Baghai et al., 2004). Finally, advances in systems biology and mathematical modeling have significantly enhanced our understanding of hormone action mechanisms. By integrating physiological information and genomic data, scientists can build predictive models explaining complex hormonal networks. For instance, with reproductive physiology, exploration of estrous behavior through the use of these models reveals the interaction between estrogen-induced gene expression and neuron signaling within particular brain regions. Through continued research here, more is learned about hormonal control of estrous behavior in animals, and this could modify breeding technique and fertility management strategy. Consequently, the integration of systems biology approaches in endocrinology will not only improve our scientific understanding but also provide useful applications to agriculture and medicine, demonstrating the significance of hormones in nature as well as in controlled environments.

9.2.2. Feedback Loops in Hormone Regulation

Feedback mechanisms play a complex role in controlling hormonal regulation in the endocrine system, and this is one of the ways of ensuring that the body has homeostasis. Mechanisms of feedback can be either positive or negative, though negative mechanisms of feedback predominate in endocrine control. Negative feedback is a response to a rise in concentration of a hormone; it responds by countering the rise in a manner that decreases the production of the hormone so as to prevent overactivity. As an example, when the level of cortisol rises due to stress, the HPA axis is inhibited, and thus the decrease in corticotropin-releasing hormone (CRH) signaling occurs. Here is an example of how the body may control itself to achieve a state of balance to guard against the negative impact of too much or too little of hormones. This kind of process shows how the endocrine system is interrelated and how feedback loops play a role in achieving body homeostasis. The role of CRH within the HPA axis is a fair reflection of the intricacy of hormone control by feedback mechanisms. CRH plays a pivotal role in the coordination of the body's reaction to stress, which is regulated by its actions upon certain G protein-coupled receptors (GPCRs). This signaling sets forth a chain of downstream effects, one of which is the stimulation of adenylyl cyclase and the related production of cAMP, which eventually leads to physiological adjustments to behave accordingly and humoral adjustments to stressors. As revealed by recent studies, investigating CRH signaling at the molecular level challenges traditional perceptions regarding GPCR function and offers possible pharmacological targets for neuroendocrine signaling disorders (Inda et al., 2017). This delicate feedback system of the CRH regulative mechanism underlines the importance of feedback mechanisms not only in hormone regulation but also in more general neuroendocrine mechanisms by which the body adjusts its reaction to internal and external factors. Moreover, the feedback mechanisms prolong their role beyond coping with stress into the essential reproductive events, and here the circadian cycle assumes a central role too. Such rhythms play a central role in the biological synchrony of various processes , such as the estrous cycle, which affect the level of hormones that decide the time of ovulation and reproduction. Over the past years, interactions between circadian timing processes and reproductive physiology have been emphasized as factors that have an effect, demonstrating that disruptions in these feedback systems lead to compromised fertility and reproductive health (Boden et al., 2013). The endocrinologic cyclic nature of processes of reproduction is tightly regulated, and there are intrinsic and extrinsic factors that stabilize such feedback loops. The combination of the interaction between hormonal regulation and circadian rhythm activity offers an insight into the science of reproductive endocrinology and points to the necessity of additional information about the interaction of these two systems, especially in the context of modern environmental imperatives (Figure 9.7).

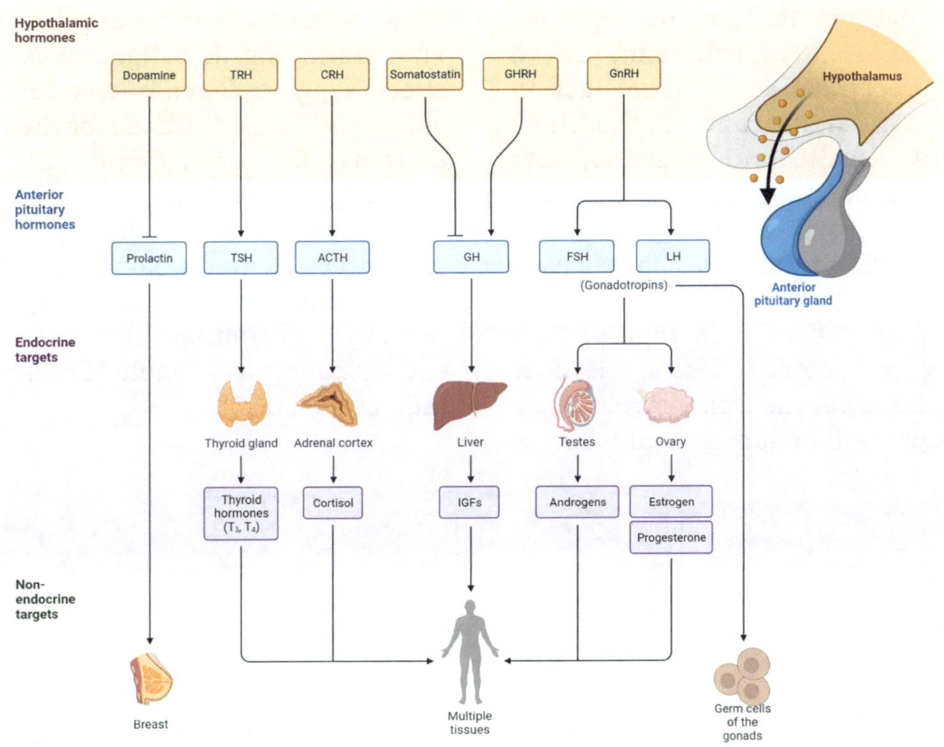

Figure 9.7. Endocrine feedback loop.

Source: https://endoconsult.b-cdn.net/wp-content/uploads/endocrine-feedback-loop-overview.png.

9.2.3. Role of Receptors in Hormone Signaling

The role played by receptors in hormone signaling is crucial for the normal functioning of endocrine systems since they act as the direct mediators through which hormones exert their physiological effects. Chemical messengers or hormones elicit their biological responses by binding to specific receptors on the cell membrane or inside target cells, which trigger cascades of biological responses. This enables cells to elicit a response to alterations in the internal and external world appropriately. For instance, in the hypothalamic-pituitary-adrenal (HPA) axis, CRH is receptor-bound to its GPCRs, CRHR1 and CRHR2, thereby initiating downstream signaling cascades that are responsible for stress reactions. Recent research emphasizes the role of how the identification of such molecular interactions can reveal new pharmacological targets for endocrine disease treatment, emphasizing the complexity and importance of receptors in hormone signaling and overall homeostasis (Inda et al., 2017). In addition, the intricate ballet of receptors and hormones emphasizes the physiological complexity of reproductive signaling. Hormones , such as estradiol (E2) and progesterone direct reproductive events with their effect on specific receptors to produce such responses as the LH surge necessary for ovulation. Importantly, this surge is transduced by the release of kisspeptin in the brain in reaction to the novel actions of E2 and neuroprogesterone. These observations of reproductive physiology illustrate the central role of many receptors in hormone action modulation with significant implications for reproductive health and future fertility treatments. Confirmation of the existence and activity of gonadotropin-inhibitory hormone (GnIH) and its effects on gonadotropin-releasing hormone (GnRH) supports the significance of receptor signaling pathways in reproductive control and suggests potential clinical relevance (Bentley et al., 2016). Aside from reproduction, hormone receptors function in a number of organ systems, helping to demonstrate endocrine interrelatedness. Coordination of reproductive and stress hormones, for instance, demonstrates coordination of states of physiology. CRH not only controls the stress response but also influences reproduction by modulating the HPA axis. This double role can lead to opposing physiological needs, particularly in the state of chronic stress. The continuing investigation of the receptor effects suggests that a clearer definition of such pathways has implications for the design of new therapies for various endocrine diseases. By detailing the mechanisms of receptor binding to hormones at the molecular level, scientists are better able to develop selective therapeutic interventions for specific receptor pathways, thereby developing our understanding of endocrinology as a whole (Bentley et al., 2016; Inda et al., 2017).

Test Your Knowledge

1. What are the main mechanisms of hormone action?
2. What is the role of receptors in hormone signaling?

9.3. Common Endocrine Disorders

Learning Outcome

1. Describe diabetes mellitus and its types;
2. Know the thyroid disorders;
3. Learn about adrenal gland disorders.

Endocrine disorders are characterized by an extensive variety of diseases caused by the malfunctioning of the release and control of hormones. An example is Cushing's syndrome, which has possibly diverse etiologies, including adrenal tumors or pituitary adenomas, and which is caused by long-term exposure to elevated levels of cortisol. Besides the fact that the disease is linked with other dangerous metabolic disorders , such as obesity and hypertension, it is also linked with dangerous comorbidities , such as musculoskeletal and neuropsychiatric manifestations. As discussed, patients suffer from cognitive impairment, depression, and cardiovascular event risk, making early detection and treatment an imperative to efficiently manage cortisol levels and avoid resulting health risks (Biller et al., 2016). To be able to enhance patient outcomes and increase the quality of life, clinicians should understand that Cushing's syndrome is a multifaceted condition. Diabetes mellitus is another common endocrine disease, and it mainly includes Type 1 and Type 2. Type 1 diabetes is generally an autoimmune disease that leads to absolute insulin deficiency, whereas

Type 2 diabetes consists of insulin resistance in combination with relative insulin deficiency. Diabetes has increased exponentially all over the world and is a major concern for public health. Diabetes complications are not limited to hyperglycemia; complications also involve CVD, neuropathy, nephropathy, and retinopathy, which are the sources of significant morbidity and mortality. Besides glycemic control, lifestyle factor control, which includes dietary factors, physical activity, and weight, is included in effective diabetes management. Therapeutic interventions, such as continuous glucose monitoring (CGM) and insulin analogs, continue to advance, providing the patient with better disease management and reducing the burden of complications for diabetes (Biller et al., 2016). Moreover, endocrine disorders should be managed using a global, multidisciplinary care strategy, especially in cases of gender identity and hormonal balance disorders. The standard is the endocrine care of transgender women and men, in the requirement by the endocrinologists to handle distinctive psychological and physiological issues that are gender-affirming. Transgender women are promoted to undergo estrogen and androgen-blocker therapy to stimulate the best physical changes that will make their lives better, whereas transgender men typically receive testosterone therapy to virilize. Current recommendations describe the necessity to research potential future areas of risk, such as venous thromboembolism in trans women and the fact that nonbinary people require individualized treatment. Moreover, the data show that there is an unprecedented decrease in the mental health impairment of the patient group receiving gender-affirming therapies, which proves the usefulness of integrated care in the practice of endocrinology. This shows the relevance of endocrinologists in the treatment of not just the biological conditions of hormone treatment but also the more general psychosocial conditions of the well-being of the patient (Figure 9.8).

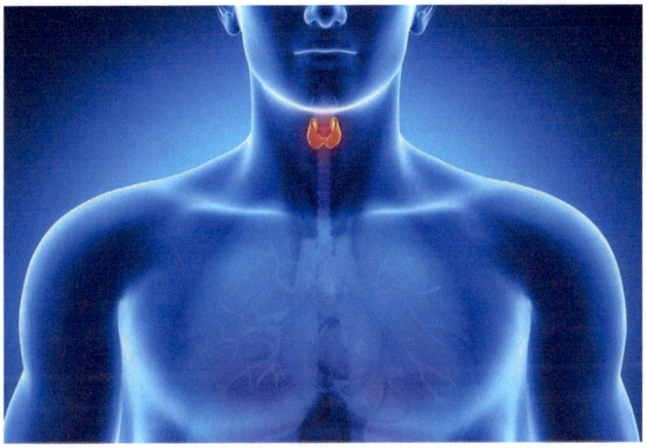

Figure 9.8. Anatomical illustration highlighting the thyroid gland.

Source: https://silverlinehospital.in/storage/treatment-details/endocrine-disorders.jpg.

9.3.1. Diabetes Mellitus and Its Types

The multifaceted nature of diabetes mellitus reveals itself by its classification into different types, primarily Type 1 and Type 2 diabetes, and gestational diabetes. Type 1 diabetes, an autoimmune condition, results from the loss of beta cells of the pancreas that secrete insulin. Without the production of insulin, there is hyperglycemia that needs to be managed with external administration of insulin. Type 2 diabetes, however, is characterized by a resistance to insulin caused by the cells of the body failing to respond to insulin. Type 2 diabetes is most often associated with obesity, physical inactivity, and genetic predisposition, as it demonstrates the intersection of lifestyle factors and endocrinological health. In addition, understanding of the pathophysiology that separates these types of diabetes is relevant to the construction of appropriate interventions and the optimization of hormonal regulation, particularly in view of the rising epidemic of obesity and its secondary impact on the incidence of diabetes. Gestational diabetes mellitus (GDM) is another important category, being gestational in nature and presenting certain challenges to both maternal and fetal health. Characterized by glucose intolerance usually in the second trimester, GDM can be complicated by macrosomia, preeclampsia, and post-delivery Type 2 diabetes risk. Treatment of GDM is best accomplished through multiple interventions using diet modification, exercise, and, at times, by insulin therapy to achieve normoglycemia. The growing GDM burden therefore, highlights the need for efficient public health interventions to address risk factors , such as obesity and inactivity during pregnancy. Stratification of healthcare services allocated to the diagnosis and treatment of diabetes in pregnant women needs calibration, as it is a complex interplay between physiological as well as situational factors, influencing the efficacy of treatment and outcomes of health (DeGaetano et al., 2019). Diabetes research extends also beyond the individual types, as in the diabetes investigations in different populations, i.e., household cats as a model for human Type 2 diabetes. The similarities discovered in the mechanisms of insulin resistance across species are offering insights into the enhanced understanding of diabetes pathology. In addition, conditions , such as feline hypersomatotropism reveal the complexities and co-founding characteristics between various categories of diabetes, including pituitary activity in maintaining insulin resistance (Dirtu et al., 2015). Such relative research not only propels veterinary endocrinology research but also expands the scope of human diabetes research, precipitating improved diagnostic methods and therapeutic approaches that can temper the disease's global dynamics. Such interdisciplinary studies are critical to furthering research in diabetes and crafting multi-pronged plans to combat this complex public health problem (Figure 9.9).

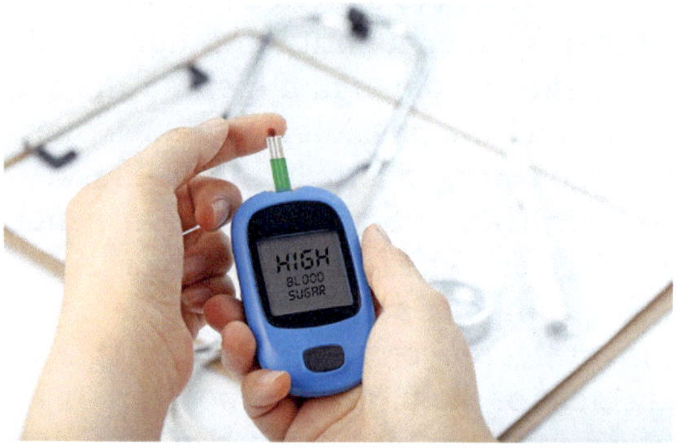

Figure 9.9. Diabetes mellitus.

Source: https://jsshospital.in/wp-content/uploads/2022/03/Blog.jpg.

9.3.2. Thyroid Disorders: Hyperthyroidism and Hypothyroidism

Hyperthyroidism and hypothyroidism are forms of thyroid disease that play a significant role in the pathology of endocrine disease and health. Hyperthyroidism, which is manifested as thyrotoxicity owing to the overproduction of thyroid hormones, is normally caused by diseases like Graves' disease or thyroid nodules. Hyperthyroidism overactivity can be expressed with loss of weight, tachycardia, restlessness, and intolerance to heat, effectively altering the patient's quality of life. Untreated hyperthyroidism does not just leave one feeling uncomfortable; it may go as far as developing some severe complications , such as heart disease and osteoporosis. Most frequently, treatment succeeds using antithyroid drugs, radioiodine treatment, or even surgery. In the meantime, the curiosity of how things work and how treatment may be most effectively accomplished is quite important to clinicians since the end result for the patient and the health of the population in general depends on it. Hypothyroidism is caused by the underproduction of thyroid hormones, the etiology of which includes autoimmune diseases like Hashimoto's thyroiditis, all the way to iodine deficiency. Hypothyroidism patients normally present with a constellation of symptoms that include tiredness, gaining of weight gain, depression, and cold intolerance. The treatment in the clinic is typically by thyroid hormone replacement therapy (HRT) with levothyroxine, which requires precise dose regulation to produce optimal levels of TSH. What is particularly interesting, though, is the smaller subgroup of hypothyroid patients who prove resistant to conventional treatment and need more than normally anticipated quantities of levothyroxine. The prevalence highlights the necessity of a comprehensive treatment modality since other factors like drugs absorption may hinder the control. Practitioners must determine potential underlying conditions that can prevent successful therapy, thus enabling better patient compliance and quality of outcome (Benvenga et al., 2017). Interaction with other disease conditions is also a developing field to study about thyroid disease. Research has been done on the possibility of an interaction between thyroid status and other types of cancer , such as endometrial and ovarian cancer. In an enormous meta-analysis of Nurses Health Study data, prior hypothyroidism or hyperthyroidism did not statistically significantly relate to risk of these cancers. However, trends were revealed, such as an inverse relationship between longstanding hypothyroidism and endometrial cancer, which suggests intricate interactions deserving of study (Alexander et al., 2013). This depicts that thyroid health is not restricted to the endocrine system but is embedded within the bigger scope of physiological wellness. These findings highlight the necessity for ongoing study on thyroid disease's impact, as knowledge about these relationships can be employed in directing preventative and therapeutic strategies in endocrinology (Figure 9.10).

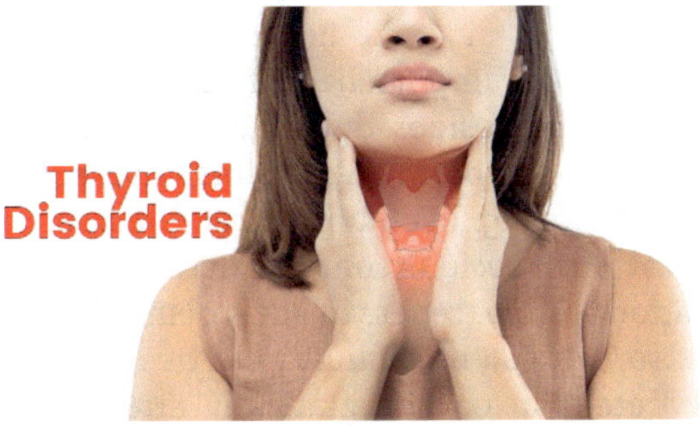

Figure 9.10. Thyroid disorders.

Source: https://diabecare.org/images/thyroid-disorder.jpg.

9.3.3. Adrenal Gland Disorders: Cushing's Syndrome and Addison's Disease

Adrenal glands are significant components of the endocrine apparatus of the body and secrete hormones that regulate metabolism, immune response, and stress. Among disorders affecting these glands, Cushing's syndrome and Addison's disease are two poles of cortisol production. Cushing's syndrome due to hypercortisolism may have more than one etiology, such as pituitary adenomas or adrenal tumors. The consequent hypercortisolism leads to a variety of presentations clinically , such as obesity, hypertension, diabetes, and skin texture changes like striae (purple stretch marks) and bruising. This dysregulation not only has physical effects but also psychological effects due to altered body image and mood, and hence the management needs to be integrated and can include surgery, drug therapy, and lifestyle modification for successful treatment. On the other hand, Addisons disease is caused by the deficiency of cortisol production, typically secondary to autoimmune destruction of the adrenal cortex or secondary adrenal insufficiency. This leads to a variety of symptoms including fatigue, weight loss, hypotension, and hypoglycemia. The patients of Addison's disease may have an adrenal crisis that may be fatal, especially in times of stress or acute illness, and therefore warranting the importance of early diagnosis and treatment. Besides, due to the nonspecificity of its early symptoms, Addisons disease will often not be diagnosed until after considerable progression of serious complications. Continued education and awareness of adrenal insufficiency are also critical in clinical practice, wherein early detection can dramatically alter patient outcomes. Patients are likely to require long-term glucocorticoid therapy to mimic physiological cortisol levels, a measure of the chronic status of the management practice employed. In understanding Cushing's syndrome and Addisons disease, it is essential to consider the broader implications on health and well-being. While both disorders originate from dysregulation of cortisol levels, their management strategies differ significantly, reflecting the paradigm of individualized care in endocrinology. For instance, while it is important to treat the metabolic and psychological consequences of hypercortisolism in Cushing's syndrome, Addison's disease is necessitating stabilizing the adrenal function and preventing adrenal crisis. Moreover, scientists are increasingly finding interest in the genetic predisposition and environmental factors in the etiology of these conditions because identification of the underlying etiology may cast light on novel therapeutic targets. Both syndromes demonstrate the pivotal function of adrenal glands in homeostasis, emphasizing the need for continued research and clinical attention in order to better enhance patient care in the field of endocrinology (Figure 9.11).

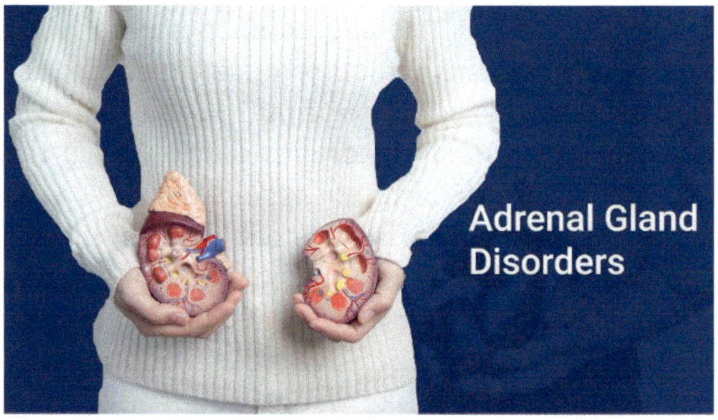

Figure 9.11. Adrenal gland disorders.

Source: https://endocrinologistinahmedabad.com/wp-content/uploads/2023/03/Adrenal-Gland-Disorders-scaled.jpg.

Test Your Knowledge

1. What are the types 2 of diabetes mellitus?
2. What are the most common thyroid disorders?

9.4. Diagnostic Techniques in Endocrinology

Learning Outcome

1. Understand the blood tests for hormone levels;
2. Describe the imaging techniques for gland assessment;
3. Know the genetic testing for hereditary endocrine disorders.

Endocrinology practice involves a broad variety of diagnostic methods that serve as the basis for effective patient management and therapeutic treatment modalities. Endocrine hormones are examined through immunoassay and mass spectrometry as key tools for quantifying hormone levels in serum, urine, or tissue. These techniques provide clinicians with the choice of assessing imbalances of endocrine disorders , such as hyperthyroidism, diabetes, and adrenal insufficiency. In addition, breakthroughs in biomarker studies have led to more precise and sensitive testing, contributing to enhanced diagnostic accuracy. For instance, use of biomarkers like anti-Müllerian hormone (AMH) in the evaluation of ovarian function has been demonstrated to increase reproductive diagnostics significantly. These advances in technology of hormonal evaluation set the need for constant adaptation to new technology in endocrinology because they can be utilized to enhance the outcome of patients and more tailored therapeutic strategies (Manisha et al., 2023). The integration of imaging techniques into diagnosing endocrine disorders has transformed diagnosis and management of hormonal disorders by endocrinologists. Modalities , such as ultrasound, computed tomography (CT), and magnetic resonance imaging (MRI) provide visual information on endocrine anatomy and potential pathologies. For example, thyroid ultrasound can easily identify nodules or structural alteration, which is most indicated in malignancy risk evaluation. Moreover, nuclear medicine imaging, or by the use of gamma cameras, is applied in all utilitarian purposes in disease diagnosis , such as hyperthyroidism and adrenal tumors through the capability of imaging physiological hormone function. This has been made possible with advancements in gamma camera technology that have improved resolution in imaging and diagnostic sensitivity, thereby ultimately leading to more knowledgeable clinical decisions (Mishra, 2024). With the progression of imaging technologies, they will further become an integral part of standard lab tests and transform the realm of endocrinology diagnosis.

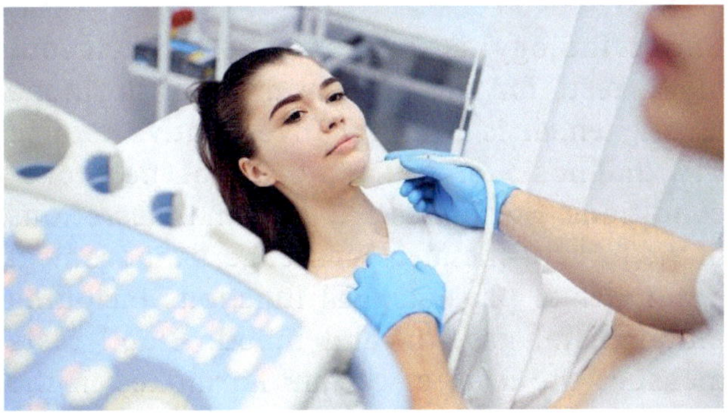

Figure 9.12. Medical professional performing a thyroid ultrasound examination.

Source: https://lirp.cdn-website.com/6fe71637/dms3rep/multi/opt/uS5IDUowRaZJJi2VMxKvoShuHpnSUoDa1623681502-1920w.jpg.

Even more new technologies ushering in the dawn symbolize convergence to even more specific and personalized diagnostic pathways in endocrinology. With technologies , such as next-generation sequencing (NGS), genetic mutations to underlying inherited endocrine disorders can be detected to facilitate targeted interventions and appropriately guided genetic counseling. Moreover, the availability of AI-driven software for data analysis is a significant possibility for increasing diagnosis accuracy through enhanced image interpretation and bioinformatics. Not only are these developments a possibility for early diagnosis, but also methods to track disease advancement and treatment response are presented in an effective way. As the discipline advances further, the application of a multi-disciplinary strategy that incorporates genetic, biochemical, and imaging data will be the key to coping with the complexity of endocrine illness and patient care in general (Manisha et al., 2023; Mishra, 2024) (Figure 9.12).

9.4.1. Blood Tests for Hormone Levels

Endocrinology is not able to do without blood tests for the measurement of hormone levels, which is a useful investigative tool in the diagnosis of the majority of hormonal conditions. Hormones are glandular secretions in the form of chemical messengers that control a number of physiological functions including metabolism, growth, and mood. Blood tests measure the level of certain hormones in the blood and provide insight into the activity of the endocrine system. For example, fluctuations of cortisol levels, which exhibit a circadian profile, can be a sign of adrenal insufficiency or Cushing's syndrome. Their quantitation permits clinicians not just to establish the presence of disorders but also their etiology, thus enabling individualized treatment that most often involves adaptation of lifestyle, replacement of hormones, or other therapy. The complexity of regulation of hormones substantiates the importance of context in interpreting test results of blood assays. Hormone concentrations vary considerably based on the hour of day, stress, and diet. Blood glucocorticoids, for instance, typically quantify their level of binding to plasma in which there is most bound protein, a state that results in low free hormone concentrations. But it's the free fraction that's biologically active, and which has been determined to have some circadian and ultradian rhythm, according to blood levels of free corticosterone research (Droste et al., 2012). Clinicians will have to consider these dynamics in interpreting tests since they can have a significant effect on diagnosis and treatment planning. Apart from that, identification of such rhythms is also required for avoiding misdiagnosis, particularly those diseases that rely on chronic stress or other environmental factors. Apart from that, additional advancements in the methods of assay and knowledge about the interaction between hormones have revolutionized endocrinology. For instance, use of combined stimulation tests, i.e., GH-releasing hormone (GHRH) and arginine, allows for finer pituitary function evaluation (Mehltretter et al., 1996).

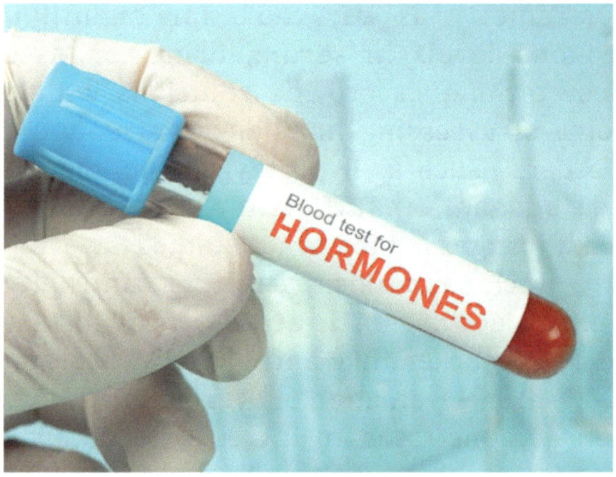

Figure 9.13. Blood tests for hormone levels.

Source: https://img.freepik.com/premium-photo/doctor-holding-blood-tube-analysis-hormones-biochemistry-lab-blood-sample-study-levels-hormone-tests_431724-9912.jpg.

These tests can detect potential endocrine axis dysregulation, particularly when normal measurement techniques yield inconclusive results. Capacity to recognize decline of hormonal response to stimulation is an expression of the presence of underlying somatostatin elevation issues or pituitary constraint. Thus, these advanced blood tests, besides making diagnosis more accurate, enable targeted therapies to be planned. As technology advances, it is likely that the blood tests will also be enhanced to provide more information regarding hormonal balance and its possible consequences on disease and health (Figure 9.13).

9.4.2. Imaging Techniques for Gland Assessment

Imaging techniques are of critical significance in the assessment of several glands in the endocrine system, and they are used to diagnose as well as treat disease. MRI is especially valuable and is utilized for the assessment of the pituitary gland. Newer techniques , such as the dynamic T1-weighted contrast-enhanced sequences, have been established as the gold standard in the assessment of this region. However, these classical approaches are deficient in assessing the intrinsic permeability properties of the pituitary. The most recent study highlights the potential of the golden-angle radial sparse parallel approach, with which the permeability properties of the individual components of the glands can be made available. With the application of this novel MRI technique, health care providers can obtain more detailed physiological information, leading to improved diagnostic accuracy and improved patient outcomes (Babb et al., 2015). In addition to MRI, other imaging techniques like scintigraphy yield unique advantages in gland assessment, particularly the thyroid gland. Scintigraphy remains the preferred method of assessment of thyroid function, especially in hyperthyroidism. Nuclear imaging through this method enables functional assessments that are indispensable in diagnosis and thyroid disease management. Unlike MRI, which primarily offers structural imaging, scintigraphy is effective in characterizing hormonal activity such that clinicians can recognize abnormal glucose uptake patterns characteristic of disease states. It is worth noting that while procedures , such as ultrasound or CT also find use in the assessment of gland anatomy, they cannot provide functional information, thereby rendering them less effective under some situations of endocrine testing (Daminet et al., 2016). The addition of newer imaging modalities to endocrine practice is a significant step towards more accurate and functional gland evaluations. The ability to differentiate between normal physiological states and pathologies with enhanced imaging modalities allows doctors to make informed decisions regarding patient treatment. For instance, use of golden-angle radial sparse parallel technique accounts for differences in signal-time curves to enable clearer differences between conditions like microadenomas and simple cysts in the pituitary gland. These advances underscore the significant role of continuing research and technology developments toward increased diagnostic potential in endocrinology. With improvements in these imaging techniques, they will necessarily determine the future of gland assessment and our overall understanding of endocrine illnesses (Babb et al., 2015) (Figure 9.14).

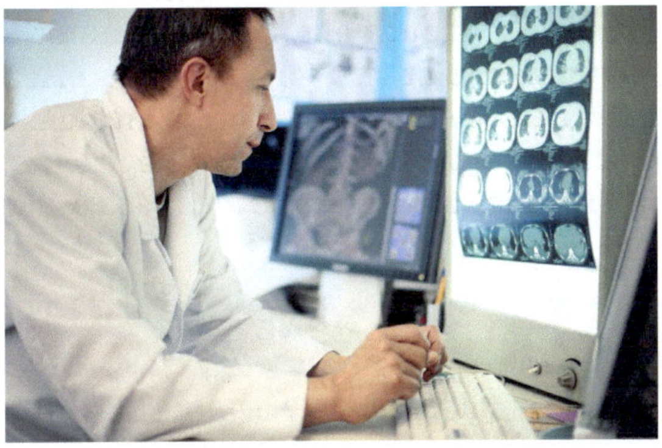

Figure 9.14. Diagnostic imaging techniques.

Source: https://www.healthimages.com/content/uploads/sites/2/2019/10/radiologist.jpg.

9.4.3. Genetic Testing for Hereditary Endocrine Disorders

Genetic testing is now the key diagnostic and management tool for inherited endocrine diseases. They present with combinations of endocrine dysfunction, influencing levels and metabolism of hormones. As more is understood about the genetics of these diseases, clinicians are increasingly employing genetic testing to obtain absolute diagnoses, which guide treatment planning. Genetic testing's power lies in its ability to shed light on the underlying attributions of endocrine disorders, especially where clinical presentation may overlap between multiple conditions. For instance, disorders , such as pseudohypoparathyroidism exhibit such subtlety and need thorough molecular examination to discern particular genetic abnormalities that hold significance for patient care and long-term health outcomes (Ahmed et al., 2018). Genetic testing not only facilitates accurate diagnoses but also facilitates the identification of at-risk individuals among family members, through appropriately informed medical genetics counseling. This is particularly important in inherited endocrine diseases, where patterns of inheritance within families may have profound health implications among relatives of index patients. By identifying genetic mutations placing patients at risk for endocrine disease, health care providers can devise individualized monitoring and intervention strategies. Aside from that, such an aggressive approach can also alleviate the psychological burden imposed on families, allowing them a clearer understanding of their risks and the potential avenues of their health. The information gathered through genetic testing thus becomes a critical element in the development of care plans that integrate, enabling early interventions that can mitigate severe endocrine-related complications among future generations (Helner et al., 2019). The application of genetic discoveries to clinical practice goes beyond diagnosis and family planning; it also improves treatment available to patients. Genetic characterization of disorders, for example, can provide information for focused therapeutic approaches that are personalized to the patient's unique genetic profile. This is illustrated in disorders , such as those with hormone resistance, where focused therapy can notably enhance patient quality of life and clinical success. In tandem with advancements in genetic technology, studies persist in finding new avenues of therapy based on genetic profiling, and hence, the treatment of endocrine disorders becomes more effective. Thus, the role of genetic testing becomes sophisticated enough to transcend diagnostic roles alone, transforming the science of endocrinology by creating the basis for precision medicine tailored to individuals with genetic endocrine disorders (Ahmed et al., 2018).

Test Your Knowledge

1. What blood tests test hormone levels?
2. What is a genetic test for hereditary endocrine disorders?

9.5. Treatment Approaches in Endocrinology

Learning Outcome

1. Learn about hormone replacement therapy;
2. Describe the medications for endocrine disorders;
3. Know the lifestyle modifications and their impact.

The discipline of endocrinology involves a range of treatment methods aimed at treating disorders of hormones, which can have a major effect on overall health and well-being. Hormonal imbalances can present themselves through symptoms that target more than one system within the body, requiring a comprehensive treatment plan. Conventional hormonal replacement treatments, for example, are frequently used to treat hypothyroidism and adrenal insufficiency. These treatments are optimized to re-establish optimal hormone levels, thereby improving symptoms and reducing the risk of any accompanying complications. Other more recent treatment approaches include the use of biologics and novel pharmacologic agents that target specific pathways of hormone control. These emerging developments emphasize the need for individualizing therapy according to the patient, taking into account the underlying pathology as well as the specific hormonal deficiencies to be treated. Outside of pharmacotherapy, lifestyle interventions play a key role in the control of endocrine disease. Combined with dietary changes, exercise therapy, and psychotherapy, they are integral to optimizing therapy efficiency. Diabetes mellitus, for example, is significantly enhanced by multidisciplinary management programs involving diet therapy and exercise therapy in combination with drug therapy. These integrated treatment practices not only address the metabolic aspect of the condition but also improve patients' quality of life overall. Furthermore, recent evidence shows the value of education in patient self-management, improving an active role in their own health process. The combination of these pharmacological and non-pharmacological approaches illustrates the evolving approach to treatment in endocrinology, emphasizing a patient-centered approach to the necessity of flexibility in therapeutic treatment. Another essential component of endocrinology treatment is continuous monitoring and evaluation of patient improvement. Return visits are indicated to confirm the effectiveness of the chosen interventions and institute corrective measures as appropriate in a timely fashion. For instance, individuals taking thyroid HRT require frequent blood tests to ensure hormone levels remain in the optimal range, with drifts leading to the symptoms of hyperthyroidism or hypothyroidism.

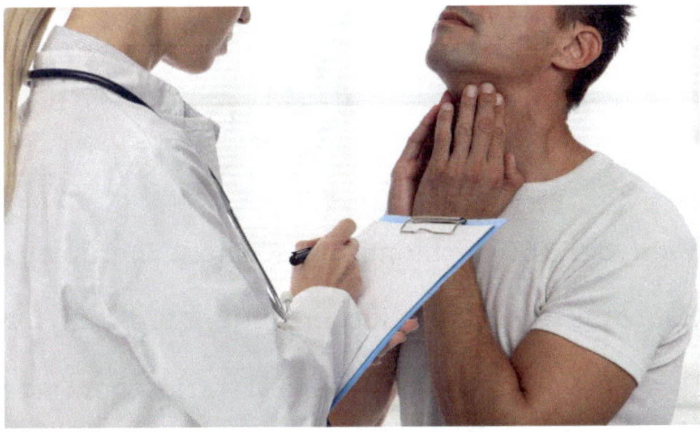

Figure 9.15. Treatment of endocrine disorders.

Source: https://ucfhealth.com/wp-content/uploads/2020/10/endoctrine-disorders.jpg.

Moreover, technological advancements, such as for diabetic patients like continuous glucose monitors, facilitate real-time assessment so that patients can actively manage their conditions. Scientific research funded by organizations , such as the Biotechnology and Biological Sciences Research Council also goes a long way in enhancing such treatment methods, leading to new treatments as well as improved patient outcomes (Allen et al., 2015). The integration of such integrated strategies emulates the adaptive and dynamic nature of care in endocrinology that responds to the multifaceted needs of a patient population (Capiau et al., 2016) (Figure 9.15).

9.5.1. Hormone Replacement Therapy

Hormone replacement therapy (HRT) has turned out to be a central treatment in the field of endocrinology, particularly among individuals with deficiencies in hormones. HRT is employed considerably to correct symptoms of testosterone or estrogen deficiency, which are characteristically seen in menopause and andropause, respectively. The treatment not only corrects bodily symptoms , such as hot flashes but also plays an important role in increasing psychological comfort and quality of life. But whereas HRT holds out vast benefits, it is also vital to balance the potential risks from long-term therapy, such as CVD and certain types of cancer.

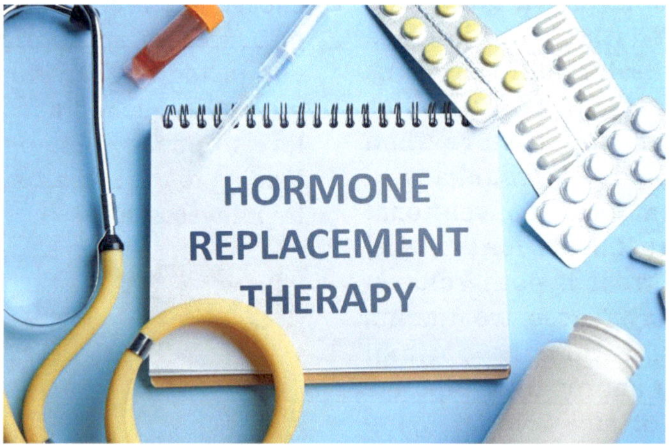

Figure 9.16. Hormone replacement therapy.

Source: https://sa1s3optim.patientpop.com/assets/images/provider/photos/2667109.jpg.

The complex risk-benefit ratio therefore necessitates that treatment protocols must be individually customized and continuous patient monitoring when patients are on HRT, so that therapeutic goals are aligned with individual health statuses. Apart from the treatment of androgen and menopausal deficiencies, HRT has also emerged in the context of pediatric populations, particularly growth hormone deficiency (GHD). Recombinant human growth hormone (rhGH) has been the treatment standard in children diagnosed with GHD with the aim of normalizing their capacity for growth and maximizing their entire pattern of health. Recent findings, however, have highlighted concerns regarding the long-term effects of continued administration of rhGH therapy into adulthood. Studies indicate that children with GHD growing up during childhood can be at risk of experiencing bone health and cardiovascular function-associated challenges if not meticulously monitored during their transition to adulthood. This lends credence to the imperative need for comprehensive, long-term studies of the safety and efficacy of continued rhGH treatment since treatment decisions must be grounded on a solid foundation in both short-term advantage and long-term health outcome (Ahmed et al., 2016). Hormone monitoring during therapy is included in optimization of HRT outcomes, particularly in children on rhGH. Current guidelines suggest serial assessment of serum insulin-like growth factor 1 (IGF-1) as a reference for adjusting GH dosage and minimizing adverse effects. It has been shown in studies that IGF-1 and binding protein changes can significantly impact clinical management to enhance growth response in children with GHD (Clayton et al., 2000). These findings suggest an extension of use in monitoring hormone levels, calling for individual dosage according to response. Furthermore, the findings indicate that a more individualized approach, possibly dose-per-body-surface-area rather than weight, can yield superior clinical results. This level of precision in HRT is a promising development in the science of endocrinology, which eventually leads to safety along with efficacy in the management of patients (Figure 9.16).

9.5.2. Medications for Endocrine Disorders

Endocrine disorders typically demand complicated medication regimens aimed at addressing the needs of the specific patient. One such example is hormone replacement therapies, which serve a critical role in replacing deficiencies resulting from several endocrine disorders. In transgender individuals, for example, hormonal therapies are needed to manifest desired physical characteristics. The Endocrine Society's practice guidelines allow for the treatment of transgender women using estrogens in combination with androgen-depressing medications, which will produce changes like breast growth and fat redistribution. Transgender men also typically require testosterone treatment for virilization, such as the gain of muscle mass and the cessation of menstruation. However, it is important to take into account potential side effects, especially cardiovascular risks, in a bid to offer informed patient decision-making during their course of treatment and thereby optimize the general efficacy and safety of such intervention (Arcelus et al., 2018). Furthermore, management of hypothyroidism is often difficult, particularly in the case of patients who are resistant to normal thyroxine replacement therapy. Some of these patients might require supratherapeutic levothyroxine doses to achieve normalization of TSH levels. This therapeutic challenge may be caused by , such as drug absorption abnormalities or even lack of adherence to prescribed therapy. Clinically, one's initial reaction tends to be an increase in the dosing of levothyroxine; nevertheless, this maneuver really unwittingly increases the risk of adverse effects due to prolonged exposure to supratherapeutic levels. Besides, unusual dosage titration leads to wasted costs and a burden of many medical visits and lab tests for patients and medical staff as well. Therefore, systematic examination of individual cases plays an essential role in identifying underlying determinants affecting the effectiveness of medication, aligning treatment methods with best practice (Benvenga et al., 2017). Apart from hormone replacement therapies, other endocrine disorders need special pharmacological care in managing symptoms or preventing complications. For instance, medications used in treating hyperthyroidism or adrenal insufficiency need precise dosages and regular monitoring to avoid complications. Hyperthyroid patients may be treated with medications , such as methimazole or propylthiouracil to inhibit thyroid hormone formation, while glucocorticoids are often employed in managing adrenal insufficiency. All these medications have specific side effects and a risk profile that must be extensively discussed with the patients. The careful consideration and customization of endocrine disorder medications not only assist in the attainment of better clinical outcomes but also in enhanced patient compliance and quality of life, highlighting the importance of personalization in endocrinology (Figure 9.17).

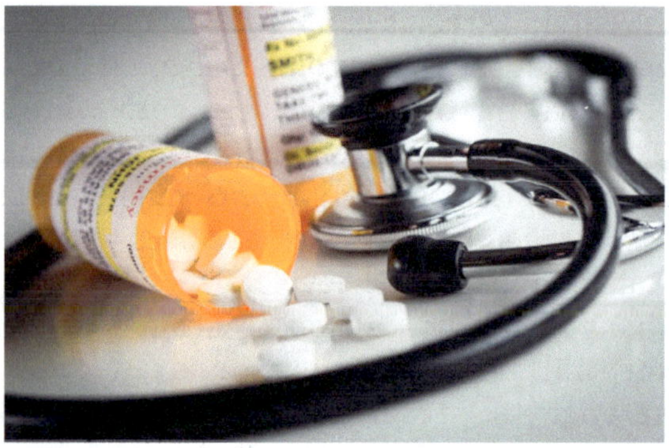

Figure 9.17. Propylthiouracil is an oral medication prescribed to help manage an overactive thyroid.

Source: https://images.ctfassets.net/yixw23k2v6vo/ew_wysiwyg_fid4968_asset/0400c9d666ed1d59ffcf19b92931cafb/69066886_M.jpg?fm=webp&fit=thumb&q=65&w=1728&h=1152.

9.5.3. Lifestyle Modifications and Their Impact

The role of lifestyle modification in the care of endocrine disorders cannot be overstressed, particularly in disorders , such as polycystic ovary syndrome (PCOS). PCOS is an extremely prevalent endocrine disorder in the women in the reproductive age group and affects a significant proportion of this population. The dynamic interaction of obesity, insulin resistance, and genes is all implicated in the pathogenesis of PCOS and its numerous health consequences, including metabolic syndrome and type II diabetes mellitus (Bernier et al., 2012). Existing literature emphasizes the reality that lifestyle modification, with dietary changes and increased physical activity, can be an important aspect in managing symptoms effectively. By addressing the reduction in insulin resistance through such modifications, women can significantly enhance PCOS symptoms, illustrating the extremely impactful role that lifestyle intervention can play for endocrine health outcomes. The same principle applies to the management of menopausal symptoms in breast cancer survivors, underlining the significance of lifestyle modification. The majority of breast cancer survivors experience symptoms of estrogen deficiency, including vasomotor symptoms and mood changes, which could affect their quality of life (Davis et al., 2017). In such cases, the implementation of non-hormonal therapeutic approaches, in addition to lifestyle therapies like exercise and mindfulness training, has been described as having beneficial effects. These modifications not only offer symptom relief for menopausal symptoms but also contribute to long-term health, reducing the risks for CVD and osteoporosis, both significant concerns in this group.

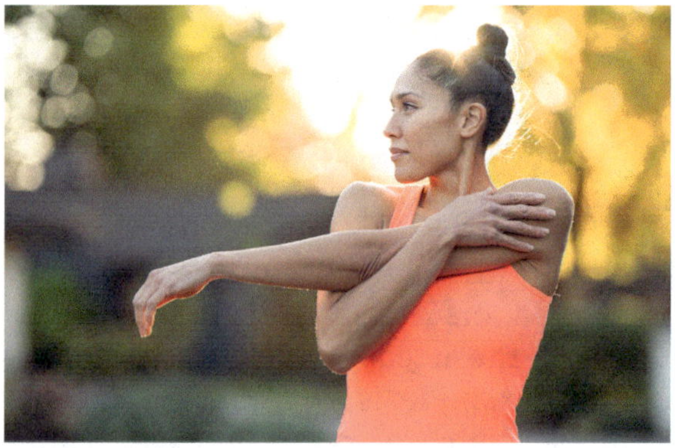

Figure 9.18. Woman stretching outdoors, representing physical activity and hormonal health.

Source: https://www.mariongluckclinic.com/wp-content/uploads/2022/09/how-does-exercise-affect-our-hormones-marion-gluck-clinic.jpg.

Growing interest in maximizing lifestyle as a first-line management strategy underscores the importance of holistic approaches in endocrine treatment. The eventual extent of lifestyle modifications is beyond immediate symptom relief to influence long-term endocrine wellness. In conditions like PCOS and management of menopausal symptoms, adoption of healthier lifestyle practices can result in sustainable metabolic and psychological changes. This preventive approach not only involves patients as active agents in managing their care but also acts as a key adjunct to drug therapy. Above all, the body of evidence supporting lifestyle interventions in such cases emphasizes its therapeutic possibility in transforming the endocrine health management scenario for the future. Thus, the inclusion of lifestyle modification into treatment plans must be considered an essential component of treatment for patients facing multiple endocrine disorders, which makes them a focal point in discussions of successful endocrinological treatment (Figure 9.18).

Test Your Knowledge

1. What is hormone replacement therapy (HRT)?
2. What is the significance of lifestyle modifications in managing endocrine disorders?

9.6. Advances in Endocrinology

Learning Outcome

1. Investigate the endocrine disruptors;
2. Describe the innovations in hormone therapies;
3. Understand the role of technology in endocrine research.

Recent advances in reproductive endocrinology have maximized the treatment choices for infertile patients. The last decade has seen significant progress in ovarian stimulation protocols and hormonal manipulation that has made assisted reproductive technologies (ART) a more personalized setting. Personalized treatment strategies through regimen personalization based on unique hormone profiles, particularly through the use of biomarkers like AMH levels, have maximized ovarian response rates and conception success significantly. These technologies not only optimize oocyte recovery but also optimize embryo quality, leading to better implantation and healthier deliveries. As further reproductive endocrinology continues to advance, these targeted approaches bring about a notable paradigm shift in the approach and delivery of fertility treatments, reflecting on the intersection of technology and personalized medicine in enhancing reproductive health (Manisha et al., 2023). Research into endocrine disease impact on fertility has also come a long way, particularly in the management of diseases , such as polycystic ovarian syndrome (PCOS) and thyroid dysregulation. Increased realization of the role this endocrine dysregulation plays in reproductive capability recognizes the necessity for full hormonal assessment in the management of fertility. Certain research indicates that the coordinated treatment approach based on hormone regulation can significantly override the adverse effects of these conditions on fertility. For instance, approaches that employ the use of GnRH analogue application have been promising to balance the hormone levels in order to facilitate better reproductive success. By targeting the imbalances of hormones that cause infertility directly, such approaches are an indication of the dynamic advancements of reproductive endocrinology that target individualized treatment to the patient and maximum treatment efficiency (Manisha et al., 2023). In oncologic endocrinology, current studies have also come to further elucidate the interactions among genetic mutation and tumor vascularization in advanced medullary thyroid carcinoma (MTC). Tumors harboring RET mutations were found to display unique angiogenic profiles, which would mean that these cancers would respond differently to antiangiogenic therapy. The upregulation of proangiogenic factors in RETmut tumors also indicates that there is a more virulent microvascular milieu that could influence treatment regimens. Understanding these mechanisms makes it possible to design specific therapies that exploit the unique vascularization characteristics of the tumor. This specificity, which may include combined therapy with PDGF inhibitors, shows growing promise for precision medicine in endocrinology to justify the need for further research to further establish therapeutic options for patients (Figure 9.19).

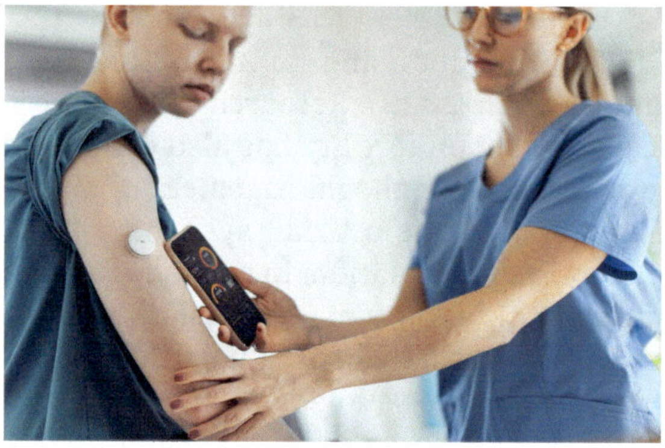

Figure 9.19. Advancements in endocrinology: Emerging trends and research.

Source: https://wp04-media.cdn.ihealthspot.com/wp-content/uploads/sites/464/2024/03/iStock-1796960382-1.jpeg.

9.6.1. Research on Endocrine Disruptors

Research on endocrine disruptors has shown their profound impact on human health as well as environmental ecosystems. Endocrine disruptors, predominantly man-made chemicals, can interfere with the body's hormonal systems and cause a myriad of problems from developmental disorders to reproductive dysfunction. Research emphasizes how these chemicals operate through a complex array of biological mechanisms, which remain outside our knowledge due to the complicated nature of endocrine signaling pathways. Notably, research has shown that certain EDCs have biological activity at startlingly low doses, refuting the conventional toxicological paradigm that "the dose makes the poison." This raises the need to enhance our knowledge on the mechanisms of action and their implications on public health and safety (Bellingham et al., 2016). Recent studies have demonstrated the impact of fetal exposure to environmental chemicals on the developing fetus and subsequent endocrine function. For example, research indicates that consistent maternal exposure to a mixture of environmental chemicals can disrupt critical mRNA expression of genes central to the hypothalamo-pituitary-gonadal (HPG) axis in developing sheep. Interestingly, duration and timing of exposure dramatically affect such important neuroendocrine regulatory gene expression as GnRH and kisspeptin, with a sex-dimorphic pattern of male fetuses exhibiting deviations towards feminized mRNA levels in certain situations. It underlines the delicate balance between endocrine function and environmental influences and points out that even exposure before conception can trigger long-term effects on neuroendocrine development, thereby questioning reproductive health in future generations (Bellingham et al., 2016). With growing evidence, researchers are increasingly worried about the long-term implications of EDCs not just on humans but also on various animals of the kingdom. Projects like the European Union's COMPRENDO project attempt to uncover the health danger posed by androgenic and antiandrogenic chemicals, evaluating both their effect on wildlife and on human beings. With this comparative approach, similarities and differences between biological responses to endocrine disruptors within a spectrum of different biological systems are hoped to be discovered, advancing the whole picture of their ecological and health impact. As more is realized about how complicated endocrine systems are, the necessity for addressing the effect of such chemicals is for tighter regulatory measures and more public awareness to safeguard not just environmental but also human health from these omnipresent dangers (Allera et al., 2006) (Figure 9.20).

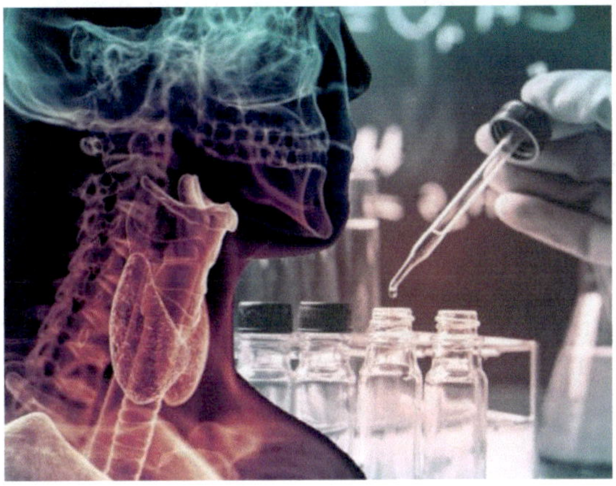

Figure 9.20. Endocrine disruptors.

Source: https://www.oecd.org/adobe/dynamicmedia/deliver/dm-aid--cd6b97f3-467d-46ec-8346-3c69938f745e/endocrine-disruptors.jpg?quality=80&preferwebp=true.

9.6.2. Innovations in Hormone Therapies

The field of hormone therapies has seen incredible progress, particularly in reproductive endocrinology. Emerging developments in ovarian stimulation regimens and the introduction of new drugs have transformed ART. Innovations , such as customized ovarian stimulation regimens focus on patient-tailored therapy, which optimizes oocyte yield and embryonic quality. These developments are leading to a dramatic enhancement in optimizing reproductive results with minimal undesirable side effects. Techniques , such as time-lapse imaging have revolutionized embryo selection techniques to facilitate enhanced implantation rates and decreased multiple pregnancies. The use of such advanced methods is a part of a broader transition toward precision medicine in reproductive medicine, reflecting the need for interventions to be tailored to each patient's unique hormonal profiles (Manisha et al., 2023). In addition to reproductive health, the management of thyroid disorders has equally had better days, especially in the cases of Hashimoto's disease. With standard therapy residing mostly in hormone replacement, there is no regard for the autoimmune predisposition of the condition. In this case, stem cell therapy is a game-changer, with the potential to regenerate thyroid tissue while modulating the immune system. Preclinical investigation has demonstrated that MSCs to be able to reduce thyroid inflammation and reinstate hormonal balance, and early-phase clinical trials are investigating the therapeutic capacity of MSCs. Immune rejection and ethical concerns are some of the issues that remain to be addressed, but studies are continuing to advance more sophisticated treatments that could be significantly beneficial to the quality of life for individuals suffering from autoimmune thyroid disease (Bochenek et al., 2024). Further, the establishment of biomarker-guided frameworks constitutes a paradigm shift in hormonal regulation, beneficially conferring benefits predominantly on couples undergoing fertility treatments. Utilizing markers , such as GnRH and AMH, doctors are able to tailor the stimulation regimens to the unique hormonal profile of each participant. This has been linked to higher conception rates and better overall outcomes, suggesting the need for precision in endocrinology. The continuous refinement of these techniques, coupled with interdisciplinary science, indicates a bright future for personalized reproductive therapies. While advancements are being achieved in this area, there has to be consideration of the ethical and social issues with huge caution so that equitable access is facilitated to these new-age therapies, thus yielding a responsible and inclusive approach to the advancement of hormone therapies (Manisha et al., 2023).

9.6.3. The Role of Technology in Endocrine Research

The application of technology in endocrine studies has transformed our knowledge about hormones and how they affect the human body at a fundamental level. The application of technologies , such as MRI and PET scans has allowed for real-time visualization of endocrine organs, improving disorders diagnosis and treatment. The development of biosensors and microfluidic devices has further facilitated real-time hormone detection, permitting precise endocrine function measurements. These technologies, not only improving clinical outcomes by having individualized treatment plans but also improving research methodology with the ability to gather and analyze improved data, are thus improving basic and applied endocrine research due to these technologies that are paving the way for new therapeutic strategies and better patient care. In reproductive endocrinology, technological progress has revolutionized fertility treatments by leaps and bounds. New ovarian stimulation protocols with customized drugs have revolutionized ART by enhancing oocyte recoveries and embryo quality. Such developments are reinforced through advancements , such as time-lapse imaging, which assists in enhanced embryo selection and thus reduced multiple gestations and increased implantation rates.

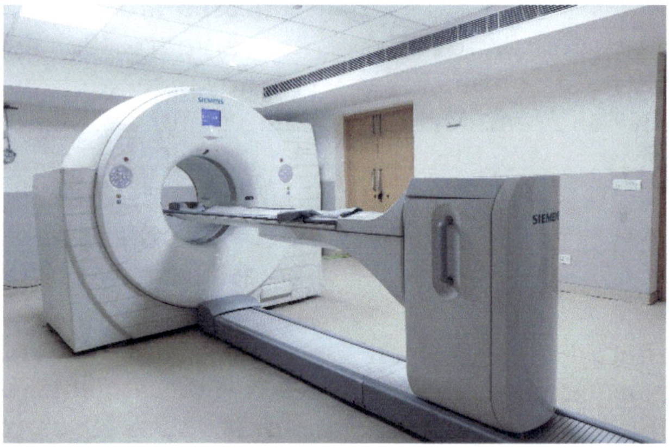

Figure 9.21. PET-CT scanner used in nuclear medicine imaging.

Source: https://www.rgcirc.org/wp-content/uploads/2023/12/Nuclear-Medicine-12-scaled.jpg.

Furthermore, biomarker-directed hormonal management unique to individuals has evolved into a vital component enhancing conception rates, especially in patients with conditions like endometriosis or PCOS. All these advances not only optimize treatment protocols but also contribute to filling gaps in knowledge about complex relationships between hormones in reproductive medicine (Manisha et al., 2023). The investigation of more specific biochemical pathways has further become a central area of study in modern endocrine research, with the function of proteins , such as the 18-kDa translocator protein (TSPO). Through the transfer of cholesterol across mitochondria, TSPO plays an essential role in neurosteroid synthesis and general endocrine regulation. New proteomic and imaging technologies have unveiled the complex interactions of TSPO with other mitochondrial proteins, implicating it in essential cellular processes , such as apoptosis and autophagy. Such discoveries open new targets for therapy since the discovery of the multidimensional role of TSPO can lead to innovative targeted drugs for targeting specific endocrine and metabolic disorders. Thus, the present research on TSPO and homologous proteins is a reflection of the growing convergence of technology and endocrinology and offers promising prospects in both diagnostics and therapeutics (Aghazadeh et al., 2016) (Figure 9.21).

Test Your Knowledge

1. What are endocrine disruptors?
2. What is the role of technology in endocrine research?

Summary

The field of endocrinology plays a key role in unraveling the intricate set of hormonal interactions controlling varying physiological functions within the body. As explained in this chapter, a deeper insight into hormones goes beyond basic biochemical processes since these substances influence behavior, metabolism, and outcomes for health profoundly. The stakes are tremendous, unveiling inherent correlations between mechanisms of hormones and disorders , such as PCOS and neurodegenerative disorders. Notably, the intricate mechanisms of action of steroid hormones, including the estrogens and progesterone, underscore the importance of a deeper understanding of their protective mechanisms and advanced signal processes in the neuroendocrine axis, as highlighted in recent studies (Deniselle et al., 2016). These findings not only serve to add to our theoretical understanding but also present possibilities for more effective therapeutic interventions against hormonal imbalance. Furthermore, the impact of CKD in the field of endocrinology cannot be overstated since it is the meeting point of endocrine systems and disease processes. CKD is characterized by a continuum of deranged hormonal and metabolic processes that contribute to increased morbidity and mortality, particularly concerning CVD risk. Research indicates that hormonal dysregulation and inflammatory markers, such as the renin-angiotensin-aldosterone system, may have key roles in the development of CKD (Slee et al., 2012). This points toward the possibility of intervention in individuals with kidney disease using an integrated model, relating endocrinological mechanisms to potential interventions that would be capable of mitigating threats from metabolic derangement as well as improving patient outcomes. Such a broad perspective not only adds to clinical assessments but also informs therapeutic modalities aimed at the underlying endocrinological disease. Summing up, application of endocrinological principles to research and clinical practice highlights an imperative need for interdisciplinary management of health. One must appreciate that hormones act extensively on the various systems of the body, influencing fertility and reproductive health, metabolic disease, and chronic disease. With the current body of research unraveling complex hormone interactions and their implications in diseases like CKD and other metabolic syndromes, future research needs to redirect focus towards the unravelling of therapeutic possibilities and prophylactic interventions based on endocrinological knowledge. The accumulated body of knowledge in the process fuels enhanced appreciation of disease mechanisms and ultimately drives innovations in treatment modalities, by which improved health gains for different groups of patients are to be expected in the future.

Endocrinology is an immense range of body processes, which are regulated by hormones, which have central functions as signaling molecules in the body. Among the characteristic aspects of endocrinology are the investigation of how interactions between hormones regulate various body functions, including metabolism, growth, reproduction, and mood. There has been a body of literature focusing on the unique endocrinological changes that women experience throughout their lives, especially with reference to the reproductive hormones. The action of female sex steroid hormones extends beyond that of reproductive health, determining more general physiological systems, and that is a key area to be explored by practitioners and researchers alike. Through the examination of these hormonal functions, the field can create knowledge that will be able to positively impact women's health results, particularly during pivotal stages in their life , such as pregnancy and menopause, thus emphasizing the need for focused research and development in this field (Elliott-Sale et al., 2024). Emphasis on female physiology within exercise and sports science presents an exciting future for endocrinological research. Despite significant advances, there is a fundamental deficiency of high-quality research that investigates the effects of female hormones on bodily health and athletic performance. Stimulating more research in this area could yield valuable data not only to enhance women's athletic training programs but also for health programs in general. Integration of female physiology in school and institutional exercise science programs matters in shaping the next generation of practice and research. Addressing this knowledge gap will facilitate researchers and educators to construct a more advanced, more knowledgeable, and more effective paradigm of how various hormonal profiles impact women and potentially revolutionize sport science and public health (Elliott-Sale et al., 2024). Finally, endocrinology as a discipline is faced with the challenge of new research paradigms that will be able to uncover the subtleties of hormonal effects in heterogeneous populations. For instance, studies on supraphysiological conditions like pregnancy or ART offer new opportunities to understand female hormone dynamics. Collaborative work and cooperative education methods can further enhance this research by exchanging resources and knowledge between different countries and cultures. Not only does this cooperative approach create opportunities for improving medical nutrition education, but it also creates opportunities for stunning public health improvements. Lastly, by encouraging teamwork and innovative thinking, the area of endocrinology can enhance our understanding of hormone action, which in turn can be used to develop new therapies and interventions for a number of health ailments.

KEY TERMS FROM THIS CHAPTER

- Adrenal glands
- Corticotropin-releasing hormone
- Endocrinology
- Hormonal imbalances
- Mood regulation
- Pituitary gland
- Thyroid dysfunction
- Triiodothyronine
- Anti-Müllerian hormone
- Cushing's syndrome
- Growth hormone
- Hormonal regulation
- Parathyroid hormone
- Reproductive health
- Thyroxine

Critical Thinking Questions

1. **Which gland is referred to as the "master gland" of the endocrine system?**
   a. Thyroid gland
   b. Adrenal gland
   c. Pituitary gland
   d. Pineal gland
2. **The hormone that regulates calcium levels in the blood is:**
   a. Insulin
   b. Parathyroid hormone (PTH)
   c. Cortisol
   d. Aldosterone
3. **The hypothalamus communicates with the anterior pituitary via:**
   a. Direct neural connections
   b. The hypothalamic-pituitary portal system
   c. Cerebrospinal fluid
   d. Hormone receptors
4. **Which of the following is a tropic hormone?**
   a. Growth hormone (GH)
   b. Thyroid-stimulating hormone (TSH)
   c. Oxytocin
   d. Antidiuretic hormone (ADH)
5. **What is the primary effect of thyroid hormones (T3 and T4)?**
   a. Regulate blood calcium levels
   b. Increase basal metabolic rate
   c. Control water reabsorption in the kidney
   d. Stimulate glucose uptake in cells

Short Answer Questions

1. What is called endocrinology?
2. What is the importance of hormones in the human body?
3. List the key components of the endocrine system.
4. What is hormonal regulation?
5. What are the most common endocrine disorders?

Answers to Critical Thinking Questions

1. (c); 2. (b); 3. (b); 4. (b); 5. (b)

References

1. Abel, M. H., Baker, P. J., Huhtaniemi, I., Morris, K. D., et al. (2009). Role of androgen and gonadotrophins in the development and function of the Sertoli cells and Leydig cells: Data from mutant and genetically modified mice. https://core.ac.uk/download/91350.pdf (accessed on 12th June 2025).

2. Acquaviva, G., Boichard, A., Casadei, G. P., Checquolo, M., et al. (2016). RET mutation and increased angiogenesis in medullary thyroid carcinomas. https://core.ac.uk/download/54537070.pdf (accessed on 12th June 2025).

3. Aghazadeh, A., Alho, C. F., Amitani, M., Anholt, J., et al. (2016). TSPO: Kaleidoscopic 18-kDa amid biochemical pharmacology, control and targeting of mitochondria. https://core.ac.uk/download/36779164.pdf (accessed on 12th June 2025).

4. Ahankari, A. S., Avdagovska, M., Ball, L., Crowley, J., et al. (2016). Proceedings of the inaugural International Summit for Medical Nutrition Education and Research. https://core.ac.uk/download/154739109.pdf (accessed on 12th June 2025).

5. Ahmed, S. F., Ahmid, M., Perry, C. G., Shaikh, M. G., et al. (2016). Growth hormone deficiency during young adulthood and the benefits of growth hormone replacement. https://core.ac.uk/download/46663961.pdf (accessed on 12th June 2025).

6. Ahmed, S. F., Bastepe, M., Bufo, R., Choplin, R., et al. (2018). Diagnosis and management of pseudohypoparathyroidism and related disorders: First international consensus statement. https://core.ac.uk/download/159136913.pdf (accessed on 12th June 2025).

7. Alexander, E., Curhan, G., De Vivo, I., Kang, J., et al. (2013). A large cohort study of hypothyroidism and hyperthyroidism in relation to gynecologic cancers. https://core.ac.uk/download/28946334.pdf (accessed on 12th June 2025).

8. Allen, T., Allende, R., Badylak, S., Bancos, I., et al. (2015). New directions for the treatment of adrenal insufficiency. https://core.ac.uk/download/30697715.pdf (accessed on 12th June 2025).

9. Allera, A., Carnevali, C., Tyler, C., van Ballegoy, C., Porte, C., Copeland, B. J., Candia Carnevali, D., et al. (2006). COMPRENDO: Focus and approach. https://core.ac.uk/download/333559.pdf (accessed on 12th June 2025).

10. Arcelus, J., Gooren, L., Klink, D., T'Sjoen, G., et al. (2018). Endocrinology of transgender medicine. https://core.ac.uk/download/162667742.pdf (accessed on 12th June 2025).

11. Inda, C., Armando, N. G., Dos Santos Claro, P. A., & Silberstein, S. (2017). Endocrinology and the brain: corticotropin-releasing hormone signaling. *Endocrine connections*, *6*(6), R99–R120. https://doi.org/10.1530/EC-17-0111 (accessed on 12th June 2025).

12. Timothy S. Gross, Beverly S. Arnold, Maria S. Sepulveda, and Kelly McDonald (2001). Relations of environmental contaminants, algal toxins, and diet with the reproductive success of American alligators on Florida lakes. USGS-Florida Caribbean Science Center and The Department of Physiological Sciences, College of Veterinary Medicine, University of Florida, Gainesville, Florida. https://core.ac.uk/download/11016994.pdf (accessed on 12th June 2025).

13. Baarendse, P. J. J., Brand, H., van den Bruggeman, V., et al. (2008). Involvement of the hypothalamic–pituitary–thyroid axis and its interaction with the hypothalamic–pituitary–adrenal axis in the ontogeny of avian thermoregulation: A review. https://core.ac.uk/

download/pdf/29259797.pdf (accessed on 12th June 2025).

14. Babb, J., Bangiyev, X. L., Block, K. T., Boada, F., et al. (2015). High-resolution DCE-MRI of the pituitary gland using radial k-space acquisition with compressed sensing reconstruction. https://core.ac.uk/download/153369857.pdf (accessed on 12th June 2025).
15. Baghai, T. C., Laakmann, G., & Schule, C. (2004). Mirtazapine decreases stimulatory effects of reboxetine on cortisol, adrenocorticotropin and prolactin secretion in healthy male subjects. https://core.ac.uk/download/16432476.pdf (accessed on 12th June 2025).
16. Beerda, B., Boer, H. M. T., Veerkamp, R. F., Woelders, H., et al. (2010). Estrous behavior in dairy cows: Identification of underlying mechanisms and gene functions. https://core.ac.uk/download/pdf/29246031.pdf (accessed on 12th June 2025).
17. Bellingham, M., Cotinot, C., Evans, N. P., Fowler, P. A., et al. (2016). Timing of maternal exposure and fetal sex determine the effects of low-level chemical mixture exposure on the fetal neuroendocrine system in sheep. https://core.ac.uk/download/74230048.pdf (accessed on 12th June 2025).
18. Bentley, G. E., Calandra, R. S., Micevych, P. E., Paredes, R. G., et al. (2016). Peripheral and central mechanisms involved in hormonal control of male and female reproduction. https://core.ac.uk/download/159295807.pdf (accessed on 12th June 2025).
19. Benvenga, S., Centanni, M., & Sachmechi, I. (2017). Diagnosis and management of treatment-refractory hypothyroidism: An expert consensus report. https://core.ac.uk/download/188829705.pdf (accessed on 12th June 2025).
20. Bergmann, M., Gratzl, M., Lahr, G., Mayerhofer, A., et al. (1992). Chromogranin A in neurons of the rat cerebellum and spinal cord: Quantification and sites of expression. https://core.ac.uk/download/12168028.pdf (accessed on 12th June 2025).
21. Bernier, D. (2012). *Polycystic Ovary Syndrome: Pathogenesis, Health Consequences, And Treatment of PCOS In Relation to Insulin Resistance*. https://core.ac.uk/download/72048051.pdf (accessed on 12th June 2025).
22. Biller, B. M. K., Colao, A., De Martino, M. C., Isidori, A. M., et al. (2016). Complications of Cushing's syndrome: State of the art. https://core.ac.uk/download/54532161.pdf (accessed on 12th June 2025).
23. Bochenek, O., Kałuża, J., Konaszczuk, A., Koper, M., et al. (2024). Stem cell therapy for Hashimoto's disease–a promising treatment method? https://core.ac.uk/download/620863157.pdf (accessed on 12th June 2025).
24. Boden, M., Kennaway, D., & Varcoe, T. (2013). Circadian regulation of reproduction: From gamete to offspring. https://core.ac.uk/download/19445268.pdf (accessed on 12th June 2025).
25. Capiau, S., Stove, C., & Velghe, S. (2016). Opening the toolbox of alternative sampling strategies in clinical routine: A key-role for (LC-)MS/MS. https://core.ac.uk/download/84043363.pdf (accessed on 12th June 2025).
26. Caro, G., Fortuna, M. C., Lenzi, A., Lolli, F., et al. (2017). Androgenetic alopecia: A review. https://core.ac.uk/download/98335500.pdf (accessed on 12th June 2025).
27. Carosa, E., Jannini, E. A., & Lenzi, A. (2018). Thyroid hormone receptors and ligand, tissue distribution and sexual behavior. https://core.ac.uk/download/160052696.pdf (accessed on 12th June 2025).

28. Clayton, P. E., Gill, M. S., Kibirige, M. S., Patel, L., et al. (2000). Monitoring serum insulin-like growth factor-I (IGF-I), IGF binding protein-3 (IGFBP-3), IGF-I/IGFBP-3 molar ratio and leptin during growth hormone treatment for disordered growth. https://core.ac.uk/download/59177.pdf (accessed on 12th June 2025).

29. Crockford, J. N., Ingram, J. R., & Matthews, L. R. (1999). Ultradian, circadian and seasonal rhythms in cortisol secretion and adrenal responsiveness to ACTH and yarding in unrestrained red deer (*Cervus elaphus*) stags. https://core.ac.uk/download/29195391.pdf (accessed on 12th June 2025).

30. Cryan, J. F., O'Riordan, K. J., Cowan, C. S. M., Sandhu, K. V., Bastiaanssen, T. F. S., Boehme, M., Codagnone, M. G., et al. (2019). The microbiota-gut-brain axis. *Physiological Reviews, 99*, 1877–2013. https://doi.org/10.1152/physrev.00018.2018 (accessed on 12th June 2025).

31. Daminet, S., Peremans, K., Saunders, J., Vandermeulen, E., et al. (2016). Hyperthyroidism in cats, part I: Anatomy, physiology, pathophysiology, diagnosis and imaging. https://core.ac.uk/download/74658457.pdf (accessed on 12th June 2025).

32. Davis, S. R., Gompel, A., Lumsden, M. A., Pinkerton, J. V., et al. (2017). Managing menopausal symptoms and associated clinical issues in breast cancer survivors. https://core.ac.uk/download/96884955.pdf (accessed on 12th June 2025).

33. DeGaetano, A., Ferrara, A., De, A. G., Hayes, A., Topp, B., Athukorala, C., Knight-Agarwal, C. R., et al. (2019). Multi-scale simulation modeling for prevention and public health management of diabetes in pregnancy and sequelae. http://arxiv.org/abs/1905.02552 (accessed on 12th June 2025).

34. Dirtu, A. C., Daly, A. F., Prahl, A. L., Wolfe, A., Capen, C. C., Reusch, C. E., Lamb, C. R., et al. (2015). Studying cat (*Felis catus*) diabetes: Beware of the acromegalic imposter. https://core.ac.uk/download/36778500.pdf (accessed on 12th June 2025).

35. Droste, S. K., Lightman, S. L., Linthorst, A. C. E., Qian, X., et al. (2012). Circadian and ultradian rhythms of free glucocorticoid hormone are highly synchronized between the blood, the subcutaneous tissue, and the brain. https://core.ac.uk/download/29026545.pdf (accessed on 12th June 2025).

36. Elliott-Sale, K. J., & Hackney, A. C. (2024). Female physiology–endocrinology: Education is lacking and innovation is needed! https://core.ac.uk/download/607977868.pdf (accessed on 12th June 2025).

37. Evans, J. A., Gasser, P. J., Klement, C., Kloehn, M., et al. (2016). Sexual differentiation of circadian clock function in the adrenal gland. https://core.ac.uk/download/213057608.pdf Kloehn, I., Pillai, S. B., Officer, L., Klement, C., Gasser, P. J., & Evans, J. A. (2016). Sexual Differentiation of Circadian Clock Function in the Adrenal Gland. *Endocrinology, 157*(5), 1895–1904. https://doi.org/10.1210/en.2015-1968 (accessed on 12th June 2025).

38. Gonzalez Deniselle, M. C., Lara, H. E., Recabarren, S. E., Roselli, C. E., et al. (2016). Developmental and functional effects of steroid hormones on the neuroendocrine axis and spinal cord. https://core.ac.uk/download/159294623.pdf (accessed on 12th June 2025).

39. Helner, N., Makukh, H., Prokopchuk, N., Sharhorodska, Y., et al. (2019). Medical genetic counseling of women with congenital heart diseases of fetus. https://core.ac.uk/download/301580705.pdf (accessed on 12th June 2025).

40. Kakcya, T., Masui, T., Oomizu, S., Sharma, R., et al. (2003). Gene expression and the physiological role of transforming growth factor-α in the mouse pituitary. https://core.ac.uk/download/12533839.pdf (accessed on 12th June 2025).

41. Laddad, M., et al. (2023). Recent advances in reproductive endocrinology: Implications for fertility treatment in gynecology. https://core.ac.uk/download/596247493.pdf (accessed on 12th June 2025).

42. Mehltretter, G., Mojto, J., Müller, O. A., Reichardt, H. M., et al. (1996). The decrease in growth hormone (GH) response after repeated stimulation with GH-releasing hormone is partly caused by an elevation of somatostatin tonus. https://core.ac.uk/download/12175988.pdf (accessed on 12th June 2025).

43. Mishra, A. (2024). *Gamma Cameras: Exploring the Technology, Applications, and Future Prospects*. https://core.ac.uk/download/617006397.pdf (accessed on 12th June 2025).

44. Potts, J. T. (2025). The control of calcium metabolism by parathyroid hormone, calcitonin and vitamin D. https://core.ac.uk/download/pdf/42878870.pdf (accessed on 12th June 2025).

45. Silva, Y. P., Bernardi, A., & Frozza, R. L. (2020). The role of short-chain fatty acids from gut microbiota in gut-brain communication. *Frontiers in Endocrinology, 11*. https://doi.org/10.3389/fendo.2020.00025 (accessed on 12th June 2025).

46. Slee, A. D. (2012). Exploring metabolic dysfunction in chronic kidney disease. https://core.ac.uk/download/17352998.pdf (accessed on 12th June 2025).

47. Steinhart, E. (2001). Persons versus brains: Biological intelligence in human organisms. https://core.ac.uk/download/287611886.pdf (accessed on 12th June 2025).

48. Sulthana, A. G. (2018). *Study of Incidence and Patterns of Adrenal Hemorrhage in All Death Cases*. https://core.ac.uk/download/235668558.pdf (accessed on 12th June 2025).

49. Syed Iqbal, S. (2016). A clinical study on the dermatological manifestations of obesity. https://core.ac.uk/download/235662077.pdf (accessed on 12th June 2025).

TECHNIQUES IN BIOCHEMISTRY

10

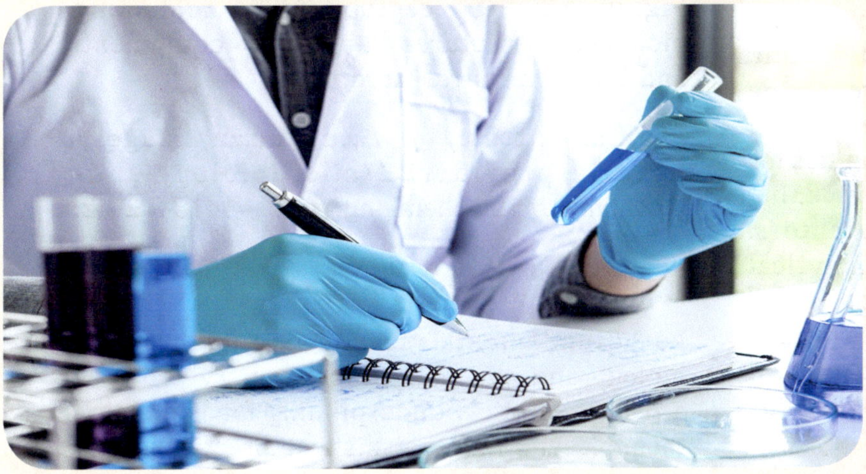

LEARNING OBJECTIVES

After studying this chapter, you will be able to:

1. Describe the principles and types of chromatography;
2. Learn about spectroscopic techniques;
3. Understand the electrophoresis;
4. Describe the mass spectrometry;
5. Know the process of molecular cloning.

Introduction

Biochemistry is a scientific discipline at the intersection of biology and chemistry, involving the molecular mechanisms that determine various biological processes. Description of such intricate biochemical processes involves the application of various methods that facilitate comprehension of biomolecules' structure, function, and interaction. These range from traditional methods , such as spectroscopy and chromatography to more recent technologies , such as NMR spectroscopy and mass spectrometry, each with its own specific use and benefit. The complexities of biological processes generally necessitate an interdisciplinary framework, with different techniques utilized in succession in the process of obtaining an integrated understanding of metabolic pathways, enzyme kinetics, and cell signaling. Such basic principles are essential to both fundamental research and applied endeavors, such as drug development and diagnostics, and thus mastery of these techniques is crucial for future biochemists. Recent advances have revolutionized the application of analytical techniques in biochemistry to make studies more efficient and accurate. For instance, NMR spectroscopy is now a handy tool in the study of solute dynamics across fluid biphasic systems. Utilizing spatially resolved NMR methods , such as spatially resolved saturation transfer difference NMR (SR-STD NMR), researchers can track exchange of solutes between immiscible phases and probe mechanisms underneath. These new techniques not only increase the scientific understanding of complex biochemical interactions but also bring new opportunities for utilization, such as pharmacological screening of binding agents to biological receptors. The ongoing evolution of such analytical tools is a significant milestone in the field, enabling scientists to overcome previously insurmountable hurdles in biochemical investigation, with far-reaching implications for various applications. In biochemistry, one must integrate novel technologies to defeat the drawbacks of traditional biophysical methods. Recent studies of epigenetics and proteomics illustrate the power of these fields to change biochemical profiling methods. For example, epigenetic biomarkers have been potential agents for measuring donors' ages and separating genetically equivalent twins, offering tangible utility in forensic investigation and other areas. In addition, enhanced mass spectrometry techniques enable complete biological sample analyses without genetic material degradation. Such investigations enhance the discriminating power of biochemical techniques, hence providing precise experimental outcomes. While the demand for more advanced procedures continues to grow, ongoing research in these areas is essential in meeting the evolving demands of biochemistry, reflecting the dynamic process nature of this ever-expanding discipline (Figure 10.1).

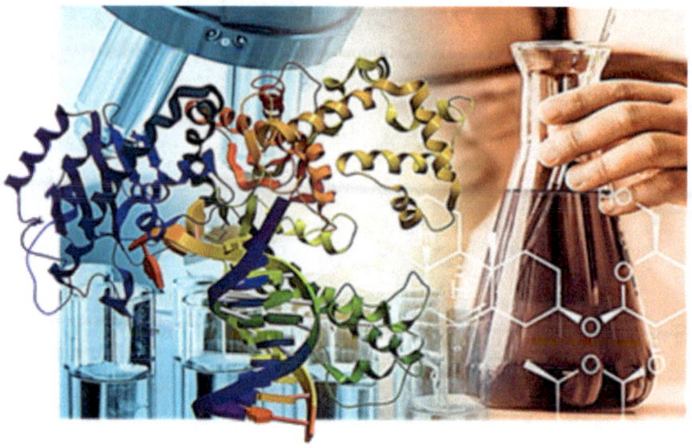

Figure 10.1. Conceptual image combining molecular structures, laboratory equipment, and biochemical research.

Source: https://www.ufs.ac.za/images/librariesprovider22/microbiology-and-biochemistry/biochem.png?sfvrsn=44184820_2.

Definition of Biochemistry

As a fundamental science sitting between biology and chemistry, biochemistry provides a firm theoretical underpinning for explaining the molecular mechanisms that direct biological occurrences. Employing a variety of approaches and techniques to study the chemical nature of cell functions, biochemistry enables scientists to probe the intricate webs of metabolism, enzyme activity, and gene expression. The relevance of biochemistry extends beyond theoretical knowledge; its applications are critical in medicine, genetics, and pharmacology. Through the explanation of biomolecules' structure and function, biochemistry gives scientists the means to manipulate biological systems and develop new remedies for health conditions. So, the definition of biochemistry as the study of chemical processes occurring and associated with living organisms not only indicates its importance but also points to its role as a foundation for the advancement of scientific inquiry and application. The study of biochemical principles typically entails the use of some of the various experimental approaches that show the discipline's multifaceted nature. Techniques , such as chromatography, mass spectrometry, and nuclear magnetic resonance (NMR) spectrometry allow analysis of biomolecules at atomic and molecular levels to identify and quantify metabolites, proteins, and nucleic acids. Additionally, the development of computationally based techniques and statistical treatment, including the modeling of estrogen receptor protein dimerization, proves the significance of mathematical techniques in biochemistry. Such modeling not only facilitates the understanding of kinetic parameters but also enhances the predictive capability of biochemistry in application contexts, particularly in drug discovery and development. Such diverse methods as a whole enrich the toolkit of biochemists and therefore encourage innovative research activities. The definition of biochemistry is further complemented by its application contexts in confronting global challenges, particularly in biotechnology. The biotechnology sector, as exemplified by what is occurring in New Zealand, demonstrates the contribution of biochemistry to innovation across various sectors. The use of biochemistry in biotechnology produces progress founded on available natural assets and creates new comparative advantages across sectors like agriculture and medicine. Furthermore, networks and institutional support are also central in the development of innovation in biochemistry because the collaboration of stakeholders, including government, industry, and researchers, is essential in the process of translating fundamental biochemical research into applied use. Understanding these dynamics not only broadens the domain of biochemistry as a discipline but also underscores its crucial contribution to societal advancement and the international economy, as is evident with research into innovation processes in this field at the moment (Marsh et al., 2000) (Figure 10.2).

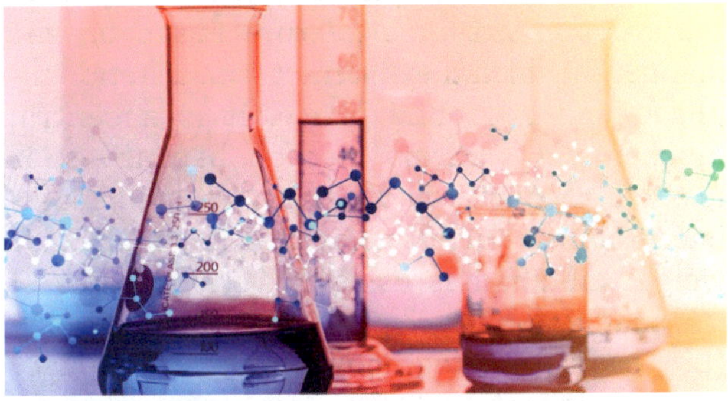

Figure 10.2. Biochemistry.

Source: https://medicalbuyer.co.in/wp-content/uploads/2022/06/Biochemistry_870x470.jpg.

10.1. Chromatography

Learning Outcome

1. Know the principles of chromatography;
2. Describe the types of chromatography;
3. Understand the applications in protein and nucleic acid separation.

As one of the central analytical methods in biochemistry, chromatography entails a set of analytical techniques applied to separate the components of a mixture based on the manner in which they interact with a stationary phase and a mobile phase. It is a central biochemical analysis method because it is feasible to purify and measure biomolecules like proteins, nucleic acids, and low molecular weight metabolites using it. Various types of chromatography, such as liquid chromatography (LC), gas chromatography (GC), and thin-layer chromatography (TLC), each serve specific purposes. For instance, LC is particularly useful in separating large biomolecules that would be destroyed upon heating, while GC can deal with volatile compounds. The effectiveness of the methods makes chromatography a valued instrument in research and clinical laboratories, where it is applied not only for the identification of compounds but also for the development of new drugs and the investigation of complex biological processes. The operation of chromatography relies on differential partitioning between phases, which can be simply explained by mathematical models and computer simulations. In the majority of cases, such systems are described by nonlinear differential equations with unknown parameters, and therefore it's impossible to analyze the corresponding chromatographic data. The models are crucial for getting information about retention times and separation efficiencies, which guide the optimization of experimental conditions. A prime example is the study of estrogen receptor protein dimerization, where mathematical calculation of parameters extracted from chromatographic data can inform the planning of future experiments (Goulet et al., 2015). By making optimal use of good analytical practice and sophisticated simulations, scientists are better able to maximize the precision of kinetic parameter estimates and hence, gain greater insight into biochemical processes and enable the improvement of biotechnological applications.

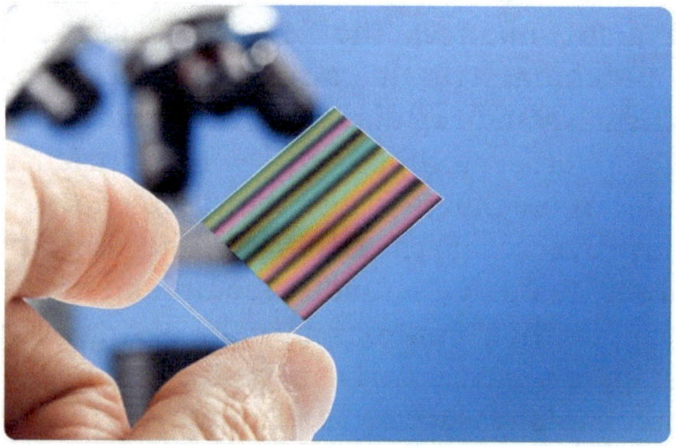

Figure 10.3. Chromatography.

Source: https://www.news-medical.net/image-handler/ts/20160809015332/ri/590/picture/2016/8/Chromatography_shutterstock_170923289.jpg.

Moreover, progress in chromatography techniques has significantly increased the sensitivity and selectivity of analysis. For instance, gas chromatography-isotope ratio mass spectrometry (GC-C-IRMS) has been a useful technique to analyze nitrogen cycling in a range of different ecosystems. It offers precise quantification of the nitrogen isotopic ratio, which is significant for distinguishing ecological and biochemical processes. Through techniques like solid phase microextraction (SPME) and purge and trap (P&T), researchers can effectively concentrate analytes to the point of being able to detect trace levels of compounds like ammonium and glycine in environmental samples (Norlin et al., 2005). The evolution of such techniques not only raises quantification abilities but also the scope of biochemical study, rendering chromatography a key component in scientific inquiry and environmental monitoring (Figure 10.3).

10.1.1. Principles of Chromatography

Chromatography is a core technique in biochemistry, and it is an important method of separation and analysis of complex mixtures of biomolecules. Chromatography fundamentally involves differential partitioning between two phases: a stationary phase and a mobile phase. The effectiveness of this separation is governed by many variables including the size, charge, and hydrophobicity of the molecules. For instance, techniques , such as high-performance liquid chromatography (HPLC) and GC utilize these principles to separate proteins, peptides, nucleic acids, and other biomolecules, allowing subsequent quantification and characterization. Chromatography's versatility is illustrated by its complementarity with mass spectrometry, where elucidation of protein structure and function is complemented by softer separation techniques, resulting in advances in proteomics and other areas of biochemistry (Rabilloud et al., 2009). One of the remarkable aspects of chromatography in biochemistry is its capacity to be customized for specific analytical purposes. Various chromatographic techniques, such as ion-exchange chromatography and affinity chromatography, require varying conditions for separation. For example, affinity chromatography allows for the purification of target biomolecules based on specific interactions with immobilized ligands and plays a crucial role in isolating proteins with unique binding specificity. Ion-exchange chromatography, in contrast, utilizes charge characteristics of biomolecules to achieve separation and enables research on protein isoforms or modifications. These modern methods are of critical significance in the era of personalized medicine, wherein understanding biomolecular interactions at the molecular level can provide more effective therapeutic interventions. Advancement and refinement of these chromatography techniques are critical in the evolution of biochemistry as a field and in furthering our understanding of complex biological systems. Finally, the integration of chromatography with new and novel analytical tools has profoundly enhanced its place in biochemistry. The partnership between chromatography and mass spectrometry, for instance, is a timeless example of how these tools can work together to elicit nuanced information about biomolecular composition and structure. For the analysis of proteins, chromatography is an analytical stepwise predecessor, enabling efficient purification of proteins before mass spectrometric analysis. This is significant, as protein mixtures are often so intricate that to need a multi-step approach for the data to lead to simplicity. Additionally, advances , such as capillary electrophoresis (CE) have more separation capability, particularly with small biomolecules , such as creatinine. The ability to eliminate interferences associated with traditional methods, such as in the determination of creatinine and creatine by CE, emphasizes ongoing progress and diversification of chromatographic techniques (Guo et al., 1998) (Figure 10.4).

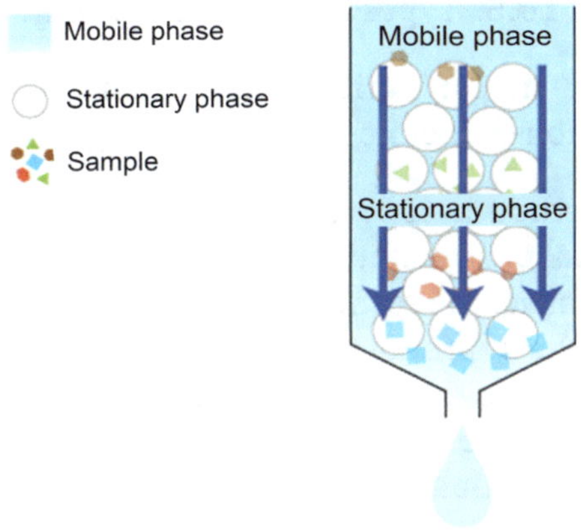

Figure 10.4. Principles of chromatography.

Source: https://ruo.mbl.co.jp/bio/e/support/method/images/chromatography-genri.png.

10.1.2. Types of Chromatography (e.g., HPLC, GC)

In biochemistry, chromatography is a basic analysis technique applied in the separation and analysis of complex mixtures. Among its various forms, HPLC is among the most widely utilized techniques. HPLC involves pumping the liquid solvent through a column packed with solid adsorbent material, where the components of the mixture are separated based on how they interact with the stationary phase. This technique is particularly appropriate for biomolecular analysis , such as proteins, nucleic acids, and low-molecular-weight metabolites, owing to its resolution and sensitivity. Moreover, HPLC can be equipped with a range of detectors, for instance, UV-Vis or fluorescence detectors, to allow for improved identification of specific analytes. Hence, the method has become pivotal in quality control, pharmacokinetics, and assessment of biological samples, which govern our understanding of biochemical processes. GC is one of the principal methods in chromatography, utilized primarily with volatile substances. Unlike HPLC, GC uses a gas as a mobile phase, typically an inert one , such as helium or nitrogen, to carry vaporized samples down a column. The stationary phase typically comprises a coated column that discriminates fractions based on boiling point and affinity for the stationary phase.

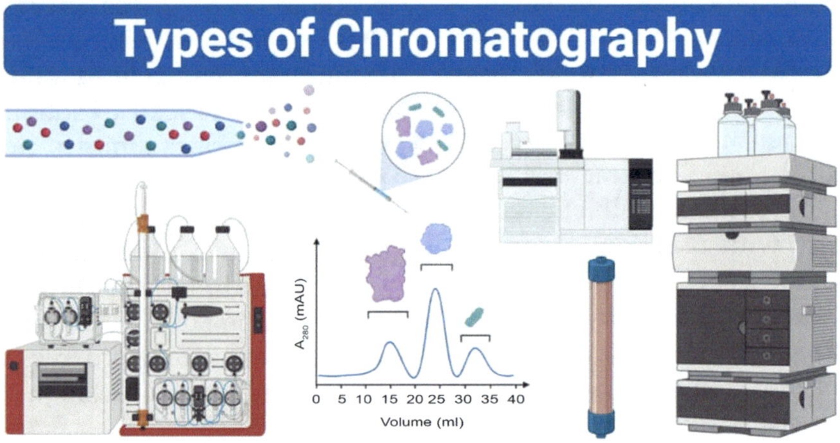

Figure 10.5. Types of chromatography.

Source: https://microbenotes.com/wp-content/uploads/2020/07/Types-of-Chromatography-Definition-Principle-Steps-Uses.jpeg.

The method is especially advantageous in the analysis of small organic molecules, fatty acids, and essential oils, providing rapid and accurate quantitation. The high-throughput nature and efficiency of GCs make the technology invaluable for various applications, including contaminant screening and metabolic byproduct analysis in environmental samples. Real-time analysis and quantitative capacity contribute to the value of GC in biochemistry, notably in toxicology and metabolic studies. Integration of newer chromatographic techniques in the study of biochemistry often calls for an explanation of their methodologies and comparative efficiency. Techniques , such as HPLC and GC have undergone advancements that enhance their performance, for instance, improved column technologies and more sensitive detectors. For instance, the development of supercritical fluid chromatography (SFC) combines the virtues of both HPLC and GC to effectively separate polar and non-polar compounds using less solvent. Additionally, methods involving the application of robust sample preparation techniques, e.g., solid-phase extraction (SPE), enhance recovery and purity of analytes to increase reliability and reproducibility in results obtained. These advances not only widen the range of chromatographic techniques but also transcend methodological biases in the measurement of biochemical characteristics. This combination of the newer methods facilitates the creation of more comprehensive profiles for substances to facilitate significant advancements in biomarker discovery and the measurement of oxidative stress by multi-angled analytical approaches, thereby enhancing biochemistry as elaborated in the academic literature (Azadmard-Damirchi et al., 2007; Marrocco et al., 2017) (Figure 10.5).

10.1.3. Applications in Protein and Nucleic Acid Separation

The applications of protein and nucleic acid separation techniques are at the core of the science of biochemistry, enabling significant studies to be carried out in molecular biology and biotechnology. From chromatography to electrophoresis, these techniques are applied for separating proteins and nucleic acids from multifarious biological mixtures. Apart from facilitating an improved understanding of molecular interactions, these techniques also purify samples for further uses, like sequencing, functional assays, and structural investigations. Progress in the separation processes continues to advance, with better specificity and efficiency, affecting therapeutic discovery and diagnostics. Advancements in electrochemical processes, particularly for protein-nucleic acid interaction, demonstrate their versatility and sensitivity, and highlight the need for further investigations and fine-tuning of these approaches in biochemical processes (Abi et al., 2015). Chromatography using resins like Sephadex G-200 illustrates a fundamental method of separation of biomolecules on the basis of size exclusion. Soluble fractions of rabbit liver homogenates, for example, showed distinct patterns of separation upon use of this technique in one recent study, marking a significant difference between liver and serum components. This size separation allows for the separation of various biomolecules like lipoproteins and nucleic acids that are crucial in establishing physiological and pathological states in living organisms. Additionally, conditions of experiments like the inclusion of ions during the separations have been discovered to affect the stability of the already-separated fractions. These resolution-level fractionation and analysis pave the way for further elucidation of cell processes and the effects of autolysis on compositional alteration in protein and nucleic acid fractions (Aizawa et al., 1966). Second, the study of protein-nucleic acid interactions by biophysical methods reveals the complex dynamics of biological systems. Techniques , such as affinity chromatography and surface plasmon resonance equip scientists with the analytical tools required to define these interactions at the molecular level, revealing transcriptional, replicational, and other vital processes. Coupling of such techniques with electrochemical tools heightens their sensitivity, enabling scientists to monitor binding reactions in real-time. As a result, the combination of these advanced biophysical methods is now capable of providing a complete understanding of protein-nucleic acid interactions, hence answering fundamental questions in biochemistry, such as gene regulation complexity and the development of effective therapeutic drugs (Abi et al., 2015).

Test Your Knowledge

1. What is the principle of chromatography?
2. What are the 2 types of chromatography?

10.2. Spectroscopy

Learning Outcome

1. Know the basics of spectroscopic techniques;
2. Describe the common spectroscopy methods;
3. Understand the role of spectroscopy in analyzing biomolecules.

Spectroscopy is a cornerstone technique within biochemistry, enabling researchers to investigate the molecular properties of biological systems through the observation of how molecules interact with different frequencies of electromagnetic radiation. Spectroscopy provides information on molecular structure, movement, and interaction through the observation of how molecules respond to different frequencies of electromagnetic radiation. Other techniques, like ultraviolet-visible (UV-Vis) spectroscopy and infrared (IR) spectroscopy, are commonly used to assess the conformation and activity of biomolecules like proteins and nucleic acids. In particular, UV-Vis spectroscopy is capable of monitoring protein folding and unfolding, and IR spectroscopy is capable of resolving secondary structures. The versatility of these techniques makes them suitable for application in varying experimental conditions, placing spectroscopy at the forefront in the field of biomolecular analysis. Its ability to furnish information that can be quantitatively analyzed further adds to its significance in biochemical research, modifying its application for accurate study of various studies that are seeking deeper insight into biomolecular interactions. In addition to traditional methods, the newer spectroscopic applications, i.e., Raman and fluorescence spectroscopies, are more commonly used in biochemistry for their specificity and sensitivity. For instance, Raman spectroscopy, particularly with carbon nanotube conjugation, is capable of interrogating protein conformation with minimal perturbation of the surrounding matrix. The immobilization of the protein on the carbon nanotubes, as described in biocompatible literature, retains significant native function and structure necessary to maintain biological activity under experimental conditions (Shah et al., 2009). The new approach not only improves the reusability and stability of the protein conjugates but also allows extensive characterization of molecular-level interactions using spectroscopic techniques. Using these advanced spectroscopic methods, researchers can deconvolute complex biochemical processes with greater precision.

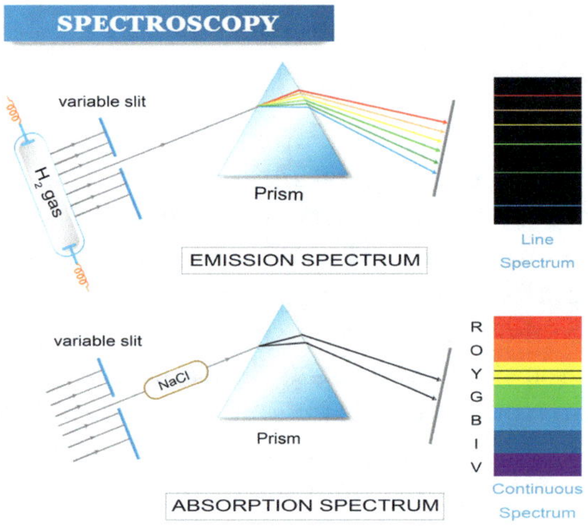

Figure 10.6. Spectroscopy.

Source: https://www.priyamstudycentre.com/wp-content/uploads/2022/11/Spectroscopy-definition-absorption-and-emission-types-of-electromagnetic-spectra-or-spectrum.png.

Chemical imaging is an emerging field for the application of spectroscopy to biochemistry wherein spatial and spectral data from a sample may be recorded simultaneously. Techniques , such as near-infrared (NIR) and IR chemical imaging allow for visual examination of biomolecular distributions and properties in tissues or cellular microenvironments (Baianu, 2011). These methods have numerous applications across various fields, ranging from medicine to agriculture, enhancing our ability to visualize biochemical processes in real-time. These developments demonstrate the marriage of spectroscopy with imaging sciences, allowing us greater insight into the spatial structure of biomolecules and their functional implications. With their improving sensitivity and resolution, these techniques are capable of reshaping our understanding of biological systems and the complex interactions between them, potentially leading to more successful therapeutic strategies and diagnostic tools in biochemistry (Figure 10.6).

10.2.1. Basics of Spectroscopic Techniques

Spectroscopic techniques have evolved as crucial tools of biochemistry whereby scientists can examine molecular structure and interactions in complex biological systems. Simply put, spectroscopy is the interaction of matter with light, where scientists can probe the electronic, vibrational, and rotational states of molecules. Techniques , such as UV-Vis, IR, and NMR spectroscopy provide us with information regarding the behavior and composition of molecules. For instance, UV-Vis spectroscopy is essential for the determination of biomolecule concentration, while IR spectroscopy is able to distinguish functional groups through vibrational transitions.

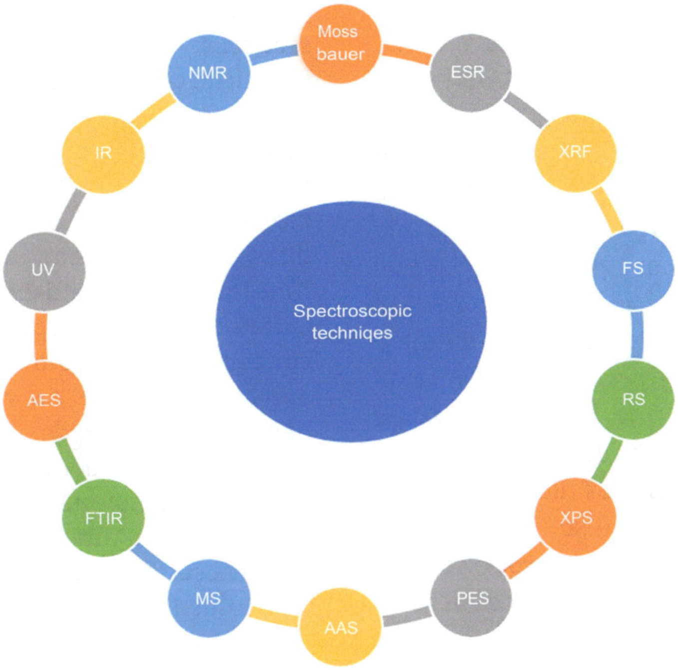

Figure 10.7. Spectroscopic techniques.

Source: https://scienceinfo.com/wp-content/uploads/2023/08/image-160.png.

The high sensitivity and versatility of these tools are critical in biochemical pathway and process investigation, thereby widening basic research and clinical application. Of significance is the fact that advanced spectroscopic techniques have proven the astoundingly great promises in medical diagnostics and treatment monitoring. A good illustration is the application of diffuse optical spectroscopic imaging (DOSI), which provides a new way of tracking treatment response in breast cancer therapy. Differing from traditional imaging methods, which are more likely to observe changes in tumor size following prolonged treatment, DOSI can quantify biophysical properties like hemoglobin concentration in real-time (Torjesen, 2016). This discussion has identified an ability to measure early response to neoadjuvant chemotherapy, using optical methods , such as DOSI, which provides valuable information that can inform treatment planning interventions. This non-invasive nature of optical methods , such as DOSI, not only offers increased patient comfort but also an opportunity for more individualized health care strategy, consistent with the current trends in precision medicine. Furthermore, glycosaminoglycan (GAG) research is another new frontier where spectroscopic techniques can uncover the complexities of carbohydrate-based biopolymers. The chemistry of glycosaminoglycans (GAGs) with variation in sulfation and epimerization renders characterization especially demanding. Recent developments in IR action spectroscopy have opened up new avenues in interrogating these complex molecules. Applying cryogenic IR spectroscopy to ion isolated in helium nanodroplets has yielded resolved and detailed spectra that are yielding precious information on sulfation patterns and monosaccharide composition (Freyse et al., 2020). This information not only improves the biochemical understanding of GAGs but also informs their roles in physiological and disease processes and therefore illuminates the impact of spectroscopic methods on basic and applied biochemistry (Figure 10.7).

10.2.2. Common Spectroscopy Methods (e.g., UV-Vis, NMR)

Spectroscopic methods are fundamental tools in biochemistry, allowing scientists to investigate molecular dynamics and structure effectively. Among the most frequently used methods is UV-Vis spectroscopy, which measures the absorbance of ultraviolet or visible light by a substance. The method is valuable in nucleic acid and protein quantitation as their aromatic amino acid and base chromophores possess specific absorbance characteristics. By relating absorbance data to concentration by the Beer-Lambert's law, researchers are able to measure the concentration of a range of biomolecules dissolved in solution. In addition, UV-Vis spectroscopy provides fast, trustworthy measurements and is therefore invaluable in enzyme kinetics as well as in metabolic research. The simplicity and effectiveness of the method allow for its widespread use in a variety of biochemical assays and thus our comprehension of living systems. NMR spectroscopy is yet another cornerstone in the biochemist's toolkit, providing high-resolution data on molecular structure and dynamics. NMR enables the identification of the three-dimensional atom arrangement in a molecule through the magnetic properties of atomic nuclei. In particular, NMR is well-suited for the study of complex biomolecules , such as proteins and nucleic acids dissolved in solution, since it can follow real-time interactions and conformational change. For instance, NMR can reveal intricate information concerning molecular dynamics, interactions, and conformations, for which reason it is of great pertinence in drug design and structural biology. Even more embracing innovative methods, such as two-dimensional NMR, have increased the resolution and interpretability of this technique, thus securing its position in demystifying biomolecular complexities and interactions crucial in biochemical research and applications. The application of spectroscopy is not merely UV-Vis and NMR and includes different methods that are appropriate for specific analysis needs in biochemistry. Molecular vibrations enable the identification of functional groups by IR spectroscopy, and Mass Spectrometry (MS) is unmatched in terms of precision in the determination of molecular masses and structure elucidation. Additionally, studies of mono-N-acyl derivatives of 2,6-diaminopimelic acid are an example of cooperation between various spectroscopic techniques, wherein IR and NMR were used to determine structural features and purity determination using CE methods (Buděšínský et al., 2014). Such mixed methodologies enable researchers to study biochemical processes as a whole, fitting their method to the individual requirements of each experimental condition. As these techniques are further developed, their use in biochemistry has the potential to increasingly uncover the intricate mechanisms behind biological systems as well as aid in our abilities within related research fields (Figure 10.8).

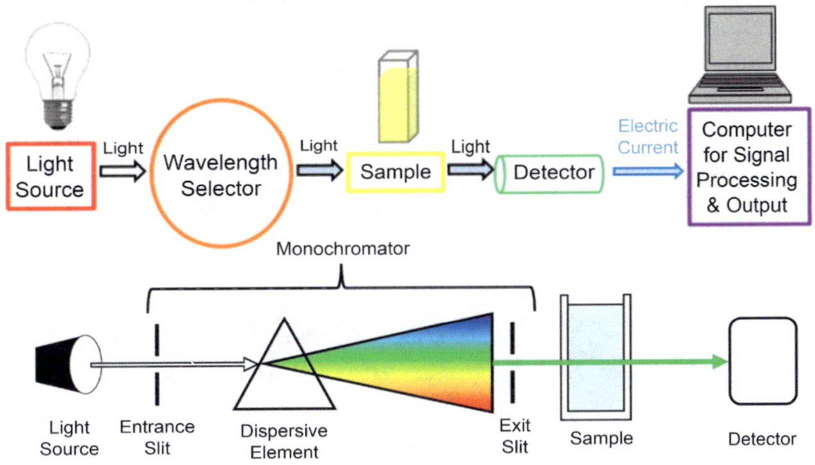

Figure 10.8. UV-spectroscopy.

Source: https://biologynotesonline.com/wp-content/uploads/2024/03/UV-Spectroscopy-Principle-Instruments-Applications.jpeg.

10.2.3. Role of Spectroscopy in Analyzing Biomolecules

Spectroscopy applied to biomolecular research is a cornerstone in biochemistry, yielding information regarding structural and conformational dynamics that are pertinent to biochemical processes. Of all the spectroscopic techniques, Raman optical activity (ROA) has been found to be a useful instrument as it is sensitive to chirality. This method detects vibrational scattering differences of biomolecules in circularly polarized light, and it provides informative information regarding secondary structures, folding motifs, and intermolecular interactions in nucleic acids and proteins. The development of ROA as a mainstream biomolecular science, as indicated by its first findings in the late 1980s, highlights the growing relevance of the method to uncover intricate structures in a biological framework. With advances in instrumentation, ROA is now standard, which allows scientists to unravel solution structural intricacies of biomolecules without crystallization (Barron et al., 2015). Spectroscopy also has application in the identification of energy landscapes of biomolecules, revealing important mechanisms involved in molecular interaction and stability. Single-molecule mechanical unfolding experiments, for example, use optical tweezers to interrogate energy landscapes of proteins in real time. Through modulation of temperature during the process of unfolding, researchers are able to measure the roughness of such landscapes and also obtain information about possible energy barriers and transition states that control biomolecular behavior. Such measurement is crucial for understanding how forces influence biomolecular stability and function. Interestingly, this does not hold for proteins only; similar principles carry over to RNA and other biomolecules, with a broader understanding of biological systems coming from it. The convergence of theoretical models and experimental measurement constitutes an effective analysis of the behavior of biomolecules under various conditions, unveiling complexities that had previously been difficult to unravel (Hyeon et al., 2006). Convergence between biochemistry and various spectroscopic techniques highlights their joint contribution to advancing the understanding of biomolecular mechanisms and structures. By examination of specific details , such as structural conformations, energy landscapes, and intermolecular interactions, spectroscopy allows scientists to study biomolecular behavior. This is particularly pertinent in drug design and protein engineering, where the physical chemistry of biomolecules can inform treatment. In addition, evolutionary adaptations and improvements in spectroscopic technology continue to make them more useful, allowing scientists to view biological phenomenon from an even closer perspective. As the technology continues to advance, the union of spectroscopy and computational modeling will continue to improve the understanding of biomolecular dynamics, paving the way for great advances in biochemistry and related sciences (Hyeon et al., 2006; Barron et al., 2015).

Test Your Knowledge

1. What is a spectroscopic technique?
2. What is the role of spectroscopy in analyzing biomolecules?

10.3. Electrophoresis

Learning Outcome

1. Know the fundamentals of electrophoresis;
2. Describe the types of electrophoresis;
3. Describe the use of advanced techniques in DNA and protein analysis.

Electrophoresis, the axial technique of biochemistry separation, exploits the movement of charged substances in an electric field. Electrophoresis is a technique of major significance in biomolecule identification as a protein separation technique as well as a tool for nucleic acid and other charged molecule separations based on size, charge, and shape. Gel electrophoresis, the most common variation, employs a gel matrix that facilitates the movement of molecules; the smaller molecules travel through the gel more quickly than large ones, and effective separation is realized. The applications are extensive, with uses , such as protein purity analysis and molecular weight determination, both critical to both research and medical settings. Further, the combination of electrophoresis with mass spectrometry has transformed protein research to allow for thorough characterization and identification of complex proteomes to emphasize its status in modern biochemical research (Rabilloud et al., 2009). Electrophoresis extends beyond the basic separation processes to encompass highly sophisticated techniques that offer improved resolution and specificity. Techniques , such as isoelectric focusing (IEF) and two-dimensional electrophoresis (2-DE) allow proteins to be separated according to size and charge. IEF exploits the unique isoelectric point (pI) of each protein, whereby they have no net charge, allowing for a highly sensitive separation. 2-DE utilizes IEF in combination with SDS-PAGE to yield comprehensive analysis of complex mixtures of proteins. These advanced methods not only increase the accuracy of proteomic studies but also enable the identification of PTMs, thereby enhancing knowledge of protein function and regulation. Thus, the versatility of electrophoresis solidifies its role as a core technique in biochemistry (Azrolan et al., 1994). Furthermore, the evolution of novel electrophoretic methods continues to revolutionize biochemistry practice, opening up new areas of creative research protocols. Electrophoresis techniques are being constructed for high-throughput analysis more and more, which allows for the simultaneous analysis of several samples, thereby streamlining experimental procedures. Furthermore, advances in microfluidics are introducing electrophoretic principles into miniaturized devices that allow for rapid analysis with incredibly small amounts of samples. This precision and automation trend in electrophoresis not only streamlines experimental procedures but introduces higher-level biochemical analysis to the masses as well. As researchers dig deeper into the intricacy of biomolecular functions and interactions, the ongoing improvement of electrophoresis remains a vital tool for releasing new scientific information and therapeutic drugs in biochemistry (Figure 10.9).

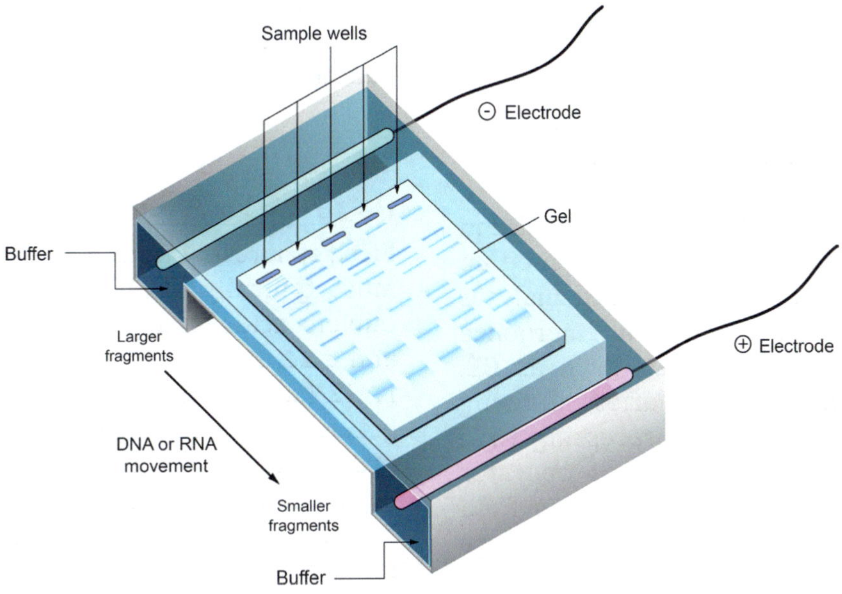

Figure 10.9. Electrophoresis.

Source: https://www.genome.gov/sites/default/files/media/images/tg/Electrophoriesis.jpg.

10.3.1. Fundamentals of Electrophoresis

The mechanism of electrophoresis relies on the movement of charged species in a medium by an electric field. The method of separation takes advantage of charge-to-mass differences of biomolecules to facilitate efficient separation of proteins, nucleic acids, and other macromolecules. A very common medium utilized is a gel composed of agarose or polyacrylamide that introduces a sieving effect. As molecules travel, their size and charge control how fast they go; smaller and more charged molecules travel faster than larger or less charged molecules. This is a vital rule for biochemists since the technique is applied widely in several subfields like proteomics and genetics to clean compounds and examine complicated mixtures. Therefore, the fundamental knowledge sets the foundation for the higher-level specific applications to deliver reliable and reproducible results in experimental scenarios. Two-dimensional gel electrophoresis is founded on the fundamental principles of classical electrophoresis with the incorporation of an additional dimension, i.e., IEF before molecular weight-based separation. First-dimensional separation separates proteins based on their isoelectric point, i.e., the pH value at which they carry no net charge. This is followed by the second dimension, where the proteins are separated by SDS-PAGE, allowing subsequent separation based on size. Application of these two in combination creates a total profiling of multi-protein mixtures, with greater information being yielded than with one-dimensional techniques. This meticulous examination is useful in various applications , such as disease biomarkers, analysis of protein expression, and PTMs. This degree of analysis can be crucial to the understanding of biological processes and the design of medical interventions, demonstrating the breadth and utility of 2-DE in biochemistry. Recent advances have opened up new avenues for electrophoresis-based analyses of biology and chemistry with the emergence of electrophoresis technologies, such as CE. CE separates in narrow capillaries, allowing higher resolution and faster processing than conventional gel electrophoresis. It operates on the same theory, using the electric field to drive the movement of analyte by charge and size. Portable CE systems have also been created, enabling field-based analysis capable of being utilized for water quality analysis, drug discovery, and counter-terrorism strategies through the identification of explosive substance. Portable platforms fuel the capability for in-situ analysis, creating the potential for real-time application in most industries. In the face of continuous innovation in electrophoresis, it is increasingly important for scientists to address challenges in system design and functionality to enable these methods to be effectively applied in response to continuing needs in biochemical analysis and research (Palhinhas, 2011; Lewis et al., 2013) (Figure 10.10).

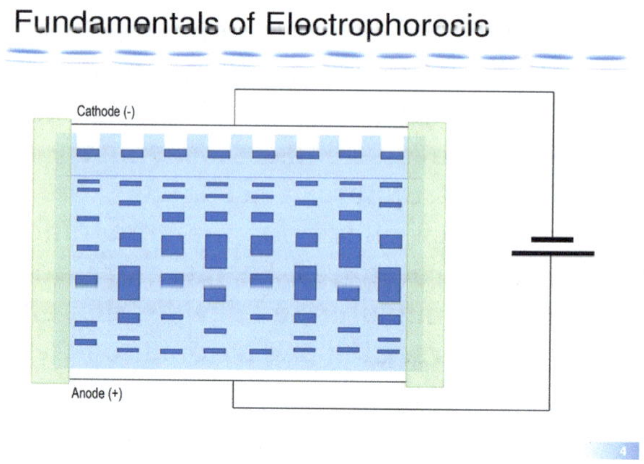

Figure 10.10. Fundamentals of electrophoresis.

Source: https://slideplayer.com/slide/16720489/97/images/4/Fundamentals+of+Electrophoresis.jpg.

10.3.2. Types of Electrophoresis (e.g., SDS-PAGE, Agarose)

Electrophoresis is a basic biochemistry technique, most typically applied to the separation of nucleic acids and proteins based on charge and size. Among electrophoresis types, SDS-PAGE (sodium dodecyl sulfate polyacrylamide gel electrophoresis) is notable as a technique of protein denaturation, facilitating standardized separation by molecular weight alone. In this method, proteins are treated with SDS, which imparts to them a charge directly proportional to their size so that when an electric field is applied, larger molecules migrate more slowly in the polyacrylamide gel compared to smaller molecules. This technique not only provides straightforward analysis and comparison of protein samples but also plays a crucial role in applications , such as the measurement of protein preparation purity and the analysis of protein expression levels in laboratory and medical research. Agarose gel electrophoresis, however, is most typically used for nucleic acid separations, particularly DNA and RNA. The gel is composed of agarose; a polysaccharide derived from seaweed that forms a network with pores through which nucleic acids can diffuse when an electric current is applied. The nucleic acid mass-to-charge ratio allows fragments of smaller size to travel faster through the gel than large fragments. This technique is central to applications like DNA fragment analysis for genetics, cloning, and forensics. Better resolution with agarose allows researchers to observe separate bands corresponding to different DNA fragments, and thus it is an effective tool for the interpretation of genetic architecture, mutation, and other applications in molecular biology. In addition, electrophoresis modifications , such as two-dimensional gel electrophoresis, make it more valuable by allowing proteins to be separated simultaneously based on both their isoelectric point and molecular weight. This is a holistic methodology that includes the complete analysis of the protein composition of a sample to facilitate the identification of isoforms and PTMs. Additionally, new techniques, such as the electrochemical detection of DNA ligase activity depicted in the most recent studies, reveal the intricate uses of electrophoresis in molecular-level understanding of biological processes. By merging electrophoretic technique with advanced analysis techniques, researchers can gain insights into higher-level biochemical processes for basic and applied sciences (Anderson et al., 1982; Vacek et al., 2008) (Figure 10.11).

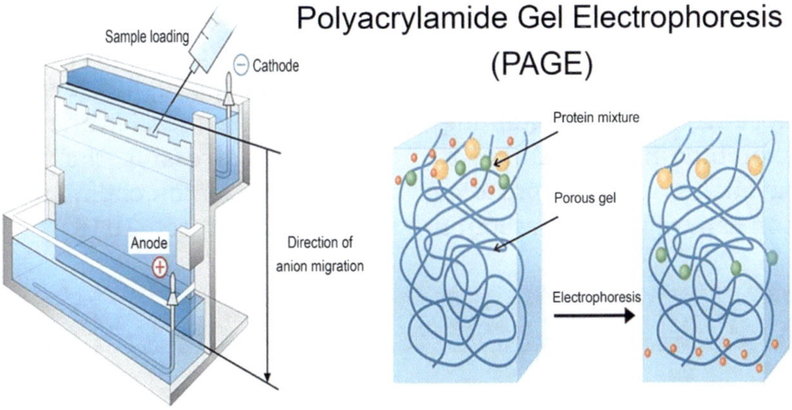

Figure 10.11. Polyacrylamide gel electrophoresis (PAGE).

Source: https://microbenotes.com/wp-content/uploads/2018/10/Polyacrylamide-Gel-Electrophoresis-PAGE.jpg.

10.3.3. Use in DNA and Protein Analysis

The use of new technology in DNA analysis has emerged as a signature aspect of modern biochemistry, providing tools for many purposes along the range from forensic science to specific therapy. Modern techniques of DNA profiling, although revolutionary, lack certain inherent limitations, particularly in terms of identifying very closely related genetic profiles. Recent studies in epigenetics offer promising possibilities for refinement. For instance, epigenetic biomarkers have demonstrated the ability to predict the age of biological samples or even differentiate between monozygotic twins, which would significantly increase the resolution of DNA evidence in forensic analysis. As pressure is increasing for more effective genetic analysis techniques, research focused on overcoming the limitations of current DNA profiling methods will prove to be vital. Further research in the fields of epigenetics and proteomics can lead to more robust methodologies, which can strengthen forensic evidence and its application in the legal process (Eilerts, 2016). Concurrently, the field of protein analysis has also benefited significantly from new biotechnological advances, especially with the development of aptamers. These oligonucleotide ligands, either single-stranded DNA or RNA, are selectively designed for high-affinity interaction with a broad range of molecular targets, including proteins. Aptamer-protein interaction characterization is significant, though to date, this has primarily been the concern of the majority of previous studies without elaborating on structural or biochemical understanding of these interactions. Knowledge extension in this area promises to release new potential applications in the field of biochemistry, like targeted drug delivery and biomarker identification. In addition, protein-aptamer complex crystallization is an area of research that continues to be committed to discovering these complex interactions with even more precision. Advances in the discipline can contribute to a more accurate understanding of the mechanisms for binding, continuing to expand the toolset available to study proteins (Baugh et al., 2012). In general, the intersection of newer tools in DNA and protein analysis is at the center of progressing biochemistry. The convergence of newer approaches , such as epigenetic profiling, with the development of aptamer-mediated interactions demonstrates the continually changing nature of the field. Not only do these advances enhance our understanding of genetic and proteomic landscapes, but they are also central to practical applications , such as forensic analysis and therapeutic identification. Continuing research in these fields is important, as it has the potential to enhance existing methods, develop new analytical instruments, and use these advances in a variety of biochemistry areas. While researchers proceed with the quest for increased discriminative power in DNA analysis and more advanced interaction studies at the higher level in protein research, the social and scientific implications are far-reaching, stressing the necessity for ongoing investment in biochemistry research (Baugh et al., 2012; Eilerts, 2016).

Test Your Knowledge

1. List the types of electrophoresis.
2. What are the techniques used in DNA analysis?

10.4. Mass Spectrometry

Learning Outcome

1. Give an overview of mass spectrometry principles;
2. Describe the mass spectrometry techniques;
3. Know the applications of metabolomics and proteomics.

Mass spectrometry (MS) is a major biochemistry technique, primarily due to its unparalleled ability to examine complex biomolecules with high sensitivity and specificity. The analytical technique operates by ionizing chemical species and discriminating between the ions based on their mass-to-charge ratio. The key components of a mass spectrometer are the ion source, mass analyzer, and detector, each having a crucial role to play in generating and quantifying molecular information. Depending on the ionization technique used, i.e., electrospray ionization (ESI) and matrix-assisted laser desorption/ionization (MALDI), researchers can now analyze an extremely wide range of biomolecules from low-mass metabolites to high-mass proteins, rendering mass spectrometry an invaluable tool in proteomics and metabolomics. Consequently, it has found invaluable use in the field of drug development, disease diagnosis, and deciphering metabolic pathways, making it a crucial aspect in contemporary biochemistry. Apart from its use in identifying and quantifying biomolecules, mass spectrometry also provides information on molecular structures using tandem mass spectrometry (MS/MS) methods. MS/MS comprises several sequential steps in mass analysis, with the ability to detail the fragmentation of ions, which assists in revealing structural details. This capability finds most value in establishing complex biomolecular architecture, such as that involved in protein PTM. As researchers strive to establish the complex networks of biochemical signaling and regulation, mass spectrometry is a tool with which to study the dynamics of such activity at the molecular level. As data analysis and instrumentation improve, mass spectrometry advances further, broadening frontiers of the scientifically feasible in the exploration of biomolecules and their interactions within living organisms. The growing applications of mass spectrometry follow an expanding quantity of literature bearing witness to its extensive set of applications within various disciplines, including forensic science, as evidenced by recent scientometric testimony. By examining publication trends associated with particular analytical techniques, researchers are able to measure the impact of mass spectrometry across disciplines. For instance, a recent literature review of publications regarding gunshot residue clearly indicates increasing research in the field, illustrating the adaptability and diversity of mass spectrometry as an analytical tool. As biochemists gain greater expertise in leveraging the power of this technique in research, it is essential to aggregate and disseminate the sheer volume of information in the literature. This not only informs further research but also enhances the teamwork nature of scientific enterprise, showcasing mass spectrometry's role in broadening our understanding of biochemical and physiological processes (Capiau et al., 2016; Cole et al., 2020) (Figure 10.12).

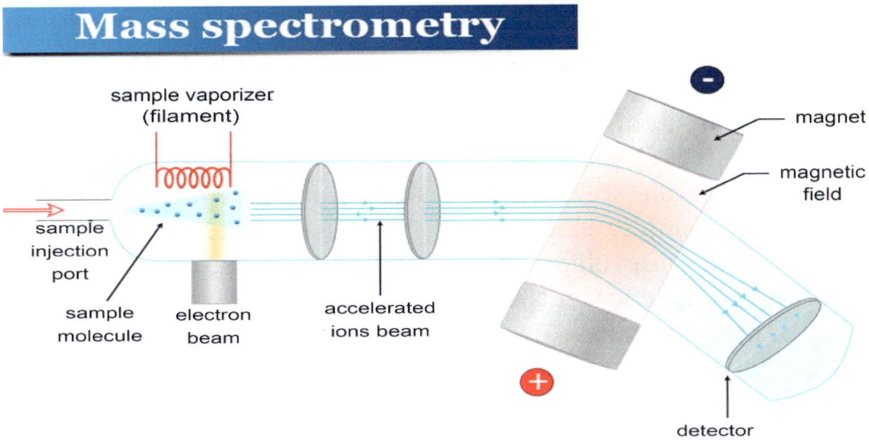

Figure 10.12. Mass spectrometry.

Source: https://www.priyamstudycentre.com/wp-content/uploads/2022/02/mass-spectrometry-instrumentation-definition-principle.png.

10.4.1. Overview of Mass Spectrometry Principles

Mass spectrometry (MS) is a cornerstone technique in biochemistry that enables the precise study of molecular structures. MS is based on the ionization of chemical species into charged particles, which are spread out as a function of their mass-to-charge (m/z) ratio. Ionization is performed by several methods, such as ESI and MALDI, depending on the nature of the sample and the requirements of analysis. Ionized, the molecules are then transferred through a mass analyzer, where their trajectories are deflected by electric or magnetic fields, such that ions can be separated from each other. This mechanistic discrimination goes on to the detection phase, where every ion's concentration is determined, providing a complete profile of the sample's constituents, which is essential for use in metabolomics through to proteomics. Mass spectrometry is of particular use for the analysis of plant metabolites. As highlighted by recent advances, numerous analytical tools, primarily mass spectrometry in combination with chromatography, facilitate the investigation of plant metabolomes. It allows for general profiling of low molecular weight metabolites significant in delineating plant growth and developmental regulation (Gullberg, 2005). An enhanced technique has been developed to enhance the throughput of metabolite analysis from complex biological samples like Arabidopsis thaliana. This approach encompasses the application of gas chromatography-mass spectrometry (GC-MS) and hierarchical data handling methodologies, thereby relieving the burden of interfering spectral peak evaluation, which is frequently encountered in complex biological matrices. These technological developments not only enhance process efficiency but also improve the accuracy of metabolomic analyses, thereby contributing significantly to the study of plant metabolism. Moreover, mass spectrometry's flexibility is not only limited to plant metabolomics but also profoundly impacts the diagnosis of inherited metabolic disorders (IEMs). With standard screening for IEMs through targeted metabolic assays, selected analytes of specific disorders were identified. Nevertheless, based on the complexity and heterogeneity of these diseases, broader analyses are required to rule out false positives and negatives (Fiehn et al., 2019). Untargeted metabolomics is a novel method that makes the simultaneous identification of an incredibly large number of metabolites in metabolic pathways possible. The technique utilizes mass spectrometry for a more comprehensive image of metabolic profiles, thereby enhancing diagnostic accuracy and facilitating improved insight into metabolic derangements. Hence, the use of mass spectrometry in clinical metabolomics will revolutionize the diagnosis of IEM, from which the significance of this technique can easily be ascertained for modern biochemistry.

10.4.2. Techniques in Mass Spectrometry (e.g., MALDI-TOF, ESI)

Mass spectrometry has entered the biochemistry field as an indispensable analysis instrument, enabling complicated characterization of biomolecules. Of its various methods, matrix-assisted laser desorption ionization time-of-flight (MALDI-TOF) mass spectrometry stands out due to its capability to analyze large biomolecules , such as proteins and polymers with great precision. By desorbing and ionizing particles trapped in a matrix with a laser, MALDI-TOF allows ions to be generated that can rapidly be characterized according to their mass-to-charge ratios. This technique is particularly useful for studying complex mixtures and has been successfully applied to resolve structures of polymers like ethylene oxide-propylene oxide copolymer, where 448 peaks were separated isotopically with identification, proving its analytical power in resolving close oligomers even if there are problems with compositional assignment (Houshia et al., 2012). Another significant technique in mass spectrometry is ESI, which is particularly good at characterizing polar molecules, including nucleic acids and low-molecular-weight proteins. In ESI, a high voltage is applied to a liquid sample to create a charged aerosol of droplets that evaporate to produce gas-phase ions. This method has several advantages like the ability to analyze compounds in their native state and ion formation over a broad mass range. ESI is also orthogonal to LC and allows complete analysis of complex biological samples. The combination of these approaches enhances their worth in biochemistry, as exemplified by breakthrough research like those investigating glutathionyl-hemoglobin (Hb-SSG) levels as a biomarker for oxidative stress, hence the relevance of mass spectrometry in clinical and environmental health (Bamonti et al., 2013). Applications involving mass spectrometry techniques like MALDI-TOF and ESI have revolutionized biochemistry, providing precious data on molecular structure and interaction.

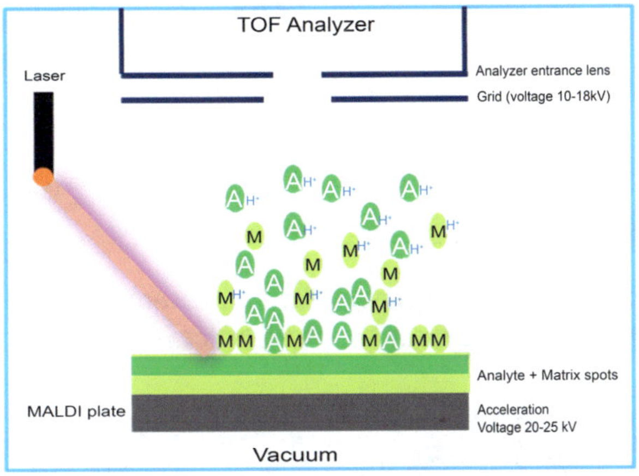

Figure 10.13. Schematic diagram of the MALDI source.

Source: https://www.chem.pitt.edu/sites/default/files/figure7.png.

MALDI-TOF's capability of offering high-resolution analysis comes in handy for analyzing complex polypeptides and oligomers, while ESIs ability to preserve integrity makes it highly suitable for measurement and identification of biologically relevant macromolecules. All these methods combined enable scientists to delve into the complexities of biological systems with the extent of accuracy that previously was not possible, presenting the potential for new possibilities in drug development, biomarker discovery, and metabolic pathway analysis. As these techniques continue to mature, they will undoubtedly bring increasingly more advances in the science of biochemistry that will help us more effectively comprehend molecular dynamics and interactions that control biological processes. In brief, the union of mass spectrometry techniques is a revolutionary step forward in the analytic capability of biochemistry that offers insight previously unattainable (Figure 10.13).

10.4.3. Applications in Metabolomics and Proteomics

Biochemistry has been completely revolutionized by the application of metabolomics and proteomics, both of which are crucial in the investigation of complex biological systems. Metabolomics involves the comprehensive investigation of metabolites, which are low-molecular-weight compounds that tell us about cellular processes, metabolic pathways, and organismal health. By applying complex analytical tools , such as mass spectrometry and NMR, researchers can develop rich metabolic profiles that can serve as biomarkers for disease as well as responses to environmental stimuli. In a clinical setting, the profiles will facilitate early diagnosis and personalized treatment regimens, and thus enable more effective healthcare treatment. Such capabilities identify the potential for metabolomic information to be complemented with other omics approaches for a more integrated understanding of biological processes. At the proteomic level, analysis of the full complement of proteins a cell or organism is producing provides insightful information regarding the functional activity of biological systems. Techniques , such as two-dimensional gel electrophoresis and LC-tandem mass spectrometry allow for separation, identification, and quantitation of proteins in complex mixtures. Proteomics thus provides a powerful tool for describing cellular function, demonstrating how proteins are connected in networks and to metabolic pathways. Moreover, the merging of proteomic data with metabolomic analysis could enhance our understanding of metabolic regulation, revealing intricate interdependencies between proteins and metabolites. This integration of data sets is particularly valuable in the study of disease, where understanding these interactions will lead to innovations in drug design and targeted therapies. Advances in technology have also propelled the application of metabolomics and proteomics in synthetic biology, particularly in microbial systems. Bioinformatics and automated high-throughput techniques aid in the discovery of new compounds, an expansion of our understanding of microbial secondary metabolism. As the majority of these compounds are of significant pharmaceutical value, the field has been pushed forward by genome mining approaches that forecast biosynthetic gene clusters of value. Metabolomics enters as a critical approach to assessing the metabolic products of constructed microbes, enabling bottlenecks in the yields of compounds to be identified. As highlighted, such discoveries can cast light on the complexities of microbial metabolism and initiate innovations in biotechnology, outlining the pivotal role of metabolomics in the biosynthesis of biologically relevant compounds (Nguyen et al., 2012; Capiau et al., 2016) (Figure 10.14).

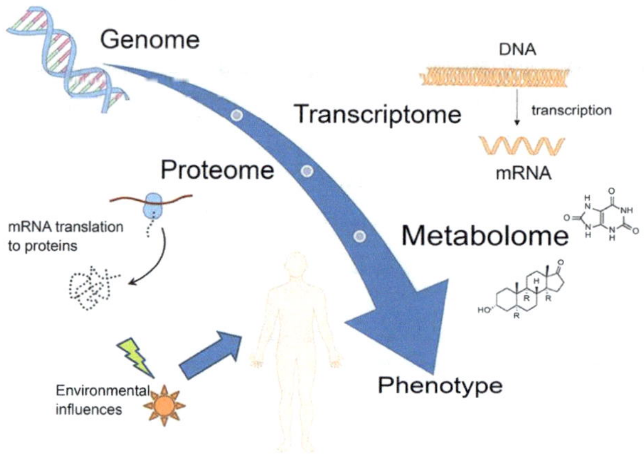

Figure 10.14. Metabolomics.

Source: https://www.creative-proteomics.com/upload/image/what-is-metabolomics-1.jpg.

Test Your Knowledge

1. What is the technique of mass spectrometry?
2. What are the applications of metabolomics?

10.5. Molecular Cloning

Learning Outcome

1. Know the basics of molecular cloning techniques;
2. Describe the steps in cloning (e.g., Vector Construction, Transformation;
3. Know the applications of genetic engineering and research.

The process of molecular cloning is a simple procedure in biochemistry by which researchers can manipulate genetic material as they wish. Molecular cloning is nothing but the separation of a single DNA sequence and inserting it into a vector, a DNA molecule with the ability to replicate itself in a host organism. The technique is important for a variety of applications, including the production of recombinant proteins, gene therapy, and the study of gene function. By employing plasmids or viral vectors, scientists can produce numerous copies of the target gene and gain in-depth complex analysis of gene expression and regulation. Gene cloning not only expands our understanding of cell mechanisms but also offers avenues for biotechnological innovation, which can be used to achieve improved crops, vaccine production, and enzymes with industrial applications. Considered to be among the most important discoveries in molecular biology, the evolution of a number of cloning protocols has increased the efficiency and consistency of the method as well. Techniques , such as restriction enzyme cutting, ligation, and transformation form the basics of cloning. Restriction enzymes are used to make molecular scissors that open DNA at predetermined sequences, thus allowing specific insertion of the target gene within a plasmid vector. Then the ligation step is the assembly of the DNA fragments into a stable recombinant molecule. The recombinant DNA is then introduced into cells of the host organism, say bacteria, where the DNA may be replicated and expressed. This multi-step process, though cumbersome, has developed significantly over time, leading to increased success with gene cloning attempts and far-reaching implications across molecular biology and biotechnology. Applications of molecular cloning are wide-ranging, and they have greatly impacted many fields , such as medicine, agriculture, and environmental science. In medical biotechnology, molecular cloning is critical in the production of therapeutic proteins , such as insulin and mAbs, which constitute the backbone of modern treatment programs. Besides, in biotechnology in agriculture, scientists employ cloning techniques in the production of genetically modified organisms (GMOs) that possess pre-defined traits , such as resistance to pests or enhanced nutritional value, hence addressing the problems of food security. Further, molecular cloning has applications in environmental applications, for example, bioremediation, where bacterial strains can be designed to degrade harmful substances. As gene functions and interactions are better understood, thanks to the cutting-edge applications of molecular cloning, the potential for novel solutions to the global problems expands even wider, with the hope for a better future owing to biotechnological progress (Figure 10.15).

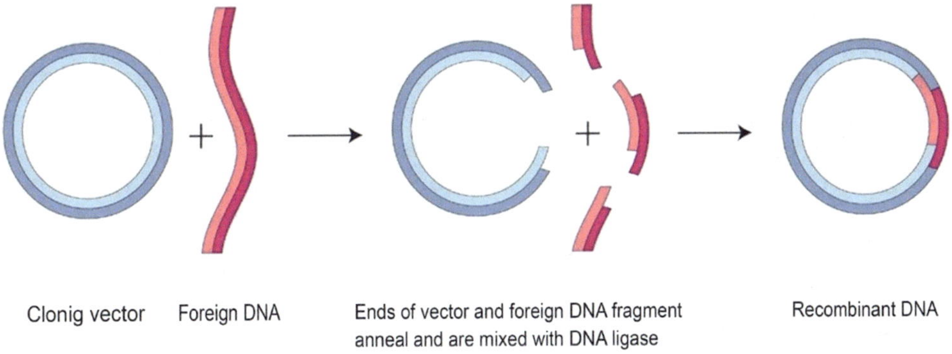

Figure 10.15. Molecular cloning.

Source: https://www.news-medical.net/image-handler/ts/20220308103905/ri/950/src/images/Article_Images/ImageForArticle_22213_16467539451682093.jpg.

10.5.1. Basics of Molecular Cloning Techniques

The principles of molecular cloning techniques are integral to gene manipulation in order to be able to comprehend and tap the potential of various organisms. The core of molecular cloning is DNA fragment isolation and amplification, which can include genes of interest. The procedure normally commences with the purification of DNA from a source organism and proceeds to the use of restriction enzymes to cut the DNA at predetermined locations. Those pieces are subsequently ligated into plasmid vectors, which in turn serve as carriers to transfer the target gene into host organisms. This simple technique not only facilitates the introduction of new genetic information but allows for the visualization of the expression and activity of the gene, hence paving the way for applications in the field of gene therapy and synthetic biology. These are steps to be learned in light of considering the moral uses and applications of genetic modification (N/A, 2021). Once the major steps of extraction and ligation are done, the most vital component of molecular cloning is the transformation of host cells with recombinant DNA. The process of transformation can occur by various means , such as heat shock or electroporation, which induce the uptake of plasmids by bacterial or eukaryotic cells. Once they get inside, the plasmids are duplicated along with the host's DNA, resulting in several copies of the foreign gene. Selection of the successfully transformed cells, usually by antibiotic resistance markers contained within the plasmid, will see only the cells with the desired genetic material survive. This is a critical step in pointing towards the versatility of molecular cloning techniques, since it allows researchers to generate large quantities of targeted DNA fragments needed for subsequent studies or for application in agriculture, medicine, and biotechnology (Goossens et al., 2020).

The application of molecular cloning techniques goes beyond mere research; it is imperative in designing new treatments as well as diagnostic processes. For instance, the ability to clone genes has made it possible to mass-produce recombinant proteins used in vaccine and enzyme therapies. Furthermore, advances in cloning have improved diagnostics, for example, DNA-based detection tools for infectious diseases, such as those caused by the neglected tropical disease, animal trypanosomosis. Methods like polymerase chain reaction (PCR) have transformed the identification and management of such diseases through rapid and efficient methodologies to identify low levels of pathogen genetic material (Vacek et al, 2008). With further advances in molecular cloning methods, their uses will continue to play greater roles in solving worldwide health issues and illuminating our knowledge of biological systems.

10.5.2. Steps in Cloning (e.g., Vector Construction, Transformation)

Cloning, a key biochemistry technique, entails a number of careful steps that allow for the successful duplication of particular DNA sequences. Vector construction, one of the key aspects of cloning, is where a virus or a plasmid is designed to be equipped with the target gene or DNA fragment. This includes the correct selection of a vector that, in addition to allowing the replication of the inserted DNA, possesses required characteristics , such as promoter sequences for the initiation of transcription and selectable markers for the screening. Construction usually comprises the use of restriction enzymes to cut both the DNA fragment and the vector so that compatible ends are ligated together, forming recombinant DNA. The advancements in recombinant DNA technology have immensely widened the frontiers of molecular biology, providing methodologies for gene expression studies, protein design, and drug production, emphasizing the exciting possibilities of this branch (Baltimore et al., 1975). Following vector assembly, transformation is the process of introducing the recombinant DNA into a host organism, commonly a yeast or bacterial cell, where it can be amplified. Transformation processes can vary, such as heat shock or electroporation, which open up the cell membrane and allow the transfer of the vector. The vector replicates with the cell's own DNA once it is engulfed by the host cell, duplicating the gene of interest multiple times. This important step opens up the way to additional analyses and applications that enable researchers to study gene function, produce recombinant proteins, or develop genetically engineered organisms. Efficient transformation of cells is fundamental for the usability of cloning in biochemistry, as it ensures the stability and integrity of introduced genetic material during subsequent generations of cells (Batiuk et al., 2017). The successful cloning of DNA sequences allows for a vast array of applications in medicine and research, making it increasingly relevant to contemporary biochemistry. Once cloned, the target gene can be expressed and characterized, opening up the potential for therapeutics, diagnostics, and synthetic biology breakthroughs. For instance, the advancements in synthetic antibody engineering, with synthetic antibodies engineered for specific biomarker engagements, are of immense potential as substitutes for traditional mAbs. This kind of development is highly entrenched in techniques adopted from cloning, showing the complementarity of these methodologies towards developing science. As the science continues to evolve, procedures like vector assembly and transformation will continue to make cloning more efficient, enabling the study of complex biological processes and the design of novel biochemicals (Batiuk et al., 2017) (Figure 10.16).

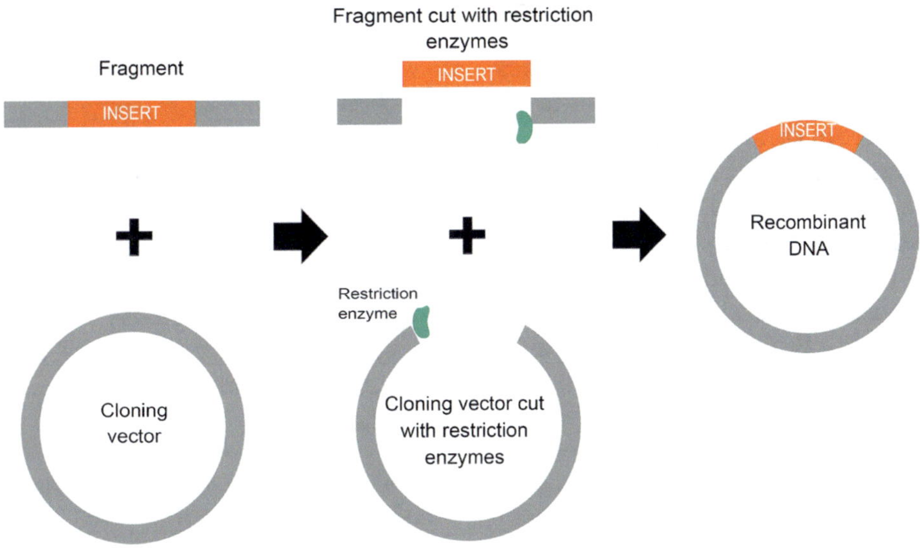

Figure 10.16. Restriction enzyme cloning.

Source: https://images.ctfassets.net/ifq1osqu2ba1/7MPbkCwfxQ0uUbJcqxRHtQ/e1a1bb16055830f59f927fabf70d3490/GN_GN_Cloning_Restriction_Enzyme-learn.png?w=1540.

10.5.3. Applications in Genetic Engineering and Research

Applications of genetic engineering are essential in advancing the growth of biochemistry, particularly in pharmaceuticals, agriculture, and environmental science. Genetic manipulation can be used to produce crops with desirable qualities, such as resistance to diseases and better nutritional content, thereby addressing food security issues worldwide. For instance, genetically modified organisms (GMOs) have been engineered to be resistant to pests and diseases, reducing the use of chemical pesticides. This not only lessens environmental stress but also enhances yield efficiency. Furthermore, these advances ensure a consistent supply of food, which is critical in a population-exploding world with global warming. With further advances in biotechnology, these applications will advance further, providing revolutionary solutions to some of the world's and humanity's challenges. The innovation of techniques in protein engineering is an example of the revolutionary potential of genetic research and engineering. With techniques , such as site-directed mutagenesis, researchers can manipulate amino acid sequences in proteins and thereby create custom proteins for specific applications in medicine and industry. The classical method is founded upon the laws of protein folding, which require a multidisciplinary understanding of biochemistry. In addition, the development of non-rational mutagenesis, or directed evolution, has revolutionized the field by allowing random mutation of encoding genes to produce massive protein variant libraries. Through the application of high-level screening methods, scientists can detect desired traits in the variants, significantly enhancing the development of new therapeutics and industrial enzymes for applications in various products, from commercial solutions to detergents used in laundry (Khan et al., 2011). The significance of collaboration and knowledge sharing in genetic engineering research is also emphasized in projects aimed at establishing networking between university personnel and industry specialists. Programs summarizing information on institutional capabilities and staff credentials ensure coordination in study activities and assist in the pursuit of funding avenues. This collaborative approach ensures that innovation in marine biotechnology and other specialist fields is complemented by a full understanding of available skills and resources (Seaman & Whitehouse, 2001). Through careful collaborations, scientists can optimize the development of innovative biotechnological products while creating the next generation of scientists. With such partnerships ongoing, the overall impact of genetic engineering on society will continue to grow, further supporting its relevance in the solution of modern problems across different sectors (Figure 10.17).

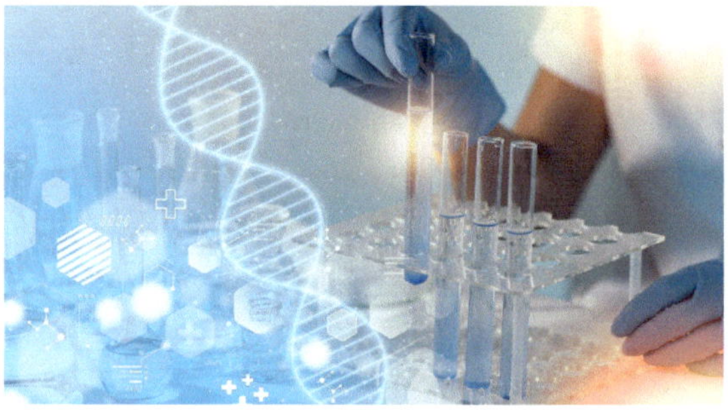

Figure 10.17. Scientist handling test tubes with a digital overlay of DNA and medical icons, representing advancements in genetic engineering.

Source: https://kahedu.edu.in/n/wp-content/uploads/2023/09/Rev.Genetic-engineering-and-CRISPR_-Revolutionizing-Biology-and-Medicine-scaled.jpg.

Test Your Knowledge

1. What are the 2 steps of cloning?
2. Which of the following are applications of genetic engineering?

SUMMARY

In outlining an investigation of the diverse methods in biochemistry, one recognizes the significant impact that new technologies, specifically AI, have made on the discipline. AI has transformed conventional methodologies, greatly advancing abilities in the analysis of data and molecular modeling. The inclusion of machine learning algorithms enables scientists to filter through large sets of data and make predictions about molecular interactions more accurately than ever before. Besides, AI-driven innovations , such as AlphaFold have greatly revolutionized protein structure prediction, demonstrating the potential of machine learning in answering challenging biological questions. Using these new methods increasingly, biochemists can push the limits of understanding towards drug discovery, enzyme design, and analysis of metabolic pathways, thus paving the way for a future generation of biochemical research and application (Junaid, 2025). Second, the increased application of stable isotope probing (SIP) techniques further substantiates advances in biochemistry. The application of 15N-DNA-SIP, among other techniques, has allowed for improved knowledge of microbial communities and how they function in ecosystems. For example, by tracing nitrogen and identifying active decomposers in different forms of organic matter, scientists can now define the ecological roles of most fungi that participate in nutrient cycling. These investigations not only provide useful information about soil health and ecosystem function but also reflect the ingenuity of biochemistry in solving complex environmental problems. The potential for incorporation of traditional biochemical techniques and cutting-edge strategies suggests a critical synergy, bringing the discipline closer to solving theoretical questions and questions of practical relevance (Rodriguez et al., 2011). Lastly, method development in biochemistry is a sign of a broader trend toward interdisciplinarity and scientific advancement. As scientists apply an eclectic toolkit of techniques, from AI-fringed models to highly advanced stable isotope techniques, opportunities for new discovery increase geometrically. Such techniques provide an integrated perception of biochemical phenomena and allow several scientific disciplines, from molecular biology to ecology, to be combined. As science advances, it will be most crucial to overcome the challenges of data integrity and ethical concerns. Not only will future scientific advances in technology and collaboration further establish our science, but it will also keep biochemistry at the cutting-edge of addressing global challenges, thus furthering its value both in educational and applied settings (Junaid, 2025; Rodriguez et al., 2011).

Technique biochemistry offers a range of new methods that significantly enhance our understanding of biological processes. Cerebral microdialysis is one of the most interesting techniques that is currently being utilized in clinical settings to monitor biochemistry of the brain in the course of neuro-intensive care. The technique allows for the online analysis of brain tissue with significant information on biochemical changes of acute brain injury. The ability to quantify multiple biomarkers through microdialysis has the potential to inform treatment and improve outcomes for patients by offering a more personalized approach to neurocritical care. While the technology is still broadly viewed as a tool of research, opportunities for widespread use are increasingly being seen with a focus on further study and validation of its clinical uses in neurobiology (Smith et al., 2006). Another significant biochemistry method is the immobilization of proteins on carbon nanotubes, which holds potential for applications across drug delivery and biosensing. It can be achieved through physical adsorption or covalent attachment, each with its own strength in protein stability and activity. The architectures of such conjugate-protein hybrids can be established by various spectroscopic methods , such as Raman and Fourier transform infrared (FT-IR) spectroscopy, which provide valuable insights into the structural stability and activity of the immobilized proteins. Studies have shown that such conjugates can retain their native structure and show significant stability, even at rigorous conditions. This flexibility demonstrates the promise of these hybrid systems to revolutionize applications in biotechnology and biochemistry by bringing theoretical research and practical applications together (Shah et al., 2009). The addition of advanced methods like microdialysis and protein immobilization is also indicative of moving towards tailored biotechnological solutions. For instance, the successful application of these methodologies hinges on their capacity to create dynamic, rich biochemical profiles, thereby allowing for more informed experimental designs and therapeutic strategies. With additional technology advancements, their combination might lead to novel platforms for monitoring cellular milieus and enhancing targeted biophysical assays. These interdisciplinarily contributed efforts are invaluable in advancing our frontiers of comprehension of intricate biochemical interactions and refining methodology across the board, from synthetic biology to drug discovery. The present research in the disciplines has the potential to advance the frontiers of biochemistry as a scientific field and as a tool of practical application in medicine and industry (Smith et al., 2006; Asuri et al., 2009).

KEY TERMS FROM THIS CHAPTER

- Agriculture
- Chromatography
- Environmental monitoring
- Healthcare
- Mass spectrometry
- Solid phase microextraction
- Supercritical fluid chromatography
- Visual Molecular Dynamics
- Biochemistry
- Ecosystems
- Gas chromatography
- Liquid chromatography
- Nucleic acids
- Solid-phase extraction
- Thin-layer chromatography

Critical Thinking Questions

1. **Which technique is commonly used to separate proteins based on their size?**
   a. Isoelectric focusing
   b. SDS-PAGE
   c. Western blotting
   d. ELISA
2. **What is the principle behind chromatography?**
   a. Separation based on charge
   b. Separation based on size
   c. Separation based on differential partitioning between stationary and mobile phases
   d. Amplification of DNA sequences
3. **Which method is used to determine the amino acid sequence of a protein?**
   a. Mass spectrometry
   b. Edman degradation
   c. Gel electrophoresis
   d. Western blot
4. **What is the main use of the spectrophotometer in biochemistry?**
   a. To measure enzyme activity by detecting light absorption
   b. To separate DNA fragments
   c. To amplify DNA sequences
   d. To visualize proteins on a gel
5. **Western blotting is used to detect:**
   a. DNA sequences
   b. RNA sequences
   c. Specific proteins
   d. Enzyme activity

Short Answer Questions

1. What is chromatography in simple words?
2. What is a spectroscopic technique?
3. What is electrophoresis?
4. What is mass spectrometry?
5. Describe the process of molecular cloning.

Answers to Critical Thinking Questions

1. (b); 2. (c); 3. (b); 4. (a); 5. (c)

REFERENCES

1. Abi, A., Aravin, A., Danhel, A., Re, A., Simonova, A., Szabo, A., et al. (2015). Biophysical and electrochemical studies of protein-nucleic acid interactions. https://core.ac.uk/download/29112106.pdf (accessed on 12th June 2025).
2. Rabilloud, T., Vaezzadeh, A. R., Potier, N., Lelong, C., Leize-Wagner, E., & Chevallet, M. (2009). Power and limitations of electrophoretic separations in proteomics strategies. *Mass spectrometry reviews*, *28*(5), 816–843. https://doi.org/10.1002/mas.20204(accessed on 12th June 2025).
3. Vacek, J., Cahova, K., Palecek, E., Bullard, D. R., Lavesa-Curto, M., Bowater, R. P., & Fojta, M. (2008). Label-free electrochemical monitoring of DNA ligase activity. *Analytical chemistry*, *80*(19), 7609–7613. https://doi.org/10.1021/ac801268p (accessed on 12th June 2025).
4. Ahmed, A., Ashraf, M., Aslam, M., Batool, A., et al. (2017). Microbial β-glucosidases: Screening, characterization, cloning and applications. https://core.ac.uk/download/188825641.pdf (accessed on 12th June 2025).
5. Aizawa, T., Matsuura, Y., Yamamoto, S., Yamamoto, T., et al. (1966). Chemical analysis of soluble fractions from normal and autolyzed rabbit liver by column chromatography. https://core.ac.uk/download/12547395.pdf (accessed on 12th June 2025).
6. Nguyen, Q. T., Merlo, M. E., Medema, M. H., Jankevics, A., Breitling, R., & Takano, E. (2012). Metabolomics methods for the synthetic biology of secondary metabolism. *FEBS letters*, *586*(15), 2177–2183. https://doi.org/10.1016/j.febslet.2012.02.008(accessed on 12th June 2025).
7. Marrocco, I., Altieri, F., & Peluso, I. (2017). Measurement and Clinical Significance of Biomarkers of Oxidative Stress in Humans. *Oxidative medicine and cellular longevity*, *2017*, 6501046. https://doi.org/10.1155/2017/6501046(accessed on 12th June 2025).
8. Anderson, D. J., Friedlander, M., Gilula, N. B., Hertzberg, E. L., et al. (1982). Comparative analysis of the major polypeptides from liver gap junctions and lens fiber junctions. https://core.ac.uk/download/9124041.pdf (accessed on 12th June 2025).
9. Angulo, J., Khimyak, Y., Monaco, S., Muñoz García, A., et al. (2019). Spatially resolved STD-NMR applied to the study of solute transport in biphasic systems. Application to protein-ligand interactions. https://core.ac.uk/download/196594938.pdf (accessed on 12th June 2025).
10. Shah, D.A, Pangule, R.C., Bale, S.S., Asuri, P., Joshi, A., Banerjee, A., ... Kane, R.S. (2009). Preparation and characterization of protein-nanotube conjugates. In Methods in Bioengineering: Nanoscale Bioengineering and Nanomedicine (pp. 1–23). Artech House. (accessed on 12th June 2025).
11. Azadmard-Damirchi, S. (2007). *Olive Oil*. https://core.ac.uk/download/11695154.pdf (accessed on 12th June 2025).
12. Azrolan, N., Boerwinkle, E., Brunner, C., Chiesa, G., Chung, B. Y., Cotten, M., Deutscher, S. L., et al. (1994). High-level expression of various apolipoprotein (a) isoforms by "Transferrinfection". The role of Kringle IV sequences in the extracellular association with low-density lipoprotein. https://core.ac.uk/download/12164944.pdf (accessed on 12th June 2025).
13. Baianu, I. C. (2011). Applications of micro spectroscopy, hyperspectral chemical imaging and fluorescence microscopy in chemistry, biochemistry, biotechnology, molecular and cell biology. https://core.ac.uk/download/pdf/290454.pdf (accessed on 12th June 2025).

14. Baianu, I. C., Charles, M., & Prisecaru, V. I. (2012). Visual molecular dynamics investigations of the impact of hydrophobic nanoparticles on prognosis of Alzheimer's disease and cancers. https://core.ac.uk/download/pdf/1570072.pdf (accessed on 12th June 2025).

15. Baltimore, D., Berg, P., Brenner, S., Roblin, R., et al. (1975). Summary statement of the Asilomar conference on recombinant DNA molecules. https://core.ac.uk/download/4879467.pdf (accessed on 12th June 2025).

16. Bamonti, F., De Giuseppe, R., De Liso, F., Della Noce, C., et al. (2013). Measurement of glutathionylated hemoglobin by MALDI-ToF mass spectrometry as a biomarker of oxidative stress in heavy smokers and in occupational obese subjects. https://core.ac.uk/download/pdf/37830718.pdf (accessed on 12th June 2025).

17. Barron, L. D. (2015). The development of biomolecular Raman optical activity spectroscopy. https://core.ac.uk/download/77601498.pdf (accessed on 12th June 2025).

18. Batiuk, E., Kiyohara, C., & Nguyen, T. (2017). Engineering synthetic antibody by expanded genetic code. https://core.ac.uk/download/84118620.pdf (accessed on 12th June 2025).

19. Baugh, C., Dijkstra, B. W., Bing, X., Bock, C., Cao, W., Chayen, N. E., Convery, M. A., et al. (2012). Characterization of aptamer-protein complexes by X-ray crystallography and alternative approaches. https://core.ac.uk/download/pdf/12960258.pdf (accessed on 12th June 2025).

20. Bottino, E., Damerow, J. L., Laubichler, M. D., Peirson, D., et al. (2017). Quantitative perspectives on fifty years of the *Journal of the History of Biology*. https://core.ac.uk/download/222886423.pdf (accessed on 12th June 2025).

21. Buděšínský, M., Gillner, D. M., Hlaváček, J., Holz, M., et al. (2014). Mono-*N*-acyl-2,6-diaminopimelic acid derivatives: Analysis by electromigration and spectroscopic methods and examination of enzyme inhibitory activity. https://core.ac.uk/download/213089545.pdf (accessed on 12th June 2025).

22. Capiau, S., Stove, C., & Velghe, S. (2016). Opening the toolbox of alternative sampling strategies in clinical routine: A key-role for (LC-)MS/MS. https://core.ac.uk/download/84043363.pdf (accessed on 12th June 2025).

23. Cole, C., Klu, J., Menard, H., Nic Daeid, N., et al. (2020). Reviewing research trends: A scientometric approach using gunshot residue (GSR) literature as an example. https://core.ac.uk/download/287601447.pdf (accessed on 12th June 2025).

24. A P Lewis *et al* 2013 *Meas. Sci. Technol.* **24** 042001

25. Eilerts, Diane F. (2016) "Beyond DNA: Epigenetics and Proteomics in Forensic Science," *Themis: Research Journal of Justice Studies and Forensic Science*: Vol. 4 : Iss. 1 , Article 10. DOI: https://doi.org/10.31979/THEMIS.2016.0410 https://scholarworks.sjsu.edu/themis/vol4/iss1/10 (accessed on 12th June 2025).

26. Fiehn, O., Ismail, I. T., & Showalter, M. R. (2019). Inborn errors of metabolism in the era of untargeted metabolomics and lipidomic. https://core.ac.uk/download/323068986.pdf (accessed on 12th June 2025).

27. Freyse, J., Grabarics, M., von Helden, G., Lettow, M., et al. (2020). IR action spectroscopy of glycosaminoglycan oligosaccharides. https://core.ac.uk/download/322846682.pdf (accessed on 12th June 2025).

28. Goossens, J., Li, Z., Magez, S., Pinto Torres, A., et al. (2020). Development of a recombinase polymerase amplification lateral flow assay for the detection of active *Trypanosoma evansi* infections. https://core.ac.uk/download/288817506.pdf (accessed on 12th June 2025).

29. Goulet, D. (2015). Modeling, simulating, and parameter fitting of biochemical kinetic experiments. http://arxiv.org/abs/1508.05359 (accessed on 12th June 2025).

30. Gullberg, J. (2005). *Metabolomics: A Tool for Studying Plant Biology*. https://core.ac.uk/download/11694915.pdf (accessed on 12th June 2025).

31. Guo, H. (1998). *Determination of Creatinine and Creatine by Capillary Electrophoresis: A Thesis Presented in Partial Fulfilment of The Requirements for The Degree of Master of Science in Chemistry at Massey University*. https://core.ac.uk/download/148645066.pdf (accessed on 12th June 2025).

32. Hansen, J., Paquette, M., Topp, R. V., Woda, A., et al. (2017). The impact of simulation sequencing on perceived clinical decision making. https://core.ac.uk/download/213086958.pdf (accessed on 12th June 2025).

33. Houshia, O. J., & Wilkins, C. (2012). Compositional analysis of the high molecular weight ethylene oxide propylene oxide copolymer by MALDI mass spectrometry. http://arxiv.org/abs/1205.6421 (accessed on 12th June 2025).

34. Hyeon, C., Thirumalai, D., Derenyi, I., Evans, E., Fisher, T. E., Hummer, G., Lide, D. R., et al. (2006). Measuring the energy landscape roughness and the transition state location of biomolecules using single molecule mechanical unfolding experiments. http://arxiv.org/abs/cond-mat/0612433 (accessed on 12th June 2025).

35. Junaid, M. A. L. (2025). Artificial intelligence driven innovations in biochemistry: A review of emerging research frontiers. https://core.ac.uk/download/648357613.pdf (accessed on 12th June 2025).

36. Khan, I., & Akhtar, M. W. (2011). Different approaches for protein engineering in industrial biotechnology. https://core.ac.uk/download/pdf/289804.pdf (accessed on 12th June 2025).

37. Marsh, D. (2000). *Fostering Innovation in A Small Open Economy: The Case of The New Zealand Biotechnology Sector*. https://core.ac.uk/download/29195694.pdf (accessed on 12th June 2025).

38. Norlin, E. (2005). *Nitrogen Isotope Analysis of Ammonium and Glycine*. https://core.ac.uk/download/11694902.pdf (accessed on 12th June 2025).

39. Palhinhas, R. M. G. (2011). *Investigation of the Effects of Weight Loss On Ovis Aries Muscle: A Proteomic Study on Three Breeds with Different Levels of Adaptation to Nutritional Stress*. https://core.ac.uk/download/12426184.pdf (accessed on 12th June 2025).

40. Provost's Office. (2013). *The Faculty Notebook, September 2014*. https://cupola.gettysburg.edu/cgi/viewcontent.cgi?article=1057&context=facnotebook (accessed on 12th June 2025).

41. Rodriguez, B., Bernard, C., Buckley, N., Cadisch, G., Cupples, C., Haichar, E. Z., et al. (2011). Assessing the effect of organic residue quality on active decomposing fungi in a tropical Vertisol using 15N-DNA stable isotope probing. https://core.ac.uk/download/44455.pdf (accessed on 12th June 2025).

42. Ryan, B. J., Batra, S., Chakrabarti, R., Chang, S., Chattopadhyay, A., Ó›Fágáin, C., Coates, N., et al. (2008). Effects of mutations in the helix G region of horseradish peroxidase. https://core.ac.uk/download/11308414.pdf (accessed on 12th June 2025).

43. Seaman, W., & Whitehouse, J. H. (2001). *Florida Marine Biotechnology: Research, Development and Training Capabilities to Advance Science and Commerce*. https://core.ac.uk/download/11016354.pdf (accessed on 12th June 2025).

44. Smith, M., & Tisdall, M. M. (2006). Cerebral micro dialysis: Research technique or clinical tool. https://core.ac.uk/download/1671050.pdf (accessed on 12th June 2025).

45. Torjesen, A. A. (2016). *An Ultra-Fast Digital Diffuse Optical Spectroscopic Imaging System for Neoadjuvant Chemotherapy Monitoring*. https://open.bu.edu/bitstream/2144/19470/1/Torjesen_bu_0017N_12323.pdf (accessed on 12th June 2025).

PROTEOMICS AND METABOLOMICS

11

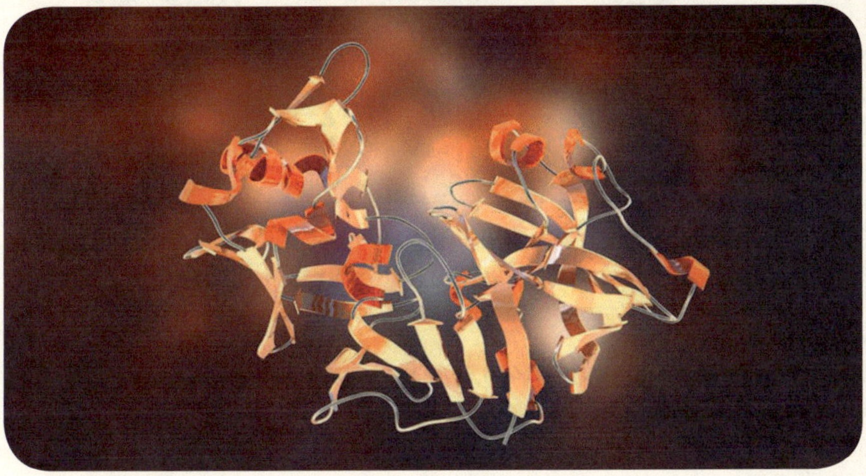

LEARNING OBJECTIVES

After studying this chapter, you will be able to:

1. Understand the techniques of proteomics;
2. Understand the techniques of metabolomics;
3. Know the applications of proteomics;
4. Know the applications of metabolomics.

Introduction

The two fields of proteomics and metabolomics have come to the forefront of the life sciences as a result of advancing technology, as well as the mounting demand for personalized medicine. Proteomics, the high-throughput analysis of proteins, explores protein structure and protein function in a defined biological context. This exploration is important given that proteins occupy pivotal roles in mediating biological processes and responses. In contrast, metabolomics examines the unique chemical signatures left behind by cell activities, as a representation of the metabolite fingerprints characterizing different states of health. These methodologies complement one another to provide a holistic picture of the molecular foundation of disease, pushing researchers towards innovations that can reshape therapeutic possibilities. In light of the focus of contemporary medicine towards precision, knowledge of protein-metabolite interactions is imperative for enhancing diagnosis accuracy and therapeutic efficacy. The significance of integrating proteomics and metabolomics is particularly evident in the context of precision medicine, where tailored therapeutic interventions are of utmost significance. Through omics approaches, clinicians are able to tailor treatment protocols with the help of molecular wisdom derived from patient data. Such adaptability is particularly valuable for diseases , such as cancer, where traditional treatment protocols often fail because they are addressing high amounts of heterogeneity and variations that are patient-specific. Through proteomics, it is now possible to detect biomarkers that have the ability to enhance patient stratification and prognosis. As recently established in the literature, the application of proteomics-guided methods can become a roadmap for individualized patient care, particularly in oncology, whereby it can guide early treatment, continuous monitoring, and the discovery of new therapeutic targets (Latosinska et al., 2017). Therefore, the application of these sciences not only addresses the existing clinical needs but also creates a path for future therapeutic breakthroughs. While proteomics and metabolomics have broad potential, some limitations have to be transcended before applying these techniques to the full extent in a clinical setting. Issues , such as data interpretation, the need for standardized methods, and dealing with huge datasets are the biggest challenges for researchers and clinicians alike. In addition, the complexity of biological systems calls for systems biology to be utilized in fully comprehending how proteins interact with metabolites. As Kamphorst & Lewis . (2017) recommend, while there is genuine enthusiasm for the promise of these omics technologies, to reach the bench-to-bedside utopia, multidisciplinary cooperation will be called for across the disciplines of bioinformatics, systems biology, and clinical research. The intersection of these areas of research is essential in the development of effective, individualized treatment programs that can ultimately lead to improved patient outcomes, making the areas of proteomics and metabolomics important areas to continue researching and developing technology in (Figure 11.1).

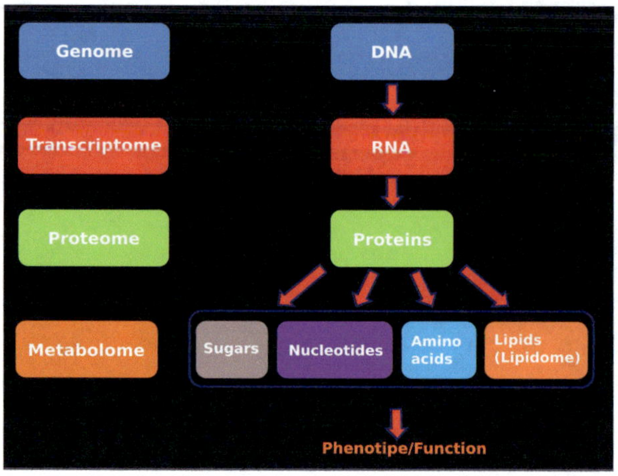

Figure 11.1. General schema showing the relationships of the genome, transcriptome, proteome, and metabolome (lipidome, glycome).

Source: https://upload.wikimedia.org/wikipedia/commons/8/8d/Metabolomics_schema.svg.

Definition of Proteomics

Proteomics, a branch of molecular biology, is concerned with the extensive exploration of proteins, particularly their structure, function, and interaction in a biological system. Proteomics encompasses various techniques designed to discover, quantify, and characterize proteins encoded by genes from an organism under defined conditions. While genomics considers the totality of an organism's genetic content, proteomics considers the dynamic nature of protein expression, which is a true reflection of real-time changes due to environmental stimulation, physiological conditions, or disease. The concerned analysis is significant because proteins are key mediators of biological processes, and their understanding is crucial to an all-encompassing investigation of cellular functions and pathways. As researchers explore the relationships between proteins and cellular functions, the field of proteomics becomes a key component of systems biology and personalized medicine, always offering insights needed to keep advancing health science and disease management. In recent years, the integration of proteomics with other omics sciences, such as genomics and metabolomics, has enhanced our understanding of complex biological systems and mechanisms of diseases. Multi-omics strategies enable the simultaneous study of multiple biomolecules, and this helps to detect potential biomarkers and targets for therapy. For example, in the case of cardiometabolic diseases (CMD), proteomics data integration can provide valuable information on protein-metabolite interactions and reveal disease pathways that would otherwise not be revealed by single-omics analysis. This connectivity emphasizes the importance of an interdisciplinary method of studying biology, wherein proteomics is utilized to augment and complement the data derived from other omics studies. The marriage of these methodologies ultimately leads to an enhanced understanding of disease advancement, which is utilized to construct more efficient diagnostic and therapeutic strategies. Moreover, the value of proteomics extends to precision medicine, an area that has a bearing on patient treatment and treatment planning. By leveraging proteomic data, clinicians can identify certain protein biomarkers indicating the presence, progression, or response to treatment of disease, particularly in oncology. For example, proteomic uses in treating bladder cancer reveal the potential of therapy regimens tailored to the patient's specific molecular profile, thus optimizing therapeutic efficiency. Proteomics not only facilitates drug target identification but also contributes to the prevention and monitoring of disease through enabling the stratification of patients according to their protein expression patterns. As this personalized medicine becomes increasingly complex, biomarker validation challenges and the need for guidelines on standardized protocols are challenges for the science, but also work to provide a firm footing for the role of proteomics in modern medical practice (Latosinska et al., 2017). The definition and application of proteomics therefore, capture a critical component of our ongoing efforts to deconstruct complex biological events and maximize health outcomes (Figure 11.2).

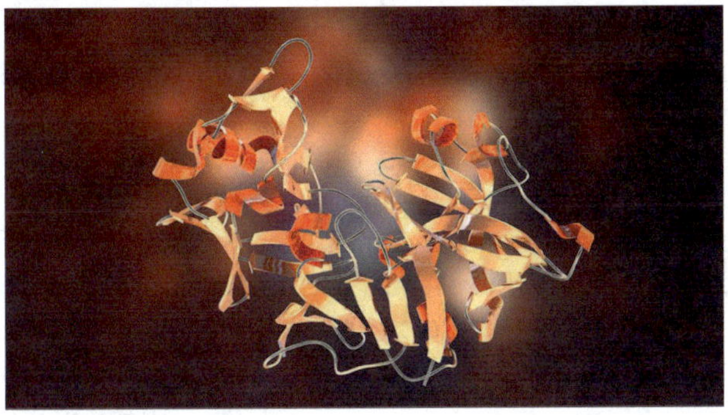

Figure 11.2. Proteomics.

Source: https://lifesciences.danaher.com/us/en/library/media_13b9e7b236b33cbe56925e5334715702becba1ac0.jpeg?width=2000&format=webply&optimize=medium.

Definition of Metabolomics

Metabolomics is an extension of systems biology and is defined as the global analysis of metabolites within a biological sample, with a view to expressing what happens in the biochemical pathways that govern cellular processes. Metabolomics is a science devoted to the discovery and quantification of low-molecular-weight organic compounds, or metabolites, that are actively engaged in metabolic processes. Through analyzing these metabolites, scientists can gain insight into the physiological state of an organism and what impact external factors, such as diet or environmental stressors, have on metabolism. Unlike genomics and proteomics, which analyze genetic data and proteins, respectively, metabolomics analyses end products of cellular processes and is therefore particularly well-suited to the study of dynamic biological systems and their response to perturbations. The complexity of metabolomics often necessitates the employment of advanced analytical techniques , such as mass spectrometry (MS) and NMR spectroscopy. These techniques allow for the high-throughput analysis of metabolites ranging from amino acids to lipids and sugars. The integration of metabolomics with the other omics technologies, as seen in pediatric pharmacotherapy, holds potential for uncovering intricate correlations between metabolic profiles and biological processes to yield better therapeutic strategies. For instance, omics profiling can facilitate the discovery of target biomarkers that correlate with various phenotypes, providing more precise medical therapies tailored to particular patients (Neumann et al., 2022). This integrative kind of analysis underscores the potential of metabolomics to revolutionize our understanding of disease and health. Metabolomics is a major technology in personalized medicine since it enables us to find individual metabolic signatures linked with individual health status. From recent research, metabolites have been found to serve as indicators of physiological alteration or pathophysiological condition and hence their implication as biomarkers. Research has reported that with a longitudinal wellness cohort, healthy individuals had distinct plasma protein profiles, which indicated that metabolomic variability is a signature of individual health stability (Tebani et al., 2020). Such stability means that a high-level understanding of metabolomics can develop more diagnostic capabilities and therapeutic interventions. Lastly, the incorporation of metabolomics in clinical research not only advances our knowledge on metabolic pathways but also provides valuable information that is necessary to develop novel and innovative treatment strategies in the field of precision medicine (Figure 11.3).

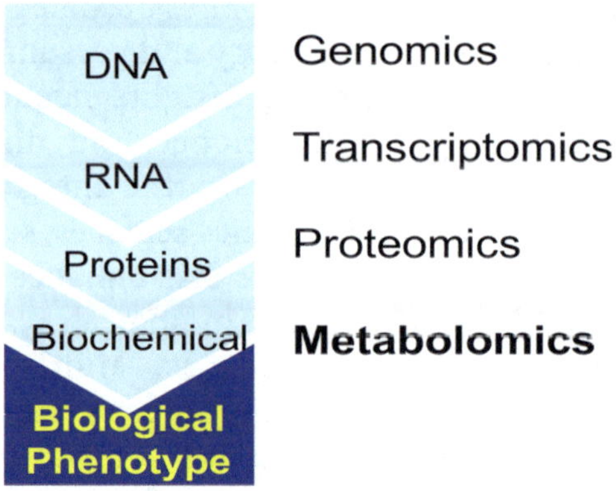

Figure 11.3. The central principle of biology showing the flow of information from DNA to the phenotype. Associated with each stage is the corresponding systems biology tool, from genomics to metabolomics.

Source: https://upload.wikimedia.org/wikipedia/commons/b/b8/The_central_dogma_of_biology_showing_the_flow_of_information_from_DNA_to_the_phenotype._Associated_with_each_stage_is_the_corresponding_systems_biology_tool_from_genomics_to_genomics_to_metabolomics.png.

11.1. Techniques in Proteomics

Learning Outcome

1. Understand the mass spectrometry;
2. Describe the technique of Two-Dimensional Gel Electrophoresis;
3. Know the protein microarrays.

Proteomics is a powerful field of post-genomic research that aims to study the large-scale analysis of proteins, their activity, and their interactions within biological organisms. Mass spectrometry (MS) is one of the most frequent instruments among the methods applied in proteomics. It allows for protein identification and quantification in complex mixtures by measuring the mass-to-charge ratio of ionized particles. Along with techniques , such as LC, MS enables high-resolution profiling of protein mixtures such that it is possible to distinguish complex proteomic profiles from different biological backgrounds. Also, advanced affinity purification and tagging methods enable protein detection in higher specificity, which is critical for elucidating functionally meaningful pathways and interactions in cellular processes. This methodological approach indicates the richness of information mass spectrometry can provide, shaping our perception of proteomics as a thrilling field of modern biological research. Another major technique used in proteomics is two-dimensional gel electrophoresis (2-DE), resolving proteins based on their isoelectric points and molecular masses. This method allows the visualization of protein mixtures that are heterogeneous and is extremely valuable in the identification of PTMs that could significantly affect protein function. The ability to create extensive protein profiles has made 2-DE a valuable tool in many different applications, such as biomarker discovery and disease diagnosis. But note the disadvantage of 2-DE, including the lack of resolution of highly hydrophobic proteins and visualization of low-abundance proteins.

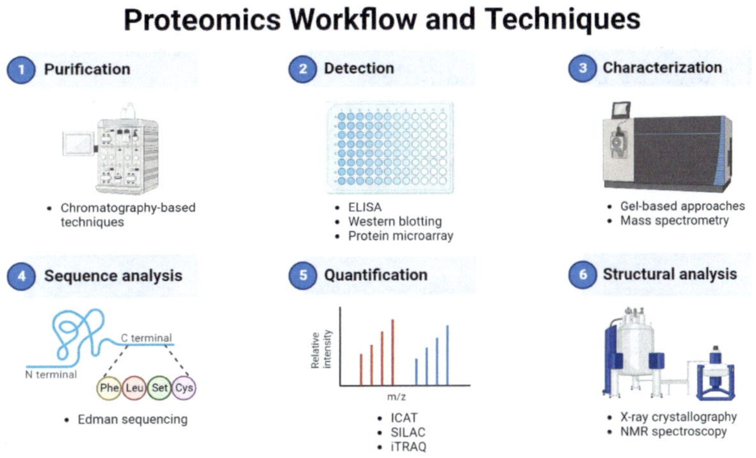

Figure 11.4. Proteomics workflow and techniques.

Source: https://microbenotes.com/wp-content/uploads/2023/06/Proteomics-Workflow-and-Techniques.jpg.

Despite these disadvantages, the integration of 2-DE with mass spectrometry and bioinformatics programs has significantly enhanced high-throughput proteomic analysis capacity, further enhancing the usefulness of conventional methods in current proteomic research. Finally, the advent of high-throughput techniques, such as tandem mass tag (TMT) labeling and bioinformatics platforms, has revolutionized proteomics. TMT labeling allows simultaneous quantitation of multiple samples in one mass spectrometry run and thereby optimizes efficiency and reproducibility. This technology is particularly critical in comparative proteomics as it allows researchers to compare changes in protein expression between multiple experimental conditions. Its interfacing with metabolomics is also becoming increasingly pertinent, as both areas endeavor to provide a comprehensive view of biological systems at more than one level. As witnessed by research currently in progress that indicates the synergistic potential of these two fields, the interfacing of proteomic and metabolomic analysis can reveal complicated dependencies among proteins and low-molecular-weight molecules, better characterizing metabolic pathways and cellular dynamics. This evolving interdisciplinary approach underscores the significance of proteomics in an increasingly integrated landscape of biological research, as reflected in recent accounts of challenges regarding data sharing in plant sciences (Alsheikh-Ali et al., 2013) and the use of metabolic profiling in synthetic microbiology (Nguyen et al., 2012) (Figure 11.4).

11.1.1. Mass Spectrometry

Mass spectrometry (MS) is a critical analytical methodology for both proteomics and metabolomics, enabling the identification and quantification of biomolecules with high specificity and sensitivity. MS is based on the ionization of chemical species and the separation of ions in accordance with their mass-to-charge ratio. With the ability to generate high quantities of quantitative information, mass spectrometry allows scientists to investigate complex biological systems and identify molecular functions responsible for propelling them. Its applications range across numerous sectors, such as clinical diagnostics, where it facilitates protein biomarker discovery, and drug discovery, providing data on metabolic pathways and interactions. The versatility of the techniques is also enhanced by some ionization techniques, such as electrospray ionization (ESI) and MALDI, which are both significant in analyzing diverse biological samples.

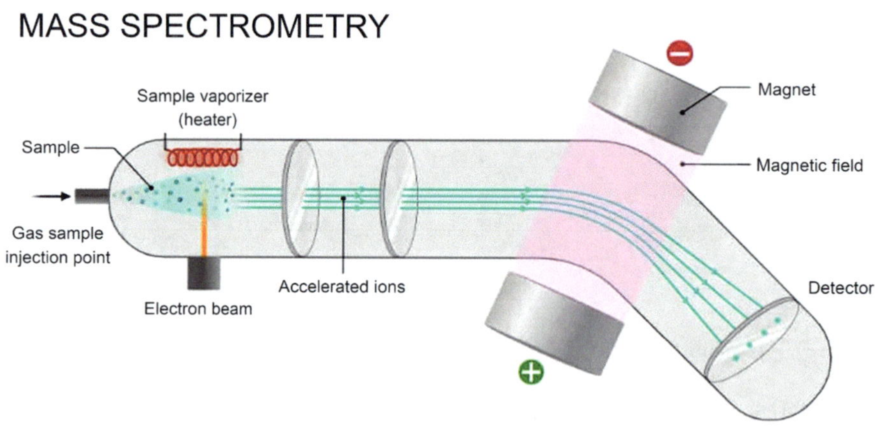

Figure 11.5. Mass spectrometry.

Source: https://microbenotes.com/wp-content/uploads/2018/12/Mass-Spectrometry-MS.jpeg.

This versatility makes mass spectrometry an essential facility in contemporary biological science. Besides identifying proteins via mass spectrometry in proteomics, their PTMs are also identified, which are central to understanding protein function and regulation. The ability to analyze protein isoforms and complexes adds depth to proteomic information to reveal cellular mechanisms at a granular. In addition, the advancement of tandem mass spectrometry, or MS/MS, increases analysis accuracy using fragmentation of ions to provide structural content to discriminate among very similar protein variants. The interaction between high-resolution mass spectrometry and bioinformatics allows the researcher to deal with and interpret data effectively and gain insights into complex biological networks. The interaction of mass spectrometry with proteomics research is continuing to give new insights into the dynamic protein-protein interactions in disease and health, improving our understanding of cellular mechanisms and possible therapeutic alternatives. Mass spectrometry is a central technique of metabolomics for global analysis of small metabolites, providing a snapshot of the metabolic status of organisms. Mass spectrometry is very highly involved in the study of microbes, with it aiding in the discovery of new secondary metabolites that have the potential to be useful in medicine and agriculture. Recent advances in metabolic profiling, facilitated by mass spectrometry technologies, are increasingly facilitating the identification of cryptic biosynthetic gene clusters and thus revealing metabolites not yet fully understood. Such complementarity of methods facilitates greater probing of metabolic pathways, discriminating bottlenecks and side products, and thus greater ability to engineer microorganisms for higher yield of the compound. The use of mass spectrometry in metabolomics highlights its crucial position in synthetic microbiology, improving the understanding of complex biochemical pathways and inspiring advances in biotechnological innovation, as recognized by Nguyen et al. (2012) (Figure 11.5).

11.1.2. Two-Dimensional Gel Electrophoresis

The technique of Two-Dimensional Gel Electrophoresis (2-DE) has been the primary vehicle for the evolution of proteomics, paving the way for all subsequent developments. The sophisticated technique excels others at separating complex mixtures of proteins based on two distinct attributes: isoelectric point and molecular weight. By employing a two-dimensional approach, this technique allows for the thorough examination of protein profiles, which is crucial to cell function and signaling cascades. 2-DE is also a very valuable tool in the detection of PTMs, further augmenting the realm of proteomics. It is fascinating that while new technologies have introduced many different alternative strategies to proteomics, 2-DE has certain particular advantages, like the fact that it can investigate intact proteins and permit integration with immunoblotting techniques, as highlighted in the literature today (Righetti et al., 2011), showing its sustained relevance within cutting-edge research. When utilized in proteomics and metabolomics, 2-DE is no longer a stand-alone method but is combined with other emerging technologies like mass spectrometry and bioinformatics. Enhanced developments of these ancillary techniques have given even higher importance to 2-DE. Mass spectrometry, for instance, provides a means of identification and quantification of proteins resolved in 2-D gels, bridging the gap between separation and identification. In addition, bioinformatics software tools are also needed to handle the resulting data, particularly owing to the high dimensionality and complexity of proteomic data sets. Integration of these techniques points towards the necessity of standardized data representations for proteomics to enhance the sharing and reproducibility of data across laboratories. By establishing such standards, researchers are also able to make data from 2-DE experiments easily comparable and re-analyzable, hence facilitating collaborative research within the area (Rabilloud et al., 2009). Despite its advantages, 2-DE does have some intrinsic limitations that researchers need to contend with. One of these is variability that may be encountered both in gel preparation and running conditions and which can compromise reproducibility and overall accuracy in protein quantification. Additionally, certain kinds of proteins, such as hydrophobic or very large proteins, will not separate well using this approach, thus making analyses challenging. Understanding these limitations is crucial for optimizing experimental design and selecting appropriate applications of 2-DE in proteomics. Despite these roadblocks, the strengths of 2-DE and ongoing improvements in technology make it an important methodology. Its ongoing improvement and advancement will most likely be pivotal in overcoming challenges in proteomic research, thus being a foundation of future research in the study of protein dynamics (Righetti et al., 2011) (Figure 11.6).

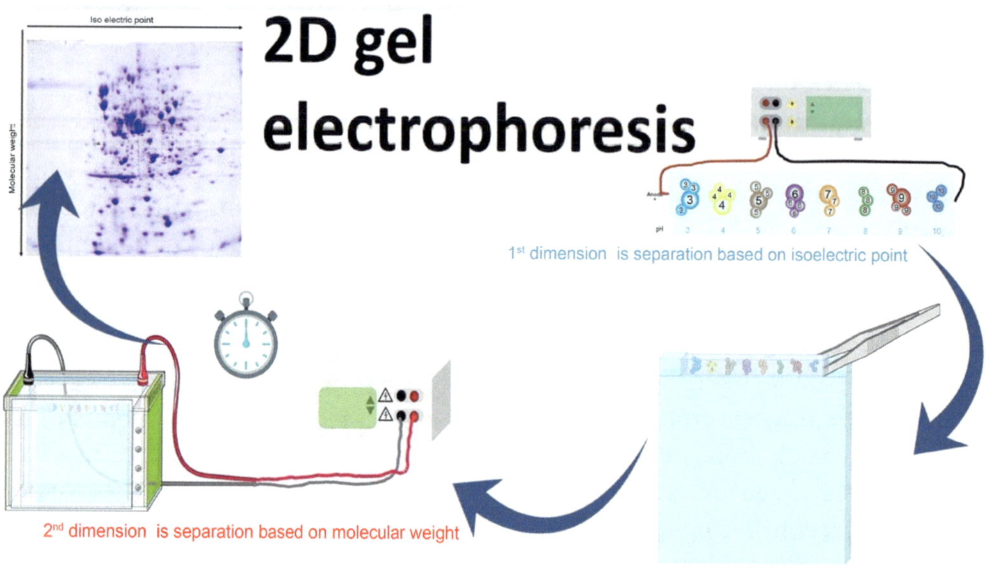

Figure 11.6. Two-dimensional gel electrophoresis.

Source: https://i.ytimg.com/vi/FHvblg338Gg/maxresdefault.jpg.

11.1.3. Protein Microarrays

Protein microarrays are a major innovation in the proteomics field, and they provide a high-throughput technique for analyzing and quantifying proteins in parallel. Immobilization of thousands of proteins onto a solid substrate is the technology, where researchers can interrogate cellular responses and disease mechanisms in an unprecedented level of detail. Such a capability is pivotal to the detection of biomarkers useful in guiding diagnostics and therapeutic intervention, especially in personalized medicine. By providing an overall view of the protein expression map, microarrays enable the quantification of protein interactions and functions within various contexts of biology. These applications highlight the potential of protein microarrays in the patient stratification based on unique molecular profiles, which might lead to more tailored treatment approaches that could have a remarkable impact on patient outcomes (Latosinska et al., 2017). Furthermore, protein microarrays offer a platform for investigating host-parasite interactions, in particular, for understanding protozoan parasite diseases. Resistance to drugs evolves and introduces complexity into the therapy regimen, emphasizing the importance of new research techniques and drug development. Microarrays offer access for high-density proteomic examination with the capacity to detect simultaneously host and pathogen proteomes and clarify infection biology dynamics. With the use of systems biology innovations, researchers can now easily analyze complex interactions, thereby paving the way for the discovery of novel drugs and more effective therapeutic interventions. Protein microarrays bridge this gap by developing large sets of data that disclose mechanisms of parasitic infection, thereby addressing the urgent need for new antiparasitic therapies (Jamshidi et al., 2015). In sum, the incorporation of protein microarrays in proteomic research represents an evolutionary step in the pursuit of comprehensive biological understanding. The technology not only improves our knowledge of protein functions and interaction but also accelerates the development of personalized medicine and disease treatment. The possibility of examining large arrays of proteins at once ensures that scientists are able to recognize pertinent biomarkers and therapeutic targets, which is critical in resolving clinical issues. With the advancing technology, the use of protein microarrays will be wider and will become an irreplaceable tool in both proteomics and metabolomics' research and clinical settings. As protein microarrays illuminate the complexities of biological systems, they can potentially revolutionize our approach to the treatment and prevention of diseases (Latosinska et al., 2017; Jamshidi et al., 2015) (Figure 11.7).

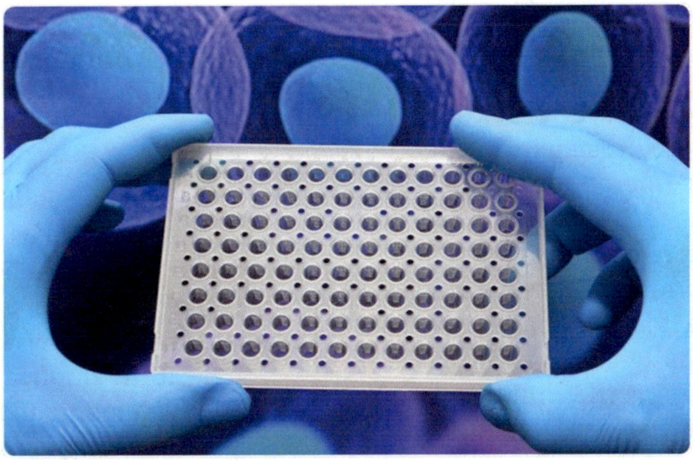

Figure 11.7. Gloved hands holding a 96-well microplate used in cell-based assays.

Source: https://www.news-medical.net/image-handler/ts/20171215060819/ri/673/picture/2017/12/shutterstock_512224762_edit.jpg.

Test Your Knowledge

1. What is mass spectrometry?
2. What is a protein microarray?

11.2. Techniques in Metabolomics

Learning Outcome

1. Learn about nuclear magnetic resonance (NMR) spectroscopy;
2. Describe the gas chromatography-mass spectrometry (GC-MS);
3. Understand the significance of liquid chromatography-mass spectrometry (LC-MS).

Metabolomic approaches are essential in identifying dynamic metabolic activities that are responsible for cellular operation and disease states. The widespread techniques applied in metabolomics include mass spectrometry (MS) and NMR spectroscopy. MS is finding its place more and more because it is extremely sensitive with the ability of handling complex mixtures, allowing scientists to profile hundreds of metabolites in a single experiment. Both targeted and untargeted metabolomic analysis can be achieved using this technique, and researchers are able to get full insight into the pathways of the metabolism. However, NMR spectroscopy is somewhat unique in its non-destructive nature and ability to quantify metabolites with no pre-separation. Both techniques have limitations and advantages, and hence it is imperative to select appropriate methodologies based on the specific research query. Lastly, the convergence of multiple techniques towards understanding changes in metabolism across different biological systems makes the metabolomics field richer. The application of standardized protocols to ensure reproducibility and data integrity is also a leading characteristic of metabolomics. Application of comprehensive experimental designs and analysis workflows is essential to enable comparison of results across studies. Sample preparation, data collection, and data processing are some of the elements that need to be controlled with care to minimize variability. Moreover, integration with other omics technologies , such as genomics and proteomics, contributes an added layer of biological interpretation as well as support for systems biology approaches. For instance, combining metabolomic profiles with proteomic data enables researchers to draw educated conclusions regarding protein-level alterations' impact on metabolic pathways, illuminating disease mechanisms. Increased collaboration and data-sharing strategies, as in the case of plant biology, are essential for advance in these methods as well as establishing good criteria for metabolomics research in the broader context (Alsheikh-Ali et al., 2013). Metabolomics is not only used in basic research but also in biotechnological innovations, particularly in synthetic biology. The recent advancement in microbial genome mining has unfolded enormous potential in the discovery of new secondary metabolites with significant implications in medicine and agriculture. Metabolomics plays a pivotal role in this regard, allowing for the global quantification of small molecules to delineate biosynthetic pathways and identify new compounds. Through the coupling of metabolomic analysis with contemporary methods in synthetic biology, scientists can optimize microbial systems for the production of valuable metabolites in high yield. By integrating these different technologies, not only is the discovery of unknown metabolic functions made easier, but also restrictions related to product consistency and compound yield optimization are corrected (Nguyen et al., 2012). Such interdisciplinary strategies prove increasingly significant for metabolomics in acquiring practical solutions for industrial purposes as well as allowing better metabolic engineering schemes.

11.2.1. Nuclear Magnetic Resonance (NMR) Spectroscopy

Nuclear magnetic resonance (NMR) Spectroscopy occupies a pivotal role within proteomics and metabolomics, as it offers a non-destructive approach to defining the structure and dynamics of biomolecules. By employing high magnetic fields and radiofrequency radiation, NMR allows researchers to perturb the molecular environment around given nuclei, mostly hydrogen, carbon, and nitrogen. This technique is particularly useful as it has the potential to provide high-resolution information about molecular conformations, interactions, and correlations between various metabolites in biostructures. As NMR technology improved, the resolution of spectra increased significantly, enabling researchers to detect and quantify a huge number of metabolites in intricate biological matrices. Also, NMR's capacity to analyze samples in their natural environment is its biggest strength in the continued pursuit of understanding the biochemical pathways that regulate cellular activity. The integration of NMR spectroscopy into metabolomics has precipitated a revolution in methodology approaches, particularly in how to approach data processing and solving problems. As highlighted by recent literature, high-throughput metabolomic experiments produced datasets whose increasing complexity demands sophisticated analytical approaches to deep interpretation. While NMR provides qualitative and quantitative data that are rich in information, researchers must undergo intense data processing to derive proper insights. Specifically, software and platforms specially designed for metabolomics have become absolutely indispensable in bridging the gap. The majority of the tools are freely available, inviting users for researchers wanting to streamline their workflows. As per the literature, it is imperative to familiarize oneself with them for enhancing data processing methods and further advancing our understanding of metabolomic landscapes and their roles in disease and health (Misra et al., 2016). Besides the identification of metabolites, the scope of NMR spectroscopy extends to entering the realm of metabolic profiling for dynamic explorations of cellular responses to shifts in the environment. This is particularly valuable in systems biology, in which mapping and modeling of metabolic pathways can offer insights into disease processes, therapeutic targets, and biomarkers. The non-destructive nature of NMR means that sampling can be repeated, allowing for longitudinal studies of the changes in metabolism over time. This is particularly useful in fields like cancer metabolism, where insights into the biochemical adaptation of tumor cells can result in the discovery of new treatments. Consequently, NMR continues to be a vital component of integrative approaches in metabolomics, enabling enhanced sensitivity towards cellular metabolism and the systemic character of changes at the metabolic level (Kamphorst & Lewis. 2017) (Figure 11.8).

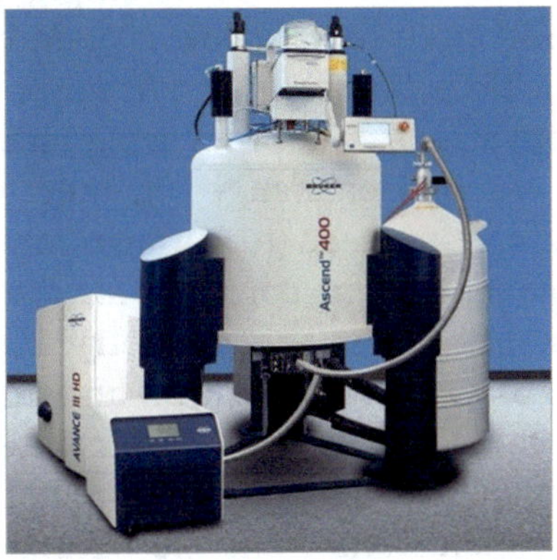

Figure 11.8. Nuclear magnetic resonance (NMR) spectroscopy.

Source: https://cpimg.tistatic.com/02531022/b/5/Nuclear-Magnetic-Resonance-Spectroscopy-NMR.jpg.

11.2.2. Gas Chromatography-Mass Spectrometry (GC-MS)

Gas chromatography-mass spectrometry (GC-MS) has become a cornerstone technique in proteomics and metabolomics, enabling researchers to analyze complex biological samples with unprecedented sensitivity and accuracy. The dual capabilities of GC for analyzing mixtures and mass spectrometry for analyzing molecular compositions allow researchers to uncover the entire scheme of metabolic pathways and protein interactions. This technology is particularly important to the analysis of volatile and semi-volatile compounds, which are critical to metabolic profiling. As researchers strive to explore the intricate relationships among metabolites and their functions in biology, GC-MS provides a solid base for quantitative detection and identification, thereby facilitating advances in areas , such as plant biology, drug discovery, and disease biomarkers. The integration of GC-MS with metabolomics has been made possible by the development of sophisticated data handling resources that enhance the strength of the methodology. The challenge of understanding complex datasets generated by employing high-throughput analyses has been found to be a stumbling block for scientists. As emphasized in recent appraisals, data processing and analysis are the principal challenges in metabolomics, emphasizing the need to implement effective algorithms and strong software for the efficient management of mass spectrometry data (Misra et al., 2016). Data visualization and annotation software tools play a vital role in interpreting metabolic profiles, allowing researchers to draw valuable conclusions from the data generated. These advancements indicate the need for continuous improvement of analytical methods to stay in line with the dynamic character of metabolomics studies. Also, GC-MS has come into being with great promise in plant metabolomics, in which it aids in disentangling the effect of various environmental factors on plant metabolism. By analyzing the metabolite profile, researchers are able to interpret regulatory patterns of growth and development in different plant species (Gullberg et al., 2005). Particularly, GC-MS-based studies have aimed at the extraction and quantification of low molecular weight metabolites from plant tissue, e.g., from Arabidopsis thaliana. The establishment of streamlined methodologies, including semi-automated data processing approaches, has considerably diminished the time and effort involved with metabolic analyses (Gullberg et al., 2005). This innovation not only enables research productivity but also provides a window for the critical comparison of metabolomic information under different conditions, paving the way toward a deeper understanding of plant physiology and reaction to external stimuli (Figure 11.9).

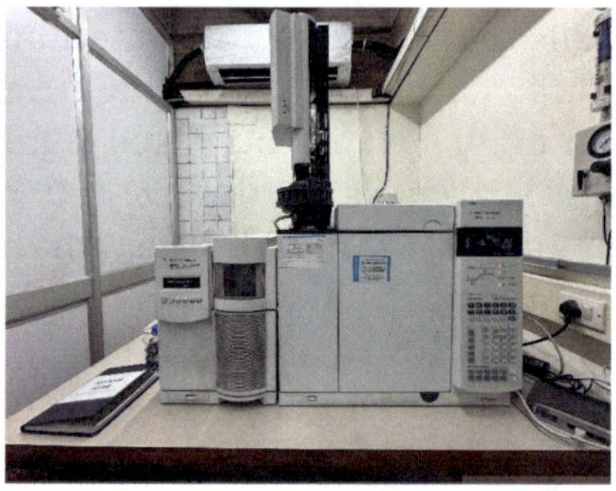

Figure 11.9. Gas chromatography–mass spectrometer (GC-MS).

Source: https://www.nii.res.in/sites/default/files/inline-images/Gas-Liquid%20Chromatography%20%28GC-MS%29_1.jpg.

11.2.3. Liquid Chromatography-Mass Spectrometry (LC-MS)

No amount of emphasis can be laid on the application of LC-mass spectrometry (LC-MS) in proteomics and metabolomics. LC-MS is an instrumental tool with the ability to identify and quantify complex biomolecules and throw light on their roles in biological processes. In proteomics, LC-MS enables the physicochemical properties, such as size and charge, to be separated from proteins before mass spectrometric analysis. This bimodal potential is significant, considering the extensive variability of proteome expression and PTM. Emerging techniques, including hydrophilic interaction liquid chromatography (HILIC), have been exploited to enhance the ability to detect metabolites so that researchers can efficiently isolate a broader variety of hydrophilic metabolites, improving overall proteomic analysis coverage of biological samples, including human plasma and urine. In the management of the complexity of metabolomics, LC-MS is a robust tool for the analysis of metabolic profiles. Metabolomics aims to establish the quantity of a group of metabolites in biological samples that will assist in the identification of metabolic markers of health and disease. Utilizing an optimized LC-MS strategy, scientists can gain global coverage of the metabolome by combining different chromatographic techniques optimized for hydrophilic and non-hydrophilic compounds. As research demonstrates, the integration of HILIC and RPLC can lead to significant improvement in metabolome coverage, detecting 44% and 108% additional metabolic features in urine and plasma samples, respectively, when these methods are integrated (Contrepois et al., 2015). Integration of these methods is important for broad metabolic profiling, ultimately leading to enhanced insight into disease mechanisms. Although the analytical capability of LC-MS is confronted with some limitations, particularly in respect to handling and interpretation of data, high-throughput metabolomics experiments with increasingly complex data sets present a further level of demand for advanced bioinformatics tools for analysis and processing. Advanced computer program solutions are required in data processing, annotation, and visualization of the metabolomics information to disentangle the intricate interactions of the metabolites and biological processes (Misra et al., 2016). This ongoing need for improved analytical tools is the marker of the importance of equipping researchers with contemporary tools that streamline data handling and enhance the interpretative platform for metabolomic research even further. As one means of overcoming these obstacles, software and databases specific to metabolomic analysis are central to the establishment of metabolomics as a research field and for creating new understanding of human disease and health (Figure 11.10).

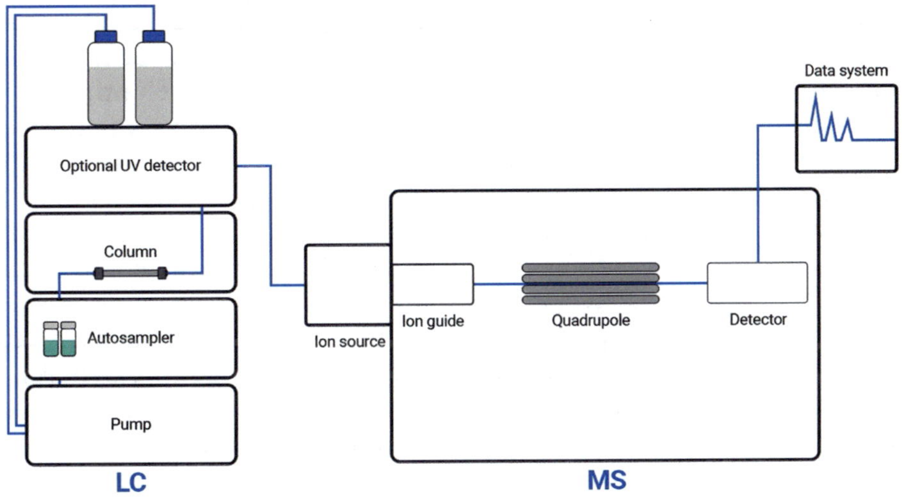

Figure 11.10. Liquid chromatography-mass spectrometry (LC-MS).

Source: https://www.agilent.com/cs/promotions/images/lc-ms-fundamentals-basic-principles-1638x950-agilent.jpg.

Test Your Knowledge

1. What is NMR spectroscopy?
2. What is gas chromatography-mass spectrometry (GC-MS)?

11.3. Applications of Proteomics

Learning Outcome

1. Discuss drug discovery;
2. Identify disease biomarker;
3. Understand the personalized medicine.

The possible applications of proteomics are vast and widespread, especially in pharmaceutical discovery and biomarker identification. Proteomics enables researchers to examine complicated protein interactions and functions, allowing them to probe disease processes more deeply. For instance, in the pharmaceutical sector, discovering potential protein targets can curtail the drug development process, offering novel treatments for conditions like cancer and neurodegenerative diseases. By the application of high-throughput proteomic approaches, scientists are capable of mapping signaling pathways for specific diseases and, subsequently, of finding biomarkers for disease progression and drug response. Ultimately, the integration of proteomic information into the biomedicine research community propels the search for personalized medicine and individualized therapeutic approaches even further, all for the purpose of improving therapeutic approaches to be more effective and disease-specific for a specific patient's needs. Besides drug discovery, proteomics is also vital in the comprehension of protein expression differences due to varying environmental and physiological conditions. This use has particular importance in fields , such as agriculture, where proteomic studies can be applied to enhance crop tolerance to stress and yield through the identification of key proteins involved in stress responses. Through techniques , such as two-dimensional gel electrophoresis and mass spectrometry, researchers have been able to examine the variations in protein abundance and modifications that reflect the adaptation of the plant to stress conditions , such as drought or pathogens. In addition, this information can be employed to drive breeding programs for raising crops more adapted to changing climate conditions. This intersection of proteomics and plant biology illustrates the broader potential of proteomic technologies for solving the most pressing global problems, such as food security and environmentally sustainable agriculture. The combination of proteomics with metabolomics is revealing pathways to comprehensive systems biology approaches that describe the intricate biochemical networks within living organisms. By concomitant examination of metabolite and protein profiles, researchers can gain a thorough view of cellular operations and how they are regulated. Such combined analyses could identify novel information on altered metabolic pathways in disease, which is of interest for the identification of diagnostic or prognostic biomarkers. For instance, integration of proteomics with metabolomics data has been utilized to identify metabolic alterations in cancer cells and reveal potential targets for novel biomarker development and therapeutic targeting. Synergistic interaction of these omics technologies is essential to advance in precision medicine as it encourages enhanced understanding of dynamic interactions between genotype, phenotype, and biochemical environment in health and disease (Kamphorst & Lewis. 2017; Misra et al., 2016) (Figure 11.11).

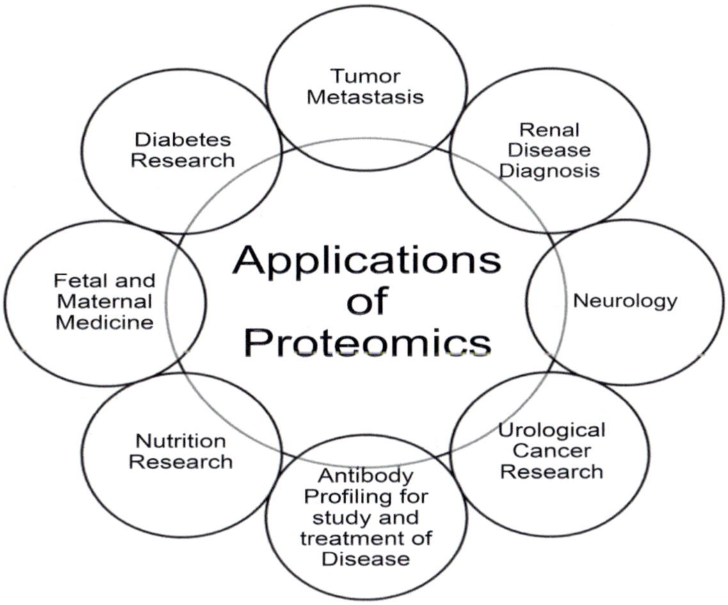

Figure 11.11. Application of proteomics.

Source: https://microbiologynotes.org/wp-content/uploads/2020/12/Application-of-Proteomics-768x575.jpg.

11.3.1. Drug Discovery

The discipline of drug discovery has undergone a revolutionary transformation with the introduction of proteomics and metabolomics. These two fields of research provide an improved understanding of biological systems at the molecular level, enabling investigators to identify novel drug targets and biomarkers. Proteomics, which examines the entire protein content of a cell or tissue, reveals dynamic protein interactions and protein modifications in response to pathological conditions. Parallel to this, metabolomics, which deals with the metabolic profiling of biological specimens, provides insight into the biochemical pathways and metabolic changes that correlate with various conditions. Together, these omics technologies enhance the recognition of the central pathways involved in pathogenesis and aid in the design of targeted therapy. As pharmacological investigation increasingly relies on these technologies, the potential for the discovery of new therapeutic agents increases, justifying the integration of proteomics and metabolomics into ongoing drug discovery programs. One of the primary means of leveraging proteomics and metabolomics in drug discovery is disease and therapeutic response biomarker discovery. Biomarkers play an extremely crucial role in stratifying patients so that the treatment can be made more individualized. By profiling the proteomes and metabolomes of the patients, researchers can identify accurate molecular signatures connected with disease states, which allows for the possibility of early detection and intervention schemes. For instance, in cancer, heterogeneity of tumors necessitates precise targeting of therapies and thus the identification of biomarkers is extremely important. Moreover, integration of these omics methodologies allows for real-time monitoring of drug responses. As exemplified by studies targeting precision medicine, the application of proteomics can elucidate tumor response to therapies and consequently inform clinical decisions and patient optimization. Lastly, this tailored strategy enhances the safety and effectiveness of therapeutic interventions. Furthermore, the uses of proteomics and metabolomics go beyond biomarker discovery and personalized medicine to enhance the ability of synthetic microbiologys in drug discovery. Genome mining technologies have revealed numerous secondary metabolite biosynthetic gene clusters in microbes that have tremendous potential for the identification of new compounds. The induction of these otherwise undefined metabolic routes has appealed to researchers interested in applying microbial biosynthesis to medicines. Metabolomics is a pivotal component in the endeavor, helping facilitate global quantitation of biomolecular compounds and identification of bottlenecks in compound production. By incorporating metabolomics and metabolic modeling, researchers can optimize microbial production systems, improving productivity and efficiency. Thus, the combination of proteomics and metabolomics not only enhances the drug discovery pipeline but also sets the stage for new therapies that address major health challenges, as shown by the potential breakthroughs outlined by Nguyen et al. (2012) and Latosinska et al. (2017) (Figure 11.12).

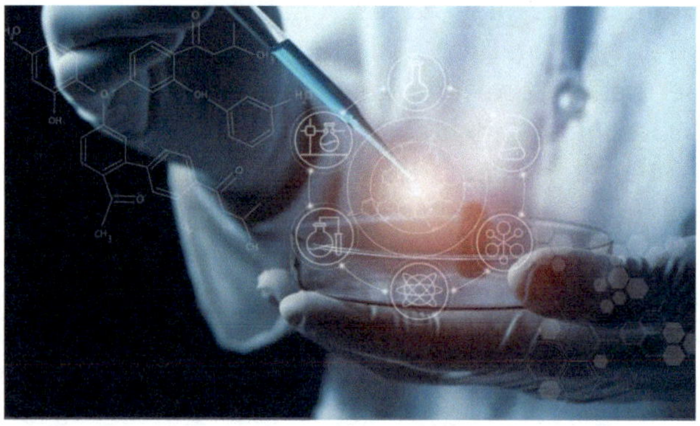

Figure 11.12. Drug discovery.

Source: https://www.ddw-online.com/wp-content/uploads/2023/01/drug-discovery-1.jpg.

11.3.2. Disease Biomarker Identification

Disease biomarker discovery is the core element of enhancing diagnostic technology and therapeutic intervention in medicine. Biomarkers are quantifiable indications of disease status and help clarify causative pathophysiologic mechanisms, especially with chronic diseases like chronic kidney disease (CKD). With the use of proteomic and metabolomic techniques, researchers can assess biological samples to prove candidate biomarkers linked with the progression of disease. From a cohort study of patients with CKD, joint application of urine and plasma analysis resulted in the discovery of 76 statistically significant peptides and metabolites. The biomarkers were significantly correlated with kidney function and had implications for improving diagnosis and treatment of CKD, demonstrating the revolutionary nature of integrative biomarker discovery for application in clinical practice (Argilés et al., 2014). Similarly, the integration of proteomics into models for personalized medicine underscores the significance of disease biomarker discovery. Proteomics, which observes the protein expression within various biological samples, provides a real-time understanding of molecular characteristics that dictate disease mechanisms. Such information is significant in guiding therapy choice with respect to individual patient profiles. The potential of proteomics to be applied in oncology, and indeed in heterogeneous disorders like bladder cancer, is one example of the potential of precision medicine. Evidence indicates that the identification of proteomic biomarkers not only facilitates stratification of patients and prediction but also their identification as potential therapeutic targets. These developments in the identification of disease biomarkers attempt to make earlier intervention more efficient and permit continuous monitoring of therapy responses. The obstacles that remain to be transcended must be overcome for the practical application of these results to become a reality (Latosinska et al., 2017). In summary, the arrival of proteomics and metabolomics has transformed the landscape of disease biomarker discovery, ushering in the possibility of rationalized disease management strategies. Through the use of the wealth of information obtained from biomarker profiling, clinicians and researchers can have more accurate diagnostic tests and more tailored treatment regimens. The combination of both proteomic and metabolomic information has the potential to uncover an integrated understanding of the mechanisms and course of disease, which will translate into improved patient outcomes. But there needs to be overcoming of the technical, biological, and clinical challenges associated with biomarker standardization and validation so that these findings can be translated into clinical practice on a day-to-day basis. Ultimately, the future of the discovery of disease biomarkers rests in collaborative efforts among various fields of science to achieve the full potential of these omics technologies for medicine (Argilés et al., 2014; Latosinska et al., 2017).

11.3.3. Personalized Medicine

The advent of personalized medicine has introduced revolutionary advancements in healthcare practice, particularly through the integration of proteomics and metabolomics. Through the study of molecular profiles at a personal level, health professionals are in a position to construct interventions customized to the specific biological characteristics of individual patients. Proteomics, or the comprehensive analysis of proteins, provides pivotal information on the proteome, which reflects the dynamic changes occurring within systems of biology. This approach not only enables disease prevention and forecasting of treatment but also enhances patient stratification for therapies. For instance, in cancer, proteomics has proven helpful in the discovery of biomarkers employed to stratify bladder cancer patients, further validating that targeted therapies lead to more effective management of complex diseases. These advances are not without hurdles as researchers work towards incorporating proteomics-guided individualized treatment into routine clinical practice (Latosinska et al., 2017). The promise of personalized medicine extends beyond oncology to encompass various chronic conditions , such as hypertension. Traditional models of treatment employ "one-size-fits-all" strategies, which fail to capture the heterogeneities and complexities of patient profiles. The reductionist paradigm has resulted in inferior blood pressure control in most instances, as variables , such as genetic susceptibility and variability in drug response both impact treatment effectiveness substantially. Through the application of knowledge from proteomics and metabolomics, medical practice can evolve towards a more sophisticated interpretation of hypertension, making it possible for individually adapted therapeutic strategies that take into account a patient's specific risk factors and biological reaction. Such evolution in treatment aims to improve drug compliance and effectiveness but also places the patient at the center, optimizing results with tailored approaches responding to their own physiological needs (Borghi et al., 2017). The future of individualized medicine relies on the continuous dialogue between technological progress in omics and practice. With increasingly advanced high-throughput technologies, the ability to assess great amounts of proteomic and metabolic data in a reasonable time period facilitates the development of personalized strategies. Further, the technologies can illuminate not only the number of biomarkers but also the pathophysiologic mechanisms of the diseases that contribute to them as well. It becomes imperative for ongoing research to overcome the challenges involved in successfully translating these advanced tools into clinical practice. The vision is to establish a health system where individualized medicine is the standard, which would facilitate improved patient handling in various medical specialties and ultimately result in higher quality health care provision (Borghi et al., 2017; Latosinska et al., 2017) (Figure 11.13).

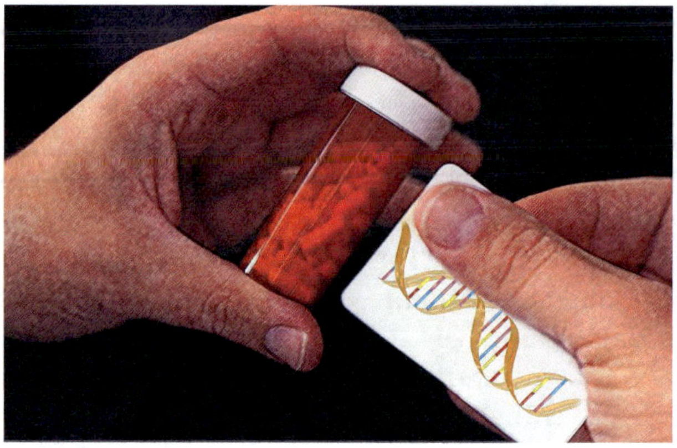

Figure 11.13. Personalized medicine.

Source: https://www.nih.gov/sites/default/files/styles/featured_media_breakpoint-medium/public/about-nih/discovery-into-health/applying-dna-to-medicine-bottle_0.jpg?itok=gq_XG1I1&timestamp=1439240671.

Test Your Knowledge

1. What is meant by drug discovery?
2. What is meant by personalized medicine?

11.4. Applications of Metabolomics

Learning Outcome

1. Learn about nutritional science;
2. Describe the environmental monitoring;
3. Describe the evolution of cancer research.

Metabolomics, the comprehensive examination of small molecules in biological systems, has a wide variety of applications in a broad number of fields , such as medicine, agriculture, and environmental science. Disease biomarker identification is one of the key applications in medicine. By examining the unique metabolic profiles of numerous conditions, researchers are able to create diagnostic tests that allow the potential for early diagnosis and a customized treatment plan. Such utility is greater than disease identification; it also enables the explanation of disease mechanisms at a molecular level. With advances in the field, the integration of metabolomics with proteomics is fast emerging, enabling the integration of a systems biology approach that enables us to better understand the intricate interaction between metabolic and proteomic alterations in health and disease (Kamphorst & Lewis. 2017). Metabolomics in agriculture has consequences for breeding crops with enhanced resistance to pests and crop improvement. Scientists can identify compounds that confer desirable traits, for example, disease or environmental stress tolerance, through metabolite profiling in plants. Such data can be employed to breed crops with superior nutrient content or under adverse conditions. Moreover, metabolomic technologies can also be applied in monitoring the efficacy of biofertilizers or biopesticides, giving insights into how these compounds affect plant metabolism and overall health. The ability to define secondary metabolites in plants can also have applications in developing sustainable, viable agricultural practices. Combining metabolomics with genomic and proteomic data can provide holistic models for enhancing plant productivity and sustainability of food production (Nguyen et al., 2012).

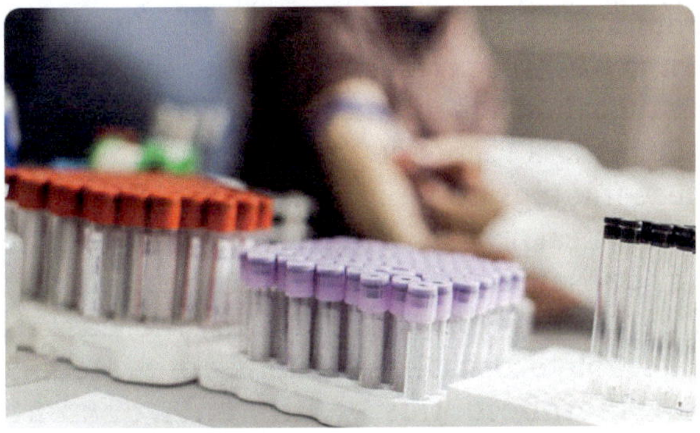

Figure 11.14. Blood collection tubes prepared for analysis with a patient undergoing venipuncture in the background.

Source: https://www.news-medical.net/image-handler/ts/20170308050755/ri/680/picture/blood%20sampling%20for%20analysis%20-%20Goran%20Bogicevic%20_thumb.jpg.

In addition, metabolomics is revolutionizing synthetic biology, in particular the discovery and design of microbial secondary metabolites. By searching for novel biosynthetic gene clusters in bacterial genomes, researchers are finding a vast set of compounds with possible biotechnological applications in medicine and industry. Metabolomics is helping in the identification of these compounds so that metabolic bottlenecks along the biosynthesis pathway of valuable secondary metabolites can be detected. Besides, the technology also optimizes the metabolic pathways using advanced modeling technologies so that microbial systems can be reprogrammed to produce pharmaceuticals or biofuels sustainably. While the promise of metabolic profiling improves, its role in synthetic microbiology keeps playing a central part, with great potential for basic research as well as available technologies (Nguyen et al., 2012) (Figure 11.14).

11.4.1. Nutritional Science

At the intersection of proteomics and metabolomics and nutritional science, it becomes evident that there are key findings regarding the impact of diet on biochemical pathways and disease. Through the observation of dynamic nutrient-biological system interactions, researchers can identify the exact molecular processes responsible for numerous metabolic processes. This is especially true in the detection of biomarkers that are associated with nutritional stress and dietary effects on health. For instance, current studies have highlighted the significance of single metabolites to act as indicators of nutritional imbalance and energy intake. Utilization of targeted and untargeted metabolomics has transformed the ability of researchers to determine subtle differences in metabolic profiles, providing a more accurate picture of nutrient utilization and energy homeostasis, particularly in organisms like Bombus terrestris, where single biomarkers were associated with dietary stress (Meeus et al., 2019). Metabolomics, when coupled with proteomics, enhances understanding of multifactorial conditions , such as CMD. Nutritional science benefits from the union by illuminating the intricate interactions of various biological molecules under the influence of dietary habits. Through this process, one can more easily comprehend the manner in which some nutrients will delay or hasten disease processes. Importantly, multi-omics integration, genomics, proteomics, and metabolomics, yields an in-depth understanding of disease mechanisms as well as of potential nutritional interventions. By integrative analysis, scientists detect highly fitting biomarkers, which lead to the prevention and control of the disease through nutrition, thus providing avenues towards personalized diets in accordance with individuals' metabolic fingerprints (Argano et al., 2019). Further, the input of gender medicine to nutritional science demonstrates the complexity of metabolic response to nutrition. There are known gender differences in metabolism that affect how individuals absorb nutrients, and it is a factor that compels the inclusion of gender-oriented analyses in nutritional research. The differences matter in creating precise dietary interventions that will help avoid CMD among individuals. Integration of information between proteomics and metabolomics allows researchers to see how certain biomolecules interact with gender-differentiated metabolism, thus augmenting the predictive accuracy of dietary recommendations. The integration of these branches of science thus not only informs us more about nutritional science but also allows for the formulation of personalized medicine in the management of long-term diseases (Argano et al., 2019) (Figure 11.15).

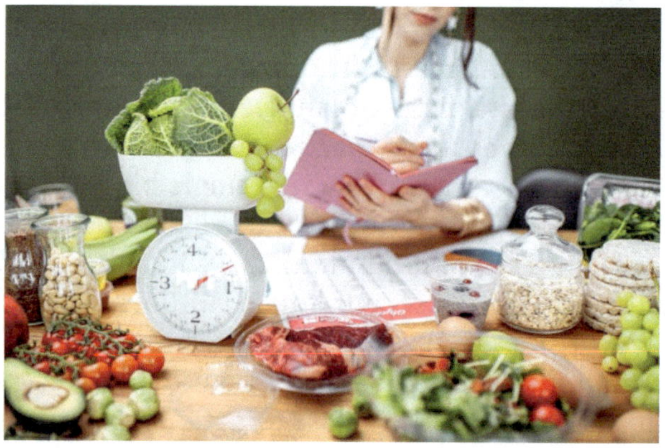

Figure 11.15. Nutritional science.

Source: https://www.nspublisher.com/wp-content/uploads/2023/03/6-1.jpg.

11.4.2. Environmental Monitoring

Environmental monitoring has emerged into greater prominence in the framework of proteomics and metabolomics due to their potential to assess the biochemical responses of ecosystems to environmental change. These omics approaches enable the integrated scrutiny of proteins and metabolites employed as environmental health indicators for the identification of pollutants and other forms of stress. For instance, changes in protein levels or metabolite profiles can reveal the physiological status of organisms exposed to environmental pollutants. Through the use of high-throughput techniques, researchers can generate vast data sets that shed light on the molecular mechanisms underlying a response to environmental stress. These findings not only enhance our knowledge of ecological processes but also inform regulation and conservation efforts directed towards safeguarding biodiversity in increasingly vulnerable ecosystems. Coupling of proteomics and metabolomics with environmental monitoring platforms offers immense innovation potential for natural resource management. Application of these technologies enables the identification of biomarkers related to stress reactions in biological systems, which is important for quantifying ecosystem health. For example, the identification of certain protein markers determining the presence of toxins in aquatic ecosystems is beneficial in monitoring the quality of water. Furthermore, metabolomics provides a holistic view of environmentally regulated metabolic processes, making it possible to determine the critical thresholds for ecosystem responses. Application of these omics tools not only advances contemporary targets of sustainable development but also supports proactive environmental resource management by increasing understanding of organism adaptability to the environment. Despite the promising applications of proteomics and metabolomics in monitoring the environment, some issues still emerge in data handling and interpretation. According to reports, the complexity of producing high-throughput data necessitates the use of new software and analytical approaches for efficient handling and interpretation of produced datasets (Misra et al., 2016). Such complexity can restrict the use of omics techniques in environmental studies, as researchers are faced with the problem of finding strong techniques for data annotation, visualization, and interpretation. Moreover, the presence of all-encompassing data that is comparable with environmental components is also important to enhance these techniques in real-world applications. Addressing these issues requires an interdisciplinary effort combining advances in computational biology with traditional ecological methods and thereby enhancing the overall efficacy of proteomics- and metabolomics-guided environmental monitoring methodologies (Figure 11.16).

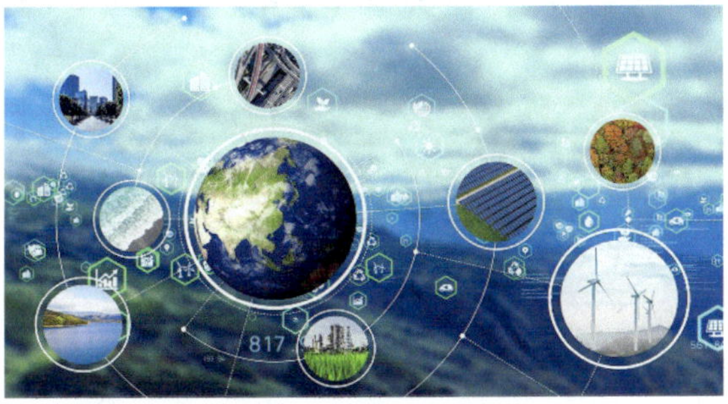

Figure 11.16. Environmental monitoring.

Source: https://www.digi.com/getattachment/Blog/post/What-Is-Environmental-Monitoring/GettyImages-1289348332-1280.jpg?lang=en-US.

11.4.3. Cancer Research

The evolution of cancer research has been revolutionized by proteomics and metabolomics, two disciplines of modern science that seek to map the intricacies of biological systems. This new approach emphasizes a move away from the traditional methods of the isolation of single proteins or genes and towards an integrative approach that assesses the entire molecular ecology of cancer. With rapid advancement in bioinformatics tools and HTS technologies, researchers now have the capacity to analyze large datasets that are representative of dynamic biological processes in real-time. In renal cancer, as a case in point, the recognition of this cancer as a multifactorial metabolic disorder with many biochemical pathway aberrations offers scientists the prospect to leverage these omics technologies to good effect, opening the way to paradigm-shifting tumour biology and drug discovery insights (Aboud et al., 2017). Proteomics, in particular, has significant potential for personalized medicine, providing for targeted therapeutic interventions on the basis of distinctive molecular signatures. This region allows researchers to monitor in real time alterations in protein expression, key markers of the disease process and response to treatment. By embracing proteomics-guided strategies, cancer treatment can progress beyond the one-size-fits-all paradigm to a patient-specific paradigm. For disease monitoring and treatment response, certain biomarkers were crucial in defining patient stratification and prognosis. The literature now includes both the potential and limitations of applying proteomics to everyday practice based on the requirement for further validation of biomarkers and therapeutic targets (Latosinska et al., 2017). With continued advances in cancer research, the confluence of proteomics and metabolomics provides fertile ground for future advancements. Through facilitation of the correlation of metabolic shifts along with protein expression signatures, deeper insight is obtained into tumor biology, which is critical to understanding the heterogeneity of cancer and resistance to treatment. In addition to making possible earlier intervention, this integrative approach also makes possible new types of therapy based on specific molecular pathways acting in various cancers. Thus, the synergy of proteomics and metabolomics in research promises to advance the precision of cancer management, ultimately leading to improved patient outcomes and the development of more effective treatment protocols. The convergence of these strategies ushers in a new generation of targeted therapy, reinforcing the pressing need for a multidisciplinary approach to addressing the complexities of cancer (Aboud et al., 2017) (Figure 11.17).

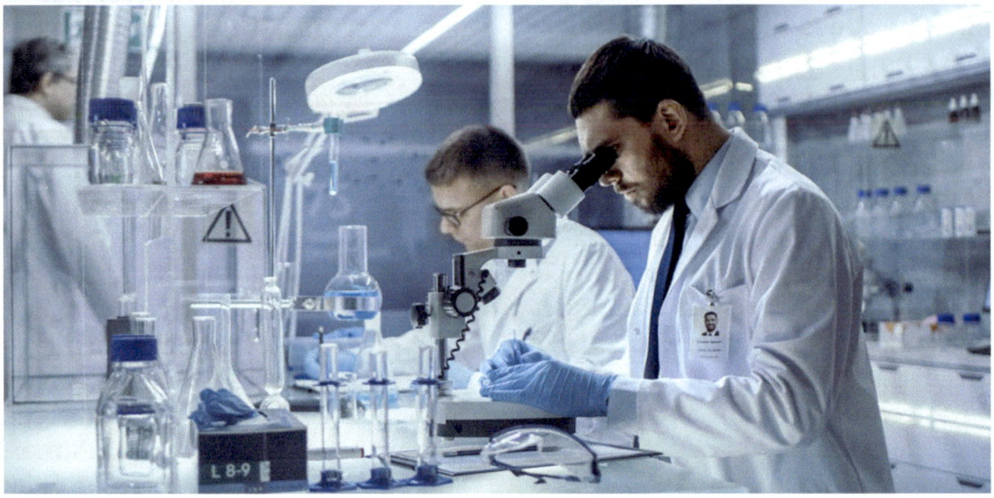

Figure 11.17. Cancer research.

Source: https://www.tfri.ca/images/default-source/page-images/research-highlights-landing-page.jpg?sfvrsn=ef7357d5_2.

Test Your Knowledge

1. What do you mean by environmental monitoring?
2. What is cancer research?

SUMMARY

The combination of proteomics and metabolomics plays a more significant role in the development of our comprehension of the complicated biological systems and diseases. The two omics sciences together are more holistic in their representation of physiological and pathological processes, as explained in this chapter. By analyzing the dynamic protein-metabolite interplay, researchers can detect biomarkers that allow for early detection, accurate diagnosis, and effective treatment for many diseases, such as CKD. The CKD study demonstrated in the findings shows the promise of an integrative approach to generate significant associations with kidney function, thereby establishing the relevance of integrative omic analyses (Argilés et al., 2014). In that regard, the convergence of the two fields can change the way we conduct disease treatment and drug search. Also, the arrival of big data in the biological sciences poses opportunities and challenges to proteomics and metabolomics. With increasing data creation, efficient data-sharing channels are required. The practice of open data sharing will have a significant effect on transparency and reproducibility of results within the scientific community, which will further stimulate the emergence of more collaborations and innovations. Limitations still exist, especially in data dissemination and use. It is crucial to find the benefits of various platforms for data sharing and to make them more user-friendly to meet researchers' needs (Alsheikh-Ali et al., 2013). By emphasizing project and community databases, the researchers will be better placed to structure and disseminate their results, which will eventually translate to the improvement of data reusability and availability. All these will together result in making the field of research a well-connected and effective working atmosphere. In general, the future of proteomics and metabolomics is more integrated and effective data sharing with the research community. Increased cooperation will not only make it possible to discover new biomarkers but also enhance the understanding of the disease mechanisms. As science advances, funders, publishers and institutions must now collaborate to offer a unified plan to make data sharing and integration sustainable. By overcoming the challenges presented and making the most of proteomics and metabolomics, the research base can speed up discoveries and make the most of health benefits worldwide. Finally, the further drive to innovation and cooperation will be required as we proceed to more personalized and efficient healthcare pathways.

Proteomics and metabolomics have now become the science that forms a pillar in the current quest to unravel the complex biological systems. Through analysis of the overall interaction of proteins and metabolites in a biological sample, researchers can infer a significant quantity of information about the molecular pathways that are at the basis of disease. In comparison to the conventional targeted methods, which deal with individual biomolecules solely, the integrative systems biology approach allows researchers to see, in a general sense, how molecular diversifications affect cellular functioning and organismal health. The strategy concurs with the growing understanding that an open-ended hypothesis-free strategy can enable novel directions of research and provide new testable hypotheses, which can ultimately enhance our understanding of dynamic biological environments (Robinson et al., 2014). Thus, the incorporation of systems biology concepts in proteomics and metabolomics studies contributes to our capability of translating molecular findings into clinically useful information. Specifically, the possibility of improved patient outcomes is of interest as far as personalized medicine is concerned. Doctors can develop treatment approaches depending on definite biological features by using proteomic profiling to define the molecular landscape of individual patients. This personalized approach covers a lot of areas in patient care, like early disease prevention, monitoring response to therapy and directing optimum intervention. Heterogeneity of tumors in cancer provides an excellent rationale for proteomics-based approaches. In the literature, it has been noted that the identification of protein biomarkers has a significant role in stratifying patients based on the outcome of the disease and treatment responsiveness (Latosinska et al., 2017). Thus, the potential of proteomics can be utilized in developing more precise and effective interventions, transforming clinicians' treatment of complex diseases, particularly in areas like cancer therapies. In addition, the organization of the large scale data analysis between proteomics and metabolomics raises the questions of the development and implementation of adequate analysis tools. As the research activities increase, the resulting data is getting more complex, demanding sophisticated computational techniques in deriving meaningful information. Our capacity to study the complex interaction of molecular components can even be improved further with the development of integrative systems analysis, which will ultimately lead to the bridging of the gap between basic discovery and clinical translation. Nevertheless, even now, there are major bottlenecks, especially when it comes to standardization and access to data. Overcoming these challenges is central to unleashing the complete strength of proteomics and metabolomics across different fields in medicine and biology so that disease mechanisms can be understood more deeply and therapeutic opportunities (Robinson et al., 2014). When this is achieved, the door is open to more powerful results that will change the treatment of patients.

KEY TERMS FROM THIS CHAPTER

- Bioinformatics
- Cancer research
- Cardiometabolic diseases
- Chronic kidney disease
- Disease biomarkers
- Electrospray ionization
- Environmental monitoring
- Genetic material
- Genomics
- Metabolomics
- Molecular biology
- Nutritional science
- Protein microarrays
- Proteomics
- Sustainability

Critical Thinking Questions

1. **Proteomics is the large-scale study of:**
   a. DNA sequences
   b. RNA transcripts
   c. Proteins
   d. Metabolites
2. **Which technique is commonly used for protein identification in proteomics?**
   a. PCR
   b. Mass spectrometry
   c. Northern blotting
   d. ELISA
3. **Two-dimensional gel electrophoresis separates proteins based on:**
   a. Size and charge
   b. Charge and isoelectric point
   c. Isoelectric point and molecular weight
   d. Size and hydrophobicity
4. **Metabolomics focuses on the study of:**
   a. Proteins
   b. Metabolites
   c. DNA
   d. RNA
5. **Which analytical technique is most commonly used in metabolomics?**
   a. Western blot
   b. Mass spectrometry and NMR spectroscopy
   c. PCR
   d. ELISA

Short Answer Questions

1. What is meant by proteomics?
2. Define the metabolomics.
3. What are the techniques of proteomics?
4. What techniques are used in metabolomics?
5. What are the applications of proteomics?

Answers to Critical Thinking Questions

1. (c); 2. (b); 3. (c); 4. (b); 5. (b)

REFERENCES

1. Abu Aboud, O., & Weiss, R. H. (2017). Translating metabolic reprogramming into new targets for kidney cancer. https://core.ac.uk/download/323071180.pdf (accessed on 12th June 2025).
2. Rabilloud, T., Vaezzadeh, A. R., Potier, N., Lelong, C., Leize-Wagner, E., & Chevallet, M. (2009). Power and limitations of electrophoretic separations in proteomics strategies. *Mass spectrometry reviews*, *28*(5), 816–843. https://doi.org/10.1002/mas.20204 (accessed on 12th June 2025).
3. Nguyen, Q. T., Merlo, M. E., Medema, M. H., Jankevics, A., Breitling, R., & Takano, E. (2012). Metabolomics methods for the synthetic biology of secondary metabolism. *FEBS letters*, *586*(15), 2177–2183. https://doi.org/10.1016/j.febslet.2012.02.008 (accessed on 12th June 2025).
4. Alsheikh-Ali, A., Ball, C. A., Barrett, T., Bastow, R., Baxter, L., Brazma, A., Breeze, J., et al. (2013). Making open data work for plant scientists. https://core.ac.uk/download/18327387.pdf (accessed on 12th June 2025).
5. Argano, V., Balistreri, C. R., Giarratana, R. M., & Lio, D. (2019). On the road to accurate biomarkers for cardiometabolic diseases by integrating precision and gender medicine approaches. https://core.ac.uk/download/268910274.pdf (accessed on 12th June 2025).
6. Argilés, À., Dakna, M., Delles, C., Duranton, F., et al. (2014). Assessment of metabolomic and proteomic biomarkers in detection and prognosis of progression of renal function in chronic kidney disease. https://core.ac.uk/download/42354001.pdf (accessed on 12th June 2025).
7. Borghi, C., Grassi, G., Rosei, E. A., Savoia, C., et al. (2017). Personalized medicine—A modern approach for the diagnosis and management of hypertension. https://core.ac.uk/download/96884785.pdf (accessed on 12th June 2025).
8. Contrepois, K., Jiang, L., & Snyder, M. (2015). Optimized analytical procedures for the untargeted metabolomic profiling of human urine and plasma by combining hydrophilic interaction (HILIC) and reverse-phase liquid chromatography (RPLC)-mass spectrometry. https://core.ac.uk/download/323062297.pdf (accessed on 12th June 2025).
9. Robinson, S. W., Fernandes, M., & Husi, H. (2014). Current advances in systems and integrative biology. *Computational and structural biotechnology journal*, *11*(18), 35–46. https://doi.org/10.1016/j.csbj.2014.08.007 (accessed on 12th June 2025).
10. Latosinska, A., Frantzi, M., Vlahou, A., Merseburger, A. S., & Mischak, H. (2018). Clinical Proteomics for Precision Medicine: The Bladder Cancer Case. *Proteomics. Clinical applications*, *12*(2), 10.1002/prca.201700074. https://doi.org/10.1002/prca.201700074(accessed on 12th June 2025).
11. Gullberg, J. (2005). *Metabolomics: A Tool for Studying Plant Biology*. https://core.ac.uk/download/11694915.pdf (accessed on 12th June 2025).
12. Jamshidi, N., Lewis, N. E., Swann, J., Winzeler, E. A., et al. (2015). Systems analysis of host-parasite interactions. https://core.ac.uk/download/323077861.pdf (accessed on 12th June 2025).
13. Kamphorst, J. J., & Lewis, I. A. (2017). Editorial overview: Recent innovations in the metabolomics revolution. *Current opinion in biotechnology*, *43*, iv–vii. https://doi.org/10.1016/j.copbio.2017.01.005(accessed on 12th June 2025).

14. Meeus, I., Rombouts, C., Smagghe, G., & Van Meulebroek, L., et al. (2019). Metabolomics-based biomarker discovery for bee health monitoring: A proof-of-concept study concerning nutritional stress in *Bombus terrestris*. https://core.ac.uk/download/227040916.pdf (accessed on 12th June 2025).

15. Misra, B. B., & van der Hooft, J. (2016). Updates in metabolomics tools and resources: 2014–2015. https://core.ac.uk/download/46559843.pdf (accessed on 12th June 2025).

16. Neumann, E., Schreeck, F., Herberg, J., Jacqz Aigrain, E., Maitland-van der Zee, A. H., Pérez-Martínez, A., Hawcutt, D., et al. (2022). How pediatric drug development and use could benefit from OMICs: A c4c expert group white paper. *British Journal of Clinical Pharmacology, 88*, 5017–5033. https://www.semanticscholar.org/paper/dbde080078ef69b6e6d1a663bbe660c348ceb76b (accessed on 12th June 2025).

17. Tebani, A., Gummesson, A., Zhong, W., Koistinen, I. S., Lakshmikanth, T., Olsson, L. M., Boulund, F., et al. (2020). Integration of molecular profiles in a longitudinal wellness profiling cohort. *Nature Communications, 11*. https://www.semanticscholar.org/paper/54d854f8f0b75527ed0965548f1c997996b37c9f (accessed on 12th June 2025).

EPIGENETICS

12

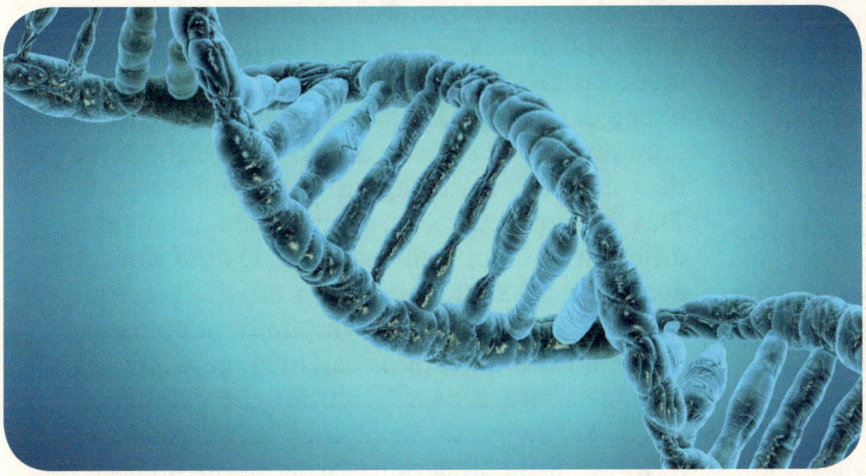

LEARNING OBJECTIVES

After studying this chapter, you will be able to:

1. Understand the mechanisms of epigenetic regulation;
2. Describe the role of epigenetics in development;
3. Understand the relationship between epigenetics and disease;
4. Describe the role of environmental influences on epigenetics;
5. Know the therapeutic applications of epigenetics.

Introduction

The field of epigenetics is a vital frontier in human biology, as it explores the complex mechanisms that regulate gene expression without altering the underlying DNA sequence. This complex level of control is crucial in normal cellular function, in addition to the manifestation of many diseases. Environmental factors, life style decisions, and even emotional states can trigger epigenetic modifications—most significantly through mechanisms , such as DNA methylation and histone modification. Such modifications can influence phenotypic traits, sometimes resulting in ailments , such as cancer, CVDs, and metabolic syndromes. As the knowledge of how genes respond to the environment improves, the complexities now reach beyond plain biology, and the prospects fall within the area of personalized medicine and therapeutic interventions. The function of epigenetics has been particularly well-illuminated in the instance of disease states like cancer, wherein it may serve as a key determinant for growth and development of tumors.

For instance, it has been shown that epigenetic alterations, i.e., abnormal DNA methylation, are at the core of human papillomavirus (HPV) carcinogenic processes. There is evidence to indicate that some methylation patterns have the ability to serve as biomarkers for the early identification of pre-invasive cervical lesions, potentially directing screening and treatment regimens. This indicates the potential value of adding epigenetic analysis to clinical diagnostics to allow for the creation of more targeted and more effective treatments. This paradigm shift not only advances our understanding of mechanistic processes but also highlights the promise of epigenetics to address key health challenges that afflict populations in the present time. In addition, epigenetic thinking extends beyond cancer to reach a wide range of health problems including CVDs. The endocrine role of the heart showcases such complexity in which biological substances , such as natriuretic peptides (NPs) are not only hormones but also epigenetically controlled entities. Examining how miRNAs and epigenetic changes affect NP production could open the door to new cardiovascular treatments, advancing our knowledge of heart failure and other related diseases.

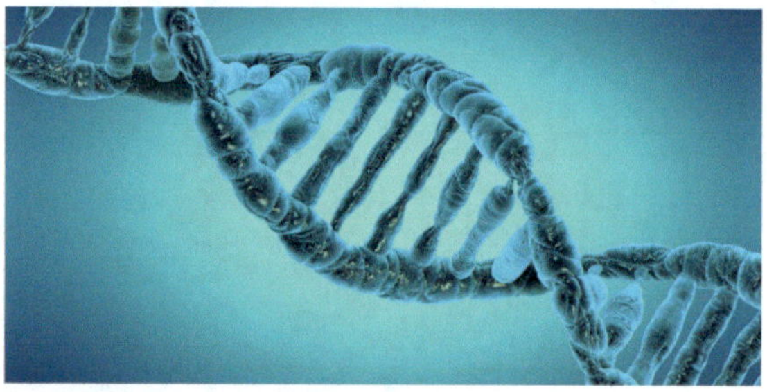

Figure 12.1. Epigenetics.

Source: https://www.niehs.nih.gov/sites/default/files/health/assets/images/epigenetics_og.jpg.

As we learn more of these epigenetic mechanisms, we discover that understanding the intricate relationship between genetic and environmental influences is the secret to new therapeutic strategies. The search for a deeper knowledge of epigenetics in man is consequently not a purely academic exercise but a vitally important one of wide relevance to health and medicine (Figure 12.1).

Importance of Epigenetics in Human Biology

Epigenetics plays a crucial role in regulating gene expression without altering the underlying DNA sequence and, therefore, influences various biological processes among human beings. DNA methylation is one of the most significant forms of epigenetic regulation whereby methyl groups are attached to specific areas of the DNA, with the majority resulting in gene suppression. This is required for proper development and differentiation of cells as it enables the correct genes to be switched on or off at the right time. For instance, in lymphoid neoplasms, epigenetic modifications can help elucidate the diagnosis and cancer evolution, as Alaggio et al. (2022) suggest. Through an investigation of how these modifications bring about disease, researchers can devise new treatments that will target epigenetic changes and enhance drug responses and customize medicine. Epigenetic mechanisms are increasingly recognized to play roles in the development of complex diseases, such as Type 2 Diabetes Mellitus (T2DM). T2DM results from the interaction between a mixture of genetic and environmental etiologic determinants that influence insulin secretion and sensitivity. Epigenetic modifications can act on these pathways, modifying the body's response to insulin regulatory processes. For instance, dietary, exercise, and gut microbiota compositional variables have been shown to cause epigenetic modifications that predispose to insulin resistance and metabolic impairment. Understandings of these mechanisms, however, not only can help explain the pathophysiology of T2DM but also can inform preventative interventions and actions to be considered that account for both genetic susceptibility as well as environmental determinants highlighted by Galicia-Garc et al. (2020). The intersection of epigenetics with metabolic disease highlights its importance in human health. The potential effects of epigenetics go beyond individual diseases, influencing more general features of human biology like development and aging. Epigenetic modifications are reversible processes which can be influenced by a variety of internal and external factors throughout an individual's lifetime, including lifestyle and environmental stressors. For example, it has been shown that epigenetic reprogramming occurs at times of significant development since this affects the gene expression throughout the individual's lifetime. Because epigenetic marks are reversible but stable, they have therapeutic potential as a mechanism for age-related decrement and chronic disease prevention. Through catalyzing increased appreciation of the ways in which epigenetics regulate human biology, researchers can access the key to optimizing health and wellbeing and creating new therapy and a better understanding of human development and disease interconnectedness (Figure 12.2).

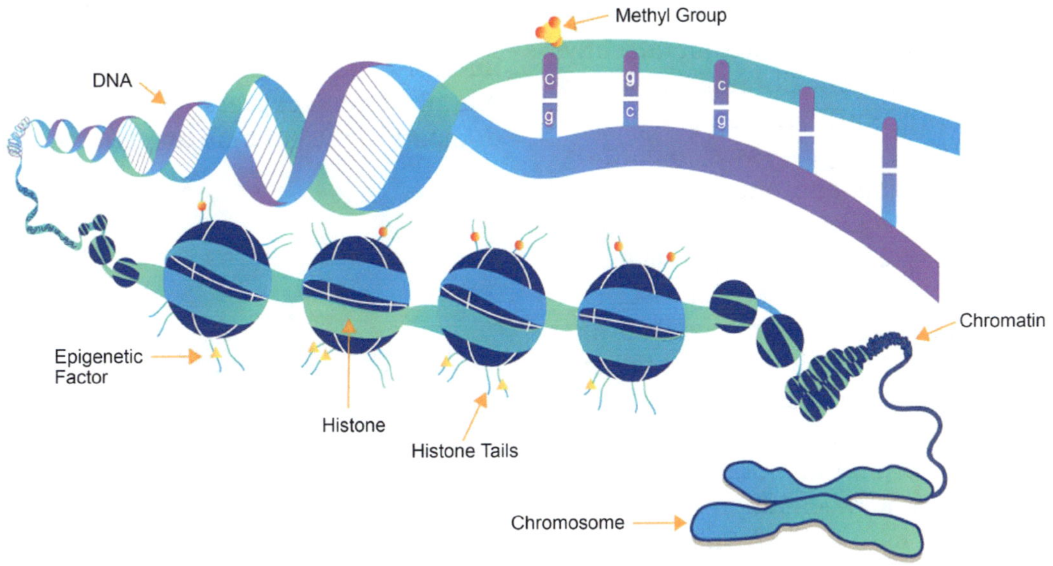

Figure 12.2. Representation of the chromatin structure, including histones and DNA, which becomes available to epigenetic marks.

Source: https://www.whatisepigenetics.com/wp-content/uploads/2013/07/dna-chromatin-histone.jpg.

12.1. Mechanisms of Epigenetic Regulation

Learning Outcome

1. Describe the DNA methylation;
2. Know the histone modification;
3. Understand the role of non-coding RNAs.

In the intricate science of epigenetics, one of the chief mechanisms of regulation is by chromatin structural alteration that directly regulates gene expression. Chromatin, which is the histone protein-DNA complex, may be modified by several processes, including acetylation, methylation, and phosphorylation. These modifications regulate the accessibility of transcription factors to the underlying DNA and thus regulate the activity of genes. For instance, the role of histone lysine demethylases has been underlined, particularly in heart failure, where their abnormal expression may disrupt fetal gene expression patterns in the adult heart. As studies go on, understanding of the finesse of how chromatin-modifying enzymes respond to cellular cues will provide valuable context on the dynamic regulatory landscape of epigenetics, highlighting the necessity of targeted intervention in diseases like heart failure, where such processes get disturbed (Deogharia et al., 2024). Another significant feature of epigenetic control is the role of non-coding RNAs, particularly miRNAs and long non-coding RNAs (lncRNAs). These molecules play essential roles in gene silencing and post-transcriptional regulation. Through the binding of complementary sequences on the target mRNAs, miRNAs can suppress translation or trigger degradation, thus inhibiting some gene expressions. In sporadic Parkinson's disease (PD), for example, environmental exposures , such as the use of pesticides have been shown to influence the expression of certain miRNAs. These changes can control the disease-specific gene regulatory networks, establishing a link between environmental exposures and genetic susceptibility. As the field advances, the exploration of non-coding RNAs in conjunction with traditional genetic analysis is essential in elucidating the pathogenesis of multifactorial diseases like PD, where genes and epigenetics interact (Tsalenchuk et al., 2023). Furthermore, the organization of the genome within the nucleus is important for epigenetic management, especially through the theory of Lamin-associated domains (LADs). The big chromatin domains are organized around nuclear edge proteins , such as Lamin A/C, that modulate gene expression by tethering specific domains of the genome to the nuclear envelope.

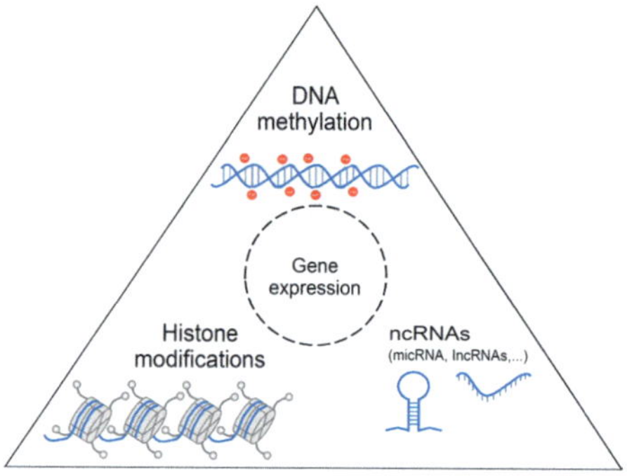

Figure 12.3. Epigenetic mechanisms contributing to gene regulation. DNA methylation, histone modifications, and noncoding RNAs (ncRNAs).

Source: https://media.springernature.com/full/springer-static/image/art%3A10.1186%2Fs13148-019-0675-4/MediaObjects/13148_2019_675_Fig1_HTML.png?as=webp.

This three-dimensional structure not only affects transcriptional activity but also participates in interactions with various epigenetic modifiers, thereby affecting cellular responses to environmental stresses and potential pathological conditions. Recent studies have clarified the intricate relationship between the three-dimensional structure of the genome and epigenetic modification in heart failure and emphasized the reality that diseases can originate from dysregulation of this spatial architecture. The ongoing research in this area is the key to knowing more about the complexities of the regulation of genes and their significance in human disease, showcasing the need for integrated methods with all aspects of genetic regulation (Deogharia et al., 2024) (Figure 12.3).

12.1.1. DNA Methylation

DNA methylation, a critical element of epigenetics, refers to the addition of a methyl group to the DNA molecule, usually to cytosine residues in CpG dinucleotides. It is a mechanism for silencing gene expression, effectively serving as a control system by determining which genes are to be activated or repressed in a particular cell type. Methylation patterns are dynamic and highly responsive to many environmental insults, including diet, stress, and toxins. These environmental factors serve to show how lifestyle can affect gene expression without always altering the underlying DNA sequence, illustrating a fundamental tenet of epigenetics. Furthermore, the heritability of methylation marks makes it clear that such epigenetic changes could be passed on through generations and affect phenotypes, as well as susceptibility to disease along the lineage. The significance of DNA methylation is underscored by its association with many health conditions, ranging from cancer and CVDs (Stanzione et al., 2020). Apart from its regulatory function in the control of gene expression, DNA methylation has emerged as a key inducer of age-related disease phenotypes, such as sarcopenia, which is a characteristic of loss of muscle strength and mass.

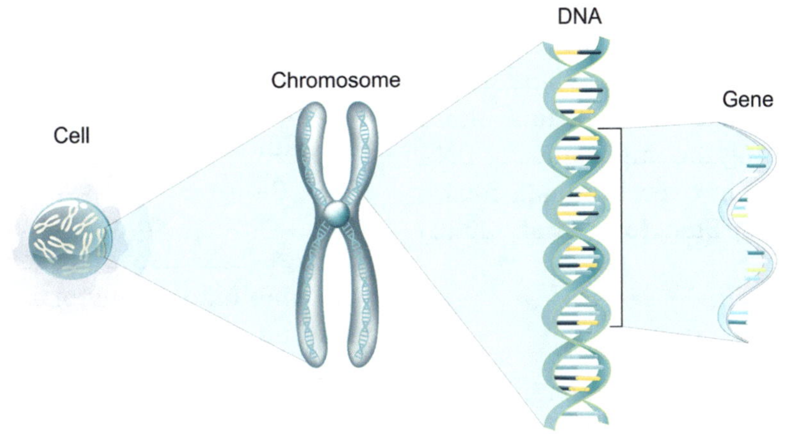

Figure 12.4. DNA methylation affects gene expression.

Source: https://biomodal.com/wp-content/uploads/2024/08/240819-how-DNA-methylation-affects-gene-expression.webp.

The methylation status of the genes that mediate muscle function has been shown to change with age, and epigenetic changes have been implicated to precipitate sarcopenia. DNA methylation has been shown to modulate muscle differentiation and maintenance pathways, leading to impaired muscle function in the elderly. Detection of mechanisms by which DNA methylation impacts sarcopenia can also shed light on its preventive and therapeutic strategies. For instance, interventions in physical exercise and diet can normalize methylation patterns and hence preclude sarcopenia effects. More research is needed to elucidate such intricate interactions and their meaning for the elderly (Gensous et al., 2019). The reversibility of DNA methylation is of great therapeutic interest, particularly for diseases related to abnormal patterns of aberrant methylation. As opposed to genetic mutations, reversible changes in the DNA sequence, epigenetic changes are reversible and can be treated with targeted therapy. It has led scientists to explore the creation of pharmacologic drugs aimed at altering methylation patterns, paving the way for new treatments for a range of diseases. In addition, the arrival of technologies that allow DNA methylation profiling throughout the genome has been a rich source of tools for dissecting complicated disease mechanisms. With each new biomarker for aging and disease progression that is revealed, e.g., epigenetic clocks, there is the possibility to transform personalized medicine by providing rationale for targeted therapeutic approaches responsive to a patient's own epigenetic landscape. These advances can also make interventions more effective, thereby citing the importance of DNA methylation research in overall human health (Gensous et al., 2019; Stanzione et al., 2020) (Figure 12.4).

12.1.2. Histone Modification

Histone modification is a fundamental aspect of epigenetic regulation, as it is one of the main mechanisms by which gene expression is controlled without altering the underlying DNA sequence. These alterations are achieved through PTMs of histone proteins, which are the core components responsible for the organization and accessibility of chromatin. The dynamic regulation of histone modifications, including acetylation, methylation, phosphorylation, and ubiquitination, allows cells to respond to various internal and external signals, thereby influencing developmental processes, cellular differentiation, and environmental response. Either through transcriptional activation or repression, depending upon their specific context and combinations, these modifications demonstrate the sophistication of epigenetic regulation in human biology. Current discoveries point to the importance of histone modification in human disease, and cancer. Aberrant histone modification patterns have been shown to destabilize physiologic gene regulatory networks, resulting in tumorigenesis and disease progression. For instance, the inhibition of histone deacetylases (HDACs) has been developed as a new anticancer strategy, which demonstrates how the targeting of histone-modifying enzymes can restore normal epigenetic landscapes.

Through the reversal of abnormal patterns of histone acetylation, these therapies have precipitated the ability to enhance the course of malignancies and have spurred continued clinical trials for epigenetic drugs that target histone modification. This dynamic between disease and histone modification illustrates the promise of epigenetic treatments to be included in traditional treatment protocols, providing a new pathway to precision medicine. Further, the progress in epigenomics over the past decade has also discovered the significance of combinatorial histone modifications, or the histone code, which characterize the unique patterns of modifications that govern specific gene expression outcomes. Such dynamics suggest that not only individual modifications but also their interactions play a crucial functional role in the regulation of genes. While studying organisms , such as *Plasmodium falciparum*, researchers have demonstrated how histone PTM landscapes regulate diverse development pathways, and this teaches us about the workings of epigenetic processes in specific biological settings (Connacher et al., 2022). These findings reiterate the necessity of rigorous research to map the intricate networks of histone modifications and thereby make inroads into their role in physiological and disease pathology and design them as optimal candidates for therapeutic development (Dai et al., 2024) (Figure 12.5).

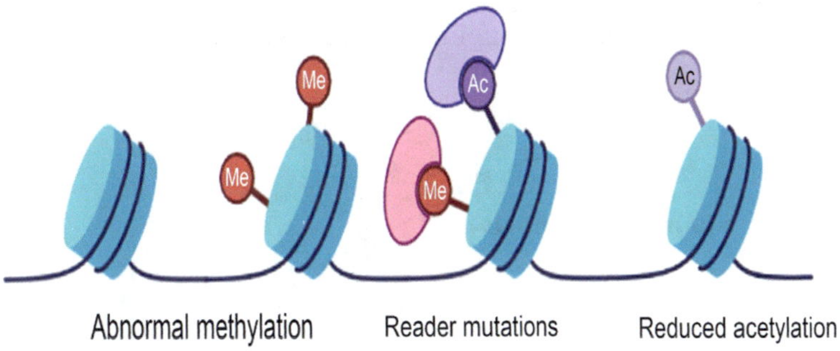

Figure 12.5. Histone modifications.

Source: https://cdn.prod.website-files.com/621e95f9ac30687a56e4297e/64a8d64171394240168f7b54_V2_1583276260194_d070d85a-44aa-4f1e-bbd4-d794cc29a375.png.

12.1.3. Non-Coding RNA Involvement

The role of non-coding RNAs in the field of epigenetics has been a focal point in research on human biology. Non-coding RNAs, particularly miRNAs and long non-coding RNAs (lncRNAs), have essential roles in controlling gene expression without functioning as protein-coding genes. miRNAs, which are small single-stranded RNA molecules, control gene expression by binding with complementary sequences in target messenger RNAs (mRNAs), resulting in their degradation or translational suppression. This is accompanied by illustration of a feed-forward circuit where miRNAs not just control the expression of target genes but also affect the enzymes participating in epigenetic changes, linking miRNA expression to massive epigenetic regulation. Therefore, dysregulation of such non-coding RNAs may trigger alterations in patterns of gene expression that lead to diseases like cancer, suggesting their function should be interpreted for diagnostic and therapeutic considerations in human health (Arif et al., 2020). In cancer, epigenetic regulation interacting with non-coding RNAs is especially significant. Dysregulation of miRNAs can alter cellular pathways during tumorigenesis, modulating gene expression for cell growth promotion or apoptosis inhibition. The interaction opens up a three-way regulatory feedback loop known as the "epi–miR–epi" feedback cycle wherein epigenetic regulators regulate miRNA expression and the latter regulates epigenetic modifying enzymes. The constant interaction may lead to lasting epigenome modifications, a key attribute of defects in cancer cells. Importantly, non-coding RNAs were also found to be potential biomarkers for cancer diagnosis and prognosis, demonstrating their importance in clinical applications. The exploration of the epigenetic regulation by miRNAs emphasizes the need for additional research in comprehending their intricate networks and therapeutic applications as cancer treatments (Arif et al., 2020). The combination of non-coding RNAs and epigenetic mechanisms also explained the prospect of utilizing dietary bioactive substances to prevent as well as cure cancer. Specifically, various phytochemicals have been found to modulate epigenetic mechanisms by influencing the expression of non-coding RNAs. For instance, certain phytochemicals re-expression silenced tumor suppressor genes by inhibiting DNA methyltransferases and HDACs, or by activating TET enzymes that reverse hypermethylation. This regulatory role is also present in non-coding RNAs, with the evidence suggesting that high dietary consumption of these molecules is able to affect miRNA expression and thereby modulate their role in the control of the human epigenome. Epigenetic modulators of dietary origin are therefore considered to be promising therapeutic targets, illustrating the indicatory role of non-coding RNAs in the broader context of human health and disease management (Figure 12.6).

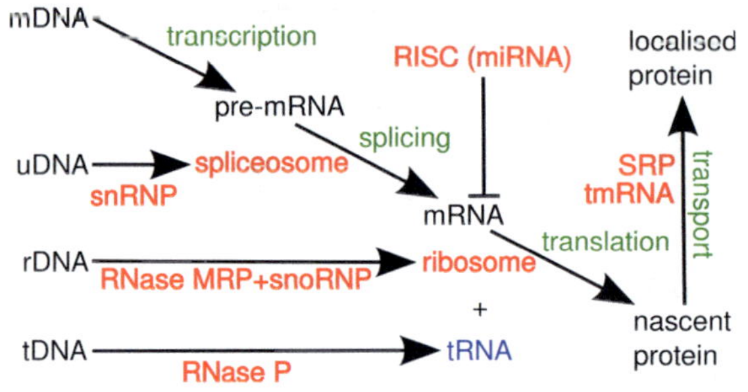

Figure 12.6. The roles of non-coding RNAs: Ribonucleoproteins are shown in red, non-coding RNAs in blue.

Source: https://upload.wikimedia.org/wikipedia/commons/e/e6/NcRNAs-central-dogma.svg.

Test Your Knowledge

1. What is the significance of DNA methylation?
2. What is the histone modification?

12.2. Epigenetics and Development

Learning Outcome

1. Understand the role of embryonic development;
2. Describe the process of cell differentiation;
3. Know the concept of epigenetic changes across the lifespan.

Epigenetics is an important force of development that acts upon genetic and environmental information to determine phenotype and function along the life course of an organism. The methylation, a basic epigenetic modification, can very well influence gene expression. For instance, during the development of an embryo, the regulation of methionine metabolism is an important aspect of enzymatic activity that maintains normal cellular function. Specific mention is made of the crucial role of methionine since it plays a role in methyl metabolism and itself undergoes complex alterations which affect DNA as well as histone modification. Furthermore, disruptions in methionine levels have a widespread impact on developmental outcomes, affecting pregnancy and resulting in a plethora of congenital abnormalities. This is a discipline that celebrates the imperative of understanding how epigenetic changes may arise from both internal metabolic states and external environmental stress, and ultimately influence human health right from early stages in life (Yan et al., 2025). The conversation between epigenetics and developmental phenomena is also illustrated through the influence of maternal diet on child health. Experiments have shown that methionine deficiency or excess at times of pregnancy when the embryo is growing will disturb patterns of methylation in the fetus, inducing gene-expression changes that can have lasting implications for health. Folate-maintained carbon metabolism is particularly significant here since vitamin deficiencies in maternal diets can hinder effective formation of methyl donors, making developmental defects more likely. This connection adds strength to one of the most important aspects of epigenetic regulation—how environmental factors, such as nutrition, are able to pass epigenetic signals to alter developmental outcomes. As more emphasis is put on such connections, nutritional therapy to optimize methionine and folate intake during preconception and pregnancy ever more appear necessary to provide optimal development and reduce the risk of late-onset illness (Yan et al., 2025).

Furthermore, as nations work to develop their human capital, epigenetic influences on health and development become crucial information in the development of ideal education and social policies. In nations that seek economic development, like Cambodia, investment in higher education can be guided by information on the influence of epigenetic influences on learning and development. Educational leaders can utilize the knowledge of methylation functions and environmental determinants, such as proper nutrition, to establish conditions that will optimize students' physical and cognitive development. Some of the challenges for higher education systems are molding curriculum to incorporate new studies of epigenetic determinants and ensuring graduates possess the competencies necessary to flourish in an era of accelerated change. These initiatives will ultimately result in a trained working population capable of driving the country's development to its goals, underlining the interdisciplinarity of understanding epigenetics in diverse contexts.

12.2.1. Role in Embryonic Development

Embryogenesis is a complex and well-coordinated process whereby one fertilized zygote gives rise to a multicellular organism. At the center of this process lies the activity of epigenetics, which regulates gene expression and cell differentiation without altering the underlying DNA code. During early development, epigenetic activities , such as DNA methylation and histone modification regulate cell identity and lineage determination. For instance, primordial germ cells (PGCs) develop as a consequence of specific epigenetic modifications that set their fate by orchestrating epigenetic regulation in managing the organism's future reproductive capacity. Understanding the epigenetic mechanisms controlling the development of PGCs can potentially offer information on reproductive health and human evolutionary past, emphasizing the intricate relationship between genetics and epigenetics during embryogenesis (Esfahani et al., 2024). As embryonic development progresses, tight gene expression control becomes increasingly important to ensure proper differentiation and growth. To this end, epigenetic controls must continuously adapt to the cellular environment to allow for the correct transcriptional activity needed to differentiate into various cell types. Studies on the epigenetic marks of embryos during development have demonstrated that these controls are not static but actively shape developmental fate. For example, in *in-vitro* fertilization (IVF) embryos, developmental arrest during early development has been associated with dysregulation of a group of significant epigenetic marks playing roles in transcriptional activity and cell cycle progression. Identifying molecular mechanisms of such arrests, especially hub genes, can enable greater insight into developmental competence and improved ART (Zhang et al., 2023). Further, the dynamic nature of epigenetic modifications illustrates the embryonic development program's plasticity toward adapting to a range of external stimuli. Epigenetic modifications can be caused by environmental factors, maternal health, and nutrition, suggesting that these stimuli have appreciable consequences on the developing embryo. Plasticity is essential, given that it enables embryos to adapt to a range of adversity in order to achieve successful implantation and continued development. Long-term research into the epigenetics of embryonic development sheds light not only on the regulation of gene expression during this most important stage but also on the gateway to resolving infertility and other developmental disease issues. As such, the nature of forces driving embryonic development is paramount to understanding reproductive medicine's advancement and unwinding human biology's mysteries (Zhang et al., 2023; Esfahani et al., 2024) (Figure 12.7).

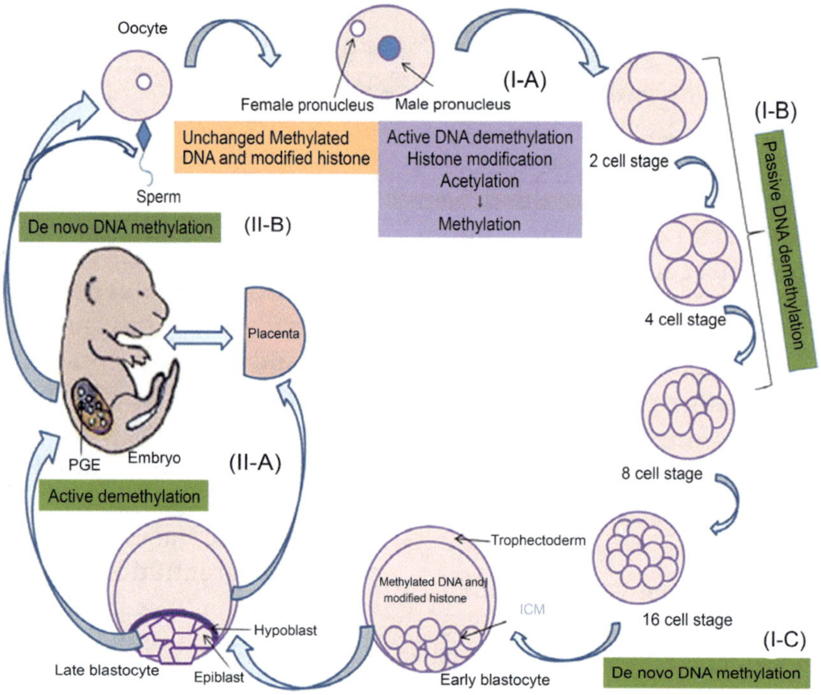

Figure 12.7. Embryo development and epigenetic reprogramming cycle.

Source: https://www.researchgate.net/profile/Moonmoon-Deb/publication/227166053/figure/fig3/AS:279971160444936@1443761734258/Embryo-development-and-epigenetic-reprogramming-cycle-Epigenetic-modifications-take.png.

12.2.2. Influence on Cell Differentiation

The intricate process of cell differentiation is profoundly regulated by epigenetic mechanisms, as they manage the expression of genes without altering the underlying DNA sequence. Through modifications , such as DNA methylation and histone acetylation, cells are enabled to specify the expression of genes required for their specific function. This form of regulation is particularly crucial in stem cells, which have the capability to develop into numerous various cell types based on what signals they receive from their environment. For instance, some signaling compounds can turn on or off particular genes, guiding stem cells along various paths of differentiation. Clarifying these epigenetic factors not only illuminates normal development processes but also sheds light on pathological processes where differentiation processes are disrupted, ultimately affecting tissue regeneration and homeostasis. Model cell line experiments have yielded critical knowledge on the epigenetic factors controlling differentiation. For example, experiments performed in HepaRG cells illustrate the role of dimethyl sulfoxide (DMSO) in triggering cell differentiation while simultaneously manipulating the epigenetic control. DMSO has been found to enhance the infectivity of such cells by human adenoviruses, and this illustrates how environmental factors can change the course of the behavior of cells. Such findings stress the importance of the realization that differentiation is not all the result of intrinsic genetic programming but can be substantially regulated by environmental agents. This cross-talk between epigenetics and environmental determinants serves to underscore the intricacy of cell identity, where cells adapt and respond to the environment yet retain the capacity for differentiation. Cellular metabolism and differentiation are starting to be appreciated as issues of interest in the field of epigenetics. Various metabolic pathways have now been realized to have significant influences on the epigenetic modifications that dictate cell fate. For instance, differentiation of skeletal cells , such as chondrocytes and osteoblasts is not only triggered by growth factors but also by changes in cellular metabolism that provide the necessary energetic and biosynthetic support to these processes. Emerging evidence suggests that quintessential metabolites of metabolism can shape epigenetic marks, thereby maintaining or altering differentiation pathways. Thus, the synergy between metabolic signaling and epigenetic regulation offers new avenues to understand how cells differentiate and mature, suggestion that therapeutic interventions in metabolic pathways would initiate tissue repair and regeneration in humans (Figure 12.8).

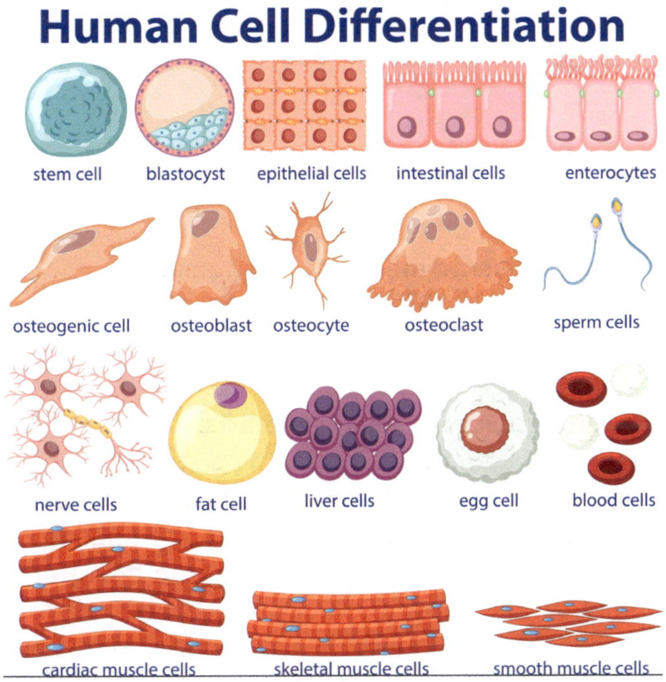

Figure 12.8. Human cell differentiation.

Source: https://cdn.vectorstock.com/i/2000v/62/23/information-poster-cellular-differentiation-vector-33806223.avif.

12.2.3. Epigenetic Changes Across the Lifespan

The concept of epigenetic changes during the lifespan has attracted a lot of attention from researchers in the science of human genetics. Epigenetics can be simply explained as chemical alterations that affect gene expression without altering the underlying DNA sequence, primarily via such mechanisms as DNA methylation and histone modification. Evidence indicates that such epigenetic modifications are dynamic in nature and can be susceptible to being influenced by intrinsic biological determinants and extrinsic environmental factors. For example, early life exposures to life, exposure to toxins, diet, and physical activity are all capable of modifying epigenetic changes that result in long-term health effects and disease susceptibility.

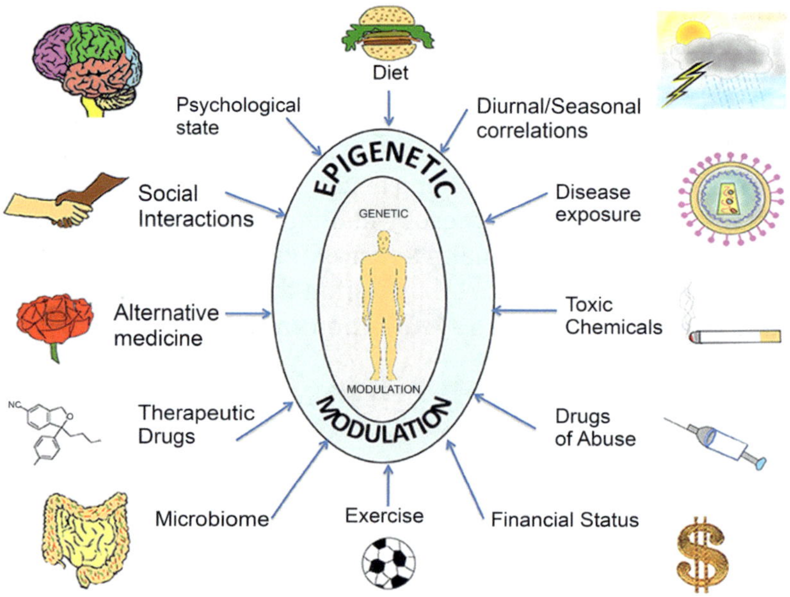

Figure 12.9. A compilation of epigenetic influences on humans.

Source: https://www.frontiersin.org/files/Articles/105911/fcell-02-00049-HTML/image_m/fcell-02-00049-g001.jpg.

This points toward the notion that our genetic potential is not just determined by heredity but also by the general experience throughout life, providing a strong interaction between nature and nurture in determining human health. Another view of epigenetic changes is found in the theory of epigenetic clocks, or biological aging biomarkers. These clocks utilize the DNA methylation pattern to estimate the age of a person and provide insight into the aging processes and individuality variations. Initial human studies have now been replicated in a number of mammalian species with the discovery that DNA methylation trajectories are approximated by a saturating exponential function, a relationship that holds for roughly a third of an organism's lifetime (Ratan et al., 2024). This finding depicts the manner in which DNA methylation changes serve as reliable biological age markers, ultimately enabling scientists to understand better age-related illnesses , such as cancer, CVD, and neurodegenerative disorders (Giannuzzi et al., 2024). In making these epigenetic clocks more accurate, scientists are now beginning to unravel the complexities of determinants of lifespan, a development that may pave the way for treatment-targeted interventions. Investigating the consequences of epigenetic modifications throughout the lifespan also applies to the study of age-related illnesses and overall health conditions. The progressive loss of organismal fitness, which is characteristic of aging, can be described in terms of epigenetic modifications that are acquired throughout a person's lifetime. These changes can make cells less resilient to responding to stressors or fixing harm, making them more susceptible to age-related illnesses. Experiments with such models as the short-lived killifish have also contributed to illuminating this association through the study of the interaction between lifespan, epigenetic aging, and regenerative capacity. Experiments indicate that in certain strains, the increased epigenetic aging is not reversed with tissue regeneration, which highlights underlying biological determinants governing lifespan and health (Giannuzzi et al., 2024). These findings not only enhance our understanding of the process of biological aging but also offer gateway possibilities for the development of epigenetically directed strategies for extending lengthening health span and quality of life improvement (Figure 12.9).

Test Your Knowledge

1. What is embryonic development?
2. What is the process of cell differentiation?

12.3. Epigenetics and Disease

Learning Outcome

1. Know the relationship between epigenetics and cancer;
2. Understand the role of epigenetics in neurological disorders;
3. Describe the impact of epigenetics on metabolic diseases.

The intricate relationship between epigenetics and disease underlies the importance of valuing how gene expression is regulated more than in the code itself. Epigenetic marks , such as DNA methylation and histone modification are important regulators of gene activity, controlling many biological processes , such as cell differentiation, development, and environmental response. These changes can decide the vulnerability of a person to diseases, such as cancer, by modifying oncogene and tumor suppressor gene expression. The dynamic character of histone modification that creates a histone code drastically impacts chromatin structure and gene accessibility, with ramifications for cellular function and disease causation. Studying these changes offers important insights into potential therapeutic avenues for prevention and treatment of human conditions and the need for continued study in this new field of epigenetic research (Liu et al., 2023). Additionally, the kynurenine pathway is a place where epigenetics and immune response intersect, that being in autoimmune disease and inflammatory illness. Indoleamine-2,3-dioxygenase (IDO) function within this pathway has been shown to be anti-inflammatory and protective in disorders , such as rheumatoid arthritis. Pathway dysregulation may be responsible for worsening of disease, suggested by the adverse consequences of IDO deletion in models. Worth mentioning is the interaction between kynurenines and regulatory T cells, which suggests that balance may be complex in influencing disease development. This intricate interaction points out the therapeutic value of epigenetic regulation, e.g., through DNA methylation, in modulating susceptibility to inflammatory diseases. Understanding such mechanisms provides valuable insight into novel therapeutic strategies for inflammatory and autoimmune diseases, paving the way for further disease control (Huang et al., 2020). Current research into the epigenome promises new treatment in the realm of precision medicine. The ability to identify specific epigenetic alterations associated with various disease conditions suggests that therapy could be tailored to the patient's specific epigenetic profile. For instance, modulation of specific histone-modifying enzymes can alter the course of cancers, while modulation of pathways like kynurenine can reframe the therapy for autoimmunity and chronic inflammatory disorders. The dynamic character of epigenetic changes creates challenges and opportunities in the area of therapeutic development, as investigators work to untangle the intricate interaction between genetic and environmental influences. Lastly, creating an advanced overarching understanding of epigenetics and disease could not only enhance disease prevention but also therapies that improve the quality of life of patients afflicted by a range of disorders, underlining the necessity of epigenetics for human well-being (Liu et al., 2023).

12.3.1. Connection to Cancer

The intricate relationship between epigenetics and cancer plays a pivotal role in unraveling tumorigenesis and therapeutic manipulation. Epigenetic modifications , such as DNA methylation and histone modification are pivotal in the modulation of gene expression and the regulation of cellular events including proliferation, apoptosis, and differentiation. Alteration of epigenetic modifications may lead to tumor suppressor gene silencing and oncogene activation, providing a cancer growth microenvironment. For instance, chronic obstructive pulmonary disease (COPD) provides an excellent example wherein environmental exposures, coupled with genetic predisposition, both cause epigenetic alterations and heightened cancer risk. COPD patients experience molecular alterations that render them vulnerable to lung cancer and wherein 0.8–1.7% of these patients develop cancer annually (Karolina et al., 2023). These findings identify the essential role that epigenetic processes have in cancer biology, demonstrating how environmental stimuli and genetic susceptibility combine to increase malignancy risk. G-quadruplex (G4) structures are yet another illustration of the convergence point of epigenetics with cancer biology. Four-stranded DNA structures, they are implicated in gene expression regulation and the preservation of genomic integrity, both to prevent tumorigenesis. Recent advances in the understanding of G4 structures show their increased incidence in cancer cell phases compared to normal cells and indicate a potential role in cancer evolution. G4s can influence transcription by interacting with a variety of proteins, including transcription factors and helicases, and thereby modulate genes of malignancy expression. Furthermore, therapeutic approaches against G4 structures are now being explored, providing hopeful avenues for cancer treatment. As further research unfolds, the identification of G4s role in cancer biology reinforces the importance of epigenetic determinants in cancerous developments even further, which still characterize the intricate relationship of genetic and environmental determinants in cancer formation (Spiegel et al., 2019). The implications of understanding such epigenetic interactions transcend basic research to practical applications in cancer therapy. By describing the machinery of epigenetic changes and how these affect gene expression, researchers are optimistic that they can create targeted therapies that can reverse tumor abnormalities. The integration of epigenetic analysis into cancer diagnosis allows for the development of personalized treatments tailored to an individual's genetic and epigenetic profiles. Additionally, ongoing research into the interactions between environmental exposures and epigenetic alterations will provide further insights into cancer vulnerability, resulting in preventive measures and new therapies. The link between epigenetics and cancer not only enlightens us on the bottom-line biology of tumorigenesis but also provides a framework for analysis for building therapeutic interventions that can profoundly impact clinical behavior in oncology (Figure 12.10).

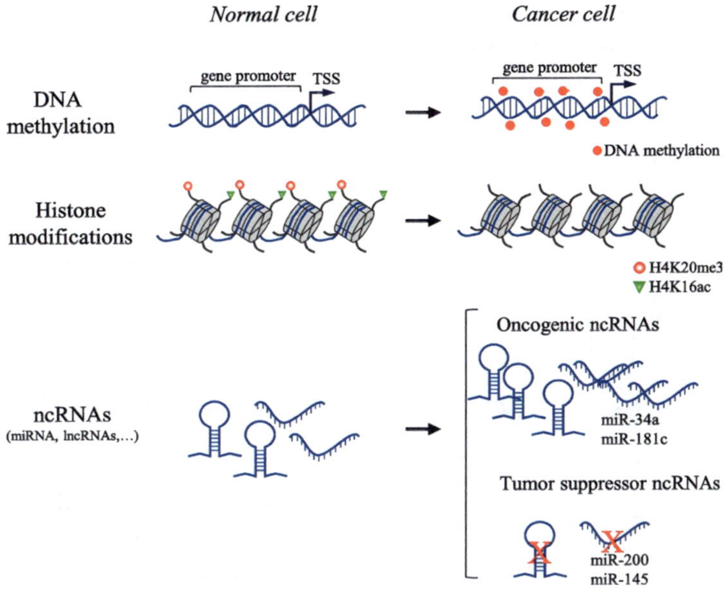

Figure 12.10. Examples of epigenetic alterations in cancer cells. Hypermethylation of promoters of tumor suppressor genes, global loss of H4K20me3 and H4K16ac, and up- or downregulation of miRNAs that target oncogenes and tumor suppressor genes, respectively.

Source: https://media.springernature.com/full/springer-static/image/art%3A10.1186%2Fs13148-019-0675-4/MediaObjects/13148_2019_675_Fig2_HTML.png?as=webp.

12.3.2. Role in Neurological Disorders

The intricate interplay between epigenetics and neurologic disease highlights the profound impact of gene regulation on brain disease and function. General control non-depressible 5 (GCN5), a histone acetyltransferase responsible for regulating gene expression through the modification of chromatin, is one of the most important members of this group. Repeated experiments have demonstrated that deregulation of GCN5 activity is associated with neurological disease. For instance, GCN5 dysregulation has been linked with neurodegenerative disease and psychiatric diseases, suggesting that proper epigenetic control is critical to maintain the health of neurons. Such mechanisms must be deciphered since inhibition of GCN5 could provide new therapeutic approaches for reversing or mitigating the manifestations of neurodegeneration and cognitive loss and thus illustrate the value of epigenetic modification in the treatment of neurological disease (Md. Haque et al., 2021). Furthermore, nutrient epigenetics has been implicated in neurological disease etiology, in the case of folate and its synthetic derivative folic acid. Folate is at the center of one-carbon metabolism, which is critical for DNA methylation and gene regulation. A deficiency of folate during developmental windows of time has been implicated in neural tube defects and neuropsychiatric disease, showing the importance of optimal dietary levels for brain function. Forced folic acid fortification in North America has substantially reduced the incidence of neural tube defects, demonstrating the use of epigenetic theory to implement preventive health intervention.

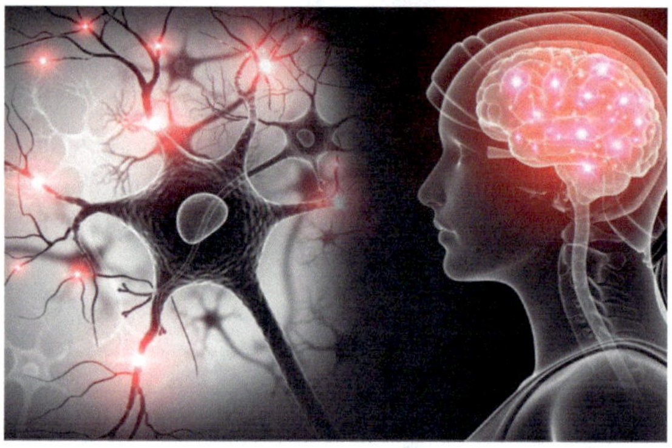

Figure 12.11. Neurological disorders.

Source: https://drrohitgupta.co.in/wp-content/uploads/2024/06/10-Common-Symptoms-of-Neurological-Disorders-Dr-Rohit-Gupta.png.

But the bifunctionality of folate in colorectal carcinogenesis, being able to potentially protect normal tissue but enable cancer growth, exemplifies the sophistication of nutritional intervention and neurological consequence (Warzyszynska & Kim, 2014). Furthermore, the coming together of epigenetics, lifestyle, and environmental determinants cannot be overlooked when thinking of neurological disease. Stress, diet, and toxins have been shown to induce epigenetic mechanisms, which can alter gene expression for neuronal function and vulnerability. For instance, oxidative stress and inflammation are known to alter the histone acetylation pattern, thereby modulating neurodegenerative pathways. Thus, epigenetic health-promoting lifestyle interventions , such as B-rich folate diets, may provide useful means of preventing the onset of neurological disease. Through public health interventions incorporating epigenetics, there is potential for achieving improved cognitive health and neurodisease resistance, which is the revolutionary promise of understanding epigenetic processes in human health (Figure 12.11).

12.3.3. Impact on Metabolic Diseases

The complicated interaction between epigenetics and metabolic disease highlights the way in which the environment induces irreparable alterations in gene expression and, as a consequence, human health. Metabolic disorders, such as obesity and type 2 diabetes, are increasingly recognized to be susceptible to epigenetic modulation, potentially induced through diet, physical activity, and chemical exposures. For instance, DNA methylation and histone modification changes can cause deregulation of genes in metabolic pathways. This underscores the therapeutic promise of epigenetic processes to convey the impact of lifestyle determinants of metabolic health so that interventions may reverse or correct these changes and improve metabolic outcomes in individuals with these issues, hence benefiting public health. SCFAs, especially those derived from gut microbiota fermentation, gained popularity in recent years due to their impact on metabolic health. SCFAs , such as acetate, propionate, and butyrate, besides serving as energy sources, help to sustain glucose metabolism and suppress inflammatory responses. Research indicates that SCFAs possess the capability to modulate epigenetic modifications by acting on the activity of histone acetylation and deacetylation enzymes, thereby regulating inflammation and metabolic gene expression. Because the Western diet is low in dietary fiber, the resultant suppressed production of SCFAs that ensues may be one contributor towards the rising incidence of metabolic diseases, an indicator of the significance of the understanding of diet impacts on the microbiome and their epigenetic effects on health (Bart et al., 2021). In addition, the topic of cardiovascular health most clearly demonstrates the manner in which epigenetics intersects metabolic diseases through aging. Epidemiological studies have shown that the aging heart undergoes a cascade of alterations in its metabolism, influencing its function and contributing to CVD risk. Reprogramming of metabolic pathways in cardiac cells results in cellular senescence, which is involved in heart failure and other CVDs. This shows that understanding the epigenetic regulation of metabolic pathways in aged hearts may provide insight into therapeutic strategies against heart disease. The continued investigation of the molecular pathways responsible for these changes will be essential in the design of novel interventions to reverse cardiac function and maximize overall metabolic well-being as one ages (Xie et al., 2023) (Figure 12.12).

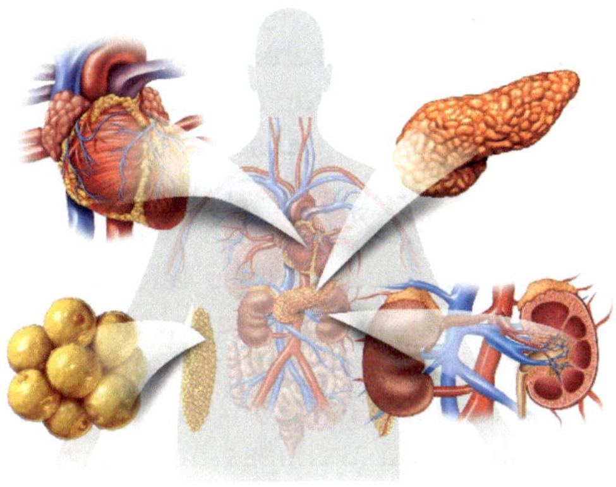

Figure 12.12. Illustration highlighting the impact of metabolic disorders on major organs, including the heart, liver, pancreas, kidneys, and adipose tissue.

Source: https://www.news-medical.net/images/news/ImageForNews_791981_17278369167506575.jpg.

Test Your Knowledge

1. What is the role of epigenetics in cancer development and progression?
2. What is the role of epigenetics in neurological disorders?

12.4. Environmental Influences on Epigenetics

Learning Outcome

1. Describe the effects of diet and nutrition on epigenetic modifications;
2. Describe the impact of stress and lifestyle on epigenetics;
3 Know the influence of toxins and pollutants.

Environmental functions on epigenetics constitute the foundation of insight into the dynamic interaction between environment and genetics in shaping human health. DNA methylation and histone modification are epigenetic processes that present mechanisms through which environmental stresses can modulate gene expression without changing the underlying sequence of DNA. As a result, exposure of an individual to elements , such as diet, toxins, and stress can initiate heritable changes that influence physiological response as well as disease susceptibility. For example, studies have shown that specific micronutrients play a primary role in the development of the brain since they influence gene function through epigenetic pathways. These findings serve to emphasize the possibility of non-genetic influences having persistent impacts, underlining the need to account for environmental interactions when investigating human health outcomes and disease courses (Bekdash, 2024). Along with diet, gut microbiota has also been identified as an important environmental influence shaping the epigenetic profile. Recent research has demonstrated that gut microbiota composition and function are shaped by various factors , such as diet, lifestyle, and geography. The host's epigenome is influenced by this microbiome, which regulates gene expression through biochemical signals and metabolites that can modulate histones and DNA. This interaction emphasizes the importance of a healthy gut microbiome in the facilitation of overall health and wellness and may also aid in further elucidating the interaction between lifestyle and epigenetic modifications. The interaction between epigenetic regulation and gut microbiota is of particular relevance in disorders , such as obesity and inflammatory bowel disease (IBD), where disruption can result in severe health implications (Kim et al., 2024). Secondly, the implications of environmental conditions on epigenetics reach far beyond the immediate health effect, as they have the potential to influence subsequent generations. The environmentally caused epigenetic changes can be transmitted by inheritance, an effect termed transgenerational epigenetic inheritance. This contradicts the conventional concept of genetics and sets debates in motion regarding why certain populations are said to be more susceptible to particular diseases based on past exposure to deleterious environmental elements, including pollution and nutritional deprivation. Thus, knowledge of environmental determinants needs to be incorporated into public health interventions so that measures to counteract risks proactively and enhance well-being across generations can be taken. Understanding such epigenetic mechanisms can lead to more personalized medical interventions and prevention strategies that take into account not just genetic vulnerabilities but also environmental contexts.

12.4.1. Effects of Diet and Nutrition

Diet and nutrition are pivotal to the control of epigenetic modifications, which have tremendous health implications during a lifetime. Gene expression is influenced by nutrition in a complex way such that each micronutrient impacts specific biological pathways that regulate cellular functions. For instance, folic acid and vitamins B6 and B12 are vital nutrients that act as central methyl donors in one-carbon metabolism, with a significant involvement in DNA and histone methylation reactions. The alterations can modulate gene expression and therefore affect susceptibility to disorders , such as mental diseases and metabolic syndromes. It is through appreciation of these connections that the importance of food selection is enhanced, particularly at key developmental stages when building blocks for health are established. Nutritional interventions that optimize micronutrient absorption can hence serve as preventive strategies against looming health problems, calling for greater sensitivity of diet impacts on genes and overall health (Bekdash, 2024).

In addition, current research is centered on the function of the gut microbiota in mediating dietary influences on epigenetic regulation. The intestinal microbiota, a live and active microbial consortium, actively interacts with the constituents of the diet to regulate metabolic pathways and immunity. Specific nutrients, including vitamins D, iron, fiber, zinc, and magnesium, have been discovered to influence the composition and function of gut microbiota, thus driving epigenetic modification. This bidirectional dynamic points to the manner in which food choices can impact gut health and, through epigenetic modification, influence gene expression along inflammatory and oxidative stress pathways. By providing an adequate diet that promotes a healthy microbiome, one may promote not only gut health but overall health as well. This complex interaction emphasizes the need for an integrative approach to nutrition that considers its far-reaching impact on both epigenome and microbiota (Ferenc et al.,

2024). Moreover, dietary implications of epigenetic changes are not only of individual health significance but also of public and social health significance. As the understanding of epigenetic mechanisms influenced by diet progresses, policies can be developed to address dietary deficits in the population. For example, promoting exposure to foods rich in nutrients and incorporating educational interventions on the importance of micronutrients could contribute significantly to public health. In addition, recognition of the epigenetic effects of early dietary intervention presents potential for reversing health disparities caused by socioeconomic determinants. Generally, it can be made possible to enhance our disease prevention and health promotion plan by considering the role of diet and nutrition in terms of epigenetics to make society healthier. Identification of the nutritional aspects that contribute to epigenetic variation will inform future research and policy development for improved health outcomes at a collective level (Bekdash, 2024; Ferenc et al., 2024) (Figure 12.13).

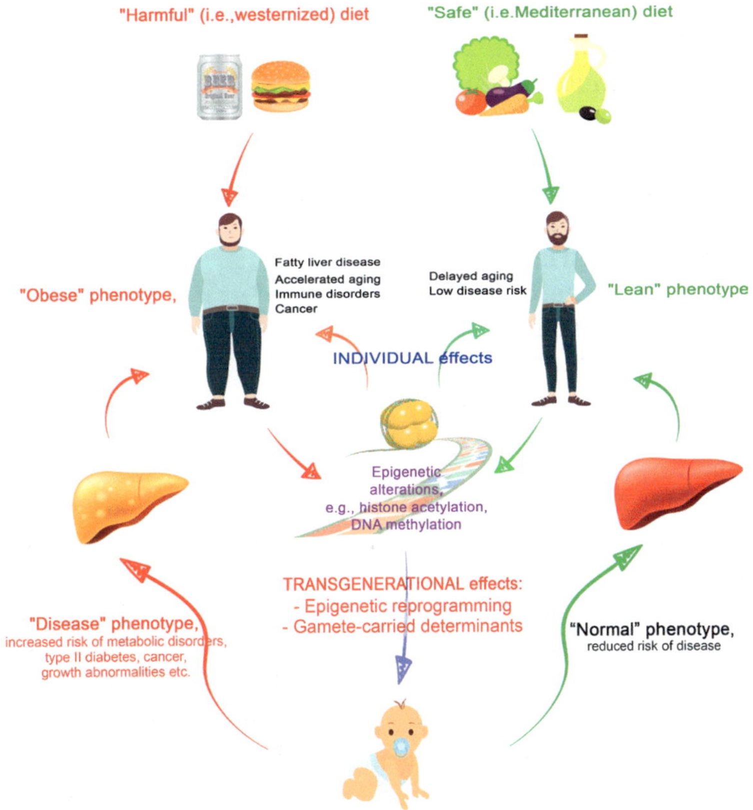

Figure 12.13. The diet affects the epigenome to modify individual and transgenerational phenotypes.

Source: https://www.mdpi.com/ijms/ijms-19-03425/article_deploy/html/images/ijms-19-03425-g001.png.

12.4.2. Impact of Stress and Lifestyle

The intersection of stress, lifestyle, and their epigenetic influence is a more applicable area of study for contemporary health science. Stress and particularly chronic stress, have become an inducer of varied biological responses with the ability to deeply alter gene expression. The epigenetic change is often achieved via changes , such as DNA methylation and histone changes, which can be equated to the onset of diseases like CVD and psychiatric disorders. Because lifestyle factors are involved in stress management, such as diet and exercise, their relevance cannot be overstated. As an example, a dietary study described the potential for employing a plant-based diet to reverse the adverse effects of biomarkers of stress to propose a mechanism of building individuals' resilience to stress via lifestyle modification (Alzughayyar et al., 2025). Furthermore, habits of lifestyle also extend to encompass the entire health outlook, including physical fitness and mental health. Research has confirmed that physical activity that is undertaken regularly is able to initiate epigenetic improvements, enhance mood and cognitive processes and reduce stress levels. This physical activity creates a feedback loop where lowered stress raises compliance with lifestyle, leading to improved overall health results. Programs aimed at total lifestyle modification, such as the Healthy Lifestyle Community Program, have established that systematic interventions can significantly enhance risk profiles for various lifestyle illnesses (Alzughayyar et al., 2025). The interdisciplinarity of addressing such dynamics highlights the importance of integrative approaches considering psychological health alongside physical health. Apart from lifestyle adjustments, the environment where one lives is also crucial in stress management and overall wellness. Some stressors have the impact of magnifying conditions, leading to maladaptive acts that influence lifestyle choices even more. The brain's reaction to such stressors, particularly where the hippocampus and its implication in approach-avoidance conflicts is in question, supports the complex relationship between environmental causes and epigenetic effects. Implications of these findings are that life choices and genetic predispositions converge at a point, reflecting on a continuum of health in relation to determinants from inside and outside the person. By integrating evidence from various disciplines, like epigenetics and behavioral sciences, we can best address the multidimensionality of health, opening up possibilities to manage stress and make healthier lifestyle decisions (Figure 12.14).

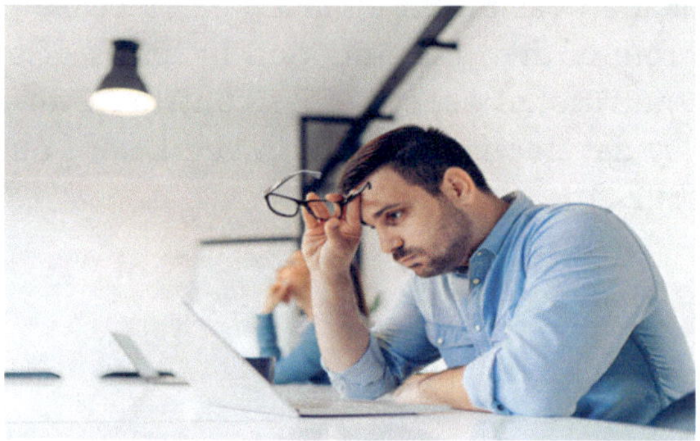

Figure 12.14. Man experiencing eye strain or fatigue while working on a laptop.

Source: https://nura.in/wp-content/uploads/2025/04/Untitled.png.

12.4.3. Influence of Toxins and Pollutants

The increasing incidence of environmental pollution and poisonous contaminants is an ominous threat to human health beyond the immediate physical environment. Among these, EDCs are noteworthy as especially cunning chemicals that interfere with normal hormone functions in order to create a vast spectrum of diseases from reproductive illness to metabolic syndrome. The long-term impact of EDCs exposure is scary because the chemicals are capable of inducing epigenetic modifications that might change the gene expression pattern without touching the genetic code itself. For example, changes in DNA methylation patterns take place when human beings are exposed to chemicals, and this makes them susceptible to conditions , such as obesity and hormone-sensitive cancers. Therefore, understanding the nuanced interactions between EDCs and human health demands an appreciation of their epigenetic impacts, which underscore the subtle dynamic between gene expression and environmental exposures (Kumar et al., 2020). Toxin exposure's impacts are not only immediate but may also be transgenerational. Such lingering calls into question how pollutants actually reach human biology, primarily through epigenetic mechanisms that are then transmitted to subsequent generations. Research has established that the effect of EDCs can be observed in children, and it implies a health risk inheritance due to the environmental conditions faced by previous generations. Such results have implications for a review of public health policy aimed at averting exposure to these harmful chemicals. Complete mechanisms for monitoring environmental poisons and implementing preventive measures are required in order to manage these problems effectively. Elucidation of the multileveled effects of toxins in gene regulation uncovers the pathways through which environmental stresses remain at the forefront of public health concerns (Kumar et al., 2020). Metabolomics has emerged as an essential method for assessing the biological impacts of toxins and toxicants. The science enables high-throughput examination of metabolites, and it unveils how chemicals like EDCs influence human physiology and result in disease processes. By characterizing metabolites produced after exposure to toxins, researchers are able to correlate environmental pollutants with alterations of metabolic pathways. Using this all-embracing view of biology, it is shown that metabolites function as crucial signaling molecules and immune response regulators, exerting significant impacts on health. The ongoing research with metabolomics reveals the intricate, systemic interactions that occur in organisms when exposed to toxins, putting the exposure versus environment and biochemical reaction into perspective. Further research along this direction will definitely add to our understanding of how toxins, metabolites, and epigenetic control interact with each other (Figure 12.15).

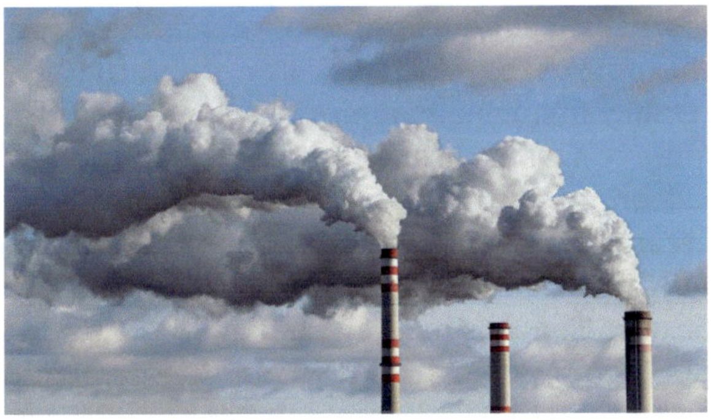

Figure 12.15. Environmental toxins and their impact on reproductive health.

Source: https://www.inovifertility.com/wp-content/uploads/2024/11/Osteen_Environmental-Toxins_1200x700-1024x597-1.jpg.

Test Your Knowledge

1. What are the effects of diet and nutrition on epigenetic modifications?
2. What is the impact of stress and lifestyle on epigenetics?

12.5. Therapeutic Applications of Epigenetics

Learning Outcome

1. Learn about epigenetic drugs and treatments;
2. Know the potential of personalized medicine;
3. Know the ethical considerations in epigenetic therapies.

The therapeutic value of epigenetics has gained great momentum in the recent past, with particular interest in neurodegenerative disorders , such as vascular dementia (VaD). VaD possesses characteristic cognitive and memory disturbances, predominantly resulting from complex interactions of genetic and environmental factors. Therapeutic strategies currently address symptomatic treatment and not the etiologic processes involved in the disease. The absence of effective therapy has opened up a door to investigate the epigenetic background of VaD. Recent studies highlight that environmental modulators of gene expression are capable of inducing a curative effect, and epigenetic modulation may potentially yield new therapies that hold the prospect of reversing cognitive impairment. Lastly, further knowledge regarding such mechanisms gives us promising avenues towards building targeted intervention strategies that have the potential to prevent or even halt VaD, emphasizing the crucial intersection of epigenetics and human health for neurodegeneration conditions (Selvaraji et al., 2025). In regenerative medicine and the bone healing in particular, the research of epigenetics has a tremendous potential. Human fetal mesenchymal stem cells (hfMSCs) are of research interest because of their specific properties that allow them to possess more regenerative potential than adult stem cells. The challenge of replicative senescence, though, has the tendency to hinder the therapeutic use of these cells. New approaches have been created that involve resetting the epigenetic condition of hfMSCs to render them more functional. Methods , such as non-integrative episomal reprogramming of amniotic fluid stem cells (AFSCs) to induced MSCs (iMSCs) hold tremendous promise. The iMSCs obtained through derivation are multipotent for long-term and show increased expression of genes that control tissue regeneration, suggesting epigenetic reprogramming may restore young stem cells and potentially increase their therapeutic efficacy in regenerative medicine (Corcelli et al., 2025). In addition, the activity of EVs released by iMSCs illustrates another exciting aspect of epigenetic drug therapy. These vesicles play an important role in intercellular communication and are increasingly found with their potential to modulate mechanisms of tissue repair. iEVs can facilitate the promotion of fibroblast migration, which is a critical element of wound healing and recovery following injury. Secretory pathways on the basis of epigenetic regulation point to cellular context influencing therapeutic outcomes.

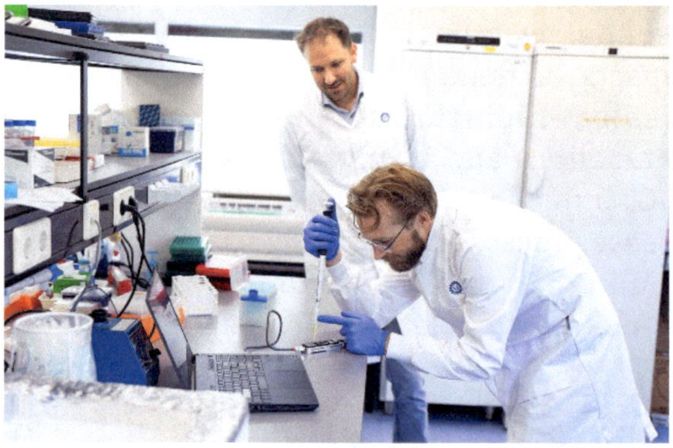

Figure 12.16. Researchers conducting an experiment using a micropipette and laptop in a molecular biology lab.

Source: https://www.genengnews.com/wp-content/uploads/2024/04/Epigenetics_UMCUtrecht_Pic1.jpg.

By identifying and manipulating these pathways, researchers can develop targeted treatments that take advantage of the therapeutic potential of stem cell-derived vesicles to enhance tissue regeneration. Further research on these epigenetic mechanisms has tremendous potential not only for regenerative medicine but also to advance our overall understanding of healing processes in human biology (Corcelli et al., 2025) (Figure 12.16).

12.5.1. Epigenetic Drugs and Treatments

The rapidly developing field of epigenetic drugs and treatments offers new vistas in the realm of disease therapy, particularly with regard to complex diseases , such as cancer. Epigenetic modifications, including DNA methylation and histone alterations, are essential in regulating gene expression without changing the underlying sequence of DNA. As these changes lie at the heart of cancer development and cancer progression in most malignancies, they present an interesting target for therapeutic intervention. The use of epigenetic drugs would aim to reverse such changes, returning normal gene operation and thereby inhibiting cancer growth. Advances have recently indicated that targeting such epigenetic dysregulation can potentially enhance the efficacy of existing therapeutic modalities, leading to an encouraging synergy in personalized medicine. Greater understanding of cancer biomarkers through extensive molecular epigenetic profiling helps to tailor such interventions to optimize therapeutic effects and minimize side effects (Yu et al., 2024). SCFAs form a highly interesting category of epigenetic modifiers that regulate gene expression and cellular functions in various tissues and organs. Synthesized during the fermentation of dietary fiber by gut microbes, SCFAs , such as acetate, propionate, and butyrate play multifaceted roles in providing intestinal homeostasis and metabolic health. Interestingly, they exert epigenetic functions by controlling histone acetylation and the activity of HDACs. Such a metabolic pathway serves as a basis for therapeutic strategies for epigenetic regulation, linking dietary intervention and health of the microbiota to disease prevention and cure. The potential of SCFAs as therapy for the prevention of metabolic disorders and inflammatory diseases is promising for the future of dietary intervention in epigenetic therapy. Through understanding how SCFAs talk to cellular processes, researchers can better utilize the molecules to develop new therapies (Bart et al., 2021). As studies continue to better define the complexities of the epigenome, the landscape of epigenetic drugs has transitioned significantly, from embryonic theoretical entities to promising therapeutic agents. A number of epigenetic inhibitors, such as DNA methyltransferase inhibitors and histone deacetylase inhibitors, have been exhaustively tried in clinical trials to evaluate their safety and efficacy in a variety of diseases, ranging from hematologic malignancies to solid tumors. These therapies not only aim to reactivate tumor suppressor-associated genes that are epigenetically modified and silenced but also attempt to shift the tumor microenvironment toward one more amenable to immune attack.

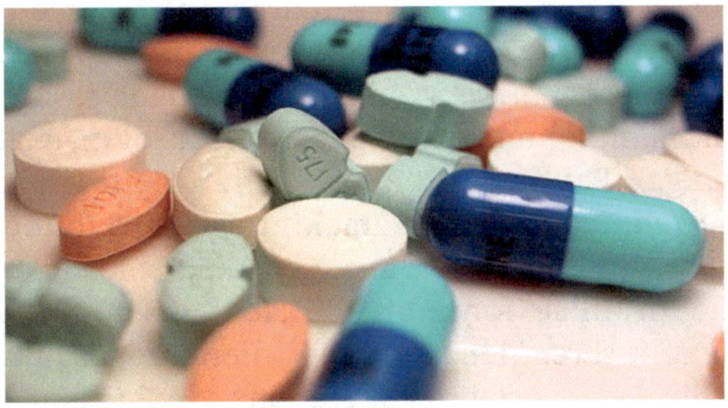

Figure 12.17. Drug discovery.

Source: https://blogs.biomedcentral.com/on-biology/wp-content/uploads/sites/5/2016/09/pills-620x342.jpg.

The success of these therapies has enabled new modalities in combinatorial treatment, where epigenetic drugs are combined with immunotherapy or traditional cytotoxic drugs with the goal of employing a more comprehensive treatment plan. Continued innovation in epigenetic drug discovery has the potential to make treatments more effective and also give more options to patients with complicated diseases (Yu et al., 2024) (Figure 12.17).

12.5.2. Potential for Personalized Medicine

The promise of personalized medicine, based on epigenetic progress, has the potential to revolutionize the delivery of healthcare. With our expanding understanding of the function of epigenetic modifications in gene expression, clinicians are better positioned to individualize therapy based on distinct epigenomic profiles. Such a shift is particularly relevant in oncology, where cancer intrinsic heterogeneity necessitates adaptive therapeutic strategies. For instance, the GDSC dataset analysis is intended to deliver accurate genomic markers that are connected to drug resistance and sensitivity in cancer cells. With the application of machine learning approaches, such as the Random Forest algorithm, this research enhances our ability to predict a patient's response to specific treatments, thereby enhancing patient results and limiting undesirable side effects of generic drugs (Pant et al., 2024). The implications for clinical decision making are profound, suggesting that personalized medicine holds the promise for more efficient, customized patient care. Along with this, there are also the ethical and social considerations of epigenetics-based personalized medicine that need to be taken into account. As we implement epigenetic information in clinical practice, discrimination and stigmatization are issues, prompting important debates on data privacy and patient autonomy. Ethical principles will be developed to deal with the complexities of the applications of epigenetic data to achieve informed consent and to protect citizens from negative social impacts. The incorporation of ethics in the application of epigenetics in personalized medicine will promote a fairer healthcare setting. Moreover, the principle of distributive justice must be applied to fair access to epigenetic interventions among populations to avoid disparities that may arise from differential access to tailored therapy on the basis of environmental and lifestyle exposures (Santaló et al., 2022). Overall, the rush toward personalized medicine based on epigenetic understanding holds both revolutionary promise and an abundance of challenges. With the elucidation of interactions between gene expression and external factors, epigenetics holds out the promise of tailored treatment protocols for the unique genetic makeup and environmental exposure of the patient. This route holds the promise of substituting the one-size-fits-all approach that has been characteristic of medicine in the past. However, the path forward is not challenge-free; ongoing research must reconcile the promise of customization with the ethical imperatives of privacy, informed consent, and social justice. Advances in this arena must thrive through collaborative efforts among scientists, clinicians, ethicists, and policymakers to ensure personalized medicine evolves responsibly and maximizes its benefits for all (Santaló et al., 2022; Pant et al., 2024) (Figure 12.18).

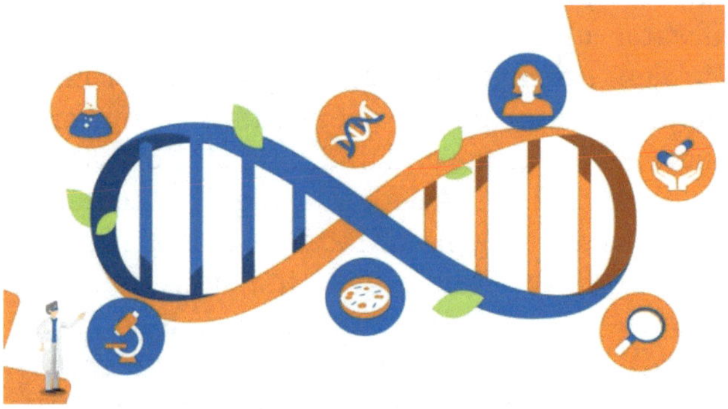

Figure 12.18. Personalized medicine.

Source: https://ispe.org/sites/default/files/styles/site_750_x_420/public/2021-10/1121_PE_SO_Valley_01.jpg?itok=YK-_K8_8.

12.5.3. Ethical Considerations in Epigenetic Therapies

The epigenetic treatments constitute a difficult terrain of ethics, primarily informed consent and patient autonomy. As these emerging treatments are capable of altering gene expression without the underlying DNA sequence being altered, this raises the question of how much the patients actually understand the implications of the treatment. The need for comprehensive education on epigenetic mechanisms is paramount because individuals must be aware of both potential benefits and harms. Researchers need to prioritize transparency in communication so that participants learn the treatment experimental design and long-term implications. This is supportive of the ethical principle of autonomy since individuals have the right to informed decisions about their health. Regulatory bodies and research communities must develop robust guidelines to underpin the ethical codes, allowing patients to have meaningful engagement with novel epigenetic therapies (Percie et al., 2020). In addition to informed consent, the ethics of epigenetic therapy can be diverse and more tailored to the risk of abuse or unexpected outcomes. Having the ability to deliberately modify epigenetic markers could bring with it enhancement therapies, in which the aim is to improve attributes , such as intelligence or physical prowess.

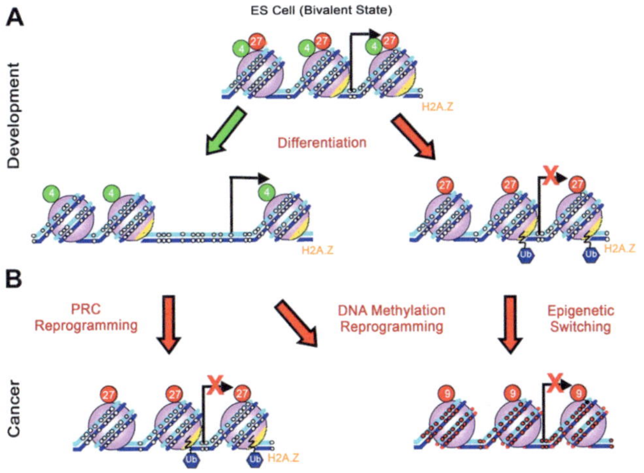

Figure 12.19. A diagram of epigenetic therapy.

Source: https://upload.wikimedia.org/wikipedia/commons/5/58/Epigenetic_therapy_diagram.jpg.

This sends extremely strong ethical messages about fairness and availability, since not every population will necessarily have access to these possibilities to the same extent. Moreover, the possibility of creating socio-economic disparities by genetic improvements undermines the founding premise of justice in medicine. Therefore, it becomes necessary for epigenetics players to engage in a discussion on how to appropriately use such technologies, not only anticipating the social implications but ensuring equal access (Zakrzewski et al., 2019). Lastly, the potential intergenerational impact of epigenetic therapies lends a layer of complexity to the ethical debate. In contrast to conventional genetic treatments that impact only the patient being treated, epigenetic modifications have the potential to be transmitted to generations to come and affect their development and health. This presents deep questions about long-term implications for society and researchers' and clinicians' responsibilities to think about the consequences of what they are doing beyond their immediate patients. Ethical stewardship in this regard necessitates ongoing debate among scientists, ethicists, and policymakers to develop guidelines that prioritize the welfare of coming generations. While scientists continue to explore the great potential of epigenetic interventions, they must be vigilant to the broader implications of their findings, ensuring that ethical considerations are integrally woven into the story of scientific advance and public health policy (Zakrzewski et al., 2019; Percie et al., 2020) (Figure 12.19).

Test Your Knowledge

1. What are epigenetic drugs used for?
2 What is the potential of personalized medicine?

SUMMARY

The study of epigenetics in man uncovers a complex dance of forces regulating gene expression and disease susceptibility. Unlike genetic mutations, epigenetic alterations are reversible and are promising sites for therapeutic intervention. Research substantiates that environmental exposures, lifestyle patterns, and even microbiome influence significantly impact epigenetic profiles, emphasizing the dynamic nature of human biology. Notably, understanding such epigenetic phenomena opens the gates to preventive therapies in medical research. For instance, as evidenced in the study of melanocytic nevi, early detection and public campaigns can significantly impact health, since treatments at an epigenetic level might enhance quality of life (Chesca et al., 2024). This adaptability practically redrafts conventional healthcare models, whereby epigenetic initiation discovery forms the foundation of new models of preventive medicine. Besides, the effects of epigenetics extend to so-called immunometabolism, which is distinctly recognized in the case of Alzheimer's disease and the like. The tasks of upcoming studies encompass the aim to unmask the effects of some epigenetic modifications on the function of myeloid cells and their intrinsic protective functions against neurodegeneration. The findings related to the expression of LACTB reveal that epigenetics could have the potential to influence lipid metabolism and protein synthesis in immune cells, providing insight into the disease process (Molina et al., 2024). As the scientific community continues to investigate these correlations, it is apparent that treating the epigenetic characteristics of diseases has the potential to revolutionize therapeutic methods. This approach illuminates a comprehensive perspective of health, emphasizing a multi-dimensional approach unifying genetic, epigenetic, and environmental factors. In summary, the study of epigenetics in humans is a critical frontier for understanding the complexities of gene expression and disease susceptibility. As researchers unfold the intricate interplay between epigenetic factors and health endpoints, the promise of developing targeted therapies expands. Merging concepts across a broad range of areas of study, genetics to immunology, may potentially make our knowledge more precise about human biology and disease processes. Preventative strategies and educational interventions cannot be overemphasized, because they are instrumental in bringing epigenetic science to real-world health interventions (Chesca et al., 2024). In an age of swift progress in biotechnology and personalized medicine, the epigenetic vision provides a paradigm shift that is based on the promise of a healthier future built on a better appreciation for our biological nature.

Of core relevance among the subject matters of epigenetics in human beings is the multifaceted role of DNA methylation in gene expression control and metabolic regulation. This epigenetic mark is a core mechanism of adipose tissue biology, a key determinant of the rising epidemics of type 2 diabetes (T2D) and obesity. Studies explain that adipose tissue dysregulation is at the root of these conditions, and it highlights the significance of understanding the epigenetic controls that govern metabolic function and energy balance. A comprehensive examination reveals that DNA methylation events not only influence adipocyte formation but are also capable of causing transgenerational transmission of metabolic issues, emphasizing the role of epigenetics in contemporary debates and interventions related to health that aim to respond to obesity-related issues (Kang et al., 2019). In addition, the environmental context in which one develops has immense effects on epigenetic alterations and health outcomes. For instance, at the time of puberty, adolescent girls are most susceptible to external environmental factors that could induce molecular changes, thereby predisposing them to many conditions, including breast cancer. Unhealthy dietary habits characterized by message-reliant media communication can exacerbate this risk, as can exposure to environmental toxins ubiquitous in lower socioeconomic communities, where healthier options may not be readily available. This convergence of environmental stress and epigenetic susceptibility underscores the relevance of targeted public health interventions that encourage advocacy for such exposure awareness and better lifestyle choices, ultimately nurturing a deeper awareness of epigenetic consequences in human health (Aljaber et al., 2020). Finally, the exploration of epigenetics in humans reveals a complex interaction between genetic and environmental influences, demonstrating the significance of understanding such dynamics in preventing risks to health. Among the major conclusions, there is a focus on how DNA methylation regulates critical physiological processes, particularly in adipose tissue, and its contribution to obesity and T2D. Additionally, personal susceptibility, especially during development stages like puberty, underscores the necessity of intervention in the aspect of environmental elements that affect epigenetic variation. Ongoing study contributes to more public awareness concerning such problems, which can incite healthy interventions and policy-making that ultimately result in a healthier population better equipped to counteract epigenetic problems (Aljaber et al., 2020; Liu et al., 2023).

KEY TERMS FROM THIS CHAPTER

- Cell differentiation
- DNA sequence
- Epigenetic alterations
- Epigenetics
- Human papillomavirus
- Lymphoid neoplasms
- Natriuretic peptides
- Primordial germ cells
- DNA methylation
- Embryonic development
- Epigenetic modifications
- Histone modification
- In vitro fertilization
- Metabolic imbalances
- Non-coding RNAs

Critical Thinking Questions

1. **Epigenetics refers to:**
   a. Changes in the DNA sequence
   b. Changes in gene expression without altering the DNA sequence
   c. Mutations in genes
   d. RNA splicing variations
2. **Which of the following is an epigenetic mechanism?**
   a. DNA methylation
   b. Point mutation
   c. RNA interference
   d. Gene duplication
3. **DNA methylation commonly occurs at which nucleotide base?**
   a. Adenine
   b. Guanine
   c. Cytosine
   d. Thymine
4. **Which of the following is NOT a type of histone modification?**
   a. Acetylation
   b. Methylation
   c. Phosphorylation
   d. DNA replication
5. **Non-coding RNAs that regulate gene expression epigenetically are called:**
   a. mRNA
   b. tRNA
   c. microRNA (miRNA)
   d. rRNA

Short Answer Questions

1. What is epigenetics?
2. Why is epigenetics important in humans?
3. What are the mechanisms of epigenetic regulation?
4. What is the role of epigenetics in development?
5. What are the environmental influences on epigenetics?

Answers to Critical Thinking Questions

1. (b); 2. (a); 3. (c); 4. (d); 5. (c)

References

1. Alaggio, R., Amador, C., Anagnostopoulos, I., Attygalle, A. D., Araújo, I., Berti, E., Bhagat, G., et al. (2022). The 5th edition of the World Health Organization classification of hematolymphoid tumors: Lymphoid neoplasms. *Leukemia, 36*, 1720–1748. https://doi.org/10.1038/s41375-022-01620-2 (accessed on 12th June 2025).
2. Aljaber, D., Au, D., Benmarhnia, T., Cardiff, R., et al. (2020). Environmental exposures during puberty: Window of breast cancer risk and epigenetic damage. https://core.ac.uk/download/323070388.pdf (accessed on 12th June 2025).
3. Alzughayyar, D., Weber, R. M., Husain, S., Schoch, N., & Englert, H. (2025). Impact of the Healthy Lifestyle Community Program (HLCP-3) on trimethylamine N-oxide (TMAO) and risk profile parameters related to lifestyle diseases during the six months following an intervention study. *Nutrients, 17*. https://www.semanticscholar.org/paper/3a312b7f43cd3907b7e8dff293eae4ba557bf228 (accessed on 12th June 2025).
4. Arif, K., Elliott, E. K., Haupt, L. M., & Griffiths, L. R. (2020). Regulatory mechanisms of epigenetic miRNA relationships in human cancer and potential as therapeutic targets. *Cancers, 12*, 2922. https://doi.org/10.3390/cancers12102922 (accessed on 12th June 2025).
5. Bekdash, R. (2024). Epigenetics, nutrition, and the brain: Improving mental health through diet. *International Journal of Molecular Sciences, 25*. https://www.semanticscholar.org/paper/d2e219abc66f8cae47b2bca5b3bc1b787f44b745 (accessed on 12th June 2025).
6. Bertels, J. C., He, G., & Long, F. (2024). Metabolic reprogramming in skeletal cell differentiation. *Bone Research, 12*. https://www.semanticscholar.org/paper/1d15ad4fa65bf0e359d4c777c652f3942dc4da12 (accessed on 12th June 2025).
7. Bhattacharjee, S., & Dashwood, R. H. (2020). Epigenetic regulation of NRF2/KEAP1 by phytochemicals. *Antioxidants, 9*, 865. https://doi.org/10.3390/antiox9090865 (accessed on 12th June 2025).
8. Chesca, A. (2024). Morphological epiderma analyze for diagnosis. *Medicine and Ecology*. https://www.semanticscholar.org/paper/dc42db9981536687a5d17d087ac919bb9866059b (accessed on 12th June 2025).
9. Connacher, J., von Grüning, H., & Birkholtz, L. (2022). Histone modification landscapes as a roadmap for malaria parasite development. *Frontiers in Cell and Developmental Biology, 10*. https://www.semanticscholar.org/paper/e06e9777e402ac2c35a05ab3fab9e41f29adcb82 (accessed on 12th June 2025).
10. Corcelli, M., Petzendorfer, E., Hawkins, K., Vlahova, F., Caruso, C., Hasan, M. M., Durrant, K., et al. (2025). Rejuvenated human amniotic fluid stem cells: A superior source of standardized induced mesenchymal stem cells for enhanced therapeutic applications. *bioRxiv*. https://www.semanticscholar.org/paper/c96cd680cf490d4bb4f06eb4b5ba1a25cecb3fbf (accessed on 12th June 2025).
11. Czarnecka, K. H., Mukherjee, D., Maryanchik, S. V., & Rudzińska, M. (2023). Biological and genetic mechanisms of COPD, its diagnosis, treatment, and relationship with lung cancer. *Biomedicines, 11*, 448. https://doi.org/10.3390/biomedicines11020448 (accessed on 12th June 2025).

12. Dai, W., Qiao, X., Fang, Y., Guo, R., Bai, P., Liu, S., Li, T., et al. (2024). Epigenetics-targeted drugs: Current paradigms and future challenges. *Signal Transduction and Targeted Therapy, 9*. https://www.semanticscholar.org/paper/3c0b020550b9e80b754c00294f225c54a57ba237 (accessed on 12th June 2025).

13. Deogharia, M., & Gurha, P. (2024). Epigenetic regulation of heart failure. *Current Opinion in Cardiology*. https://www.semanticscholar.org/paper/72fabe3f13b827f807082eea6eb148f36e03eaf9 (accessed on 12th June 2025).

14. Esfahani, S., Zheng, Y., Arabpour, A., Resto Irizarry, A. M., Kobayashi, N., Xue, X., Shao, Y., et al. (2024). Derivation of human primordial germ cell-like cells in an embryonic-like culture. *Nature Communications, 15*. https://www.semanticscholar.org/paper/1f7154f2f5d900e92b6f6689fd47de0918c0e4e0 (accessed on 12th June 2025).

15. Ferenc, K., Sokal-Dembowska, A., Helma, K., Motyka, E., Jarmakiewicz-Czaja, S., & Filip, R. (2024). Modulation of the gut microbiota by nutrition and its relationship to epigenetics. *International Journal of Molecular Sciences, 25*. https://www.semanticscholar.org/paper/a1628aefc3b9f4980fe6c13364cb1136ad4a8eca (accessed on 12th June 2025).

16. Forastieri, C., Romito, E., Paplekaj, A., Battaglioli, E., & Rusconi, F. (2024). Dissecting the hippocampal regulation of approach-avoidance conflict: Integrative perspectives from optogenetics, stress response, and epigenetics. *Hippocampus, 34*. https://www.semanticscholar.org/paper/af652f12e05dc4eae9e6a6e02c02775c70ac31c1 (accessed on 12th June 2025).

17. Galicia-García, U., Benito-Vicente, A., Jebari, S., Larrea-Sebal, A., Siddiqi, H., Uribe, K. B., Ostolaza, H., et al. (2020). Pathophysiology of type 2 diabetes mellitus. *International Journal of Molecular Sciences, 21*, 6275. https://doi.org/10.3390/ijms21176275 (accessed on 12th June 2025).

18. Gensous, N., Bacalini, M., Franceschi, C., Meskers, C., Maier, A., & Garagnani, P. (2019). Age-related DNA methylation changes: Potential impact on skeletal muscle aging in humans. *Frontiers in Physiology, 10*. https://www.semanticscholar.org/paper/37c3689a51fd1c1df32f50ee3f3421950294f888 (accessed on 12th June 2025).

19. Giannuzzi, C., Baumgart, M., Neri, F., & Cellerino, A. (2024). Epigenetic clock and lifespan prediction in the short-lived killifish *Nothobranchius furzeri*. *bioRxiv*. https://www.semanticscholar.org/paper/fbd9154ebae0e9e587ee9967794c4f7c53941361 (accessed on 12th June 2025).

20. Haque, M. E., Jakaria, M., Akther, M., Cho, D. Y., Kim, I. S., & Choi, D. (2021). The GCN5: Its biological functions and therapeutic potentials. *Clinical Science, 135*(1), 231–257. https://www.semanticscholar.org/paper/1f21674e3a33394b286bc4659174b616d188dfd5 (accessed on 12th June 2025).

21. Hofmann, K., Hofmann, S., Weigl, F., Mai, J., & Schreiner, S. (2024). DMSO and its role in differentiation impact efficacy of human adenovirus (HAdV) infection in HepaRG cells. *Viruses, 16*. https://www.semanticscholar.org/paper/b2ca347d591582eb909fba47987c8b3aac1cdfbe (accessed on 12th June 2025).

22. Huang, Y. S., Ogbechi, J., Clanchy, F. I. L., Williams, R., & Stone, T. W. (2020). IDO and kynurenine metabolites in peripheral and CNS disorders. *Frontiers in Immunology, 11*. https://doi.org/10.3389/fimmu.2020.00388 (accessed on 12th June 2025).

23. In, C. (2025). The role of higher education institution leaders in building human capital in Cambodia: Challenges and strategies. *Journal of Social Sciences and Humanities*. https://www.semanticscholar.org/paper/9de522b01fd2f3347d434e48269cb38a9716c2a8 (accessed on 12th June 2025).

24. Kang, S., & Ma, X. (2019). Functional implications of DNA methylation in adipose biology. https://core.ac.uk/download/323080862.pdf (accessed on 12th June 2025).

25. Kim, B., Song, A., Son, A., & Shin, Y. (2024). Gut microbiota and epigenetic choreography: Implications for human health: A review. *Medicine, 103*. https://www.semanticscholar.org/paper/1a13cbaedc9353eb247c7a71b89dc5a002e025ab (accessed on 12th June 2025).

26. Kumar, M., Sarma, D. K., Shubham, S., Kumawat, M., Verma, V., Prakash, A., & Tiwari, R. (2020). Environmental endocrine-disrupting chemical exposure: Role in non-communicable diseases. *Frontiers in Public Health, 8*. https://doi.org/10.3389/fpubh.2020.553850 (accessed on 12th June 2025).

27. Liu, R., Wu, J., Guo, H. H., Yao, W., Li, S., Lu, Y., Jia, Y., et al. (2023). Post-translational modifications of histones: Mechanisms, biological functions, and therapeutic targets. *MedComm, 4*. https://doi.org/10.1002/mco2.292 (accessed on 12th June 2025).

28. Meza-Menchaca, T., Albores-Medina, A., Heredia-Mendez, A., Ruíz-May, E., Ricaño-Rodríguez, J., Gallegos-García, V., Esquivel, A., et al. (2024). Revisiting epigenetics fundamentals and its biomedical implications. *International Journal of Molecular Sciences, 25*. https://www.semanticscholar.org/paper/63d95143e930f9759529d2eb02d359dc5d641be6 (accessed on 12th June 2025).

29. Pant, L., Al Mukaddim, A., Rahman, M. K., Al Sayeed, A., Hossain, M. S., Khan, M. T., & Ahmed, A. (2024). Genomic predictors of drug sensitivity in cancer: Integrating genomic data for personalized medicine in the USA. *Computer Science & IT Research Journal*. https://www.semanticscholar.org/paper/2a3597d32cedd5f2f5690112a3136db0246ef249 (accessed on 12th June 2025).

30. Percie du Sert, N., Ahluwalia, A., Alam, S., Avey, M. T., Baker, M., Browne, W. J., Clark, A., et al. (2020). Reporting animal research: Explanation and elaboration for the ARRIVE guidelines 2.0. *PLoS Biology, 18*, e3000411. https://doi.org/10.1371/journal.pbio.3000411 (accessed on 12th June 2025).

31. Ratan, P., Devaskar, S. U., & Pellegrini, M. (2024). Defining mammalian lifespan through epigenetic aging timescales. *Medical Research Archives*. https://www.semanticscholar.org/paper/4d49fe601514d2a34a00bb60481cfc876ff8c992 (accessed on 12th June 2025).

32. Romero Molina, C., See, W. Y., Patel, T., Liu, Y., Marcora, E., & Goate, A. M. (2024). Basic science and pathogenesis. *Alzheimer's & Dementia, 20*(Suppl 1), e086622. https://www.semanticscholar.org/paper/62c9d8cd992b8312dab75b20cb7e29564dddbd3a (accessed on 12th June 2025).

33. Santaló, J., & Berdasco, M. (2022). Ethical implications of epigenetics in the era of personalized medicine. *Clinical Epigenetics, 14*. https://www.semanticscholar.org/paper/b57a0219fc400a8f056ad22f83b840ad57e0b5fc (accessed on 12th June 2025).

34. Selvaraji, S., Mosberger, J., Fann, D., Lai, M. K. P., Chen, C. L. H., & Arumugam, T. (2025). Unveiling the therapeutic promise of epigenetics in vascular cognitive impairment and vascular dementia. *Aging and Disease*. https://www.semanticscholar.org/paper/

f270583efd37fe2261dde7cc8e42e791e94c079a (accessed on 12th June 2025).

35. Siegel, E., Berglund, A., Riggs, B. M., Eschrich, S., Kristen, M., Ajidahun, A., Shibata, D., et al. (2013). Abstract PR08: Identification of novel methylated genomic regions in invasive cervical cancer using a genome-wide approach. *Cancer Prevention Research, 6.* https://www.semanticscholar.org/paper/915d7d164effb69a1f8f863732f699b40acccaf7 (accessed on 12th June 2025).

36. Spiegel, J., Adhikari, S., & Balasubramanian, S. (2019). The structure and function of DNA G-quadruplexes. *Trends in Chemistry, 2,* 123–136. https://doi.org/10.1016/j.trechm.2019.07.002 (accessed on 12th June 2025).

37. Stanzione, R., Cotugno, M., Bianchi, F., Marchitti, S., Forte, M., Volpe, M., & Rubattu, S. (2020). Pathogenesis of ischemic stroke: Role of epigenetic mechanisms. *Genes, 11.* https://www.semanticscholar.org/paper/ed9ad8ee1c489b3ebbd1d853c318b39b26d68fae (accessed on 12th June 2025).

38. Tolera, M. (2023). The "smart city" between urban narrative and empty signifier: Shaggar in focus. *World Journal of Education and Humanities.* https://www.semanticscholar.org/paper/25ed3db34ce39d30521eba05eecbd2b01cff1a4f (accessed on 12th June 2025).

39. Tsalenchuk, M., Gentleman, S., & Marzi, S. (2023). Linking environmental risk factors with epigenetic mechanisms in Parkinson's disease. *NPJ Parkinson's Disease, 9.* https://www.semanticscholar.org/paper/6ec57e35ca530e663a41af958883c5f3c499450c (accessed on 12th June 2025).

40. van der Hee, B., & Wells, J. M. (2021). Microbial regulation of host physiology by short-chain fatty acids. *Trends in Microbiology, 29,* 700–712. https://doi.org/10.1016/j.tim.2021.02.001 (accessed on 12th June 2025).

41. Volpe, M., Gallo, G., & Rubattu, S. (2022). Endocrine functions of the heart: From bench to bedside. *European Heart Journal.* https://www.semanticscholar.org/paper/43b453f81ab271a7c7f955cd8e2e06f39005e8bd (accessed on 12th June 2025).

42. Warzyszynska, J., & Kim, Y. I. (2014). Folate in human health and disease. https://www.semanticscholar.org/paper/35f82e57d116405167feb86265c1fb97d75ceb20 (accessed on 12th June 2025).

43. Wishart, D. S. (2019). Metabolomics for investigating physiological and pathophysiological processes. *Physiological Reviews, 99,* 1819–1875. https://doi.org/10.1152/physrev.00035.2018 (accessed on 12th June 2025).

44. Xie, S., Xu, S. C., Deng, W., & Tang, Q. (2023). Metabolic landscape in cardiac aging: Insights into molecular biology and therapeutic implications. *Signal Transduction and Targeted Therapy, 8.* https://doi.org/10.1038/s41392-023-01378-8 (accessed on 12th June 2025).

45. Yan, C., He, B., Wang, C., Li, W., Tao, S., Chen, J., Wang, Y., et al. (2025). Methionine in embryonic development: Metabolism, redox homeostasis, epigenetic modification and signaling pathway. *Critical Reviews in Food Science and Nutrition.* https://www.semanticscholar.org/paper/3cca7781304fbc3258f652000aba2db6b1e8b9c0 (accessed on 12th June 2025).

46. Yu, X., Zhao, H., Wang, R., Chen, Y. Y., Ouyang, X., Li, W., Sun, Y., et al. (2024). Cancer epigenetics: From laboratory studies and clinical trials to precision medicine. *Cell Death Discovery, 10.* https://doi.org/10.1038/s41420-024-01803-z (accessed on 12th June 2025).

47. Zakrzewski, W., Dobrzyński, M., Szymonowicz, M., & Rybak, Z. (2019). Stem cells: Past, present, and future. *Stem Cell Research & Therapy, 10*. https://doi.org/10.1186/s13287-019-1165-5 (accessed on 12th June 2025).

48. Zhang, W., Li, K., Li, S., Lv, R., Ma, J., Yin, P., Li, L., et al. (2023). High-throughput sequencing reveals hub genes for human early embryonic development arrest in *in vitro* fertilization: A pilot study. *Frontiers in Physiology, 14*. https://www.semanticscholar.org/paper/60bbb3bf0e217a1c0bc9406cbef0d596bfebaa31 (accessed on 12th June 2025).

BIOCHEMICAL PHARMACOLOGY

13

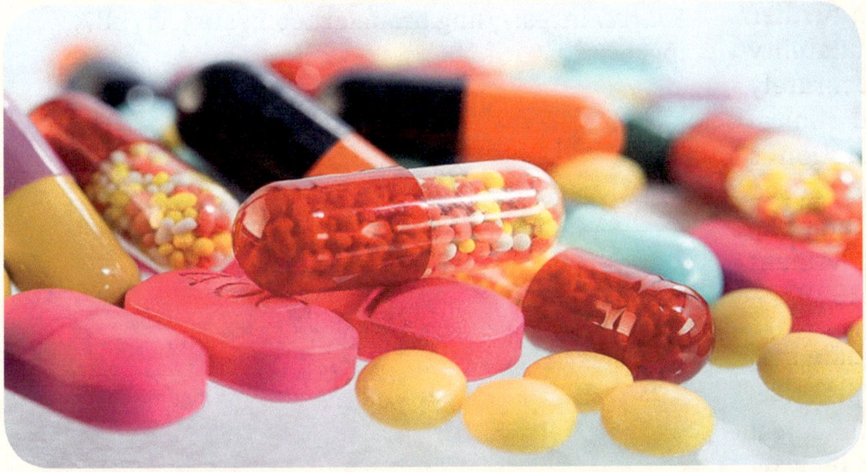

LEARNING OBJECTIVES

After studying this chapter, you will be able to:

1. Describe the basic principles of pharmacology;
2. Describe the drug development process;
3. Understand the mechanisms of drug action;
4. Describe the types of biochemical drugs;
5. Know the drug interactions and their associated side effects;
6. Discuss the current trends in biochemical pharmacology.

Introduction

The field of biochemical pharmacology is a bridge discipline between biochemistry principles and pharmacological practice. Biochemical pharmacology focuses primarily on understanding the processes by which biological molecules affect drug action, such as the effects of drug molecules on enzymes, receptors, and signal transduction mechanisms. Through the study of these interactions at the molecular level, researchers are better able to design more effective therapeutic interventions tailored to an individual patient's specific needs. With the intricacy of biochemistry in human beings, it is crucial to acknowledge that the final potency of a drug depends on factors , such as chemical structure, mode of administration, and biochemical properties. These factors underscore the significance of integrating biochemical data into drug design, leading to more precise and optimized therapies. Understandings of drug bioavailability form the core of the discipline of biochemical pharmacology as it directly influences the therapeutic efficacy of a drug. Drug bioavailability describes the extent and speed of an administered dose reaching the systemic circulation and subsequently influencing the target site of action. Bioavailability is influenced by phenomena , such as gastrointestinal absorption, first-pass metabolism, and distribution in the tissues of the body, which in turn influence the clinical efficacy of drugs. The significance of research here is apparent, with the optimization of bioavailability potentially leading to increased therapeutic efficacy. Moreover, the role of advancements in technology in further defining our understanding of bioavailability and enabling scientists to more accurately assess these factors in laboratory and clinical settings is equally significant. This evolution is significant in overcoming the challenges caused by the poor bioavailability of drugs, a stumbling block for the provision of effective treatment modalities in patients (Stielow et al., 2023).

No more important is the role that guidelines play in biochemical pharmacology practice, where they are the template by which medical professionals can steer the art of drug therapy through its complexity. An example is the ESC/EAS Guidelines, emphasizing the necessity to balance clinical judgement with today's scientific understanding and individual patient-specific circumstances. These guidelines are a significant resource for health practitioners to guarantee that pharmacological interventions are conducted ethically and effectively with regard to the specific health conditions of patients. Moreover, these guidelines continuously aid updates in consideration of continuously evolving research as a reflection of the dynamic character of pharmacological science. Harmonizing these guidelines with individual patient treatment enhances therapeutic strategies in addition to supporting the responsibility of healthcare providers to remain vigilant with respect to traditional and new pharmacological concepts (François et al., 2019) (Figure 13.1).

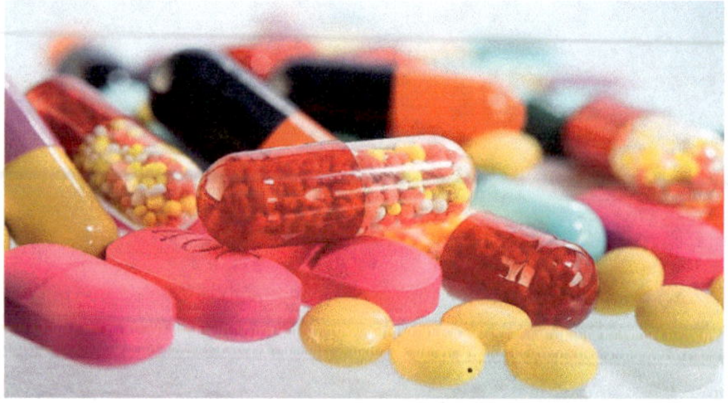

Figure 13.1. Biochemical pharmacology.

Source: https://img.brainkart.com/subject/287.jpg.

13.1. Basic Principles of Pharmacology

Learning Outcome

1. Describe the pharmacokinetics and pharmacodynamics;
2. Understand the therapeutic index and drug safety.

The fundamental concepts of pharmacology are the foundation to understanding drug action and its effects on biochemical pathways in the body. The underlying principle of this science is the rule of pharmacokinetics, which dictates drug absorption, distribution, metabolism, and excretion. These processes dictate how a drug acts on the body to influence its efficacy and safety profiles. For instance, understanding the rate at which a drug is absorbed can inform clinical personnel on when to administer clinical intervention, for example, in critical care conditions. This critical link between pharmacokinetics and patient care is typically highlighted in study materials applied in teaching medical practitioners on the usage of pharmacological agents in disease management, especially in managing critically ill patients, as cited by Nuho et al. (2021). In addition to pharmacokinetics, the second fundamental principle is pharmacodynamics, where it deals with the biochemical and physiological actions of medications and how they work. It studies the action of drugs on cellular activity and produces therapeutic effects. Pharmacodynamics is used in predicting the efficacy and duration of drug action, which is essential in enhancing treatment protocols. In addition, inclusion of methods like microdialysis (Nuho et al., 2021) adds to the understanding of the local effect of pharmacological agents in the targeted tissues, hence gaining more knowledge about their therapeutic value. Such an investigative approach makes pharmacology describe a biocomplexity of drug structure and function, further establishing applicability of biochemical principles to clinical practice. Furthermore, translation of pharmacological principles does not merely cover fundamental research to practice but also is the underlying relationship between the two. Therefore, comprehension of the physiological context, i.e., electrolyte balance or the activity of neurotransmitters, is essential for clinical practitioners to diagnose and treat most conditions. Such blending of basic biochemical principles and clinical practice ensures that medicine is grounded on a firm understanding of human physiology, as seen in the example of the treatment of acute conditions like pulmonary insufficiency or cardiac arrhythmias (Barondess, 1968). Therefore, the study of pharmacology not only enhances the efficacy of therapy but also gives a key foundation towards the concept of personalized medicine whereby medications are both efficacious and tailored to the patient's requirements (Figure 13.2).

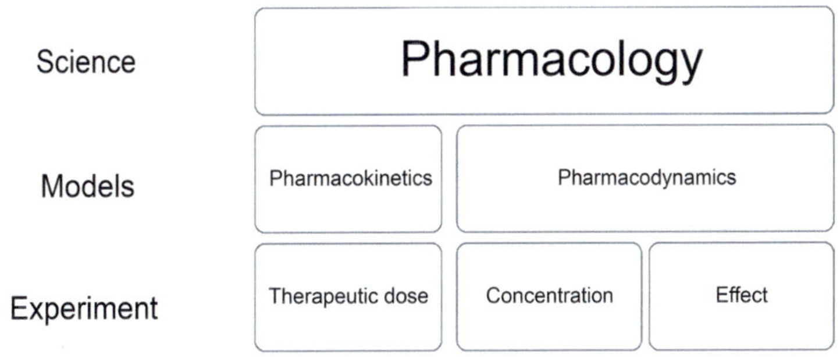

Figure 13.2. Schematic representation of the different components acting in human pharmacology and their classification.

Source: https://learning.eupati.eu/pluginfile.php/668/mod_book/chapter/350/image.png.

13.1.1. Pharmacokinetics: Absorption, Distribution, Metabolism, and Excretion

Pharmacokinetics entails the complex interplay of procedures required to understand the drug absorption, distribution, metabolism, and excretion by the body. Absorption is the initial step, where a drug travels from the administration site to the systemic circulation. Absorption is influenced by the formulation of the drug, the administration route, as well as physiological barriers like the gastrointestinal tract. A perfect example of that includes savolitinib, an oral MET inhibitor. In a phase 1 clinical trial, the oral bioavailability of the drug was noteworthy at 69%, highlighting its excellent absorption characteristics (Miah et al., 2023). It is pertinent information as they not only demonstrate the capacity of a drug for systemic circulation but also provide likely dosing regimens to maximize the therapeutic effects. Once absorbed, the distribution phase determines where the drug is distributed in the body organs and tissues. This is a critical phase, as it determines the amount of a drug that reaches its destination. Distribution can be influenced by tissue perfusion, drug solubility, and plasma protein binding. For instance, RGLS4326, a microRNA inhibitor, exhibits preferential renal accumulation, which is desirable for its therapeutic action (Kamel et al., 2023). The pharmacokinetics of RGLS4326 revealed a long half-life and minimal residual liver and kidney accumulation after repeated dosing.

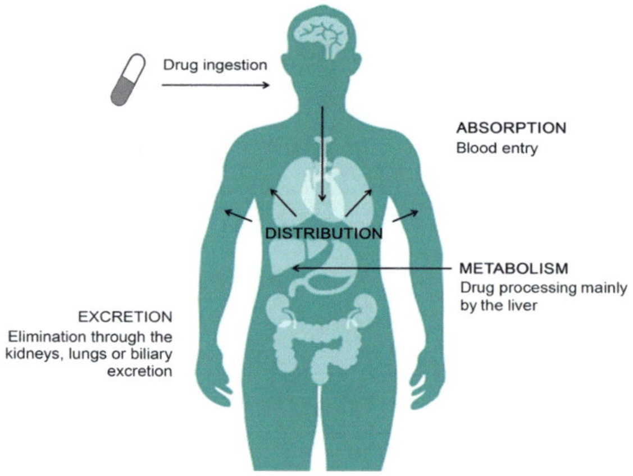

Figure 13.3. The four stages of pharmacokinetics are represented by the acronym ADME.

Source: https://static.wixstatic.com/media/160a9f_e46c0d673cd24d1d825e8c14b075d2f8~mv2.jpeg.

These patterns of distribution are central to how drugs become effective and produce side effects, making the production of site-directed therapy with maximal effect and minimal systemic exposure feasible. Metabolism and excretion are the terminal processes in pharmacokinetics and are critical in defining a drug's duration of action and toxicity. Metabolism, which occurs primarily in the liver, is the process by which enzymatic conversion the drug is enzymatically converted into more hydrophilic products for easy excretion. For savolitinib, broad elimination was through metabolic pathways, illustrating the contribution of metabolism to pharmacokinetics (Miah et al., 2023). In comparison, RGLS4326 showed minimal metabolism, with renal excretion being the primary route of elimination, allowing for extensive recovery in urine as intact drug at high percentages (Kamel et al., 2023). Understanding these profiles of excretion not only directs the dosing schedules but also permits the prediction of drug interaction, which assists in the effective and safe use of pharmacological drugs in the clinical setting (Figure 13.3).

13.1.2. Pharmacodynamics: Drug-Receptor Interactions

The complex branch of pharmacodynamics primarily discusses the aspects of drug-receptor interactions, which are the framework of the mechanism of drug effect on the biological system. Pharmacodynamics, simply put, examines how drugs affect the body, i.e., with which other receptors they interact. Such receptors are usually proteins on cell membranes that transmit the physiological effects of endogenous substances or pharmacological agents. The drug-receptor binding process can lead to conformational changes that stimulate cellular actions. This interaction is of importance because it will determine the efficacy and safety of drug-like compounds in therapy for ailments from chronic diseases to acute diseases. Such a discussion cannot go on without invoking the concept of selectivity and specificity of receptor interactions. The drugs can bind with different affinities for their target receptors and produce either therapeutic effects or side effects. Triptans are a family of medications employed in the treatment of migraines and selectively activate serotonin 5-HT1B/1D receptors, inducing vasoconstriction and headache relief. In recent studies, it has been demonstrated that among the triptans, eletriptan is a complex pharmacokinetic and dynamic agent. It demonstrates enhanced efficacy and tolerability, especially among patients who are likely to bear cardiovascular risk factors. Such interactions underscore the role of pharmacodynamics in optimizing drug design and individualizing treatment modalities in clinical practice, as evidenced by current studies and evidence supporting the same. Pharmacodynamics further encompasses the study of dose-response relationships, providing insight into the minimum effective dose as well as potential levels of a drug's toxicity. When drugs bind to their receptors, the action may vary with different drug concentrations, thereby influencing clinical outcomes.

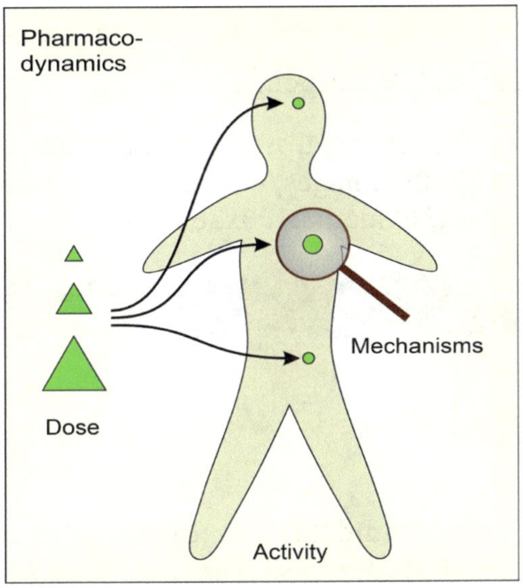

Figure 13.4. Pharmacodynamics.

Source: https://upload.wikimedia.org/wikipedia/commons/thumb/c/c5/Pharmacodynamics.svg/800px-Pharmacodynamics.svg.png.

The law is invoked when referring to polypharmacy; multidrug administration at the same time, where interactions might lead to complex effects. In some cases, simultaneous use of some drugs enhances therapeutic effects, while in others, adverse effects are observed. For instance, the coadministration of serotonergic drugs with triptans , such as eletriptan necessitates vigilance to prevent the risk of serotonin syndrome due to probable drug–drug interactions (DDIs) (Boothroyd et al., 2011). The knowledge of such drug-receptor interactions adds more meaning to the pharmacodynamics in biochemical pharmacology, pointing towards the necessity of thorough research during drug development and therapeutic applications (Boothroyd et al., 2011) (Figure 13.4).

13.1.3. Therapeutic Index and Drug Safety

The therapeutic index is essential to drug safety and effectiveness in biochemical pharmacology. The therapeutic index of a drug refers to the ratio of the toxic dose and the effective dose and is a key index of safety. A large therapeutic index suggests that there is a large range of effective doses and dangerous doses, thus suggesting greater safety when a drug is prescribed. In contrast, low therapeutic index drugs require close monitoring and dosage adjustment in order to minimize toxicity while ensuring therapeutic effects. Such a differential therapeutic index requires extensive pharmacokinetic and pharmacodynamic assessment in the course of drug development, along with ongoing risk-benefit analysis in the clinic to ensure patient safety. The therapeutic index plays a pivotal role in the scenario of traditional and modern pharmacological therapies as well. For instance, the use of Xuebijing, a traditional Chinese medicine, has been promising in the control of infections with an acceptable safety profile. In clinical trials for its efficacy against Acinetobacter baumannii infections, meta-analyses reported impressive reductions in clinical outcomes and bacterial elimination with no serious adverse drug events (Li et al., 2025). Such evidence highlights the need for a study of the therapeutic index of herbal therapy and demonstrates that they can be of therapeutic benefit with no excessive risk to the patient. This integration of ancient and modern tactics in biochemical pharmacology not only contributes more knowledge to the field of therapeutic effectiveness but also facilitates the identification of safer treatment regimens. Relative to herbal therapy, drugs like levothyroxine sodium typify the issue of narrow therapeutic indices with modern-day pharmacotherapy. Levothyroxine, critical in hypothyroidism management, needs to be dosed carefully since it possesses a narrow therapeutic index, where small changes create toxicity. New advances in analytical methods, such as FT-IR spectroscopy, help in proper quantitation of the drug to ensure maximum drug safety (AlBathish et al., 2024). Such new methods enable quality control and supplement the rigid monitoring for patients who are dependent on narrow therapeutic index drugs. Thus, additional R&D in drug safety protocols is the most critical area in addressing the complexities associated with both traditional and novel pharmacological interventions in biochemical pharmacology (Figure 13.5).

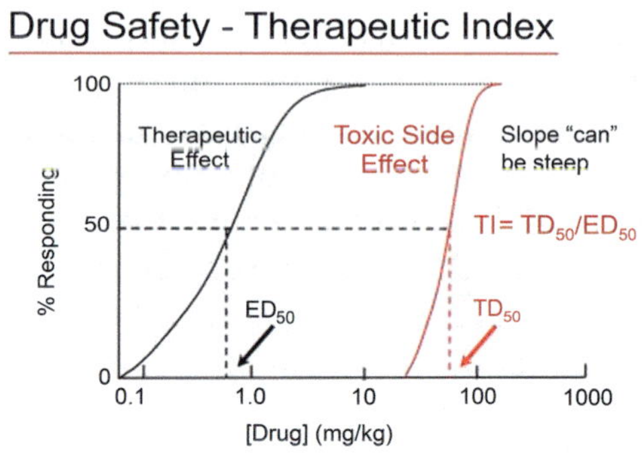

Figure 13.5. Therapeutic index.

Source: https://upload.medbullets.com/topic/107009/images/6e49bfae2c1b79c8cd7415fbdd8a23f0.media.400x284.jpg.

Test Your Knowledge

1. What are the four stages of pharmacokinetics?
2. What is the pharmacodynamics?

13.2. Drug Development Process

Learning Outcome

1. Understand the preclinical research and testing;
2. Know the process of clinical trials;
3. Describe the post-marketing surveillance and drug approval.

The drug development process is a complex and multidisciplinary process of extensive research, rigorous testing, and critical evaluation to determine the safety and effectiveness of new drugs. The process initiates with initial research to identify potential drug targets, which generally involves biochemical studies defining the molecular mechanisms of disease. The good candidates are then subjected to preclinical studies using *in vitro* and *in vivo* models. Traditional *in vitro* models, such as two-dimensional cell culture, are inclined to fail to accurately imitate the physiological status of humans, which is a big challenge to interpret safety and efficacy outcomes. To solve such bottleneck issues, novel technologies , such as FRESH™ 3D bioprinting are employed to create more physiologically relevant human cardiac tissues, bridging the gap between laboratory finding and clinical application, and enabling early pharmacology screens of drug candidates (Finkel et al., 2023). Following successful preclinical trials, the drug development proceeds to clinical trials, which are critical for identifying the safety and effectiveness of the drug in humans. The trials are structured in phases, commencing with small-scale Phase I trials to establish safety and dose, followed by large Phase II and III trials to establish efficacy and monitor side effects. The application of computational methods has become unavoidable in this stage, particularly with the evolution of the complexity of drug regimens in clinical practice. The identification of potential drug–drug interactions (DDIs) employing sophisticated computational platforms enhances the screening process by approximating the probability of interactions, thus avoiding adverse effects. These include tools , such as the BioChemDDI model, which are leaders in this advancement and use machine learning methods to evaluate and forecast possible DDIs successfully (Ren et al., 2022). This success culminates in drug trial completion, regulatory submissions, where information that has been collected during the drug development process is thoroughly evaluated by agencies like the FDA. This process is vital in ensuring that the new medication has strict safety and efficacy standards before its approval for public use. After approval, post-marketing surveillance does not cease, but instead, there is a necessity to follow up on the long-term safety and efficacy of the medication in the general populace. The continuous feedback loop generated from both clinical trials and practical usage guides following improvements in drug formulation and usage instructions to maximize pharmacological effectiveness and safety. With the field of drug development continuing to advance with new technology, the integration of biochemical understanding remains a cornerstone of successful pharmacological innovation (Figure 13.6).

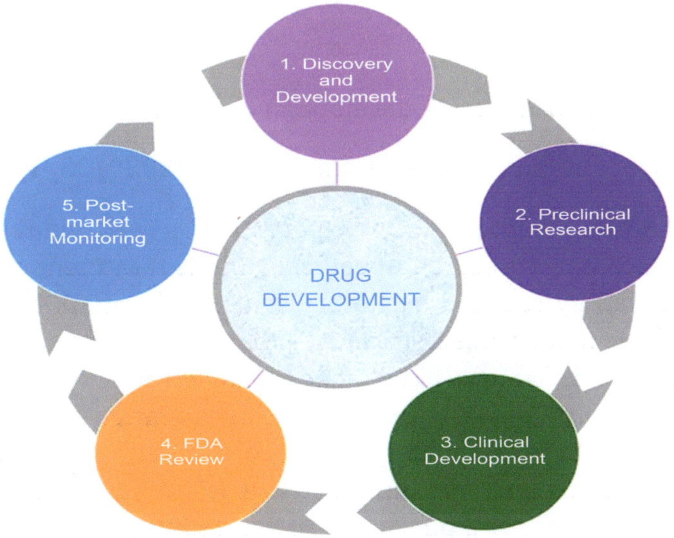

Figure 13.6. Drug discovery and development process.

Source: https://thesciencenotes.com/wp-content/uploads/2023/04/Drug-Development-Phases-Stages.webp.

13.2.1. Preclinical Research and Testing

Preclinical investigation and testing are a crucial part of the drug development process that aims to identify the safety and efficacy of new therapeutic agents before they are given to human patients. Traditionally, this has been done primarily through animal models to estimate pharmacodynamics and pharmacokinetics, which provides extremely useful information on how a candidate drug behaves within a biological system. Although they contribute generally to medical science, animal research is more and more criticized on grounds of ethics and varying predictive accuracy in mimicking human response. The criticisms have spurred the application of the 3Rs: Replacement, Reduction, and Refinement which encourage the utilization of alternative approaches for the minimization of animal use in research. This change is representative of a sustained focus on the development of ethical standards together with scientific excellence in pursuit of treatments that can successfully shift from the preclinical to clinical environments (Roy et al., 2025).

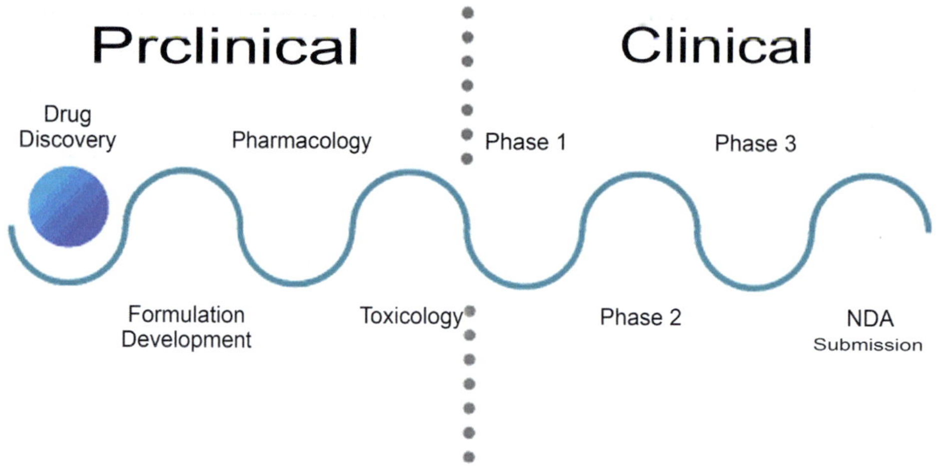

Figure 13.7. Preclinical phase of the drug development process.

Source: https://www.fiosgenomics.com/wp-content/uploads/2020/05/1-512x256-1.png.

The investigation of AMPA receptor allosteric potentiators (AMPAkines) is but one example of the innovative nature of preclinical research, specifically in the treatment of neurodegenerative and psychiatric disorders marked by reduced excitatory synaptic function. In other work, the type of compounds like CX1837 have had promising results, enhancing synaptic transmission and cognitive performance in rodent models. While CX1837 had demonstrated widespread improvements in cognition-dependent behavior, its clinical usefulness has been limited by adverse effects , such as the potential to induce seizures with higher dosing. This dynamic between efficacy and safety serves to underscore the inherent preclinical testing limitations, as it is observed that favorable outcomes in models of animals are not necessarily a guarantee of success in clinical application. Consequently, the rigor of preclinical trials remains crucial in valuing the therapeutic window and optimization of dosing, as seen in the varying responses of CX1837 across doses (Daniel et al., 2025). As the face of preclinical research evolves, what is needed now is to create new methodologies that will enhance the validity of predictive models without sacrificing ethics. Advances in computational models, *in vitro* assays, and the development of organ-on-a-chip technology are moving towards reducing animal testing. They have the potential to better replicate human biological responses, which can enable faster translational research. Further deployment of these alternatives is in favor of regulatory efforts, such as the newly enacted FDA Modernization Act, which places emphasis on current scientific alternatives to traditional animal testing. Implementation of these kinds of methods not only helps address ethical concerns but could ultimately lead to faster drug development timelines, thereby enhancing the overall preclinical research productivity and providing a more humane approach to pharmacological innovation (Roy et al., 2025) (Figure 13.7).

13.2.2. Clinical Trials: Phases and Regulations

The process of clinical trials is key to producing effective and safe medicines, conducted in special phases that facilitate systematic testing of a drug for safety and efficacy. The Phase I trials primarily focus on assessing the safety of a drug and employ a small number of people to determine the pharmacokinetics of the drug and identify any side effects. As the trials progress to Phase II, attention shifts to determining efficacy in a larger group of subjects, with ongoing safety monitoring. Notably, Phase III trials are essential in that they involve a larger sample and aim to confirm the efficacy of the drug while comparing it to current therapies. These official phases ensure that any new medicines are well tested, ultimately leading the way for the regulatory filings in front of the likes of the FDA and EMA, which lay onerous requirements to safeguard patient safety and data integrity during the research. Regulatory bodies play a central role in overseeing clinical trials to ensure compliance with guidelines established to protect participants and enable advances in medical science. The International Council for Harmonization (ICH) has established extensive rules, such as those outlined in its E17 guidelines, to control multi-regional clinical trials (MRCTs). Such rules will facilitate streamlining since they will allow trials conducted in numerous regions to be conducted under one protocol, thereby ensuring there is increased efficiency in the drug approval process and removal of duplication. The use of MRCTs not only facilitates international cooperation but also provides regulatory authorities with the opportunity to review full data, thus benefiting drug sponsors and patients equally. By creating a framework of global cooperation, regulatory authorities ensure that new therapies are made available in a timely fashion across different populations. In the ongoing advancement of drug development, there can be no exaggeration about the importance of flexibility in clinical trial design. The recent advances emphasize the need to make protocols responsive to accommodate unique patient populations and differential genetic patterns that could influence drug activity. Trials like studies of epithelial sodium channel (ENaC) blockers are typical examples of adaptive tendencies, with researchers exploring the minutest responses evoked by such molecules in individual disease contexts. As clinical trials transition into progressively challenging diseases, such as acute respiratory distress syndrome and primary biliary cholangitis, regulatory agencies must keep pace with novel methodologies to enable the generated data to be solid and informative. This balance between clinical progress and regulatory oversight is still relevant, with new treatments not only achieving standards of safety but also catering to extensive numbers of patients' requirements as laid out in dominant trial timetables (Jang, 2018; Lemmens-Gruber & Tzotzos, 2023) (Figure 13.8).

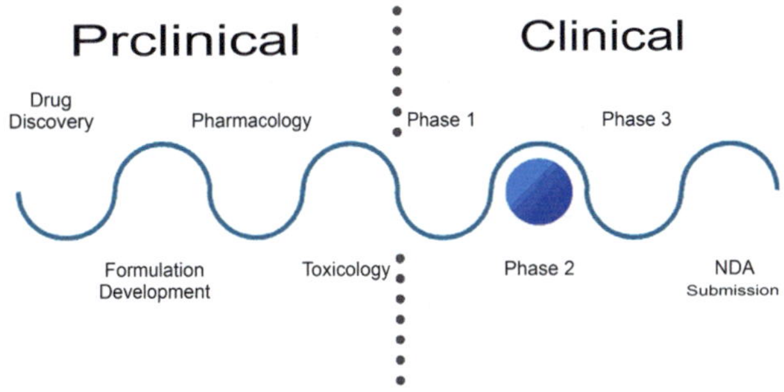

Figure 13.8. Phase 2 of the clinical drug development process.

Source: https://www.fiosgenomics.com/wp-content/uploads/2020/06/Phase-2-of-Clinical-Drug-Development-compressed.png.

13.2.3. Post-Marketing Surveillance and Drug Approval

The approval process for drugs is a critical phase in the life cycle of pharmaceutical innovation, a strict process to ensure efficacy and safety. While pre-marketing clinical trials test the impact of a drug within a controlled setting, they do not usually mirror the entire spectrum of conditions that may arise when the drug hits the market for a wider population. Post-marketing surveillance is essential to bridge this gap because it enables post-marketing surveillance of adverse events and long-term outcomes that were not possibly identifiable in the trials. The history of drug approvals teaches significant lessons, most significantly after the thalidomide tragedy, emphasizing the necessity for intensive post-marketing evaluation. Hence, regulatory bodies have put in place strict regulations that provide transparency and facilitate ongoing monitoring of drug safety to guarantee public health and maintain confidence in medical advancements (Reynolds et al., 2008). The post-marketing surveillance is not merely data collection on adverse drug reactions (ADRs); it serves as a vehicle for continuous improvement in drug formulation and utilization. This ongoing surveillance can lead to modification of drug use directions, adjustments in dosage, and even market removal where there is high risk. Pharmaceutical firms and regulators collaborate in this sense towards the development of an environment that promotes data sharing. As illustrated by today's drug development initiatives, the use of technological advancements, such as data analysis and patient registries, enhances the efficacy of surveillance activities to accelerate response to emerging safety concerns. In addition, the integration of patient feedback into surveillance work ensures that real experience with drug use among patients shapes ongoing regulatory responses, thus affirming patient-centered direction for pharmaceutical regulation (Donnelly et al., 2006). During an era when the innovation rate in drugs is high, active post-marketing surveillance is essential to get the best drug safety. National and international regulatory systems assist in enabling an integrated strategy to monitor drugs even after marketing authorization. Initiatives , such as the Joint Technology Initiative on Innovative Medicines highlight the necessity of combining efforts in drug research and surveillance, with public-private partnerships being proposed to enhance the efficacy of monitoring practices in the pharmaceutical industry. The involvement of a wide variety of stakeholders, such as regulatory authorities, academia, and the pharmaceutical industry, guarantees that there is a multi-faceted approach to post-marketing surveillance and therefore, improved patient safety and responsible treatment choices. Collectively, these actions not only reinforce the credibility of drug approval processes but also highlight the continuous obligation of all involved to safeguard public health (Reynolds et al., 2008) (Figure 13.9).

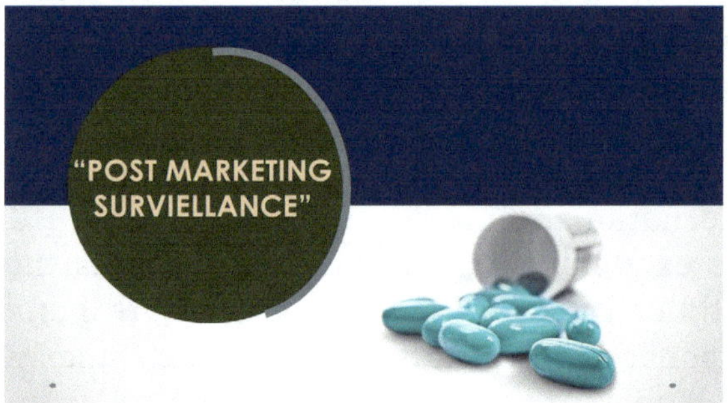

Figure 13.9. Post marketing surveillance: Monitoring drug safety after approval.

Source: https://media.licdn.com/dms/image/v2/D5612AQEc9-DfwqPp-w/article-cover_image-shrink_720_1280/article-cover_image-shrink_720_1280/0/1725386813956?e=2147483647&v=beta&t=2VwZYrpkGq2fRuhofjWLLeIpOcHWHKV0PCQdX3ZJfVc.

Test Your Knowledge

1. What is the process for clinical trials?
2. What is the post-marketing surveillance?

13.3. Mechanisms of Drug Action

Learning Outcome

1. Understand the enzyme inhibition and activation;
2. Describe the receptor signaling pathways;
3. Describe the genetic factors influencing drug response.

Understanding mechanisms of drug action is at the core of biochemical pharmacology because it acts as a foundation for the development of therapy plans. The pharmacodynamic aspect of drug action is the interaction that occurs between a drug and biological targets of the body , such as receptors, enzymes, and nucleic acids. These interactions lead to a variety of physiological and biochemical changes that provide the basis of drug therapy and toxicity. Careful examination of these mechanisms not only describes how drugs exert their actions but also how these events can be optimized for increased therapeutic effects. Therefore, their identification provides the possibility of designing more effective and safer medication regimens, enabling more precise treatment protocols in different medical specialties. In addition, drug-drug interaction (DDI) studies have become more important in light of difficulties related to polypharmacy, particularly where there is high comorbidity within the population. The identification of likely DDIs necessitates new techniques underpinned by the utilization of computational methods to predict interaction probabilities. For instance, applying machine learning algorithms and natural language processing can prove to be critical here. In this context, the BioChemDDI model integrates various biological and biochemical information to predict interaction risks sufficiently well. It highlights the significance of not only understanding the immediate effects of a drug but also the effects of continued co-administration on the pharmacological context. Through the improvement of our predictive power for DDIs, such computational systems are handy tools for clinicians and scientists in preventing drug-related adverse effects, in the wake of findings from research on the significance of effective predictive approaches (Ren et al., 2022). Finally, an explanation of the mechanisms of action of chemotherapeutic drugs is critical in guiding cancer treatment strategies. Molecular-level knowledge of tumor cell kill by these drugs through apoptosis or necrosis is important in order to fine-tune the therapy regimens. Studies that combine biochemical methods with cell biological approaches offer valuable insights into cellular responses caused by chemotherapeutic drugs. A combination of two disciplines facilitates more direct recognition of drug action pathways and potential resistance mechanisms that arise under therapy. Supported by recent studies, the fruitful implementation of multi-methodological approaches has successfully demonstrated tumor cells' pathophysiological directions under pharmacotherapy, highlighting the value of comprehensive comparative analyses in improving therapeutic efficiency and minimizing toxicity (Sazonova et al., 2022) (Figure 13.10).

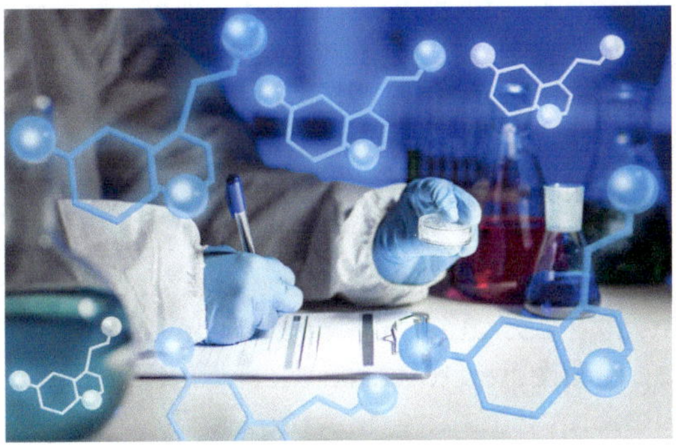

Figure 13.10. Scientist documenting laboratory findings with molecular structure overlays, representing mechanisms of drug action.

Source: https://ptcbtestprep.com/wp-content/uploads/2020/05/top-mechanisms-of-action.jpg.

13.3.1. Enzyme Inhibition and Activation

The mechanism of enzyme inhibition and activation is an important feature in biochemical pharmacology, particularly in view of its importance in drug design and disease treatment. Enzymes are biochemical catalysts that catalyze various metabolic pathways. They must be precisely regulated, otherwise aberrations will lead to states of disease. Inhibitors play their part by binding to enzymes and dampening their activity, like disconnecting a circuit. This procedure is very relevant in cancer treatment, where specific enzyme targets can be involved in tumor growth or drug resistance. A good example is the phosphoglycerate dehydrogenase (PHGDH) enzyme that has been linked with glioma stem-like cells, which are involved in radiotherapy resistance, and the utility of specific enzyme inhibition strategies in cancer combat and in enhancing therapy outcomes (Liu et al., 2025). However, enzyme activation is needed in the case of several physiological processes, and augmentation of enzyme activity may confer therapeutic benefit. Some activators are able to raise enzyme efficiency, thereby supporting favored biochemical pathways that may be compromised in disease states. For example, underactive enzymes in disease states can be overcome by restoring homeostasis and improving the metabolic profile by using activating agents. With targeted therapy, understanding the transcriptional regulation of regulatory enzymes becomes important. In medulloblastoma, the Sonic Hedgehog (SHH) pathway illustrates how activation of an enzyme can be redirected towards therapeutic advantage; the deubiquitinating enzyme Usp7, for instance, stabilizes the protein Atoh1, a tumor growth driver that is central to the disease (Cigna et al., 2024). The increasing insight into such molecular interactions further accentuates the importance of enzyme activation in the therapeutic area. Integration of the concepts of enzyme inhibition and activation is a foundation for novel forms of therapeutic approaches in biochemical pharmacology. With further study shedding light on intricate regulation mechanisms governing enzyme function, possibilities of designing new pharmacological agents persist as tremendous. With the specific inhibition or stimulation of enzyme mechanisms, drugs may be designed that are more targeted and less likely to cause adverse effects. Furthermore, personalized approaches to medicine become increasingly practical as greater knowledge of patient-specific genomic profiles is offered through advances in genomic technology. Enzyme activity manipulation in a strategic way could provide more therapeutic benefits tailored to the individual patient. Ultimately, a subtle comprehension of these enzymatic reactions will be critical to enhancing patient outcomes in a wide range of diseases and conditions in future pharmacologic innovation (Figure 13.11).

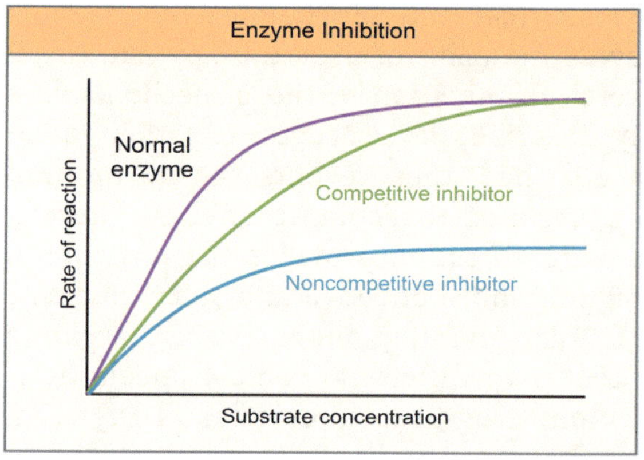

Figure 13.11. Enzyme inhibition: Competitive and noncompetitive inhibition affect the rate of reaction differently.

Source: https://assets.coursehero.com/study-guides/lumen/images/boundless-biology/enzymes/figure-06-05-042.jpeg.

13.3.2. Receptor Signaling Pathways

Signaling mechanisms of receptors are the hallmark of biochemical pharmacology because they regulate the physiological activities of various chemicals, including drugs. Receptors embedded in cell membranes are the focus of these signaling mechanisms because, upon binding by a ligand, they undergo conformational change, which activates a series of intracellular signals. Receptors can be broadly classified into ion channel-linked receptors, GPCRs, and enzyme-linked receptors. Each type acts in isolation, but all converge on common signaling molecules , such as second messengers and kinases, leading to cell responses that could be gene expression modifications, metabolic change, or cell proliferation. It is this understanding that leads to the establishment of therapeutic drugs that block specific receptors to produce the desired effects with minimum side effects, a main agenda in pharmacological progress. CRH is a fine example of a GPCR-mediated pathway, particularly with respect to response to stress. Receptor activation initiates both the generation of cAMP and the MAPK pathway, which are vital for physiological adaptation. Recent reports have revealed some complexities in this classic model of GPCR signaling. For instance, CRH binding to its receptors triggers extracellular signal-regulated kinases (ERK1/2) upon stress, demonstrating the fine interplay between hormonal signaling and cell response. Furthermore, the understanding of the function of CRH goes beyond mere physiological response in that it is also involved in various pathophysiological states ranging from anxiety disorders to metabolic syndromes. This multidimensional nature of receptor signaling pathways highlights the requirement for precise molecular definitions to direct therapeutic intervention and pharmacologic intervention to restore balance in deranged systems (Inda et al., 2017). In addition, the phenomenon of multidrug resistance (MDR) for cancer chemotherapy illustrates how receptor signaling pathways are paramount in pharmacology. Tumor cells can modify their receptor expression, particularly those that transport drugs, leading to futile chemotherapy regimens. The redox mechanisms regulating MDR have been shown to interact substantially with such pathways. For instance, chemotherapeutic agents that first enter the tumor microenvironment can induce activity in several drug transporters , such as MDR1, essentially reducing their intracellular concentrations. This redox-regulated process is highly linked with the Nrf2 pathway that regulates the induction of antioxidants and detoxification enzymes upon oxidative stress. The complexity of these interactions warrants research into new paradigms, such as redox-active drugs, in the treatment against MDR, thus emphasizing the dynamic and central role of receptor signaling within biochemical pharmacology (Cort et al., 2016).

13.3.3. Genetic Factors Influencing Drug Response

The interaction between genetic factors and drug action is a central aspect of biochemical pharmacology with crucial consequences to the efficacy and safety of pharmacotherapy. Genetic differences between individuals account for variability in drug metabolism, action, and susceptibility to toxicity. Such variations are mainly caused by polymorphism in genes encoding drug metabolizing enzymes, transporters, and drug targets. For instance, variations in cytochrome P450 genes can have a tremendous impact on the metabolism of most drugs, altering drug levels within the body. Such diversity underlines the importance of personalized medicine, where genetic testing is employed to tailor drug therapy to an individual patient to enhance treatment efficacy and minimize toxicities resulting from inappropriate dosing. Further, the emergence of MDR in cancer therapy is a classic example of how genetic considerations can significantly affect therapeutic outcomes. Genetic alteration of tumor cells can cause overexpression of transport proteins like MDR1, which are capable of pumping chemotherapeutic agents out of the cells before they become cytotoxic. This condition not only diminishes the effectiveness of these treatments but also highlights the paramount significance of redox mechanisms, which are intimately linked to inherited traits and adaptation processes. The under-stressed Nrf2 pathway, responsible for antioxidant defense, demonstrates this complex relationship as well, as it gets stimulated by oxidative agents induced during chemotherapy. Subsequently, the understanding of the genetic mechanisms of MDR is fundamental in a bid to develop approaches that can circumvent or exploit the resistance mechanisms. Lastly, the evolving field of pharmacogenomics tries to overcome challenges precipitated by genetic variation in drug response. By identifying specific genetic markers associated with drug metabolism and effect, researchers are able to design individualized therapies that are more effective and associated with fewer side effects. Genomic integration into practice has the potential to transform treatment plans by allowing patients to be identified who will derive the most benefit from individual drugs and avoid life-threatening side effects. As observed in the literature, the complex interaction between genetic factors, drug metabolism, and resistance mechanisms necessitates further research in the pharmacogenomic field to provide future therapeutic interventions that are effective and safe across different patient populations (Aghazadeh et al., 2016; Cort et al., 2016) (Figure 13.12).

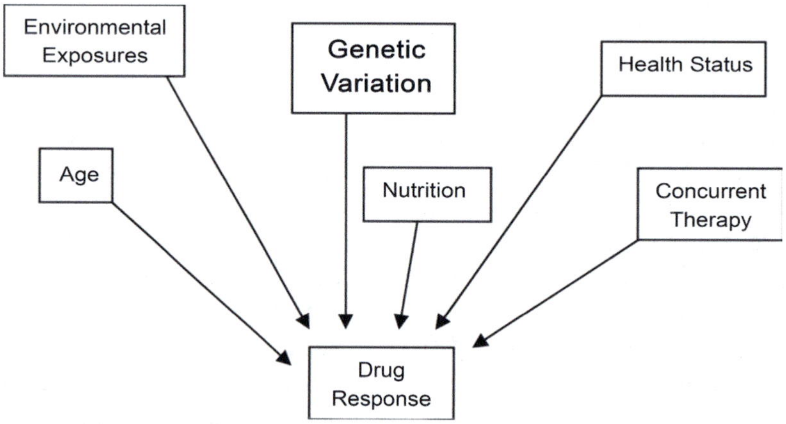

Figure 13.12. The major factors that affect a person's response to a drug.

Source: https://www.researchgate.net/profile/Michael-Waddell-3/publication/220604647/figure/fig3/AS:670010989096963@1536754476092/The-major-factors-that-affect-a-persons-response-to-a-drug.png.

Test Your Knowledge

1. What is enzyme inhibition and activation?
2. What are the genetic factors influencing drug response?

13.4. Types of Biochemical Drugs

Learning Outcome

1. Know the small molecule drugs;
2. Describe the biologics and monoclonal antibodies;
3. Explore gene therapy and RNA-based therapeutics.

Categorization of biochemical drugs is mostly based on their mode of action and the biological pathways they target. Biochemical drugs can be broadly classified as small molecules and biologics. Small-molecule drugs are typically low-molecular-weight substances that readily penetrate the cell and thereby modulate intracellular events. These types of drugs act most commonly by means of receptor interaction, enzyme inhibition, or altering certain biochemical pathways. In contrast, biologics are larger and more complex molecules produced through biological means, i.e., proteins or nucleic acids. They are largely comprised of mAbs, recombinant proteins, and gene therapies, which can provide targeted therapy to diseases through immune regulation or the replacement of defective genes. It is essential to distinguish between these two categories to understand their use, therapeutic action, and side effects in treating different medical conditions. One of the most important applications of biochemical drugs is in the treatment of chronic disease, including diabetes, cardiovascular conditions, and cancer. A case in point is antidiabetic medication , such as insulin and metformin, which illustrates the impact of biochemical drugs on glucose metabolism and insulin sensitivity. These medications are pivotal in controlling blood sugar levels, illustrating the relationship between biochemical pharmacology and disease management. Moreover, cancer drugs, such as chemotherapeutics and targeted therapies, are designed to exploit specific molecular characteristics of cancer cells. For example, growth factor receptor inhibitors or blockers of oncogenic pathways can deliver great benefits for patients. This also highlights the need for continued research and development in biochemical pharmacology to make more effective and individualized regimens of treatment, ultimately to provide improved disease control and patient quality of life. While the benefits of biochemical drugs in treating many conditions are obvious, the potential adverse effects thereof cannot be overlooked. The therapy with these drugs may lead to severe metabolic abnormalities, as evident in pediatric epilepsy studies with antiepileptic drugs (AEDs). The research revealed that different types of epilepsy might influence hematological and biochemical parameters, like serum ionized calcium and concentration of hemoglobin, which require special monitoring regimens in such children (Asmaa et al., 2024). Similarly, studies on plant-based biochemical drugs , such as *Ricinus communis* extracts, show the presence of various active phytochemicals with therapeutic potencies, albeit with their toxicity requiring extensive examination (Mittal, 2024). These areas must be appreciated in the practice of biochemical pharmacology because they reflect the fine balance between patient safety and therapeutic activity and individual health needs.

13.4.1. Small Molecule Drugs

Small-molecule drugs are a characteristic feature in the practice of biochemical pharmacology, founded primarily on their ability to engage with biological processes at the molecular level. Typically characterized as low-molecular-weight organic molecules, small-molecule drugs are recognized for their capacity to control biological action by binding with high specificity to proteins, enzymes, or receptors. Their synthesis and design employ an extensive depth of molecular interaction knowledge to facilitate highly specific therapeutic actions. Ongoing improvement in drug discovery methods, such as HTS and structure-based drug design, accelerates the identification of potent small molecules. As discovered, these molecules can profoundly affect disease pathways, thereby facilitating more effective treatment strategies. Lastly, their clinical use demonstrates their central role in advancing the boundaries of personalized medicine since tailored therapies are aimed at optimizing patient response. The drug industry has dramatically changed over the last several decades, and small-molecule drugs have been at the center of therapeutic options. Their advantages include oral use, optimal pharmacokinetic profiles, and the potential for combinations in polypharmacy, particularly in disease states , such as cancer and CVD. Compared to large biologics, which can be expensive and time-consuming to produce, small molecules are often cheaper and easier to produce. Furthermore, the development of network pharmacology has provided opportunities to investigate the pleiotropic effects of small molecules and better understand their mechanisms of action in biological networks. As highlighted in current research, such an approach not only maximizes drug discovery but also reinforces targeted medicine initiatives through delivering intelligence regarding how several pathways can be simultaneously addressed to reach therapeutic targets (Marsh et al., 2010). Despite their numerous advantages, the use of small molecule drugs is not problem-free or constraint-free. Problems like drug resistance, side effects, and the intricacies of polypharmacy make it imperative to have a complete grasp of pharmacodynamics and pharmacokinetics. Moreover, although small molecules can be highly beneficial therapeutically, they tend to run into regulatory issues in relation to their safety and efficacy profile. There is a relevant discussion in the scientific community, which pits the pharmacology of small molecules against other methodologies, like homeopathy, which has completely different concepts of treatment. This difference allows the thorough exploration of therapeutic efficacy and the scientific rationale of various drug modalities. Hence, the understanding of the multidisciplinary nature of small molecule drugs is key to progressing towards efficient and effective therapeutic interventions in modern medicine (Aabel et al., 2017) (Figure 13.13).

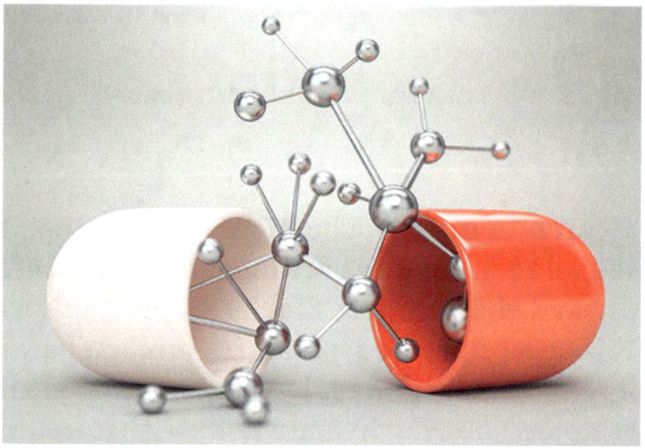

Figure 13.13. Small molecule drugs.

Source: https://cdn.the-scientist.com/assets/articleNo/65652/aImg/31245/small-molecule-therapeutics-treat-cancer-and-other-diseases-m.png.

13.4.2. Biologics and Monoclonal Antibodies

Monoclonal antibodies (mAbs) and biologics are a pharmacological breakthrough that employs biological materials to engineer therapeutic products targeted specifically at combating a number of diseases, particularly autoimmune diseases and cancers. Biologics are distinct from traditional small-molecule medications in that they are large, complex molecules composed of living organisms, making very selective interaction with biological targets possible. This selectivity decreases off-target actions and enhances therapeutic effectiveness, positioning biologics , such as mAbs at the heart of individualized medicine. The complex process of generating these biologics involves thorough preclinical testing and clinical trials to guarantee their efficacy and safety in patients. Moreover, the availability of biologics is capable of modifying treatment paradigms, revolutionizing standard-of-care regimens for chronic disease. With the progress of research, biologics in treatment protocols reflect an evolving understanding of mechanisms of disease and individual response to treatment. mAbs, a type of biologic, are engineered to bind specific antigens on the surface of pathogens or tumor cells. This focused approach enables the triggering of immune reactions against these targets, offering an effective therapeutic modality in cancer and infectious disease. In cancer, mAbs can induce direct cytotoxicity, inhibit tumor growth, or deliver cytotoxic agents with specificity for malignant cells, thereby maximizing therapy with minimal systemic toxicity. The role of mAbs has emerged in the past decade with the advent of immunotherapy, using the body's immune system to fight cancer. The increasing demand for mAbs in the market today, the research now delves into combination therapies to increase efficacy in treating multicomponent disease conditions, a rising dependency on biologicals in contemporary pharmacological intervention. Apart from this, new developments in biotechnology have introduced novel formulations and delivery systems, expanding the use of biologics and mAbs in the clinic. Techniques , such as drug delivery systems using nanoparticles have entered the scene, taking advantage of the principles of nanomedicine to enhance the bioavailability and targeting efficiency of these drugs. By improved pharmacokinetics and biodistribution of the mAbs, such delivery systems facilitate more effective treatment strategies, particularly for long-term diseases where constant release of the drug is beneficial. Problems caused by the cost of biologics and complexity of their production are yet primary subjects of concern for scientists and producers. As prophesied in the therapeutic guideline discussion, practitioners must navigate such volatile environments with patient-centered care. Through the provision of guarantees for the use of state-of-the-art research and regulation models, the future of biologics in pharmacology looks good with the promise of treating an expanded array of health problems targeted (François et al., 2019; Patra et al., 2018) (Figure 13.14).

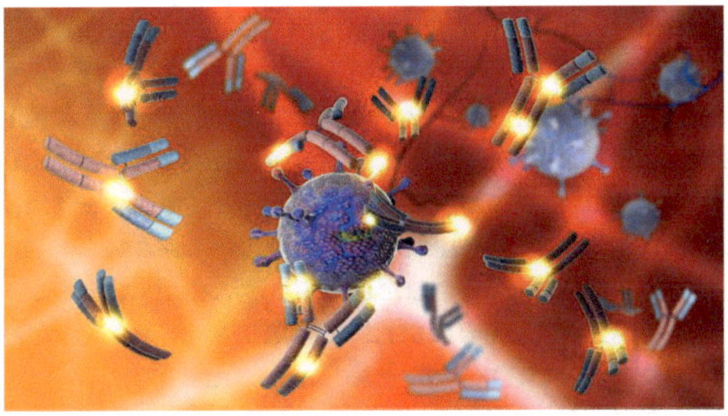

Figure 13.14. Illustration of antibodies targeting viral particles, representing an immune response.

Source: https://www.europeanpharmaceuticalreview.com/wp-content/uploads/shutterstock_1918936286.jpg.

13.4.3. Gene Therapy and RNA-Based Therapeutics

The advent of gene therapy and RNA therapies represents a powerful advance in biochemical pharmacology, revolutionizing disease treatment at the genetic level. The underlying assumptions of such treatments are the manipulation of genetic factors to restore normal function. A significant finding was the discovery of ribonucleic acid interference (RNAi), which has revolutionized paradigms in functional genomics as well as translational medicine. The ability to control gene expression with precision is used for the treatment of pathological conditions that are related to deregulated gene function. Through the use of reagents , such as small interfering RNA (siRNA), researchers and drug companies are now equipped with novel methods for developing therapeutics to treat a wide range of diseases, including genetic diseases and cancers, with significantly enhanced efficacy and specificity (Ayers et al., 2009). The application of RNA-based therapeutics is observed most strongly in the area of cancer therapy, where the alteration of gene expression can potentially result in considerable therapeutic effect. Cancer cells commonly exhibit dysfunctional gene control, such as the overexpression of cyclin-dependent kinases (CDKs), to ensure tumor growth and survival. Inhibition of such unbalanced signaling pathways through RNA-based medicine, particularly those involving siRNA technology, is a highly attractive field of therapeutic prospect. For instance, the CDK4/6 inhibitor palbociclib, which has been FDA-approved, illustrates the way in which the inhibition of specific molecular pathways results in improved clinical responses in breast cancer. These examples illustrate the potential for RNA-based therapeutics to optimize targeted therapies and enhance the prognosis of patients by repressing the oncogenic causes of cancer (Duan et al., 2016). With studies advancing, the union of gene therapy with RNA therapeutics into treatment regimes will more and more shape treatment paradigms for various diseases. The ability to leverage genetic uniqueness to tailor therapy is paving the way for tailored medicine, where effectiveness becomes paramount with reduced side effects. Also, ongoing research on long-term effects and safety profiles of these therapeutic modalities will be of prime significance for their effective use. Even as scientists further clarify the complex interactions of gene expression, the promise of RNAi technology and gene therapy to cure previously incurable illnesses remains clear, ushering in a new biochemical pharmacology era. The future of medicine lies not only in its immediate therapeutic effects but also in its potential to shape the future of medicine (Figure 13.15).

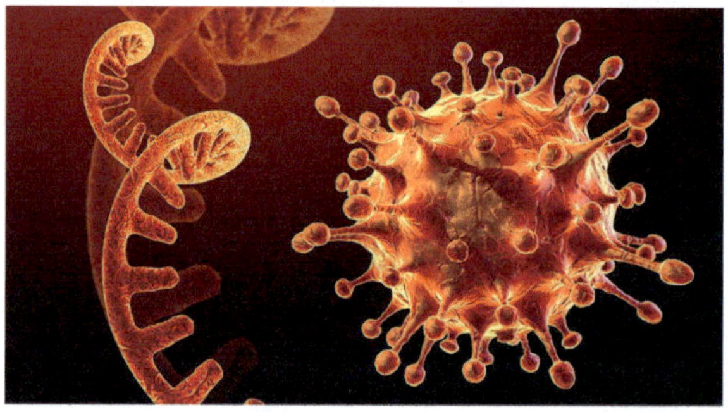

Figure 13.15. Gene therapy and drugs based on RNA technology.

Source: https://www.rna-genetherapy.eu/wp-content/uploads/2023/12/RNA_gene-theraphy.png.

Test Your Knowledge

1. What are small-molecule drugs?
2. What are monoclonal antibodies?

13.5. Drug Interactions and Side Effects

Learning Outcome

1. Describe the types of drug interactions;
2. Describe the adverse drug reactions and their management;
3. Know the strategies to minimize drug interactions.

The description of DDIs and their resulting side effects is a central concept of biochemical pharmacology since DDIs have significant effects on patient safety and the efficacy of treatment. DDIs are a consequence of the alteration of the pharmacologic effect of a given drug when another drug is present, an effect that can lead to adverse effects or failure of therapy. For instance, the utilization of multiple drugs—known as polypharmacy—can make medication regimens complex, particularly in vulnerable patients with hematological malignancies. The prevalence of polypharmacy among such patients is considerable, as becomes clear from a study that revealed that 22.7% of the individuals, prior to hospitalization, were already taking a quantity of medications, thus exposing them to toxic interactions. Insight into the mechanisms and implications of these interactions is important for clinicians to develop effective and safe treatment strategies. Secondly, drug interaction complexity could give rise to significant variation in clinical outcomes, necessitating stringent assessment methods. Different studies have documented numerous antimicrobial-related possible drug–drug interactions (pDDIs), and thus it has become more pertinent to utilize reliable databases for monitoring such interactions. Research has established that over 72.5% of hematology malignancy patients experienced at least one clinically relevant antimicrobial-related pDDI in the course of their hospitalization (Calzetta et al., 2024). This highlights the paramount importance of health professionals paying attention to the potential for dangerous interactions since there exists a direct correlation between such interactions and prolonged hospital stay. Lack of concordance among disparate interaction databases, which is evident by low concordance between UpToDate and other databases, exemplifies the complexity of being able to accurately predict drug interactions (Calzetta et al., 2024). Moreover, the effects of drug interactions are not only of direct clinical significance but also on overall health outcomes. By affecting the pharmacokinetics and pharmacodynamics of the co-administered drugs, DDIs not only produce adverse effects but also potentially decrease the therapeutic action of necessary treatment. The theory of synergy in pharmacology is within the possible road to bettering the outcomes of treatment, as explained in current literature. Pairing drugs with various mechanisms may offer greater therapeutic benefit, possibly with no side effects, enhancing the quality of patient care (Calzetta et al., 2024). Application of the same in this instance of such pairing would require systematic assessment in order to define good pairs based on concentration-response and administration timing. Lastly, a synergistic approach of understanding and controlling drug interactions is important for the evolution of clinical practice in biochemical pharmacology (Figure 13.16).

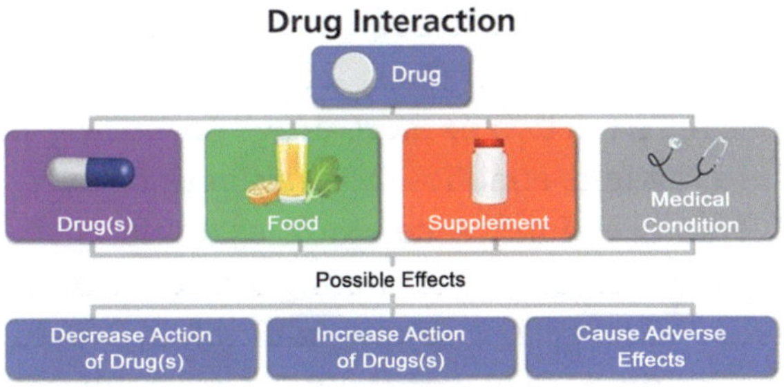

Figure 13.16. Drug interaction.

Source: https://hivinfo.nih.gov/sites/default/files/inline-images/DrugInteraction.jpg.

13.5.1. Types of Drug Interactions: Pharmacokinetic and Pharmacodynamic

Understanding drug interactions in biochemical pharmacology, particularly the distinction between pharmacokinetic and pharmacodynamic interactions, is essential since their effects on patient safety and therapeutic efficacy are of utmost importance. Pharmacokinetic interactions occur when a drug alters the absorption, distribution, metabolism, or excretion of another drug, thereby affecting its level and efficacy in the body. For instance, such drugs that either inhibit or induce cytochrome P450 enzymes would have a profound impact on other drug metabolism, thus exposing a patient to increased risk of toxicity or therapeutic failure.

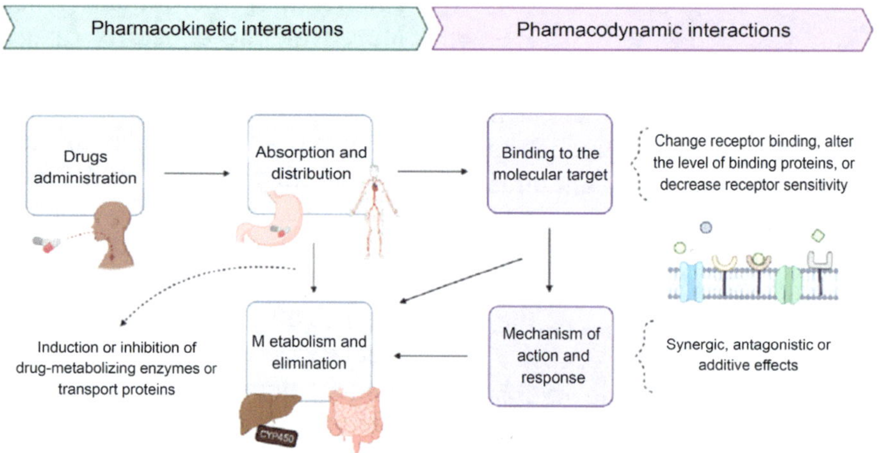

Figure 13.17. Pharmacokinetic and pharmacodynamic drug interactions.

Source: https://www.researchgate.net/profile/Lucas-Maciel-8/publication/360278432/figure/fig2/AS:1170120298762247@1655989827151/Pharmacokinetic-and-pharmacodynamic-drug-interactions-In-pharmacokinetic-interactions.png.

A classic example of this is seen when duloxetine is administered with citalopram, and duloxetine has a tremendous impact on citalopram pharmacokinetic profile, significantly raising the area under the concentration-time curve as well as influencing peak plasma concentrations. These modifications necessitate rigorous observation and dosage adjustments not to result in adverse effects and to exert therapeutic efficacy, which underscores the pharmacokinetic interaction complexities in clinical practice (Elgawish et al., 2024). Pharmacodynamic interactions, on the other hand, are effects resulting from two or more drugs producing similar or opposite pharmacological actions. These kinds of interactions enhance the therapeutic effect, which may give rise to synergistic effects or exacerbate adverse reactions. A common example is the simultaneous use of anticoagulants and antiplatelet drugs, which can generate high risks of bleeding and necessitate careful monitoring of patients to ensure efficacy and safety. Additionally, factors like the patient's genetic makeup can influence the interaction of drugs at the pharmacodynamic level. The warfarin example illustrates this; genetic polymorphism between targets and metabolizing enzymes leads to highly variable drug responses, with the challenge of being able to control anticoagulation therapy. This variability illustrates why the understanding of both pharmacological action and genetics is essential, particularly when therapies are being combined (Geng et al., 2024). With better healthcare, the need for an understanding of drug interaction grows more pertinent, particularly in polypharmacy. With the increasing complexity of treatment regimens, especially in the elderly and in individuals with complex chronic diseases, the risk of exposure to drug interactions increases. This reality necessitates a clear knowledge of both pharmacokinetic and pharmacodynamic mechanisms to avoid risks and maximize therapeutic benefits. Secondly, the development of high-tech models of computation for anticipating drug interaction, such as in studies of warfarin dynamics, serves to demonstrate the ongoing search to modify medication schedules based on the patient's unique characteristics and genes. The models can forecast interaction, which has the potential to inform clinical decisions and enhance drug therapy. Lastly, these strategies demonstrate the overruling significance of integrated pharmacological knowledge in driving patient outcomes and safety innovation within the evolving paradigm of pharmacotherapy (Geng et al., 2024) (Figure 13.17).

13.5.2. Adverse Drug Reactions and Their Management

The management of ADRs is a critical field of biochemical pharmacology because it emphasizes the complex relationship between drug activity and patient safety. It is in most biological systems prone to drug agents' activity, resulting in a variety of unwanted effects that compromise the efficacy of treatment. Understanding the biochemical pathways in which drugs get metabolized and the body's response to these drugs is imperative for health professionals in trying to avoid harm. Multidisciplinary management is required as ADRs are extremely variable across individuals according to genetic, environmental, and lifestyle factors. With the use of individualized therapeutic interventions, medical professionals can enhance the safety profile of the prescribed medication without inappropriately treating the etiologic conditions to which they were initially targeted. The multimodal treatment is combined with aggressive patient monitoring, a thorough understanding of drug interactions, and therapeutic adaptations accordingly. Recognition of the manifestations and manifestations of ADRs holds the highest significance for adequate management. Health practitioners are tasked with the critical responsibility of separating usual side effects from toxic reactions, requiring immediate action. For instance, medications used in chronic disease treatment, such as diabetes, tend to cause a multitude of cutaneous side effects, compromising clinical practice among practitioners. This is particularly so, given that diabetes now touches around 537 million adults globally; a number set to rise exponentially. Identification of specific ADRs that are specific to oral hypoglycemic therapy and insulin therapy is significant as it informs the clinical decision-making process of patient care. Identification of such adverse events early is what may have a dramatic impact on treatment protocols and patient outcomes, which means ongoing education and vigilance of drug therapy practice is essential (George et al., 2024). The philosophical underpinning of traditional medicine, for instance, Ayurveda, yields wealth of knowledge concerning patient safety in addition to preventing adverse reactions. While ADRs are not mentioned in ancient texts, the fundamental axioms allow caution when preparing and administering drug preparations. The Charaka Samhita, for instance, stresses taking into consideration numerous patient-specific factors—, such as constitution and digestive strength—when examining potential responsiveness to treatments. Traditional art of personalized medicine resonates in modern-day pharmacological practice, further encouraging fuller understanding of patient profiles, as well as environmental impacts on health. In both historical and current contexts, shared knowledge and understanding of ADRs and their management remain most critical to ensure more effective therapy regimens that are sensitive to safety and efficacy in patient care (Haryan et al., 2024) (Figure 13.18).

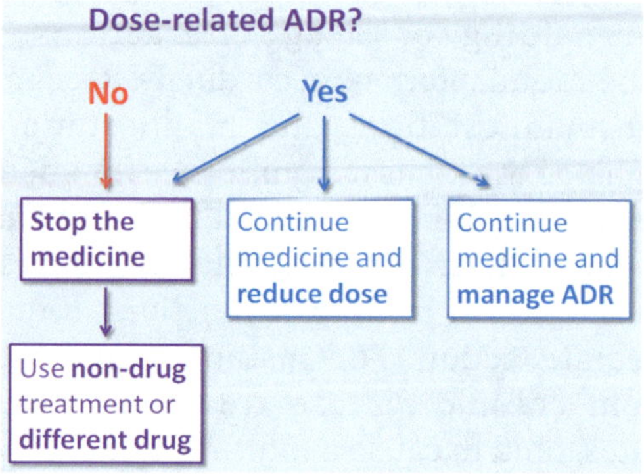

Figure 13.18. Management of adverse drug reactions.

Source: https://filestore.medicineslearningportal.org/images/ADR%20management%20algorithm%202.png.

13.5.3. Strategies to Minimize Drug Interactions

In the realm of biochemical pharmacology, the biggest issue facing healthcare providers is managing drug interactions. With a growing population of older adults and high levels of polypharmacy in patients, particularly older adults, drug interaction poses an exponentially high risk. Comprehensive medication reviews (CMRs) have become an essential practice in preventing these risks. CMRs involve a holistic review of the entire drug regimen of a patient in which clinicians can identify potential DDIs and adjust prescriptions. By the integration of systematic review results and drug interaction analyses in older patients, healthcare providers can enhance therapeutic efficacy and patient safety (Khan et al., 2025). These pre-emptive measures not only guard patient health but also make treatment regimens sense, so drugs live together in harmony in the big picture of patient healthcare. Apart from CMRs, the deployment of clinical decision support systems (CDSS) is another important role in drug interaction prevention. CDSS are computerized platforms providing evidence-based recommendations to health professionals regarding drug prescriptions. These systems match patient-specific data and cross-match this with evidence-based pharmacological knowledge to determine possible DDIs. By using CDSS, clinicians are able to make good, informed choices that reduce unwanted side effects, particularly in complex polypharmacy cases. Current studies have shown that training in geriatric pharmacology and the availability of up-to-date screening tools are most important to healthcare professionals' effective implementation of CDSS within practice (Khan et al., 2025). Therefore, by expanding both the utilization and availability of such systems, health professionals are able to significantly minimize the occurrence of adverse interactions and maximize patient outcomes. Yet another important method for minimizing drug interactions is through the implementation of individualized prescription methods. The customization of medication regimens to the individual needs and metabolic properties of the patient can tremendously reduce the risk of adverse interactions. An accurate assessment of patient-specific variables like age, weight, kidney and liver function, and the existence of comorbidities allows clinicians to customize treatments for individual requirements. Also, ongoing education about mechanisms of MDR, including that provided by ATP-binding cassette (ABC) transporters, can provide hints toward potential pharmacokinetic interactions. For instance, understanding how certain drugs may impact the efficacy of chemotherapy drugs helps in the formation of more effective therapeutic strategies while avoiding life-threatening drug interactions. As advanced as personalized medicine continues to advance, the aspect of personalized care remains a progressive step in the manner in which drug prescribing is managed, ultimately in an attempt to safeguard patients from the dangers of drug interactions (Figure 13.19).

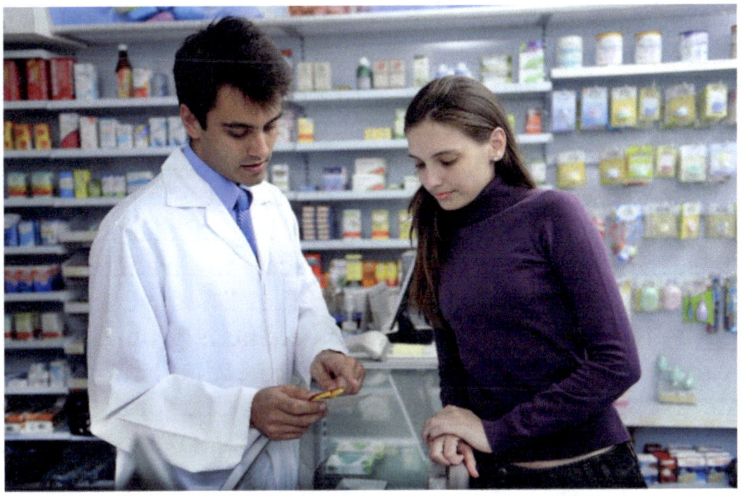

Figure 13.19. Pharmacist counseling a patient on medication use at a pharmacy counter.

Source: https://www.bemedwise.org/wp-content/uploads/2019/11/shutterstock_64389427-scaled.jpg.

Test Your Knowledge

1. What are the 2 types of drug interactions?
2. What are the strategies to minimize interactions?

13.6. Current Trends in Biochemical Pharmacology

Learning Outcome

1. Describe the personalized medicine and pharmacogenomics;
2. Know the advances in drug delivery systems;
3. Understand the role of artificial intelligence in drug discovery.

The emerging field of biochemical pharmacology is controlled by the developments in personalized medicine, which tailors the therapeutic approach to the individual patient's genetic and biochemical profile. This maximizes efficacy with fewer side effects, fundamentally altering the paradigm from one-size-fits-all to one-skin-fits-all therapy. This advancement is made possible by the more sophisticated techniques in genomic sequencing and biochemistry that allow a better understanding of disease mechanisms. By integrating pharmacogenomics into practice, health care professionals are able to select drugs that are particularly efficacious in certain groups of patients who share a specific genetic profile, thereby optimizing the therapeutic effect. Further, with the growing evidence base for such practices, it attests to the role of biochemical pharmacology as it guides drug development and application, and ultimately to more effective treatment regimens for a variety of diseases, including cancer and metabolic disorders. Another major trend in biochemical pharmacology is growing emphasis on drug repurposing as an economic strategy to advance the availability of effective treatments. As there is so much failure in drug development, researchers are increasingly using authorized drugs in an effort to discover further therapeutic uses. Not only does this save money and time on the creation of new medications, but it also takes advantage of established safety profiles, which can dramatically enhance patients' access to treatments. By applying bioinformatics and molecular modeling, scientists can rapidly evaluate the effectiveness of known compounds against a wide range of illnesses. The method has already been effective in such fields as oncology, where compounds created to be used against one type of cancer are being reused to treat others, reflecting the variety and usefulness of existing pharmacologic agents in addressing unmet medical needs (François et al., 2019). Moreover, the employment of biotherapeutics like mAbs and gene therapy is also gaining application in biochemical pharmacology. Such advanced drugs are designed to address the causative basis of disease biological processes rather than mere relief from symptoms, a change in paradigm towards more effective interventions. For instance, the production of mAbs has been used to accelerate the therapy of autoimmune diseases and cancer by being directed particularly against the pathogenic cells or proteins. Gene therapies also aim to correct aberrant genes responsible for disease progression, with the hope of providing curative treatments rather than palliation only. The expanding horizon of biotherapeutics underscores the importance of ongoing research and development in biochemical pharmacology, as it heralds new opportunities for therapeutic interventions that can benefit patient outcomes in chronic and multifactorial conditions (Wai et al., 2017).

13.6.1. Personalized Medicine and Pharmacogenomics

Pharmacogenomics-based development of personalized medicine is an important step towards more individualized healthcare solutions. It was pioneered by the Human Genome Project, whose culmination provided a glimpse of the human genome that had never been seen before. Unlike the traditional models of medicine that follow a one-size-fits-all approach, personalized medicine promises to classify patients into various groups as per genetic susceptibility and response to therapy. This individualized strategy not only attempts to enhance the efficacy of treatments but also tries to minimize side effects by tailoring drugs directly to an individual's unique biochemical profile. Effective implementation of personal medicine is grounded on two main objectives: accurate distinction of disease into subtypes and existence of drugs that target these specific conditions (Wang et al., 2023). Also, the use of big data analytics in personalized medicine has already radically changed the pharmacogenomics paradigm. Exponential growth in biomedical omics data, like genomics, proteomics, and metabolomics, has created problems as well as avenues for interpretation of data, as well as deployment in the clinical arena. By leveraging advanced computational techniques and machine learning algorithms, researchers can interpret large data sets to identify patterns that result in unique drug responses or potential side effects. Such a data-driven approach enables the formulation of customized therapy plans that correlate better with a person's genetic profile, thereby enhancing treatment effectiveness. According to existing studies, the application of big data not only improves discovery rates within pharmacogenomics but also facilitates the development of robust models capable of effectively linking genetic variation to clinical decision-making (Hassan et al., 2022). The future of personalized medicine and pharmacogenomics will be of great significance to biochemical pharmacology. The research initiative that is presently directed towards enhancing such a methodology underscores the necessity of continued interchange among genomics, computational biology, and clinical practice. In the future, the emphasis on individual differences and their influence on drug metabolism and drug action will be critical. Personalized medicine has the potential to revolutionize treatment regimens, not just making them more effective but also much more patient-centered. For this to be realized, however, there must be ongoing efforts to overcome existing hurdles, such as data interoperability and ethical concerns surrounding genetic testing. With advances in the field, the personalized medicine approach will become a standard clinical practice that redefines treatment paradigms in terms that optimize both efficacy and safety (Wang et al., 2023) (Figure 13.20).

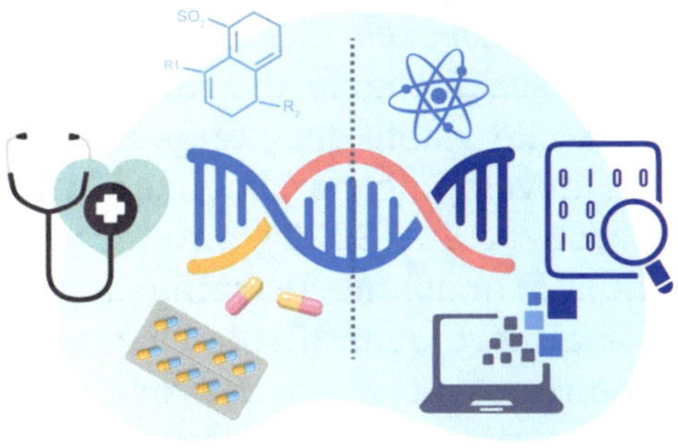

Figure 13.20. Pharmacogenomics: The role in personalized medicine.

Source: https://coreprescribingsolutions.co.uk/wp-content/uploads/2024/03/PHARMACOGENETICS-VS-PHARMACOGENOMICS-1024x679.jpg.

13.6.2. Advances in Drug Delivery Systems

Drug delivery systems have evolved and have been a major development in biochemical pharmacology to mark the beginning of a new era of more effective and personalized therapeutic interventions. The traditional drug delivery systems are marked with bioavailability, specificity, and toxicity-based dose limitations and thus have contributed to the development of more sophisticated systems. With newer developments, the advent of nanotechnology has enabled it to deliver drugs at the cellular level with specificity. By encapsulating pharmaceuticals in nanoparticles, researchers can optimize their therapeutic efficiency and minimize side effects. This model not only rationalizes the pharmacokinetics of drugs but also personalizes therapies to individuals' unique requirements, thereby fulfilling the promise of personalized medicine. Such novel modalities have highlighted the critical intersection of drug design, delivery routes, and therapeutic responses in favor of improved therapeutic intervention (Marsh et al., 2010). Additionally, developments in drug delivery systems are increasingly being led by increased understanding of biological and physiological processes, thus embracing multi-target network pharmacology paradigms. This approach recognizes that diseases are predominantly caused by complex interactions in biological networks rather than by the single-drug-single-target paradigms. With this understanding, scientists have been developing multi-targeted delivery systems that can modulate entire signaling pathways, a more holistic strategy to treatment. These advances also appreciate the role of patient-specific factors, including genetic variations and co-morbidities, in determining the appropriateness of a particular therapeutic intervention. Thus, the new methods based on network pharmacology not only promise improved drug efficacy but also bring along a paradigm shift that is in harmony with personalized medicine, thus facilitating the development of safer and more effective drugs designed with improved precision in mind (Tasn Aádi et al.). Furthermore, the economic implications of such drug delivery technologies also tend to underscore the necessity for updating traditional models of drug administration. As the population faces increasing rates of chronic disease and diseases requiring extended therapy, rational drug use has become a priority. Economically viable systems of drug delivery are required to improve compliance, conserve healthcare expenses, and maximize patient benefit. Identification of the psychological and behavioral aspects of addiction, including the case of habit-forming drugs, places emphasis on the need for control of drug delivery pathways. New systems that can evolve dosing based on real-time patient inputs have the potential to capture the dynamic variability of human behavior and hence create a need to bridge the gap between user experience and biochemical features in the health industry (Tasn Aádi et al.). These technologies present challenges and opportunities for improving drug administration practice to maximize efficacy while considering patient dynamics and the overall healthcare economics (Figure 13.21).

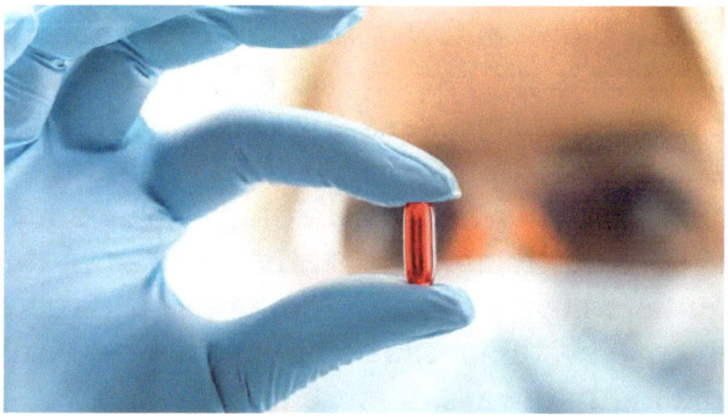

Figure 13.21. Advances in drug delivery systems.

Source: https://blog.bccresearch.com/hubfs/Advanced-Drug-Delivery.webp.

13.6.3. Role of Artificial Intelligence in Drug Discovery

The application of AI for drug discovery is a cutting-edge approach that can have the capability to accelerate the discovery of therapeutic leads considerably. One of the major advantages of applying AI is its ability to handle vast volumes of data, like genomic, proteomic, and metabolomic data, which are typically multi-dimensional and complex in nature. As researchers seek to untangle the complexities of human disease, the ability of AI to rapidly scan and interpret that information is invaluable. Applying machine learning algorithms, AI can discern patterns not readily evident to traditional methods, thereby enhancing the efficiency of drug design and optimizing lead compounds in the early development pipeline. This paradigm shift is not merely a question of speed; it also optimizes the precision of target identification and validation, pointing to AI's key role in modern biochemical pharmacology. Aside from this, utilizing AI is not simply a matter of information processing; it is also the application of sophisticated algorithms to uncover novel anticancer targets that can lead to novel therapies. For instance, through the integration of biological networks into its computational modeling, AI can enlighten the relationship between the components of cellular systems, especially in diseases like cancer. Network-based approaches enable the identification of biomarkers and viable drug targets, which are crucial in developing personalized medicine. Also, as You et al. (2022) put forward, the application of machine learning approaches allows for a more quantifiable examination of the relationships between network attributes and disease states. This possibility to forecast and rank druggable targets on the basis of empirical facts makes AI a worthy ally in overcoming the challenges faced during drug discovery. Besides, new findings in biomolecular condensates offer new opportunities for AI to speed up drug discovery. These membraneless organelles play a key role in cellular processes because they compartmentalize the biomolecules needed for various physiological processes. The comprehension of how and why condensates are created and function introduces new therapeutic possibilities, e.g., developing condensate-modifying therapeutics (c-mods) as proposed by Diana et al. (2022). AI has the potential to facilitate the identification of c-mods by the exploration of biological interactions within biomolecular networks, hence making it easier to identify new drugs for these intricate targets. This integration of AI with biochemical pharmacology illustrates an anticipatory approach to addressing human diseases, transforming traditional paradigms of drug discovery, and offering unprecedented opportunities for therapeutic intervention (Figure 13.22).

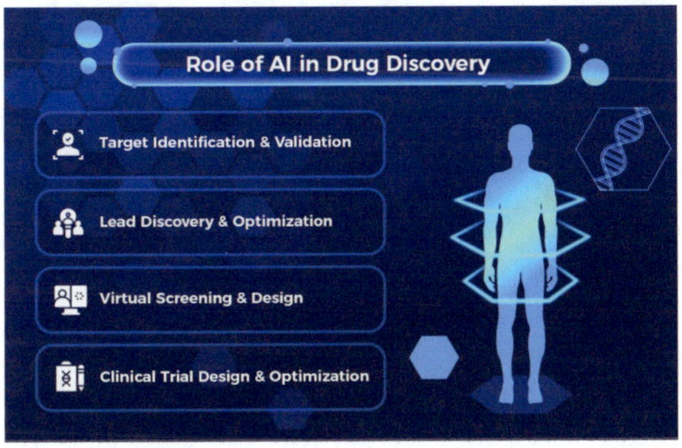

Figure 13.22. Role of artificial intelligence in drug discovery.

Source: https://assets.bacancytechnology.com/blog/wp-content/uploads/2024/05/01083614/Role-of-Artificial-Intelligence-in-Drug-Discovery.webp.

Test Your Knowledge

1. What is personalized medicine and pharmacogenomics?
2. What is the role of artificial intelligence in drug discovery?

SUMMARY

In concluding biochemical pharmacology's implications, note that the science of biochemical pharmacology exists with a multidimensional aspect to interpret drug action and design. Conjoining the molecular mechanisms and protein interaction analysis allows scientists to design therapies for intervening in specific pathways, which can significantly boost the treatment outcome. For instance, experiments indicate that drugs , such as those found in YuShu Soup can modulate critical pathways involved in the cellular stress responses. This targeted approach describes how specific proteins, like HSP90 and components of the Akt/Bcl-xL pathway, are therapeutic targets that reverse cell damage in conditions like exertional heatstroke, leading to better patient management. Thus, continued study of drug agents through biochemical insights is imperative in progressing with therapeutic approaches, as evidenced by the traditional drugs findings. Moreover, the application of natural products in biochemical pharmacology justifies the necessity for blending ancient wisdom with modern scientific methods. The investigation of Huperzine A as a neuroprotectant is an example and suggests its therapeutic application in blocking diabetic retinopathy-associated retinal neurodegeneration. Based on network pharmacology integrated with biochemical experiments, researchers have identified pathways, including HSP27-regulated pathways, that are implicated in the apoptosis of retinal cells. This bidirectional strategy not only vindicates the efficacy of ancient treatments but also creates new doorways for new treatments that can fight serious health conditions. Therefore, the intersection of ancient practices and contemporary science enriches the subject, driving the frontiers of newer pharmacological methodologies. Finally, research in biochemical pharmacology cannot be overemphasized. As the field advances, the prospect of discovering new therapeutic agents that exploit established biochemical pathways becomes increasingly important. The charting of complex relationships in biological systems will support the precision of drug design, such as that seen with YuShu Soup and Huperzine A, both of which alter key signaling pathways to produce their beneficial effects. By addressing the biochemical processes underlying the therapeutic effects, scientists can maximize efficacy and reduce side effects, informing prospective clinical use. In conclusion, the summation gleaned from the existing research is a compelling future for drug discovery, with an overriding framework proposing innovative science paired with ancient medicinal traditions, which will provide an overall approach towards pharmacological progress.

A central role in biochemical pharmacology is the individualized treatment of ailments , such as inflammatory bowel disease (IBD), i.e., ulcerative colitis and Crohn's disease. The diseases are a difficult challenge due to their long-term course and variability of symptoms presented by patients. The recommendations presented by an array of stakeholders, including patient representatives and medical professionals, point to the importance of patient-centered care plans based on rigorous evidence-based practices. The review of 88,247 publications and including multidisciplinary insight, the consensus presents highly valuable recommendations for both pharmacological and non-pharmacological interventions. This systematic approach not only addresses the management of illness but also emphasizes the central role of patient-clinician partnership in optimizing the effectiveness of treatment, highlighting the complex management of IBD as discussed in biochemical pharmacology (Christopher et al., 2019). The role of cellular signaling networks cannot be overemphasized in discussions of pharmacological interventions either. The Hippo pathway is a classic illustration of the ability of biochemical reactions to regulate cell proliferation and cell differentiation, with direct implications for therapeutic applications. The Hippo pathway is critical during organ development and acts as a master sensor of biochemical and biomechanical stimuli within the cellular context. By activating the LATS kinases, Hippo signaling inhibits the function of major transcriptional coactivators , such as YAP and TAZ and ensures cellular homeostasis. Dysregulation of this pathway may lead to aberrant cell proliferation and differentiation, making the cells susceptible to malignancy. Hence, advancements in the regulation of Hippo signaling are giving vital insights toward the design of targeted therapies in the field of cancer therapeutics as well as other biochemical pharmacology areas (Jyoti et al., 2018). Based on such insights, the development of biochemical pharmacology is defined by a harmonious blend of clinical practice and molecular biology. Integration of diverse research creates a potential for end-to-end comprehension of disease mechanisms, affecting the development of new drugs. Example includes recognition of the cross-talk among immune reactions in IBD treatment and exploitation of cell pathways , such as Hippo, indicating the importance of an integrative pharmaceutical strategy. Emphasis on interdisciplinarity maximizes the capacity to innovate and revolutionize clinical interventions tailored to the unique profile of every individual. Thus, with advancement in biochemical pharmacology, there is the need to leverage collective efforts across different disciplines to tackle disease complexity, so that pharmacological development remains effective and sustainable for patient care (Lamb et al., 2019).

KEY TERMS FROM THIS CHAPTER

- Adverse drug reactions
- Biochemical drugs
- Drug bioavailability
- Hypothyroidism
- Multidrug resistance
- Pharmacokinetics
- Phosphoglycerate dehydrogenase
- Therapeutic index
- Antiepileptic drugs
- Biochemical pharmacology
- Drug–drug interactions
- Infrared spectroscopy
- Pharmacodynamics
- Pharmacology
- Post-marketing surveillance

Critical Thinking Questions

1. **What is the primary focus of biochemical pharmacology?**
   a. The clinical application of drugs
   b. Mechanisms of drug action and interaction at the molecular and cellular levels
   c. Drug manufacturing processes
   d. Drug distribution and marketing
2. **What is the role of cytochrome P450 enzymes in drug metabolism?**
   a. Protein synthesis
   b. Phase I reactions , such as oxidation, reduction, and hydrolysis
   c. Drug excretion through urine
   d. Transport of drugs across membranes
3. **What does the term "bioavailability" mean in pharmacology?**
   a. The fraction of the drug that is metabolized
   b. The proportion of the drug that reaches systemic circulation unchanged
   c. The rate at which a drug is excreted
   d. The ability of a drug to cross the blood-brain barrier
4. **Which of the following factors can affect drug metabolism?**
   a. Age
   b. Genetic polymorphisms
   c. Liver function
   d. All of the above
5. **A drug with a high therapeutic index is:**
   a. More toxic and less effective
   b. Safer with a wide margin between therapeutic and toxic doses
   c. Only used for severe conditions
   d. Easily metabolized

Short Answer Questions

1. What is biochemical pharmacology?
2. What are the basic principles of pharmacology?
3. What are the mechanisms of drug action?
4. List the types of biochemical drugs.
5. What are drug interactions?

Answers to Critical Thinking Questions

1. (b); 2. (b); 3. (b); 4. (d); 5. (b)

REFERENCES

1. Aabel, A., Ahn, A., Anick, B., Bekelman, B., Bell, B., et al. (2017). Comparison of veterinary drugs and veterinary homeopathy: Part 1. https://core.ac.uk/download/96600356.pdf (accessed on 12th June 2025).
2. Abdelfatah, A. A., Ahmed, A., Hassan, M. H., & Bakry, A. H. (2024). Hematological and biochemical parameters in various clinical and pharmacological types of childhood epilepsy. *SVU-International Journal of Medical Sciences*. https://www.semanticscholar.org/paper/b707548d92304ea1d6e87e762bf04a4bfebebf0a (accessed on 12th June 2025).
3. Aghazadeh, A., Aghazadeh, A., Alho, A., Amitani, M., Anholt, R., Anholt, R., et al. (2016). TSPO: Kaleidoscopic 18-kDa amid biochemical pharmacology, control and targeting of mitochondria. https://core.ac.uk/download/36779164.pdf (accessed on 12th June 2025).
4. AlBathish, M., Gazy, A., Al Jamal, M., & Bejjani, A. (2024). Utilization of the FTIR spectroscopic method for the quantitative determination of the narrow therapeutic index levothyroxine sodium in pharmaceutical tablets. *Pharmacia*. https://www.semanticscholar.org/paper/9687c33607f3f69e685568d24a3457e8ee9ee091 (accessed on 12th June 2025).
5. Inda, C., Armando, N. G., Dos Santos Claro, P. A., & Silberstein, S. (2017). Endocrinology and the brain: corticotropin-releasing hormone signaling. *Endocrine connections*, *6*(6), R99–R120. https://doi.org/10.1530/EC-17-0111(accessed on 12th June 2025).
6. Ayers, D., & Day, P. J. R. (2009). Unlocking the potential of RNA interference as a therapeutic tool. https://core.ac.uk/download/46602227.pdf (accessed on 12th June 2025).
7. Barondess, J. (1968). Care of the critically ill. *JAMA Internal Medicine, 121*, 577–578. https://www.semanticscholar.org/paper/f5389ba6a75191ee2fcfa0dad000d1e4e31987bd (accessed on 12th June 2025).
8. Boothroyd, D. (2011). *Pharmacology*. https://core.ac.uk/download/29175462.pdf (accessed on 12th June 2025).
9. Calzetta, L., Page, C. P., Matera, M., Cazzola, M., & Rogliani, P. (2024). Drug-drug interactions and synergy: From pharmacological models to clinical application. *Pharmacological Reviews, 76*, 1159–1220. https://www.semanticscholar.org/paper/ef37bca029116239fa36d9b1e00dfeb6956e78fd (accessed on 12th June 2025).
10. Capi, M., Curto, M., De Andrés, F., & Gentile, G., et al. (2016). Eletriptan in the management of acute migraine: An update on the evidence for efficacy, safety, and consistent response. https://core.ac.uk/download/74319151.pdf (accessed on 12th June 2025).
11. Cigna, S. M., Basili, I., Bernardi, F., Lospinoso Severini, L., Forget, A., Chang, C. H., Yu, H., et al. (2024). MDB-79. The deubiquitinating enzyme USP7 cooperates with sonic hedgehog signaling to promote medulloblastoma. *Neuro-Oncology, 26*, 0–0. https://www.semanticscholar.org/paper/85f383c282a485658954eafcb3992ae3996bc335 (accessed on 12th June 2025).
12. Cort, A., De Luca, C., Korkina, L., Ozben, T., et al. (2016). Redox control of multidrug resistance and its possible modulation by antioxidants. https://core.ac.uk/download/74320865.pdf (accessed on 12th June 2025).
13. Dong, J., Yang, Z., & Fan, C. (2023). Network pharmacology study on mechanism involved in the use of YuShu Soup for the treatment of exertional heatstroke. *Tropical Journal of*

Pharmaceutical Research. https://www.semanticscholar.org/paper/4a394d00adb8ce0c66ae6cd2ade3cbac0e490c12 (accessed on 12th June 2025).

14. Donnelly, F. (2006). Innovative medicines for Europe. https://core.ac.uk/download/83019707.pdf (accessed on 12th June 2025).

15. Duan, Z., Hornicek, F. J., Kan, Q., Shen, J., et al. (2016). The emerging roles and therapeutic potential of cyclin-dependent kinase 11 (CDK11) in human cancer. https://core.ac.uk/download/323080349.pdf (accessed on 12th June 2025).

16. Elgawish, M., Atta, A. M., Hafeez, S. M., Abdel Mageed, S. S., Mahmoud, A. M. A., Moustafa, M. A., & Ali, M. A. (2024). Investigation of pharmacokinetic and pharmacodynamic interactions between citalopram and duloxetine: An integrated analytical, computational, behavioral, and biochemical approach. *ACS Pharmacology & Translational Science, 7*(12), 4032–4042. https://www.semanticscholar.org/paper/de9599aa77f0da54adc28ebb7f5b9e1b652d1f93 (accessed on 12th June 2025).

17. Finkel, S., Sweet, S., Locke, T., Smith, S., Wang, Z., Sandini, C., Imredy, J., et al. (2023). FRESH™ 3D bioprinted cardiac tissue, a bioengineered platform for *in vitro* toxicology and pharmacology. *bioRxiv*. https://www.semanticscholar.org/paper/603bfe7e47f320fb931938df22a18c78e04c2d44 (accessed on 12th June 2025).

18. Geng, K., Shen, C. Y., Wang, X., Wang, X., Shao, W., Wang, W., Chen, T., et al. (2024). A physiologically-based pharmacokinetic/pharmacodynamic modeling approach for drug–drug-gene interaction evaluation of S-warfarin with fluconazole. *CPT: Pharmacometrics & Systems Pharmacology, 13*, 853–869. https://www.semanticscholar.org/paper/b80530cb3f5c98b6fc75e1b2433ce67ec99ba3a1 (accessed on 12th June 2025).

19. George, N. M., Sangolli, P. M., Thulaseedharan, A., & Dominic, S. (2024). Cutaneous adverse drug reactions to antidiabetic medications and medical devices used in management of diabetes mellitus. *Journal of Skin and Stem Cell*. https://www.semanticscholar.org/paper/7c2a64f6d9968a55e513b7d930e7da4026ec4b64 (accessed on 12th June 2025).

20. Haryan, J. K., Haryan, T. J., Mohapatra, S., Inamdar, M., & Priya, P. (2024). Navigating adverse drug reactions in Ayurvedic pharmacology: A comprehensive analysis. *International Journal for Research Publication and Seminar*. https://www.semanticscholar.org/paper/3751c664ee68e09708acbd787ddc269c52615194 (accessed on 12th June 2025).

21. Hassan, M., Awan, F. M., Naz, A., deAndrés-Galiana, E. J., Álvarez-Machancoses, Ó., Cernea, A., Fernández-Brillet, L., et al. (2022). Innovations in genomics and big data analytics for personalized medicine and health care: A review. *International Journal of Molecular Sciences, 23*, 4645. https://doi.org/10.3390/ijms23094645 (accessed on 12th June 2025).

22. Jang, I. (2018). Regional clinical pharmacology trials for multi-regional clinical trials. *Translational and Clinical Pharmacology, 26*, 101–102. https://www.semanticscholar.org/paper/96feb8edae38ae30656b27dd0170e5bf8598b607 (accessed on 12th June 2025).

23. Kamel, A., Owen, T., Cole, I., Valencia, T., & Lee, E. C. (2023). Pharmacokinetics and absorption, distribution, metabolism and excretion of RGLS4326 in mouse and monkey, an anti–miR-17 oligonucleotide for the treatment of polycystic kidney disease. *Drug Metabolism and Disposition, 51*, 1536–1546. https://www.semanticscholar.org/paper/010a44af26169d3bbf68b799baf3d7f9b5d2e21b (accessed on 12th June 2025).

24. Khan, E., Ijaz, A., Jan, F., Rashid, S., & Mercado Mercado, G. (2025). Investigating specific

drug-drug interactions and their clinical implications in polypharmacy, particularly in elderly patients. *Journal of Medical & Health Sciences Review*. https://www.semanticscholar.org/paper/dd62153842c39c65f32b46d753442d68f8c62567 (accessed on 12th June 2025).

25. Lamb, C. A., Kennedy, N. A., Raine, T., Hendy, P., Smith, P. J., Limdi, J. K., Hayee, B., et al. (2019). British Society of Gastroenterology consensus guidelines on the management of inflammatory bowel disease in adults. *Gut, 68*, s1–s106. https://doi.org/10.1136/gutjnl-2019-318484 (accessed on 12th June 2025).

26. Lemmens-Gruber, R., & Tzotzos, S. (2023). The epithelial sodium channel—An underestimated drug target. *International Journal of Molecular Sciences, 24*. https://www.semanticscholar.org/paper/fc58fe71b521f1ab1a830b603f0b73fd6d476985 (accessed on 12th June 2025).

27. Li, J., Sun, Y., Wen, H., Xiao, B., Wang, J., Li, Z., Wang, L., et al. (2025). Therapeutic efficacy and mechanisms of Xuebijing in *Acinetobacter baumannii* infection based on meta-analysis and integrated pharmacology approaches. *Frontiers in Pharmacology*. https://www.semanticscholar.org/paper/6a38e992a0df66cb4a48618b9f85f30b08c5219f (accessed on 12th June 2025).

28. Liu, X., Liu, B., Wang, J., Liu, H., Wu, J., Qi, Y., Liu, Y., et al. (2025). PHGDH activation fuels glioblastoma progression and radio resistance via serine synthesis pathway. *Journal of Experimental & Clinical Cancer Research: CR, 44*. https://www.semanticscholar.org/paper/79665fb5238328831fc9167f47ee17f44b289fb6 (accessed on 12th June 2025).

29. Mach, F., Baigent, C., Catapano, A. L., Koskinas, K. C., Casula, M., Badimón, L., Chapman, M. J., et al. (2019). 2019 ESC/EAS guidelines for the management of dyslipidemias: Lipid modification to reduce cardiovascular risk. *European Heart Journal, 41*, 111–188. https://doi.org/10.1093/eurheartj/ehz455 (accessed on 12th June 2025).

30. Madrid, M. F., Mendoza, E. N., Padilla, A. L., Choquenaira-Quispe, C., Guimarães, C. J., Pereira, J. V. de M., Barros-Nepomuceno, F. W. A., et al. (2024). *In vitro* models to evaluate multidrug resistance in cancer cells: Biochemical and morphological techniques and pharmacological strategies. *Journal of Toxicology and Environmental Health, Part B, 28*, 1–27. https://www.semanticscholar.org/paper/9c20f3a94197c575cfeffed46e723d3593f1211b (accessed on 12th June 2025).

31. Marsh, A., Singer, D. R. J., Taylor, P. C., Watkins, D., et al. (2010). Personalized medicine: The impact on chemistry. https://core.ac.uk/download/45676.pdf (accessed on 12th June 2025).

32. Miah, K., Vishwanathan, K., Scarfe, G., Li, Y., Hara, I., Cantarini, M., Argue, J., et al. (2023). A phase 1 study to evaluate absolute bioavailability and absorption, distribution, metabolism, and excretion of Savolitinib in healthy male volunteers. *Clinical Pharmacology in Drug Development, 12*, 1536–1546. https://www.semanticscholar.org/paper/a7e731d1e7369a8c50398f85dc4780385270a583 (accessed on 12th June 2025).

33. Misra, J. R., & Irvine, K. D. (2018). The Hippo signaling network and its biological functions. *Annual Review of Genetics, 52*, 65–87. https://doi.org/10.1146/annurev-genet-120417-031621 (accessed on 12th June 2025).

34. Mitrea, D. M., Mittasch, M., Gomes, B. F., Klein, I. A., & Murcko, M. A. (2022). Modulating biomolecular condensates: A novel approach to drug discovery. *Nature Reviews Drug Discovery, 21*, 841–862. https://doi.org/10.1038/s41573-022-00505-4 (accessed on 12th June 2025).

35. Mittal, A. (2024). Computational screening and biochemical analysis of *Ricinus communis*

Linn root. *African Journal of Biological Sciences*. https://www.semanticscholar.org/paper/b510053c4019a8cd9121ac7b761a85c883ba8ed1 (accessed on 12th June 2025).

36. Oktay, Z., Güner, R., Kayaaslan, B., Hasanoğlu, I., Kaya Kalem, A., & Özet, G. (2024). Investigation of polypharmacy, antimicrobial-related potential drug-drug interactions in patients with hematological malignancies. *Journal of Oncology Pharmacy Practice: Official Publication of the International Society of Oncology Pharmacy Practitioners*. https://www.semanticscholar.org/paper/889d2f7e9d334829d9822dfcb43e7b14d3ec0e2e (accessed on 12th June 2025).

37. Patra, J. K., Das, G., Fraceto, L. F., Campos, E. V. R., Rodriguez-Torres, M. P., Acosta-Torres, L. S., Díaz-Torres, L. A., et al. (2018). Nano based drug delivery systems: Recent developments and future prospects. *Journal of Nanobiotechnology, 16*. https://doi.org/10.1186/s12951-018-0392-8 (accessed on 12th June 2025).

38. Radin, D. P., Zhong, S., Cerne, R., Shoaib, M., Smith, J. L., Witkin, J. M., & Lippa, A. (2025). Preclinical pharmacology of CX1837, a high-impact ampakine with an improved safety margin: Implications for treating Alzheimer's disease and ischemic stroke. *Current Alzheimer Research*. https://www.semanticscholar.org/paper/35bd5fed4555e612dd38f2b6e72d36cca673efcb (accessed on 12th June 2025).

39. Ren, Z. H., Yu, C., Li, L., You, Z., Pan, J., Guan, Y., & Guo, L. X. (2022). BioChemDDI: Predicting drug–drug interactions by fusing biochemical and structural information through a self-attention mechanism. *Biology, 11*. https://www.semanticscholar.org/paper/c428b372d38772d7d2f9c745a4b63820cea3c1ad (accessed on 12th June 2025).

40. Reynolds, L. A., & Tansey, E. M. (2008). Clinical pharmacology in the UK, c.1950–2000: Industry and regulation. https://core.ac.uk/download/30696180.pdf (accessed on 12th June 2025).

41. Roy, S., Parveen, M., Bala, A., & Sur, D. (2025). The 3C (cell culture, computer simulation, clinical trial) solution for optimizing the 3R (replace, reduction, refine) framework during preclinical research involving laboratory animals. *ACS Pharmacology & Translational Science, 8*(5), 1188–1204. https://www.semanticscholar.org/paper/b4e281b1e7ce5dffcc96af3cbdd612bede9aa413 (accessed on 12th June 2025).

42. Sazonova, E., Chesnokov, M., Zhivotovsky, B., & Kopeina, G. (2022). Drug toxicity assessment: Cell proliferation versus cell death. *Cell Death Discovery, 8*. https://www.semanticscholar.org/paper/34ae89d6b265414d12964228d2cb161590dafcdf (accessed on 12th June 2025).

43. Stielow, M., Witczyńska, A., Kubryń, N., Fijałkowski, Ł., Nowaczyk, J., & Nowaczyk, A. (2023). The bioavailability of drugs—The current state of knowledge. *Molecules, 28*, 8038. https://doi.org/10.3390/molecules28248038 (accessed on 12th June 2025).

44. Tasnádi, A., & Smith, T. G. (2025). A theory of natural addiction. https://core.ac.uk/download/pdf/9316270.pdf (accessed on 12th June 2025).

45. Wang, R., & Wang, Z. (2023). Precision medicine: Disease subtyping and tailored treatment. *Cancers, 15*, 3837. https://doi.org/10.3390/cancers15153837 (accessed on 12th June 2025).

46. Wong, V. W. S., Chan, W. K., Chitturi, S., Chawla, Y., Dan, Y. Y., Duseja, A., Fan, J. G., et al. (2017). Asia–Pacific Working Party on Non-alcoholic fatty liver disease guidelines 2017—Part 1: Definition, risk factors and assessment. *Journal of Gastroenterology and Hepatology, 33*, 70–85. https://doi.org/10.1111/jgh.13857 (accessed on 12th June 2025).

47. You, Y., Lai, X., Pan, Y., Zheng, H., Vera, J., Liu, S., Deng, S., et al. (2022). Artificial intelligence

in cancer target identification and drug discovery. *Signal Transduction and Targeted Therapy, 7*. https://doi.org/10.1038/s41392-022-00994-0 (accessed on 12th June 2025).

48. Zhang, Y., Huang, W., Tian, Q., Bai, G., Wu, W., Yin, H., Hu, L., et al. (2023). Network pharmacology and biochemical experiments reveal the antiapoptotic mechanism of huperzine A for treating diabetic retinopathy. *British Journal of Ophthalmology, 108*, 989–998. https://www.semanticscholar.org/paper/d9d01d2d75cccb9bc94714a769051105853273fa (accessed on 12th June 2025).

INDEX

C

D

E

F

R

S

T